NEUROPSYCHOLOGICAL REHABILITATION

STUDIES ON NEUROPSYCHOLOGY, DEVELOPMENT, AND COGNITION

Series Editor:

Linas Bieliauskas, Ph.D.
University of Michigan, Ann Arbor, MI, USA

NEUROPSYCHOLOGICAL REHABILITATION: THEORY AND PRACTICE

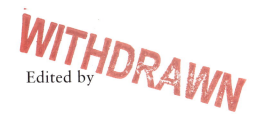

Edited by

Barbara A. Wilson

Medical Research Council, Cognition and Brain Sciences Unit, Cambridge, UK

and

The Oliver Zangwill Centre for Neuropsychological Rehabilitation, Ely, UK

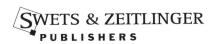

SWETS & ZEITLINGER
PUBLISHERS

LISSE   ABINGDON   EXTON (PA)   TOKYO

Library of Congress Cataloging-in-Publication Data

Neuropsychological rehabilitation : theory and practice / edited by Barbara A Wilson.
   p. cm. – (Studies on neuropsychology, development, and cognition)
   Includes bibliographical references and index.
   ISBN 90-265-1951-6
   1. Brain damage--Patients--Rehabilitation. I. Wilson, Barbara A.
   II. Series.

RC387.5.N485 2003
617.4'810443--dc21

2003045683

Cover design: Magenta Grafische Producties, Bert Haagsman
Typesetting: Grafische Vormgeving Kanters, Sliedrecht, The Netherlands

Published by: Swets & Zeitlinger Publishers
www.szp.swets.nl

ISBN 90 265 1951 6

Contents

From the Series Editor

In teaching students, I have always stressed that reporting of the results of assessment of cognitive deficit is only a first step. A Clinical Neuropsychologist must also address 'the bottom line,' which is to address the question 'Now that we know what is wrong, so what?'. It does not much good to answer a referral to evaluate speech difficulties in a young patient by informing the referring source that the patient has aphasia. Our series is intended to integrate scientific, theoretical, and applied aspects of neuropsychology and this is done superbly by Barbara A. Wilson in this volume.

Dr. Wilson has organized some of the best minds in the field of Neuropsychological Rehabilitation to answer the question 'So What?'. The development of the field is reviewed and rehabilitation approaches are described for a wide spectrum of neuropsychological disorders ranging from traditional areas of focus such as language and memory to current advances in helping patients with dementia or brain injury in childhood. The authors present not only state-of-the art techniques and approaches, but also the theoretical rationale for their development. As such, this contemporary text will be of significant value to understanding the practical implications of cognitive impairment and how to put forth the best effort at remediation or compensation. *Neuropsychological Rehabilitation: Theory and Practice* will be a welcome addition to the library of students who are developing their intervention skills, neuropsychologists in rehabilitation settings, and clinicians who seek to increase the usefulness of the recommendations in their assessment reports to meet 'the bottom line' needs of our patients.

Linas A. Bieliauskas
Ann Arbor, January, 2003

Foreword

My earliest exposure to patients with brain injury came as a result of a request to consult with a small community rehabilitation hospital in developing more effective rehabilitation programs. It seems the social work staff, in conducting routine surveys of former patients and their families a year post-discharge from inpatient rehabilitation, were surprised and very concerned about their contacts regarding individuals affected by traumatic brain injury. Reports of failed attempts to return to school and work, changes in behaviour and personality, and generally far less successful adjustment in this primarily young adult group had not been anticipated. After all, 'they had seemed to be doing so well when they left the hospital,' after a traditional rehabilitation focus on recovery of motor, self-care, and communication skills. This was in the early 1980s, and the long term, often devastating effects of brain injury in young adults resulting from trauma had just begun to be recognized. Armed with backgrounds in clinical neuropsychology, speech pathology, occupational therapy, and the neurosciences, many clinicians turned their attention to the rehabilitation of individuals with cognitive impairments. Surely the collected experience and wisdom of the traditional rehabilitation therapies, and the exciting new developments in understanding functional brain organization could be mined to reveal the fundamental nature of the problems and indicate the essence of what could and should be done.

In the two decades since, those of us working in rehabilitation have been humbled in our recognition of the impact of brain injury on our most basic cognitive capacities and functional abilities – to concentrate, to learn and remember, to think ahead, and to plan and organize one's behaviour to reach the simplest of everyday functional goals. Equally important and frequently disabling are the losses in self-confidence, and the ability to feel in control of one's actions and emotions. It became clear that effective interventions would require creativity, a deeper understanding of the impact of brain injury on everyday abilities, and an appreciation for the context in which individuals were living and working.

Barbara Wilson and her colleagues have consistently been at the forefront of this effort. Their contributions include the development of psychometric measures that began to address everyday functioning, the systematic incorporation of basic findings from experimental and cognitive psychology into rehabilitation practices, and an emphasis on clinical efficacy. In an impressive collection of books, monographs, clinical research studies, and position papers, Barbara and many of the authors in this volume have disseminated information and stimulated discussion about the theories and models underlying brain injury rehabilitation, best clinical practices, and the use of emerging technologies.

This latest edited text includes current research findings and thinking of some of the best researchers and clinicians working in neuropsychological rehabilitation today. It highlights and exemplifies the major shifts in the field: the focus on everyday functioning, the involvement of clients and families in developing and implementing treatment plans and strategies, the incorporation of activities to address behavioural and emotional responses to cognitive impairment, and the critical importance of seeing clients not strictly as individuals, but as imbedded in a social context which has tremendous power for change. It also reflects the broadening of neuropsychological rehabilitation to include children and individuals with progressive neurological disorders. There is an emphasis on scientific rigor, but in the service of developing practical and effective rehabilitative approaches, tools and techniques.

Clinical experience shines through this volume written by clinical researchers who have developed and then tested their theories and approaches to treatment within the context and realities of real-life rehabilitation programs, families, and communities. In a field that has come under great scrutiny, and for which doubters abound, this volume, reflecting the work of researchers on three continents, provides a foundation for realistic, yet optimistic expectations that neuropsychological interventions can make a difference in people's lives that is meaningful, practical, and cost-effective. It will be a great practical resource and rewarding read for anyone involved in rehabilitation.

Catherine A. Mateer
University of Victoria
Victoria, British Columbia
Canada

Chapter 1

THE THEORY AND PRACTICE OF NEUROPSYCHOLOGICAL REHABILITATION: AN OVERVIEW

Barbara A. Wilson

MRC Cognition and Brain Sciences Unit, Cambridge and the Oliver Zangwill Centre, Ely, UK

Introduction

Neuropsychological rehabilitation is concerned with the amelioration of cognitive social and emotional deficits caused by an insult to the brain. Like other kinds of rehabilitation, the main purposes of neuropsychological rehabilitation are to enable people with disabilities to achieve their optimum level of well being, to reduce the impact of their problems on everyday life and to help them return to their most appropriate environments.

Because of the complexities of the difficulties facing people with brain injury, neuropsychological rehabilitation must draw on a number of theoretical approaches. As Gianutsos said of cognitive rehabilitation (a part of neuropsychological rehabilitation) in 1989, it is a hybrid born of a mixed parentage including neuropsychology, occupational therapy, speech and language therapy and special education. Others draw from different fields. Wilson (1987) believed that three areas from within psychology are important namely neuropsychology to help us understand the working of the brain, cognitive psychology from which we obtain models of cognitive functioning that help us explain and predict phenomena and behavioural psychology to provide us with treatment strategies that can be modified or adapted for people with brain injury. McMillan and Greenwood (1993) believed that rehabilitation should draw on clinical neuropsychology, behavioural analysis, cognitive retraining and group and individual psychotherapy. Diller (1987) believed that it was important to take into account several theoretical bases.

In a recent paper Wilson (2002) attempts to put together a comprehensive model of cognitive rehabilitation. Starting with the belief that no one model is sufficient to address the complex problems facing people with brain injury, the comprehensive model includes models of cognition, assessment, recovery, behaviour, emotion, compensation and learning. Many of these models are addressed in this volume.

Theories of Neuropsychological Rehabilitation

Some early theoretical influences on neuropsychological rehabilitation

One of the earliest attempts to provide paradigms or models of treatment for people with brain injury was provided by Powell (1981). He suggested there were six treatment paradigms:

1. The non-intervention strategy (letting nature take its course).
2. The prosthetic paradigm whereby patients are helped to make the most effective use of prostheses.
3. Practice or stimulation, which is probably the most widely used treatment technique, although there is little evidence to support the notion that, on its own, it is effective for many of the problems faced by people with brain injury (Miller, 1984).
4. The maximizing paradigm in which therapists tend to maximize the extent, speed, and level of learning by such procedures as positive reinforcement and feedback.
5. Brain function therapy, or directed stimulation which aims to focus or direct tasks at certain regions of the brain to increase its activity or re-establish functions in new areas.
6. Medical, biochemical, and surgical treatments which, although beyond the brief of this chapter can sometimes be combined with other therapeutic treatments (Durand, 1982).

Although these paradigms may describe the various situations in rehabilitation they seem to be more a list of headings than they are theoretical models. Closer to models in the sense of providing theories of treatment are the five models of neuropsychological interventions suggested by Gross and Schutz (1986). These are:

1. The environmental control model
2. The stimulus-response (S-R) conditioning model

3. The skill training model
4. The strategy substitution model
5. The cognitive cycle model

Gross and Schutz claim that these models are hierarchical so that patients who cannot learn are treated with environmental control techniques; patients who can learn but cannot generalize need S-R conditioning; patients who can learn and generalize but cannot self-monitor should be given skill training; those who can self-monitor will benefit from strategy substitution; and those who can manage all of the above and are able to set their own goals will be best suited for treatment that is incorporated within the cognitive cycle model.

Although such a hierarchical model has a neatness about it, a rigid adherence to its parameters could lead to some spurious conclusions. It is highly unlikely, for example, that absolute agreement would be found between therapists who were asked to make decisions about whether a particular patient could learn or generalize. These models imply that an inability to learn can be recognized with relative ease, yet we know that even comatose head-injured patients are capable of some degree of learning Boyle and Greer (1983); Shiel, Wilson, Horn, Watson and McLellan (1993). Furthermore, it is possible to teach generalization in many instances (Zarkowska, 1987). Despite these, and possibly other reservations, it can be argued that Gross and Schutz's models are useful in encouraging therapists to think about ways of tackling problems in rehabilitation.

An interesting analogy model, 'Sinfonia Hemispherica', was presented by Buffery and Burton in (1982). They compared the brain to a symphony orchestra and brain damage to the situation which might arise should several members of the orchestra develop food poisoning and die a few hours before a concert. From their analogy we can derive several possible approaches to cognitive rehabilitation (Wilson, 1989). First there are three factors affecting the overall performance of the orchestra.

1. The *size* of the lesion – the more violinists who have died the worse will be the performance.
2. The *position* of the lesion – some violinists, such as the leader, are more important than others.
3. *Shock* – although the remaining members of the orchestra are not ill themselves, initially they will be affected by the sudden demise of their colleagues.

Buffery and Burton suggest several ways the orchestra might cope with its predicament. First, the orchestra could recruit new members to replace those who have died. Second, the orchestra could change its repertoire so that missing members are not required to perform. Third, the leader of the orchestra could ask some other members to learn the violin. These members would not be learning from scratch because they would be able to read music and follow the conductor. However, the subsequent decrease in the number of other instruments would lead to an overall decline in the orchestra's performance. Fourth, the leader could ask other instrumentalists to play the violin parts on their instruments. The resulting sound would not be perfect but would probably be reasonably acceptable.

How do these approaches translate into cognitive rehabilitation practice? Recruiting new members to replace those who have died is equivalent to restoring or repairing damaged tissue. Mechanisms of recovery will be addressed later in the chapter. Changing the repertoire is equivalent to changing the living situations and demands on people with brain injury in order to avoid problem areas and is similar to the environmental control model. Asking other members of the orchestra is equivalent to anatomical reorganization based on the idea that undamaged areas of the brain can take on the skills or functions of the damaged areas. Again, this topic will be considered below. Asking other instrumentalists to learn the violin parts is equivalent to functional adaptation or, in other words, if you cannot do something one way, find another way to do it.

Although the 'Sinfonica Hemispherica' model is a useful way of thinking about cognitive rehabilitation there are limitations to the model. In particular it does not take into account the situation which often occurs in brain injury, namely that isolated focal lesions rarely occur. Widespread diffuse damage is more likely after certain conditions such as traumatic head injury so the orchestra would not lose *all* the violinists, nor would it lose *only* violinists. Treatment in this case might involve teaching members of the orchestra to use their residual skills more efficiently, perhaps through extra rehearsal or slowing down the performance.

Rehabilitation derived from theories of cognitive functioning

In 1984 Coltheart argued that rehabilitation programmes should be based on a theoretical analysis of the nature of the disorder to be treated. He expanded on this in 1991 arguing that in order to treat a deficit one had to fully understand its nature and to do this one needed to know how the function is normally achieved. Without this model, said Coltheart, it would be impossible to determine the appropriate treatment. Although it is necessary to understand the nature of the deficit, models of cognitive functioning do not in themselves inform us on the method of treatment. Knowing *what* to treat does not tell us *how* to treat. In the words of Caramazza (1989)

'There is nothing specifically about our theory of the structure of the spelling system (or the reading system, the naming system, the sentence comprehension system, and so forth) which serves to constrain our choice of therapeutic strategy. Merely 'knowing' ... the probably locus of a deficit ... does not, on its own, allow us to specify a therapeutic strategy. To do so requires not just a theory of the structure of the system, but also, and more important, a theory of therapeutic intervention

– a theory of the ways in which a damaged system may be modified as a consequence of particular forms of intervention' (p.392).

We can conclude from this that theories of cognitive functioning are necessary but not sufficient in cognitive rehabilitation.

Are there theoretical models of Cognitive Rehabilitation?

Some people claim to be following a theoretical approach without actually doing so. An influential book by Sohlberg and Mateer (1989) appeared in 1989 in which we are told that cognitive rehabilitation should be grounded in theory. Robertson (1991), however, believes the authors do not follow their own advice. He writes, somewhat harshly... 'the theories of neuropsychological functioning which Sohlbeg and Mateer present as underlying their treatment and assessment methods are frankly facile. They are not theoretical models but collections of headings to guide assessment and treatment' (p. 88). Robertson accepts that many of the approaches make intuitive sense but he objects to them being called 'theoretical models'. A later book by Sohlberg and Mateer (2001) does much to redress these criticisms.

Gianutsos (1991) argues that cognitive rehabilitation is the application of theories of cognitive sciences to traumatic brain injury rehabilitation. Apart from the fact that it is not only people with TBI who receive cognitive rehabilitation (people with stroke, encephalitis and hypoxic brain injury are frequently seen in rehabilitation programmes), Gianutsos' approach does not appear to be at all influenced by theories from cognitive science. She favours an approach that stresses exercise and repeated practice in which clients are engaged, for the most part, in computerized exercises (Gianutsos, 1981, 1991; Gianutsos, Cochran, & Blouin, 1985; Gianutsos & Matheson, 1987). There is little, if any, evidence in these papers of theories of cognitive neuroscience.

Models and theories of cognitive rehabilitation then are hard to come by (but see Wilson, 2002). This is not to say that people are uninfluenced by theories. The models of cognitive functioning particularly those from language and reading have been very influential in the assessment and understanding of disorders (see for example Berndt & Mitchum (1995) and Basso, Cappa & Gainotti (2000). The point to be made here is that they are limited in the contribution they make to treatment. As stated before they tend to tell us what is wrong rather than what to do about it. In addition, people rarely have isolated deficits. They may have widespread cognitive problems together with emotional, social and behavioural problems. They will probably required help with everyday difficulties resulting from their impairments rather than help with a particular deficit caused by a failure in one part of the cognitive model. It is not only theories of language that have been helpful other theories from cognitive psychology have influenced rehabilitation and are frequently used, perhaps implicitly, in the assessment and management of neuropsychological impairments. The working memory model, for example, (Baddeley & Hitch, 1974), allows us to understand why someone with a normal immediate memory has problems after a delay or distraction. The dual-route model of reading (Coltheart, 1985), has revolutionised reading assessments over the past 15 years. The Supervisory Attentional System of Norman and Shallice (Norman & Shallice, 1986) has influenced the rehabilitation of people with attention and executive deficits. The list is extensive but it is still the case that in order to address the many problems faced by people with brain injury, other theoretical approaches are essential (Wilson, 2002).

Other theories relevant to cognitive rehabilitation

One of the major tasks of a clinical neuropsychologist is to undertake assessments. These are carried out in order to understand the cognitive strengths and weaknesses of our patients and clients. For this purpose standardised tests are often sufficient. They are not sufficient, however, when we want to know about the nature of everyday problems, how families cope and what treatment to offer. In these circumstances we may need to carry out a functional or behavioural assessment. Several theoretical approaches are likely to be involved in our assessments. These include psychometric models, assessments derived from models of cognitive functioning, ecologically valid assessments, localisation models and behavioural models concerned with the observation of real life problems.

Those engaged in rehabilitation will also need some understanding of theories of recovery as some of our patients/clients may be in the natural recovery period. People who survive a severe, traumatic brain injury may show recovery over a period of several years. Robertson and Murre (1999) discuss theories of recovery in some detail and Wilson (1998) considers the evidence for recovery of cognitive function after brain injury.

The management and remediation of the emotional consequences of brain injury and cognitive impairment has become increasingly important over the past decade or so. Prigatano (1999) argues that rehabilitation is unlikely to be successful if we do not deal with the emotional issues. Perhaps the most successful theoretical model for treating emotional disorders is Cognitive Behaviour Therapy (Beck, 1976; 1996). Although it is certainly one of the most important and best validated psychotherapeutic procedures (Salkovskis, 1996), less has been published about cognitive behaviour therapy with survivors of brain injury than with neurologically intact people. Williams et al. (2003), however, describe a combination of cognitive rehabilitation and cognitive behaviour therapy with two such survivors. Both had post traumatic stress disorder together with cognitive impairments. The combined treatment resulted in a reduction of their PTSD symptoms and improvement in both psychosocial and cognitive functioning (see Williams, this volume). Others, particularly Prigatano (1999) favour a milieu-orientated psychotherapeutic approach, developed from Ben-Yishay's milieu holistic approach (Ben-Yishay, 1996).

Compensating for cognitive deficits is one of the major strands of neuropsychological rehabilitation and has been for many years (Zangwill, 1947). It is akin to what Luria called Functional Adaptation (Luria, 1963). A theoretical framework for understanding compensatory behaviour was published by Bäckman and Dixon (1992) and further modified by Dixon and Bäckman (1999). Applying this framework to people with memory impairment following brain injury, Wilson and Watson (1996) found that much of the framework applied but that some modifications were required. Wilson (2000) discussed the framework in relation to a wider range of cognitive problems including language, reading and visuo-spatial deficits while Evans et al. (in press) consider factors that predict good use of compensatory strategies. The main predictors appear to be age, severity of impairment, specificity of deficit and premorbid use of compensations.

Theories and models of behaviour and learning are also necessary in understanding problems and designing neuropsychological rehabilitation programmes. Early behavioural models such as those of Kanfer and Saslow (1969) and more recent ones such as Wood (1990) enable us to incorporate the physical and neurological status of the individual together with behaviour, motivation and other factors. Wilson (1999) provides an example of how the Kanfer and Saslow (1969) model helped both in the understanding and treatment of the problems faced by a man who survived a traumatic head injury.

Learning theory, arguably one kind of behavioural theory, is of paramount importance in achieving change. Baddeley (1993) said 'A theory of rehabilitation without a model of learning is a vehicle without an engine' (p. 235). In recent years the principle of errorless learning (i.e. avoiding trial-and-error learning) has been highly influential in memory rehabilitation (Baddeley & Wilson, 1994; Wilson, Baddeley, Evans, & Shiel, 1994). Errorless learning is discussed in more detail in chapter 10 (this volume).

Although the theories and models described here are among the most important ones in neuropsychological rehabilitation, the list is not exhaustive. Wilson (2002) makes an attempt to put a number of theoretical models together to provide a comprehensive model of rehabilitation but even this model omits some aspects such as motor functioning and physical recovery.

Combining theory and practice

In our clinical work theoretical models can only take us so far. We have to adapt to the individual's needs and circumstances. The work on errorless learning, for example, has established that trial-and-error learning is not a good principle to follow for people with significant memory impairments. In order to benefit from our mistakes, we need to be able to remember them otherwise we may strengthen the incorrect response. In practice, however, the way we apply the principle will vary depending on the goals set. Clare et al's work with people with Alzheimer's Disease illustrates the point well (Clare, Wilson, Breen, & Hodges, 1999; 2000). One man wanted to remember the names of people at his social club, another woman needed to check a memory board so that she did not pester her husband with questions ad nauseam. Thus the way the principle was applied differed each time. If theories are going to be clinically useful then we need to use our clinical experience and common sense to apply the research findings. The contributors to this book illustrate some of the ways we can integrate theory and practice in neuropsychological rehabilitation.

References

Bäckman, L., & Dixon, R.A. (1992). Psychological compensation: A theoretical framework. *Psychological Bulletin, 112*, 259-283.

Baddeley, A.D. (1993). A theory of rehabilitation without a model of learning is a vehicle without an engine: A comment on Caramazza and Hillis. *Neuropsychological Rehabilitation, 3*, 235-244.

Baddeley, A.D., & Hitch, G. (1974). Working memory. In G.H. Bower (Ed.), *The psychology of learning and motivation, Vol. 8* (pp. 47-89). New York: Academic Press.

Baddeley, A.D., & Wilson, B.A. (1994). When implicit learning fails: Amnesia and the problem of error elimination. *Neuropsychologia, 32*, 53-68.

Basso, A., Cappa, S., & Gainotti, G. (Eds.). (2000). *Cognitive neuropsychology and language rehabilitation* Hove (UK): Psychology Press.

Beck, A.T. (1976). *Cognitive therapy and emotional disorders*. New York: International Universities Press.

Beck, A.T. (1996). Beyond belief: A theory of modes, personality, and psychopathology. In P.M. Salkovskis (Ed.), *Frontiers of cognitive therapy* (pp. 1-25). New York: The Guilford Press.

Ben-Yishay, Y. (1996). Reflections on the evolution of the therapeutic milieu concept. *Neuropsychological Rehabilitation, 6*, 327-343.

Berndt, R.S., & Mitchum, C.C. (Eds.). (1995). *Cognitive neuropsychological approaches to the treatment of language disorders* Hove (UK): Lawrence Erlbaum Associates Ltd.

Boyle, M.E., & Greer, R.D. (1983). Operant procedures and the comatose patient. *Journal of Applied Behavior Analysis, 16*, 3-12.

Buffery, A.W.H., & Burton, A. (1982). Information processing and redevelopment: Towards a science of neuropsychological rehabilitation. In A. Burton (Ed.), *The pathology and psychology of cognition*. London: Methuen.

Caramazza, A. (1989). Cognitive neuropsychology and rehabilitation: An unfulfilled promise? In X. Seron & G. Deloche (Eds.), *Cognitive approaches in neuropsychological rehabilitation* (pp. 383-398). Hillsdale, NJ: Lawrence Erlbaum Associates.

Clare, L., Wilson, B.A., Breen, E.K., & Hodges, J.R. (1999). Errorless learning of face-name associations in early Alzheimer's disease. *Neurocase, 5*, 37-46.

Coltheart, M. (1985). Cognitive neuropsychology and reading. In M. Posner & O.S. M. Marin (Eds.), *Attention and Performance XI* (pp. 3-37). Hillsdale, NJ: Lawrence Erlbaum Associates.

Diller, L. (1987). Neuropsychological rehabilitation. In M.J. Meier & A.L. Benton & L. Diller (Eds.), *Neuropsychological rehabilitation* (pp. 3-17). Edinburgh: Churchill Livingstone.

Dixon, R.A., & Bäckman, L. (1999). Principles of compensation in cognitive neurorehabilitation. In D.T. Stuss & G. Winocur & I.H. Robertson (Eds.), *Cognitive neurorehabilitation: A comprehensive approach* (pp. 59-72). New York, NY: Cambridge University Press.

Durand, V.M. (1982). A behavioral/pharmacological intervention for the treatment of severe self-injurious behavior. *Journal of Autism and Developmental Disorders, 12*, 243-251.

Evans, J.J., Needham, P., Wilson, B.A., & Brentnall, S. (in press). Which people make good use of memory aids? Results of a survey of people with acquired brain injury. To appear in *Journal of the International Neuropsychological Society*.

Gianutsos, R. (1981). Training the short- and long-term verbal recall of a post-encephalitis amnesic. *Journal of Clinical Neuropsychology, 3*, 143-153.

Gianutsos, R. (1991). Cognitive rehabilitation: A neuropsychological specialty comes of age. *Brain Injury, 5*, 363-368.

Gianutsos, R., Cochran, E.E., & Blouin, M. (1985). *Computer programs for cognitive rehabilitation. Vol. 3: Therapeutic memory exercises for independent use.* Bayport, NY: Life Science Associates.

Gianutsos, R., & Matheson, P. (1987). The rehabilitation of visual perceptual disorders attributable to brain injury. In M. Meier & A. Benton & L. Diller (Eds.), *Neuropsychological rehabilitation* (pp. 202-241). London: Churchill Livingstone.

Gross, Y., & Schutz, L.E. (1986). Intervention models in neuropsychology. In B.P. Uzzell & Y. Gross (Eds.), *Clinical neuropsychology of intervention* (pp. 179-205). Boston: Martinus Nijhoff.

Kanfer, F.H., & Saslow, G. (1969). Behavioral diagnosis. In C. Franks (Ed.), *Behavior therapy: Appraisal and status* (pp. 417-444). New York: McGraw Hill.

Luria, A.R. (1963). *Restoration of function after brain injury*. New York: Pergamon Press.

McMillan, T.M., & Greenwood, R.J. (1993). Models of rehabilitation programmes for the brain-injured adult - II: Model services and suggestions for change in the UK. *Clinical Rehabilitation, 7*, 346-355.

Miller, E. (1984). *Recovery and management of neuropsychological impairments.* Chichester: John Wiley & Sons.

Norman, D.A., & Shallice, T. (1986). Attention to action: Willed and automatic control of behaviour. In R.J. Davidson & G. E. Schwartz & D.E. Shapiro (Eds.), *Consciousness and self-regulation, Vol. 4* (pp. 1-18). New York: Plenum Press.

Powell, G.E. (1981). *Brain function therapy*. Aldershot: Gower Press.

Prigatano, G.P. (1999). *Principles of neuropsychological rehabilitation*. New York: Oxford University Press.

Robertson, I.H. (1991). Book review. *Neuropsychological Rehabilitation, 1*, 87-90.

Robertson, I.H., & Murre, J.M.J. (1999). Rehabilitation of brain damage: Brain plasticity and principles of guided recovery. *Psychological Bulletin, 125*, 544-575.

Salkovskis, P.M. (Ed.). (1996). *Frontiers of cognitive therapy*. New York: The Guilford Press.

Shiel, A., Wilson, B.A., Horn, S., Watson, M., & McLellan, L. (1993). Can patients in coma following traumatic head injury learn simple tasks? *Neuropsychological Rehabilitation, 3*, 161-175.

Sohlberg, M., & Mateer, C. (1989). *Introduction to cognitive rehabilitation: Theory and practice*. New York: The Guilford Press.

Sohlberg, M.M., & Mateer, C.A. (2001). *Cognitive rehabilitation: An Integrative Neuropsychological Approach*. New York: Guilford Press.

Williams, W.H., Evans, J.J., & Wilson, B.A. (2003). Neurorehabilitation for two cases of post-traumatic stress disorder following traumatic brain injury. *Cognitive Neuropsychiatry, 8*, 1-18.

Wilson, B.A. (1987). Neuropsychological rehabilitation in Britain. In M.J. Meier & A. L. Benton & L. Diller (Eds.), *Neuropsychological rehabilitation* (pp. 430-436). London: Churchill Livingstone.

Wilson, B.A. (1989). Models of cognitive rehabilitation. In R.L. Wood & P. Eames (Eds.), *Models of brain injury rehabilitation* (pp. 117-141). London: Chapman & Hall.

Wilson, B.A. (1998). Recovery of cognitive functions following non-progressive brain injury. *Current Opinion in Neurobiology, 8*, 281-287.

Wilson, B.A. (1999). *Case studies in neuropsychological rehabilitation*. New York: Oxford University Press.

Wilson, B.A. (2000). Compensating for cognitive deficits following brain injury. *Neuropsychology Review, 10*, 233-243.

Wilson, B.A. (2002). Towards a comprehensive model of cognitive rehabilitation. *Neuropsychological Rehabilitation, 12*, 97-110.

Wilson, B.A., Baddeley, A.D., Evans, J.J., & Shiel, A. (1994). Errorless learning in the rehabilitation of memory impaired people. *Neuropsychological Rehabilitation, 4*, 307-326.

Wood, R.L. (1990). Towards a model of cognitive rehabilitation. In R.L. Wood & I. Fussey (Eds.), *Cognitive rehabilitation in perspective* (pp. 3-25). London: Taylor & Francis.

Zangwill, O.L. (1947). Psychological aspects of rehabilitation in cases of brain injury. *British Journal of Psychology, 37*, 60-69.

Zarkowska, E. (1987). Discrimination and generalisation. In W. Yule & J. Carr (Eds.), *Behaviour modification for people with mental handicaps* (pp. 79-94). London: Croom Helm.

Chapter 2

STAGES IN THE HISTORY OF NEUROPSYCHOLOGICAL REHABILITATION

Corwin Boake

The Institute for Rehabilitation and Research and
Department of Physical Medicine and Rehabilitation
University of Texas-Houston Medical School
Houston, Texas, USA

Introduction

Neuropsychological rehabilitation can be defined as the use of all available means to improve the independence and the quality of life of persons with neuropsychological impairments (Jefferson, 1942). This chapter briefly reviews the history of neuropsychological rehabilitation, emphasizing general trends and identifying a few major historical figures. Other publications with more detailed information about the history of neuropsychological rehabilitation are available (Boake, 1989, 1991, 1996; Ducarne de Ribaucourt, 1997; Howard & Hatfield, 1987; León-Carrión, 1997; Prigatano, 1999).

Early Neuropsychological Rehabilitation

Neuropsychological rehabilitation is probably as old as neuropsychology itself. The French physician Paul Broca, in one of his papers describing cerebral localization of language, presented a rehabilitation program for an adult patient who was unable to read words aloud (Broca, 1865; Berker, Berker & Smith, 1986). Broca reported that the rehabilitation program began with a kind of phonics approach in which the patient was sequentially taught to read letters, then syllables, and finally to combine syllables into words. Broca reported that the program succeeded to a limited extent, in that the patient learned to read letters and syllables, but 'failed completely' to read words of more than one syllable. The rehabilitation program then switched to a whole-word approach, in which Broca 'tried then to show him these words without breaking them up into syllables, and I succeeded in teaching him a good number of them' (Berker et al., 1986, p. 1070). Broca expressed surprise that when the patient read words aloud, 'he did not recognize them through their syllables or letters,' and that 'it was only their general form, their length, their appearance that registered' (p. 1070). To check whether the patient used a whole-word reading strategy, Broca presented the patient with misspelled words created by changing 'one or two letters within a word, by replacing them with letters of the same length, as *m* for *n*, *e* for *s*, *p* for *q*, *l* for *t*' (p. 1070). Broca reported that when reading these misspelled words, the patient 'did not even notice it' (p. 1070). Broca concluded that the patient 'was learning to read through a process that was essentially different from that he went through during his youth' and that he 'could recognize a word as one would a face or landscape, the details of which had never been analyzed' (p. 1070).

In attempting to restore the reading skills of his patient, Broca was not setting a precedent. Howard and Hatfield (1987), in their historical review of aphasia therapy, cite several publications from the 1600s and 1700s that describe persons with aphasia who were helped to relearn speech and language skills. Beginning in the 1800s, Edouard Séguin and other French physicians pioneered techniques to improve the cognitive skills of children with developmental cognitive disorders. Among the tools used in this form of cognitive retraining were wooden form boards with pieces cut out in the shapes of different geometric forms. First intended as training tasks, these form boards were later adapted to serve as performance tests of intelligence (Pichot, 1948). It is unknown how and when the first steps were taken in training cognitive skills of persons with acquired brain injury. As suggested by Broca's case study, it is likely that initial attempts at neuropsychological rehabilitation of persons with acquired brain injury were aimed at language disorders. Indeed, Howard and Hatfield (1987) discuss several case studies from the late 1800s and early 1900s that used various techniques to improve communication skills of patients with aphasia. While the number of aphasia therapy publications from this period was small by current standards, the content of these publications appears to emphasize language skills relative to other cognitive domains.

One of the prominent individuals from the early period of neuropsychological rehabilitation is the American psychologist Shepherd Franz. Among Franz's many contributions are his use of psychological methodology to study the efficacy of aphasia therapy and his studies of motor learning in hemiparesis. It is possible that Franz's interest in neuropsychological rehabilitation was linked to his belief that localization of cognition in the brain was exaggerated by contemporary neurologists. In 1905 Franz reported a rehabilitation program for a patient with aphasia secondary to stroke. Following a habit-learning approach, the patient was drilled on multiple trials of naming colors and numbers, and rehearsing a prayer and poem. This type of bottom-up relearning program was typical of early attempts at aphasia therapy, termed 'speech gymnastics' by Howard and Hatfield (1987). Franz noted that the patient's gradual course of improvement was more in keeping with acquisition of a new habit than with relearning of an old habit (e.g., ice skating). Franz speculated that 'new brain paths are opened in the reeducation process' and that 'it is probable that the right side of the cerebrum takes part' in this process (Franz, 1905, p. 597). In 1917 Franz reported a study of motor relearning in monkeys with hemiparesis produced by surgical lesions (Ogden & Franz, 1917). The monkeys, who underwent a kind of rehabilitation program involving restraint of their intact forelimb, improved their motor performance in their affected forelimb. These monkey studies later helped to inspire current research into forced-use and constraint-induced therapy for hemiparesis.

First World War

Major developments in neuropsychological rehabilitation took place during the First World War, when dedicated brain injury rehabilitation centers were created for the first time. Probably the greatest development of these centers was in Germany and Austria, where a group of centers was created for medical care and rehabilitation of soldiers with brain wounds (Poser, Kohler & Schönle, 1996) (see Table 1). The Frankfurt center included a residential program or hospital, a psychological evaluation unit, and a special workshop for patients to practice and be evaluated in vocational skills. Today we are more familiar with the activities at the Cologne and Frankfurt centers because of the writings of the centers' directors, Kurt Goldstein and Walther Poppelreuter (Poppelreuter, 1917/1990).

Goldstein's writings include specific recommendations about therapy for impairments of speech, reading, and writing (Goldstein, 1919, 1942; Goldstein & Reichmann, 1920). The therapy techniques generally followed the strategy of using preserved skills to substitute for lost skills. For example, a

Table 1. Brain Injury Centers in German and Austria during World War I.

Country	City	Director
Germany	Cologne	Walther Poppelreuter
	Frankfurt	Kurt Goldstein
	Munich	Max Isserlin
Austria	Graz	H. Hartmann
	Vienna	Emil Froeschels

strategy used with patients who could not make certain speech sounds was to elicit a similar movement (e.g., blowing out tobacco smoke) and then to shape this movement into the desired speech sound. Since Goldstein did not state the source of these substitution or compensation strategies, it is possible that he deserves credit for creating or elaborating this approach. In discussing prediction of a patient's potential to return to work, Goldstein stressed the need for clinical assessments to be combined with direct observation in special vocational workshops.

The history of neuropsychological evaluation during and after World War I is less well documented. After the war, there was a clear falling off of publications about neuropsychological rehabilitation in the medical literature, probably due to the decreased incidence of traumatic brain injury in the postwar years. The neurosurgeon Harvey Cushing (1919) complained that in the USA, many veterans with brain wounds had been evaluated for disability determination, awarded a pension that was inadequate for their degree of disability, and then discharged home without further rehabilitation. Franz (1917) proposed the creation of a national institute to develop more effective interventions for veterans with nervous system injuries. Unfortunately the plan was not funded and the potential of this proposal was never realized.

Second World War

The continuity of neuropsychological rehabilitation was restored by Alexander Luria, a Russian psychologist who had earned the medical degree in order to facilitate his neuropsychological research with medical patients. When the Soviet Union entered the Second World War, Luria was assigned to a special hospital for brain-wounded veterans (Luria, 1979). Luria's synthesis of his findings with veterans with selective neuropsychological deficits due to penetrating brain wounds served as the basis for his theory of functional systems, which provided a rationale for neuropsychological rehabilitation. Therapy strategies based on this model reached beyond aphasia therapy to include interventions for disorders of motor planning, visual perception, and executive functions (Christensen & Castano, 1996). Fortunately, some of Luria's most important works were translated into other European languages. In English, the books *Restoration of function after brain injury* (Luria, 1948/1963) and *Traumatic aphasia* (Luria, 1947/1970) present Luria's work with brain-wounded veterans of the Second World War.

Developments in neuropsychological rehabilitation in other countries during and immediately after the Second World War continued the focus on aphasia. In the UK, a group of brain injury treatment centers was created, each providing both medical and rehabilitation services. The centers in Oxford and Edinburgh were sources of important discoveries in clinical neuropsychology. At the Oxford center, the neurologist W. R. Russell demonstrated the value of post-traumatic amnesia duration in predicting functional outcome from traumatic brain injury (Russell, 1971). In Edinburgh, Edna Butfield and the psychologist Oliver Zangwill carried out an uncontrolled study of outcome from aphasia therapy, using therapy techniques largely adapted from Goldstein. The authors noted that, while the results showed that patients' speech 'was judged to be much improved after re-education,' the lack of a control group limited the conclusions that could be reached because 'we possess no definite standards whereby to assess spontaneous recovery of cerebral function as opposed to the effects of re-education' (p. 75). In an attempt to control for spontaneous recovery, Butfield and Zangwill carried out a separate analysis of the outcomes of patients who had started therapy at least 6 months after the onset of illness, 'when relatively little further spontaneous improvement was to be expected'.

Zangwill made a number of theoretical and clinical proposals that are still relevant to neuropsychological rehabilitation. He proposed that neuropsychological rehabilitation could follow either of two strategies, one of 'direct retraining' and the other of 'substitution' (Zangwill, 1947). He speculated that direct retraining might be more effective with impairments, such as those of speech articulation and arithmetic, that could be addressed through drill exercises. In discussing the use of psychological testing in brain injury rehabilitation, Zangwill (1945) stressed the need for comparing psychological test results with performance in vocational workshops, in order to reach a more valid prediction of vocational outcome.

Possibly in imitation of the UK model, a group of brain injury centers was established in the USA to provide specialist medical and rehabilitation services to brain-wounded veterans (Spurling & Woodhall, 1958). In the center at Dewitt General Hospital in California, Joseph Wepman (1951) carried out an uncontrolled study of outcome from aphasia therapy. It is interesting to note that some of the psychological tests (e.g., Wechsler intelligence scales) administered to veterans in this study remain in use today, a half-century later (Boake, 2002).

In contrast to the decline in activity in neuropsychological rehabilitation after the First World War, the period after the Second World War witnessed the large-scale creation of rehabilitation programs in different countries. The profession of speech-language pathology dramatically expanded in order to meet the need for aphasia therapy in new rehabilitation facilities (e.g., Veterans Administration hospitals in the USA). The professions of occupational therapy, physical therapy, psychology, and vocational rehabilitation counseling also underwent rapid development in order to meet the needs of veterans with disabilities.

Postwar Developments

The beginning of the current period of neuropsychological rehabilitation was rooted in the postwar growth of neuropsychological research and in the increasing incidence of traumatic brain injury from motor vehicle accidents (Jennett & Teasdale, 1981). Discoveries in neuropsychological research helped to identify the specific impairments responsible for perceptual and memory disorders, implying that remediation of these underlying deficits could improve performance in a wide range of activities.

A seminal event in the history of neuropsychological rehabilitation was the rehabilitation program developed by neuropsychologists at New York University (NYU) Medical Center for patients with left visual neglect due to stroke. Research analyzing the difficulties experienced by these patients pointed to an underlying deficit in visual scanning, such that the patients made relatively fewer attempts to scan toward their left side (Diller, Ben-Yishay, Gerstman, Goodkin, Gordon, & Weinberg, 1974). Based on this research, a rehabilitation program was created to train patients to scan toward their left side. The rehabilitation program began with relatively simple scanning tasks in which patients were provided with multiple verbal and visual cues to respond correctly. With progress, patients were provided with fewer cues and presented with more difficult tasks (e.g., paragraph reading). The NYU neuropsychologist Leonard Diller and colleagues carried out a small controlled trial evaluating the visual-motor performances of patients who received scanning training on cancellation and visual search tasks (Diller et al., 1974) (see Fig. 1). Later studies by the NYU group extended the scope of training to include visual construction and body awareness (Gordon et al., 1985; Weinberg, Diller, Gordon, Gerstman, Lieberman, Lakin, Hodges, & Ezrachi, 1977, 1979). The therapy model of scanning training has inspired a large number of research studies in neuropsychological rehabilitation and appears to have influenced clinical practices of neurorehabilitation therapists (Bergego, Azouvi, Deloche, Samuel, Louis-Dreyfus, Kaschel, & Willmes, 1997; Kerkhoff, 2000; Pizzamiglio, Antonucci, Judica, Montenero, Razzano, & Zoccolotti, 1992; Robertson & Halligan, 1998; Wagenaar, Van Wieringen, Netelenbos, Meijer, & Kuik, 1992; Wiart, Saint Côme, Debelleix, Petit, Joseph, Mazaux, & Barat, 1997).

Signs of increased interest in rehabilitation of persons with traumatic brain injury became evident in the late 1960s and early 1970s, in the form of meetings devoted to this topic (Höök, 1972; Walker, Caveness, & Critchley, 1969). Accompanying this interest was a shift in the focus of research on neuropsychological consequences of traumatic brain injury, away from the functional versus organic dichotomy toward establishing an objective basis for cognitive and behavioral problems.

The development of specialized brain injury rehabilitation programs in Israel after the Yom Kippur War in 1973 is yet another example of how wartime casualties have stimulated progress in neuropsychological rehabilitation. The NYU neuropsychologist Yehuda Ben-Yishay developed a day treatment program in Tel-Aviv, where small groups of veterans with brain wounds participated in a program comprising cognitive exercises, psychotherapy, and therapeutic community activities for a duration of several months (Ben-

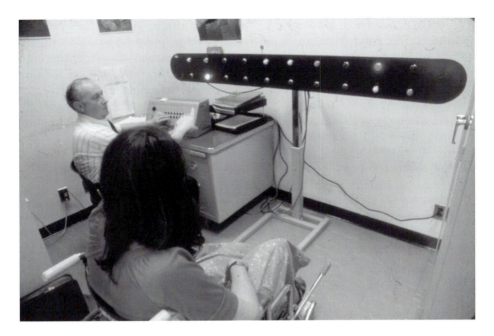

Fig. 1. Dr. Joseph Weinberg (left) operating a visual scanning apparatus (or 'scanner')
at Rusk Institute of Rehabilitation Medicine, New York University Medical
Center. The scanner was used during the 1970s and 1980s in a neuropsychological rehabilitation program for patients with visual neglect (Gordon, Hibbard,
Egelko, Diller, Shaver, Lieberman, Shaver, & Ragnarsson, 1985). The scanner
consisted of a stimulus board with two rows of colored light bulbs, controlled from a console operated by the therapist. Patients were trained to visually
scan the stimulus board from left to right, in order to detect which lights were
illuminated. In the first stage of training, patients detected single lights in the
unaffected visual field. Scanning tasks were gradually increased in difficulty
until the patient detected multiple lights on both sides of the stimulus board.
(Photo reproduced by permission of Dr. Weinberg).

Yishay, Ben-Nachum, Cohen, Gross, Hofien, Rattok, & Diller, 1978). A
major focus of therapy activities was to increase the patients' awareness of
injury-related impairments and acceptance of realistic outcomes, particularly
vocational goals (Ben-Yishay, 1996). The day treatment program model was
recreated at NYU in a form adapted to young adults with closed head injuries,
generally the result of civilian motor vehicle accidents. The basic model of his
program has been emulated in many countries (Christensen, Pinner, Møller-
Pederson, Teasdale, & Trexler, 1992; Prigatano, Fordyce, Zeiner, Roueche,
Pepping, & Wood, 1986; Scherzer, 1986).

During the 1970s and 1980s several new models of neuropsychological
rehabilitation programs were created. In a transitional learning center or
residential rehabilitation program, patients reside at the center while receiving interventions for behavior and self-care that would be more difficult to

address in a day treatment setting (Boake, 1990). The newest type of rehabilitation program attempts to directly improve the patient's adjustment to a
particular residence, community, and job, while providing few or no services
in a center. For example, a supported employment program attempts to place
a patient into a job and then provide services (e.g., job-specific memory aids)
at the actual job site (Wehman, West, Kregel, Sherron, & Kreutzer, 1995).

Alongside the holistic and vocational programs there developed a number
of interventions directed at specific cognitive deficits, many of which involved
the use of computer programs to administer repetitive drill exercises. Among
the earliest computer programs were those developed by Rosamond Gianutsos
for remediation of memory and visual impairments. For example, Gianutsos
(1981) reported a case study of a rehabilitation program for a professor with
amnesia caused by encephalitis. The rehabilitation program aimed to directly
improve his memory for new spoken information by using mass practice in
memorizing word lists. Similar treatment programs, also based on computer
software, were developed for retraining of deficits in language and visual
perception. During the 1980s a debate occurred between advocates of direct
retraining of cognitive deficits and those who maintained that, because direct
retraining was impossible, therapies should address concrete goals such as
performing a specific job (Mateer & Sohlberg, 1988).

A recent development in neuropsychological rehabilitation is the concern
with providing hard data about the efficacy of neuropsychological rehabilitation. In the USA, where clinicians have encountered increasing difficulty
obtaining insurance funding, reviews of treatment efficacy studies have
reached conflicting conclusions about the efficacy of neuropsychological
rehabilitation (Chesnut, Carney, Maynard, Mann, Patterson, & Helfand,
1999; Cicerone, Dahlberg, Kalmar, Langenbahn, Malec, Bergquist, Felicetti,
Giacino, Harley, Harrington, Herzog, Kneipp, Laatsch, & Morse, 2000;
Consensus Conference on Rehabilitation of Persons with Traumatic Brain
Injury, 1999). However, one conclusion shared by most reviewers is that
methodological flaws in existing research on neuropsychological rehabilitation limit the specific treatment recommendations that can be made in terms
of intensity, duration, and cost-effectiveness (Chesnut et al., 1999). Therefore, the future of neuropsychological rehabilitation may be shaped not only
by research showing that patients' outcomes need to be improved, but also
by research showing that interventions are effective in doing so.

Acknowledgments

I am grateful to Mary Nowak for manuscript preparation, to Sean Little for
maintaining the reference database, and to Drs. Leonard Diller and Joseph
Weinberg for the photo.

References

Ben-Yishay, Y. (1996). Reflections on the evolution of the therapeutic milieu concept. *Neuropsychological Rehabilitation, 6, 327-343.*

Ben-Yishay, Y., Ben-Nachum, Z., Cohen, A., Gross, Y., Hofien, A., Rattok, Y., & Diller, L. (1978). Digest of a two-year comprehensive clinical rehabilitation research program for out-patient head injured Israeli veterans (Oct. 1975-Oct. 1977). In *Working approaches to remediation of cognitive deficits in brain damaged persons (Rehabilitation Monograph No. 59)* (pp. 1-61). New York: New York University Medical Center Institute of Rehabilitation Medicine.

Bergego, C., Azouvi, P., Deloche, G., Samuel, C., Louis-Dreyfus, A., Kaschel, R., & Willmes, K. (1997). Rehabilitation of unilateral neglect: A controlled multiple-baseline-across-subjects trial using computerized training procedures. *Neuropsychological Rehabilitation, 7, 279-293.*

Berker, E.A., Berker, A.H., & Smith, A. (1986). Translation of Broca's 1865 report: Localization of speech in the third left frontal convolution. *Archives of Neurology, 43, 1065-1072.* (translation of Broca, 1865).

Boake, C. (1989). A history of cognitive rehabilitation of head-injured patients, 1915 to 1980. *Journal of Head Trauma Rehabilitation, 4(3),* 1-8.

Boake, C. (1990). Transitional living centers in head injury rehabilitation. In J.S. Kreutzer & P.H. Wehman (Eds.), *Community integration following traumatic brain injury* (pp. 115-124). Baltimore: Paul H. Brookes.

Boake, C. (1991). History of cognitive rehabilitation following head injury. In J. S. Kreutzer & P.H. Wehman (Eds.), *Cognitive rehabilitation for persons with traumatic brain injury: A functional approach* (pp. 3-12). Baltimore: Paul H. Brookes.

Boake, C. (Ed.) (1996). Historical aspects of neuropsychological rehabilitation [special issue]. *Neuropsychological Rehabilitation, 6(4),* 241-343.

Boake, C. (2002). From the Binet-Simon to the Wechsler-Bellevue: Tracing the history of intelligence testing. *Journal of Clinical and Experimental Neuropsychology, 24,* 383-405.

Broca, P. (1865). Sur le siège de la faculté du langage articulé. *Bulletin de la Société Anthropologique, 6,* 377-393. [reprinted in H. Hécaen & J. Dubois (Eds.) (1969). *La naissance de la neuropsychologie du langage 1825-1865* (pp. 108-121). Paris: Flammarion].

Butfield, E. & Zangwill, O.L. (1946). Re-education in aphasia: A review of 70 cases. *Journal of Neurology, Neurosurgery, and Psychiatry, 9,* 217-222.

Chesnut, R.M., Carney, N., Maynard, H., Mann, N.C., Patterson, P., & Helfand, M. (1999). Summary report: Evidence for the effectiveness of rehabilitation for persons with traumatic brain injury. *Journal of Head Trauma Rehabilitation, 14,* 176-188. (available on-line http://hstat.nlm.nih.gov/hq/Hquest/db/local.epc.ex.tbi/screen/Toc Display/S/63982/action/Toc)

Christensen, A.L. & Castano, C. (1996). Alexander Romanovitch Luria (1902-1977): Contributions to neuropsychological rehabilitation. *Neuropsychological Rehabilitation, 6,* 279-303.

Christensen, A.L., Pinner, E.M., Møller-Pederson, P., Teasdale, T.W., & Trexler, L.E. (1992). Psychosocial outcome following indivdualized neuropsychological rehabilitation of brain damage. *Acta Neurologica Scandinavica, 85,* 32-38.

Cicerone, K.D., Dahlberg, C., Kalmar, K., Langenbahn, D.M., Malec, J.F., Bergquist, T.F., Felicetti, T., Giacino, J.T., Harley, J.P., Harrington, D.E., Herzog, J., Kneipp, S., Laatsch, L., & Morse, P. A. (2000). Evidence-based cognitive rehabilitation: Recommendations for clinical practice. *Archives of Physical Medicine and Rehabilitation, 81,* 1596-1615.

Cushing, H. (1919). Some neurological aspects of reconstruction. *Transactions of the Congress of American Physicians and Surgeons, 11,* 23-41.

Diller, L., Ben-Yishay, Y., Gerstman, L.J., Goodkin, R., Gordon, W., & Weinberg, J. (1974). *Studies in cognition and rehabilitation in hemiplegia (Rehabilitation Monograph No. 50)*. New York: Institute for Rehabilitation Medicine, New York University Medical Center.

Ducarne de Ribaucourt, B. (1997). La naissance et le développement de la rééducation neuropsychologique. In F. Eustache, J. Lambert, & F. Viader (Eds.), *Rééducations neuropsychologiques: historique, développements actuels et évaluation* (pp. 9-38). Brussels: De Boeck Université.

Franz, S.I. (1905). The re-education of an aphasic. *Journal of Philosophy, Psychology, and Scientific Method, 2*, 589-597.

Franz, S.I. (1917). Re-education and rehabilitation of cripples maimed and otherwise disabled by war. *Journal of the American Medical Association, 69*, 63-64.

Gianutsos, R. (1981). Training the short- and long-term verbal recall of a post-encephalitic amnesic. *Journal of Clinical Neuropsychology, 3*, 143-153.

Goldstein, K. (1919). *Die Behandlung, Fürsorge und Begutachtung der Hirnverletzten. Zugleich ein Beitrag zur Verwendung psychologischer Methoden in der Klinik.* Leipzig: F.C.W. Vogel.

Goldstein, K. (1942). *After effects of brain injuries in war: their evaluation and treatment; the application of psychologic methods in the clinic.* New York: Grune & Stratton.

Goldstein, K. & Reichmann, F. (1920). *Über praktische und theoretische Ergebnisse aus den Erfahrungen an Hirnschußverletzten. Ergebnisse der inneren Medizin und Kinderheilkunde, 18*, 405-530.

Gordon, W., Hibbard, M., Egelko, S., Diller, L., Shaver, M., Lieberman, A., & Ragnarsson, K. (1985). Perceptual remediation in patients with right brain damage: a comprehensive program. *Archives of Physical Medicine and Rehabilitation, 66*, 353-359.

Höök, O. (Ed.) (1972). International symposium on rehabilitation in head injury, Göteborg, 1971 [special issue]. *Scandinavian Journal of Rehabilitation Medicine 4(1)*.

Howard, D. & Hatfield, F.M. (1987). *Aphasia therapy: Historical and contemporary issues*. Hillsdale, NJ: L. Erlbaum Associates.

Jefferson, G. (1942). Discussion on rehabilitation after injuries to the central nervous system. *Proceedings of the Royal Society of Medicine, 35*, 295-299.

Jennett, B. & Teasdale, G. (1981). *Management of head injuries*. Philadelphia: F. A. Davis.

Kerkhoff, G. (2000). Neurovisual rehabilitation: recent developments and future directions. *Journal of Neurology, Neurosurgery, and Psychiatry, 68*, 691-706.

León-Carrión, J. (1997). A historical view of neuropsychological rehabilitation: the search for human dignity. In J. León-Carrión (Ed.), *Neuropsychological rehabilitation: Fundamentals, innovations, and directions* (pp. 3-39). Delray Beach, FL: GR/St. Lucie Press.

Luria, A.R. (1963). *Restoration of function after brain injury* (B. Haigh, trans.). New York: Macmillan (originally published 1948).

Luria, A.R. (1970). *Traumatic aphasia: Its syndromes, psychology, and treatment* (M. Critchley, trans.). The Hague: Mouton (originally published 1947).

Luria, A.R. (1979). *The making of mind: A personal account of Soviet psychology* Cambridge, Mass.: Harvard University Press.

Mateer, C.A. & Sohlberg, M.M. (1988). A paradigm shift in memory rehabilitation. In H.A. Whitaker (Ed.), *Neuropsychological studies of non-focal brain damage* (pp. 202-225). New York: Springer.

NIH Consensus Conference on Rehabilitation of Persons with Traumatic Brain Injury. (1999). Rehabilitation of persons with traumatic brain injury. *JAMA, 282*, 974-983. (available on-line http://consensus.nih.gov/cons/log/log-intro.htm).

Ogden, R. & Franz, S.I. (1917). On cerebral motor control: the recovery from experimentally produced hemiplegia. *Psychobiology, 1,* 33-47.

Pichot, P. (1948). French pioneers in the field of mental deficiency. *American Journal of Mental Deficiency, 53,* 128-137.

Pizzamiglio, L., Antonucci, G., Judica, A., Montenero, P., Razzano, C., & Zoccolotti, P. (1992). Cognitive rehabilitation of the hemineglect disorder in chronic patients with unilateral right brain damage. *Journal of Clinical and Experimental Neuropsychology, 14,* 901-923.

Poppelreuter, W. (1990). *Disturbances of lower and higher visual capacities caused by occipital damage; with special reference to the psychopathological, pedagogical, industrial, and social implications* (J. Zihl, trans.). New York: Oxford University Press (originally published 1917).

Poser, U., Kohler, J.A., & Schönle, P.W. (1996). A historical review of neuropsychological rehabilitation in Germany. *Neuropsychological Rehabilitation, 6,* 257-278.

Prigatano, G.P. (1999). *Principles of neuropsychological rehabilitation.* New York: Oxford University Press.

Prigatano, G.P., Fordyce, D.J., Zeiner, H.K., Roueche, J.R., Pepping, M., & Wood, B.C. (1986). *Neuropsychological rehabilitation after brain injury.* Baltimore: Johns Hopkins University Press.

Robertson, I.H. & Halligan, P.W. (1998). *Spatial neglect: A clinical handbook for diagnosis and treatment.* Hove: Psychology Press.

Scherzer, B.P. (1986). Rehabilitation following severe head trauma: Results of a 3-year program. *Archives of Physical Medicine and Rehabilitation, 67,* 366-373.

Spurling, R.G., & Woodhall, B. (1958). *Neurosurgery (Medical Department, United States Army, Surgery in World War II, vol. 1).* Washington, DC: Office of the Surgeon General.

Russell, W.R. (1971). *The traumatic amnesias.* London: Oxford University Press.

Wagenaar, R.C., Van Wieringen, P.C., Netelenbos, J.B., Meijer, O.G., & Kuik, D.J. (1992). Transfer of scanning training effects in visual inattention after stroke: Five single case studies. *Disability and Rehabilitation, 14,* 51-60.

Walker, A.E., Caveness, W.F., & Critchley, M. (Eds.) (1969). *The late effects of head injury.* Springfield, IL: C.C. Thomas.

Wehman, P.H., West, M.D., Kregel, J., Sherron, P., & Kreutzer, J.S. (1995). Return to work for persons with severe traumatic brain injury: A data-based approach to program development. *Journal of Head Trauma Rehabilitation, 10(1),* 27-39.

Weinberg, J., Diller, L., Gordon, W.A., Gerstman, L.J., Lieberman, A., Lakin, P., Hodges, G., & Ezrachi, O. (1979). Training sensory awareness and spatial organization in people with right brain damage. *Archives of Physical Medicine and Rehabilitation, 60,* 491-496.

Weinberg, J., Diller, L., Gordon, W.A., Gerstman, L.J., Lieberman, A., Lakin, P., Hodges, G., & Ezrachi, O. (1977). Visual scanning training effect on reading-related tasks in acquired right brain damage. *Archives of Physical Medicine and Rehabilitation, 58,* 479-486.

Wepman, J.M. (1951). *Recovery from aphasia.* New York: Ronald.

Wiart, L., Saint Côme, A.B., Debelleix, X., Petit, H., Joseph, P.A., Mazaux, J.M., & Barat, M. (1997). Unilateral neglect syndrome rehabilitation by trunk rotation and scanning training. *Archives of Physical Medicine and Rehabilitation, 78,* 424-429.

Zangwill, O.L. (1945). A review of psychological work at the Brain Injuries Unit, Edinburgh, 1941-1945. *British Medical Journal, 2,* 248-250.

Zangwill, O.L. (1947). Psychological aspects of rehabilitation in cases of brain injury. *British Journal of Psychology, 37,* 60-69.

Chapter 3

REHABILITATION FOR DISORDERS OF ATTENTION

Tom Manly

MRC Cognition and Brain Sciences Unit, Cambridge, UK

Summary

The scientific study of attention is a relatively new and rapidly developing field. Insights from this work are already influencing clinical practice in terms of improved assessment and rehabilitation of people with brain injuries. After briefly introducing some conceptual issues, a major section of this chapter concerns one of the most striking and surprisingly common acquired disorders of attention, unilateral spatial neglect. Six very different approaches to ameliorating this condition are considered, including recent results using prism lens adaptation. In the second section, the chapter focuses on difficulties in non-spatial attention faced by adults who have suffered a brain injury. Disorders of attention are associated with slowed recovery and reduced outcome. It is clear that in addition to any direct impediment to everyday activities, problems at this level can compromise the useful expression/recovery of other capacities. Although theory, assessment and rehabilitation in this important clinical area are at an early stage, the reviewed evidence provides some optimistic pointers for future development.

Introduction

Looking around, there are probably numerous objects that you could choose to examine, pick-up, prod or just think about. If you close your eyes, you can become aware of a startling number of background sounds – the wind out-side, the whirring of the ventilation system, the distant swearing of children. If you move your focus to the sensations on your skin – you may be able to feel your watchstrap or become conscious of the pressure of your shoes against your feet. Finally try to think about the last time you were on a boat – Why were you there? Who else was present? In each case, objects, sensations or thoughts that lay largely outside awareness a moment ago can be promoted to dominate current experience by a mere expression of will. In general, we would view this capacity to selectively focus and to suppress competing information as a useful thing – allowing us to prioritise our processing and to get a job done. At other times, we can become aware that this selection is not simply a matter of choice. If we are desperately trying to listen to the sports results on the TV, for example, while maintaining a polite conversation about a friend's recent gardening triumphs, maintaining an even distribution of attention between the two competing inputs is extremely difficult.

William James (1890) wrote of attention:

'Everyone knows what attention is. It is the taking possession by the mind, in clear and vivid form, of one out of what seem several simulta-neous possible objects or trains of thought. Focalisation, concentration of consciousness are of its essence. It implies withdrawal from some things in order to deal effectively with others.'

Crucial aspects of this definition remain central to contemporary views, in particular the notions of *selection* from between potential targets, that attend-ing to one thing is likely to be at the expense of another *(capacity limitation)* and the close relationship between attention and conscious experience.

In the 1940s and 50s, attention came to some prominence as a topic ame-nable to empirical as well as introspective investigation. Psychologists would, for example, ask experimental participants to try to divide their attention between two streams of information presented using headphones to different ears (Broadbent, 1958). In other studies, deterioration in performance over long periods of performing the same, dull monitoring task was taken as the variable of interest (Mackworth, 1948). This early work has been hugely influential. The explosion in scientific investigation over recent decades has been so great that it is now, by common consent, almost impossible to provide an exclusive definition of the term 'attention'.

The application of these experimental techniques to people with brain inju-ries, and, increasingly, to healthy individuals in brain scanning studies, has led to a developing understanding of how our brains might perform 'atten-tion'. Reviewing this area in the 1990s Posner and Petersen (1990) proposed a provisional set of principles. The first was that the brain has networks or systems that are somewhat specialised in attention – that is, they are separable from basic perceptual and motor processes. Clinically, this means that it is possible to acquire a deficit that is predominantly or exclusively attentional in nature. Secondly, in experimental studies, researchers had generally referred to the 'type' of attention required in terms of the particular task demands (e.g. 'focused attention', 'spatial attention', 'sustained attention' and so forth). Posner and Petersen argued that these functional distinctions might be mirrored, to a degree, in the brain, with different areas performing rather specific attentional processes. In particular they highlighted potential separation between *'orienting'* or *'spatial attention'* – the capacity to prioritise information from one region of space; *'focused'* or *'selective attention'* – the capacity to prioritise relevant information and suppress irrelevant information regardless of its location in space; and *'alertness'*, *'vigilance'* or *'sustained attention'* – the capacity to maintain a general 'ready-to-respond' receptive state. Clinically, this again means that, depending on the location of damage, very different profiles of attentional impairment may be apparent (for other taxonomies see Mirsky, Anthony, Duncan, Ahearn, & Kellam, 1991; Van Zomeren & Brouwer, 1992).

Problems in attention and concentration are among the most commonly reported consequences of traumatic brain injury (e.g. Oddy, Coughlan, Tyerman, & Jenkins, 1985; Brooks & McKinlay, 1987). Impairments in attention, particularly spatial attention, have also been documented in over 50% of patients who have suffered a stroke in the immediate post-lesion stage (e.g. Ogden, 1985; Stone, Halligan, & Greenwood, 1993; Leclerk & Zimmermann, 2002). As our understanding of attention improves, its importance in recovery from brain injury is increasingly apparent. This applies both to attention as a useful skill in its own right and to its potential role in mediating recovery in ostensibly very separate systems, such as motor function (Ben-Yishay, Diller, Gerstman, & Haas, 1968; Denes, Semenza, Stoppa, & Lis, 1982; Fullerton, McSherry, & Stout, 1986; Sea, Henderson, & Cermack, 1993; Blanc-Garin, 1994; Robertson, Ridgeway, Greenfield, & Parr, 1997c; Cherney, Halper, Kwasnica, Harvey, & Zhang, 2001; de Seze et al., 2001; Paolucci, Antonucci, Grasso, & Pizzamiglio, 2001a; Paolucci et al., 2001b). Interventions that can lead to improvements in attentional function – or which ameliorate the effect of impairments – are therefore important clinical aims.

This chapter considers various attempts to work with patients in 'rehabilitating' these disorders. It is important, however, to issue a few words of caution at this stage:

Firstly, rehabilitation is used in inverted commas because the term should really refer to improvements in a patient's capacity to achieve important functional goals in everyday life. As we shall see, this has only been assessed in a few of the studies presented. Many of the concepts of attention that we use clinically have been imported from the 'normal' experimental literature. This offers some advantages in terms of conceptual clarity but the extent to which these relate to the difficulties that patients actually report often remains an open question. Although it is difficult to believe that we have functions that are only tapped by neuropsychological measures and untouched by real life, whether any change actually contributes to complex everyday activities should be evaluated rather than assumed. Measuring such changes amid the 'noise' of real life is, of course, a far from easy business. Many of the studies discussed here should therefore be considered as optimistic pointers to what may be possible, rather than rehabilitation per se.

Secondly, the study and assessment of attention are at a very early stage. Attention cannot be observed directly and must be inferred from the performance on tasks that require many other abilities – features that make it both a somewhat approximate exercise and one that is vulnerable to swings in the theoretical pendulum. The attention taxonomies proposed are provisional and subject to continual revision. It may well be that in a few years we will have a quite different view of the problems presented by patients and, if rehabilitation has been very closely linked to, and evaluated by, particular paradigmatic approaches, will need to rethink our interventions.

The final point, which almost goes without saying, is that rehabilitation is optimally conducted in a manner that takes into account the individual goals and circumstances of a patient, and which operates at a number of levels, including psychosocial support for the patient and his or her family. Many studies quite rightly attempt to control out such factors as 'nuisance variables' in order to examine specific effects (e.g. more general supportive rehabilitation will be offered to both the experimental and the control group). This emphasis can sometimes be misinterpreted and clearly the techniques described here are best explored as part of a broader, holistic rehabilitation framework.

Spatial Attention

Unilateral spatial neglect

Unilateral spatial neglect is probably the most striking manifestation of an *attentional* disorder. It refers to a difficulty in detecting, acting on or even imagining information from one side of space, that cannot be fully accounted for by basic perceptual loss. Patients with neglect may, for example, fail to detect food on the left side of their plate, fail to notice someone approaching from the left, miss words from the left side of a page, forget to wash or dress the left side of their body, and collide with objects when moving around. In principal, neglect can be assessed on any task that has a spatial component, as the key issue is the *difference* between performance on one side and another. In addition to observing difficulties in everyday activities, widely used standardised measures include cancellation tasks (in which patients are asked to find and cross out stimuli distributed over a sheet), line bisection (in which patients are asked to find and mark the centre of a line), and varieties of drawing and copying tasks. It is important to note at this stage, however, that spatial neglect is a rather heterogeneous condition or syndrome, with many dissociations being noted between manifestations in different patients. This means that, whilst performance on any task that shows a lateralised attentional bias may be considered definitive of neglect, it does not necessarily follow that neglect will be apparent on all other measures. Similarly, the absence of neglect on a task can not be used to completely rule out bias in other activities – or indeed to convincingly demonstrate recovery or rehabilitation.

Although neglect can occur in a variety of neurological conditions, its most frequent cause is cerebro-vascular disease, where it has been observed in up to 82% of patients with right hemisphere stroke and 65% of left hemisphere patient in the immediate post-stroke stage (Ogden, 1985; Stone et al., 1992; Stone et al., 1991; Stone et al., 1993). This almost even distribution in risk following damage to either side of the brain is followed by a strikingly asymmetrical pattern of recovery. Although the majority of patients with left or right sided damage show quite rapid spontaneous improvement in this aspect of their condition, almost all patients with chronic forms of neglect will have right hemisphere lesions and neglect the left side of space (Ogden, 1985; Stone et al., 1992; Stone et al., 1991).

In terms of the location of lesions that can lead to neglect, the disorder has classically been associated with damage to the parietal cortex (Brain, 1941; Vallar & Perani, 1986). Subsequent studies have shown, however, that neglect can be observed following damage to a variety of cortical regions (including temporal and frontal) and subcortical structures (Mesulam, 1981; Damasio, Damasio, & Chui, 1980; Bradshaw & Mattingley, 1995; Chung et al., 2000; Hier, Davis, Richardson, & Mohr, 1977; Kumral, Evyapan, & Balkir, 1999; Velasco, Velasco, Ogarrio, & Olvera, 1986; Samuelsson, Jensen, Ekholm, Naver, & Blomstrand, 1997; Karnath, Ferber, & Himmelbach, 2001). These observations suggest that aspects of the disorder can emerge following damage to a widely distributed network responsible for attention and action within space.

The *attentional* nature of the disorder is perhaps best characterised through comparison with unilateral visual field deficits, basic perceptual losses that often co-occur with neglect and which can be difficult to distinguish from the condition. Like neglect, *hemianopia* (loss of information from the majority of one visual field – and, hence, side of space) or *quadraniopia* (loss of information from one quadrant of the field) are primarily caused by cerebro-vascular disease (Hier, Mondlock, & Caplan, 1983; Zihl, 2000).

Important distinguishing features include the fact that that visual field disorders are retinotopically based, meaning that information reaching a particular *area of retinal cells* will simply not get though.[1] In contrast, neglect generally affects awareness of information because of *where it is in space*

---

[1] The situation can be slightly more complicated, depending on the precise locus of the damage. Processing in the visual system is conducted in a parallel and hierarchical fashion and it is possible to lose specific elements of information (e.g. colour, form, motion) from particular regions of the visual field. See, for example Zihl, (2000) for more detailed discussion of visual field disorders and their rehabilitation.

rather than where it falls on the retina. The neglected space may be defined relative to the head, the body midline (Karnath, Schenkel, & Fischer, 1991) or (in the case of tactile stimuli) by the location of the limbs (Mattingley & Bradshaw, 1994). Neglect can also operate along spatial co-ordinates that have little to do with the relative location of one's body. This is sometimes apparent in multiple object drawing tasks in which patients may successfully copy the right side of *each* of the presented objects, even those that lie to the left of details of another object that they omit. In a striking demonstration of such 'object-based' neglect, Driver and Halligan (1991) used drawings of skyscraper-like buildings that had a clear principle axis. They found that, as they rotated the building (causing it, for example, to lean to the right) the patient's neglect 'rotated' with it – they continued to ignore the 'left-side' of the building, despite it now being on the right side of 'space'.

Neglect, unlike visual field cuts, can be modulated by attentional cues (Posner & Walker, 1984; Riddoch & Humphreys, 1983; Halligan & Marshall, 1994b), simultaneously affect different modalities (vision, hearing, touch), and show interactions between modalities (for example, the presence of a right sided visual stimulus can modulate patients' ability to detect a touch to their left; Mattingley, Driver, Beschin, & Robertson, 1997). Bisiach and Luzzatti (1978) demonstrated that neglect could affect mental imagery as well as current perceptual input – famously showing that Milanese patients' ability to recall the buildings in the Piaza del Duomo was significantly modulated by where they imagined themselves standing – again a feature that would not be observed with basic visual loss.

As discussed, the great majority of neglect patients show rather rapid recovery from their spatial bias – and this process disproportionately favours patients with left hemisphere damage. The reasons for the assocation between chronic neglect and right hemisphere damage remain somewhat open. Weintraub and Mesulam (1987), for example, have argued that the left hemisphere is responsible for the allocation of attention to the right half of space while the right hemisphere is capable of driving attention to the left or the right. Consequently, damage to the right hemisphere leads to domination of a rightward bias from the intact left hemisphere, while an intact right hemisphere is able to compensate for damage to the left. Given recent evidence for a primary role of the temporal cortex in mediating neglect, it has been suggested that the specialisation for language within this region on the left may account for this asymmetry and differences with the animal literature (Karnath et al., 2001). Another model suggests that each hemisphere may be somewhat specialised for particular forms of processing, with the right hemisphere being better adapted to take in the whole scene and the left hemisphere better adapted to focus on local details. Again, the consequence would be that damage to the right hemisphere would lead patients to focus on specific details within right space. In contrast, damage to the left hemisphere may impair detailed processing but leave a gross representation of the spatial characteristics of a scene intact (Halligan & Marshall, 1994a).

An alternative view, emphasises the role of damage to non-spatial right hemisphere capacities that may form the setting conditions that allow neglect to *persist* (see Heilman & Valenstein, 1979; Heilman, Schwartz, & Watson, 1978; Posner, 1993; Robertson et al., 1997b; Samuelsson, Hjelmquist, Jensen, Ekholm, & Blomstrand, 1988; Robertson & Manly, 1999). In line with this view, a recent study has shown that neglect can re-emerge in apparently recovered patients as they performed a spatial test, if they were given a second attentionally demanding task to perform at the same time (Bartolomeo, 2000; see also Robertson & Frasca, 1992). Similarly, Lazar et al. (2002) have shown that administering a sedative (midazolam) to 'recovered' neglect patients could also unmask residual spatial biases – again suggesting that the availability of non-spatial limited capacity attentional resources may be important in mediating recovery.

These findings have a number of implications for how rehabilitation should be conducted with people who show a protracted form of unilateral neglect, and how the results should be assessed. The first is that rehabilitation techniques that rely on patients being aware of their deficit and using conscious (attentionally demanding) strategies to overcome it are unlikely to be effective for anything more than a brief period (see Halligan & Marshall, 1994b). The more successful techniques (see below) should be those that effectively *oblige* (rather than *encourage*) patients to become more aware of left space. The second is that – in assessing recovery and rehabilitation – if we rely exclusively on tests that are conducted in a quiet atmosphere and which implicitly focus the patient's attention on a single task, we may miss residual deficits that will be apparent in the complex, demanding and noisy setting of many everyday activities.

Rehabilitation for unilateral neglect

Prism lens adaptation
Prism lens adaptation based therapy for unilateral neglect is a relatively recent development. If the promise of these initial studies is realised, this easily administered technique is set to become a key element in programmes addressing the disorder.

Most readers are probably familiar with the distorting effects of prism lenses. If such lenses are worn as spectacles, the visual world can be shifted to the left or right, up and down, or even completely inverted. If, when first wearing such glasses, we are asked to reach out to touch an object, we will almost certainly be inaccurate – quite reasonably reaching to where we see the object rather than where it actually is. Quite rapidly, however, our motor system takes account of the shift and accuracy is restored. Although such changes could be strategic, ('I must point to the left of where I think the object is'), the effect of removing the spectacles suggests that a much more automatic correction is occurring. When the lenses are removed, pointing now tends to be inaccurate in the opposite direction – that is, the correction

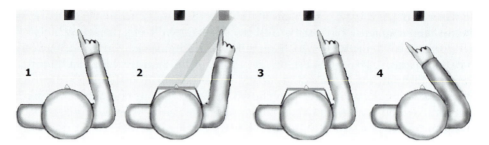

Fig. 1. Normal prism adaptation effect. 1) Before wearing the prism lenses, pointing to the object is accurate. 2) Wearing lenses that distort space to the right
initially leads to inaccurate reaching towards the apparent location. 3) Experience of errors leads to correction. 4) Removal of the lenses leads to a distortion
in the opposite direction.

for the presence of the lenses is still in place. This 'rebound' is called the *negative after-effect* (see Fig. 1). If healthy individuals are prevented from seeing
their reaches during the negative after-effect period (and therefore quickly
re-adapting), the distortion may last from minutes to hours (Redding & Wallace, 1997).

On the face of it, prisms could have a use as a prosthetic aid in visual
neglect – shifting objects located on the neglected left side to the right and into
awareness. Remarkably, however, the greater therapeutic effect appears to
emerge not when the prisms are worn permanently, but when they are briefly
used to create the negative after-effect.

Rossetti and colleagues (1998) asked a group of patients with right hemisphere lesions and left neglect to wear prim spectacles that caused a 10-degree
rightward distortion. The training involved less than five minutes of pointing
towards targets. During this phase, the reaching hand (and, hence, the error)
was visible to the patients. When the spectacles were removed there was the
expected negative after-effect. The patients' 'straight ahead' reaches now
deviated to the left relative to the pre-prism exposure baseline. Although Rossetti et al. report that the negative after-effect was much reduced in patients
showing neglect when wearing prim lenses that caused a leftward deviation,
the most striking result concerned the effect of this brief exposure to rightward distorting prisms on subsequent spatial tests. Significant improvements
were apparent in the patients' line bisection, line cancellation, drawing and
reading performance. These benefits were maintained for at least two hours
after the prisms had been removed.

In healthy people, the negative after-effect of wearing prism lenses tends
to be restricted to the 'prism-trained' hand, and, as discussed, is quite quickly
corrected if they are allowed to see their reaches during the post-prism phase.
The results of research with patients who show neglect suggests that something
rather different and more powerful is occurring. Rossetti et al. (1998) showed
that the benefits were apparent on a *reading* test – a task that clearly does not

require reaches from the trained hand (a result recently confirmed by Farnè, Rossetti, Tonolio, & Ladavas, 2002). Subsequent research has also shown improvements in general postural control (Tilikete et al., 2001), wheelchair navigation (Rossetti et al., 1999), and even mental imagery (Rode, Rossetti, & Boisson, 1999). In accounting for these apparently pervasive and lasting benefits, Rossetti et al. (1998) have suggested that the mismatch between the seen and actual location of objects acts – in some manner – to 're-calibrate' the pathological system in a more adaptive way. Mattingley (in press), citing work from Duhamel, Colby, and Goldberg (1992) and Heide and Kompf (1997), draws attention to the potential role of this strong 'error signal' in updating information from extra-retinal sources in the posterior parietal cortex.

In the largest clinical study on prism lens adaptation so far reported, Frassinetti, Angeli, Meneghello, Avanzi, and Ladavas (2002) examined the effects of a two week programme of prism exposure (20 minutes per day, 5 days per week). As with the original Rossetti et al. study, patients were instructed to point to (90) visual targets presented centrally or to the left and right, while wearing prisms that created a 10-degree rightward shift. Compared with a control group (who, although in a different hospital, were otherwise well matched on age, time-since injury and neglect severity) the prism-exposed group showed significant improvements across a range of tasks. These included both the Conventional and Behavioural subtests of Behavioural Inattention Test (Wilson, Cockburn, & Halligan, 1987), a reading measure (Ladavas, Shallice, & Zanella, 1997) and tasks requiring patients to name objects located around a room and to reach for objects on a table. As would be predicted from the earlier studies, these improvements were of much greater longevity than the negative after-effect itself, and were still present or even strengthened 5 weeks after the end of the training period.

Eye-patching
The superior colliculi in each hemisphere have a role in controlling eye-movements and shifts of attention into contralateral space. They also exist in somewhat of a dynamic relationship, activity in the right hemisphere serving to suppress activity in the left, and vice versa. As the colliculi primarily receive input from the contralateral eye (rather than visual field), Butter and Kirsch (1992) predicted that preventing stimulation to the unimpaired left colliculus by patching the right eye, may allow residual function in the right hemisphere to be better expressed.

In a study that attempted to strengthen this effect by presenting flickering light stimulation to the left eye (and therefore right colliculus), this prediction appeared to be well supported. Approximately 70% of the patients showed significantly reduced bias on a line bisection test performed while the patch was in place (although a number of other measures were unaffected).

Subsequent evaluations have, however, produced more varied results. Serfaty, Soroker, Glicksohn, Sepkuti and Myslobodsky (1995) found that, while approximately half of their sample showed benefits from right-eye patching, an almost equal number showed no benefit, and two patients were actually worse. Walker, Young and Lincoln (1996) found improvement in three patients, poorer performance in four patients and no change in two. In a case study, Barrett, Crucian, Beversdorf and Heilman (2001) reported that, whilst right eye patching produced a poorer performance, patching the *left* eye was associated with a significant reduction in neglect. It is clearly premature to rule out what might be a powerful and easily applied technique simply because it does not work for everybody. As discussed, neglect is a very heterogeneous condition. As with all the other rehabilitation interventions described here, much more work in required in examining which patients – or which forms of neglect – are most likely to benefit.

Beis, Andre, Baumgarten and Challier (1999) considered the effect of blocking input from one spatial hemifield, rather than one eye. This technique may be effective because of a behavioural training effect, effectively forcing patients to make leftward scans (or at least not let their gaze deviate to the right) if they are to 'see' at all. Reducing cortical visual stimulation to the left hemisphere may also provoke an effect similar to that outlined above, namely through allowing residual function in the damaged right hemisphere to be better expressed.

Twenty-two patients with neglect were randomly allocated to one of three groups. The first received no treatment. The second, as with Butter et al.'s study, were asked to wear glasses with patches over the entire right lens. The third group wore glasses that, due to the masking of the right side of each lens, obscured the right visual hemifield. Patients in each of the treatment conditions were asked to wear the adapted glasses for approximately twelve hours a day over a three-month period.

When re-tested at the end of the treatment (without the glasses), the hemifield group showed significantly increased spontaneous eye-movements into left space relative to the untreated control group. They also showed significant gains on a measure of functional independence in everyday activities, although the higher level of performance of the control group at the outset (leading to possible ceiling effects) means that this result should be interpreted cautiously. In contrast, the right eye patched group showed no significant benefits.

While further evaluation is warranted, including on the usefulness and safety of the treatment in the context of a dense left hemianopia, this technique is certainly easy to implement and, importantly, does not require patients to remember a strategy or consciously adjust their behaviour. If the gains in everyday activities prove reliable, the fact that the patients were exposed to the treatment as they went about their normal routine for well over 1000 hours may also be valuable in understanding this generalisation.

Visual scanning training

Attempts to increase leftward visual scans through progressive training and reinforcement have been explored since at least the 1960s. Lawson (1962), for example, describes a systematic attempt to reduce the number of left-sided word omissions made by a patient when reading a book. The procedure involved repeated reinforcement for finding the left margin of the page before beginning to read each line – in essence creating an 'object' on the left which re-contextualises the beginning of the text line as being on the 'right'. The intervention was indeed effective in reducing the frequency of left sided word omissions. The difficulty highlighted by Lawson and subsequent researchers was that such improvements could often be highly specific to the trained context – in this case not even generalising to a different edition of the same book.

Weinberg et al. (1977) and Diller and Weinberg (1977) developed a different and more abstract technique for training leftward scanning. In their procedure, patients would be asked to look at an array of lights and to track the 'movement' of the light as adjacent bulbs were sequentially illuminated. The technique was to begin with movement predominantly within right space and then progressively increase the frequency of scanning into left space. As with the reading training, patients performance on the task tends to improve but, again, generalisation to other activities has unfortunately proved rather elusive (see Webster et al., 1984; Wagenaar, Wieringen, Netelenboss, Meijer, & Kuik, 1992; Ross, 1992; Robertson, Gray, & McKenzie, 1988). This lack of generalisation does not mean that such techniques have no value in rehabilitation but does suggest that training is best conducted on activities that patients want or need to perform. Webster et al. (2001), for example, have shown that systematic training related to navigating an electric wheel-chair can produce tangible real-life advantages for patients.

Given that neglect exerts an influence over so many activities of daily living, the goal of a more general rehabilitation technique that may produce benefits across different contexts and on untrained tasks remains important. In this respect, more recent incarnations of leftward scanning training give grounds for optimism. Pizzamiglio et al. (1992) describe a programme in which patients were offered approximately 40 hours of highly systematic training. Using a variety of tasks, patients were initially given highly salient cues and encouragement for even moderate visual scans into left space. As performance improved these were progressively faded. The results suggested that, in addition to enhancing performance on the trained tasks, the programme was associated with improvements on untrained tests and, crucially, on structured everyday activities. The results were subsequently replicated in a fully randomised trial (Antonucci et al., 1995). The reasons for the success of the generalisation in comparison to previous scanning training studies remain unclear, although the authors suggest that the extended duration of the programme may have been an important factor.

Optokinetic Stimulation, Caloric Vestibular Stimulation, and Neck Muscle Vibration
A number of techniques that induce a distortion in the perception of space have been used to correct the bias of neglect. These are; *optokinetic stimula-*

tion (where a background pattern of moving dots induce involuntary eye-movements and a subjective shift in midline; Pizzamiglio, Frasca, Guariglia, Incoccia, & Antonucci, 1990); *caloric vestibular stimulation* (where a difference in temperature between the ears induced by hot or cold water induces a distortion via the vestibular system; Rubens, 1985; Cappa, Sterzi, Vallar, & Bisiach, 1987); and *posterior neck muscle vibration* (which is thought to create the illusion that the head is somewhat turned; Karnath, 1994; Karnath, Christ, & Hartje, 1993). Although these effects have been theoretically illuminating, the relatively brief duration of the improvements, in combination with the practicalities of administration, have led to pessimism about their role in rehabilitation. However, it may be that, in giving patients experience of 'the left' without requiring voluntary exertion of effort, such interventions may have value as part of broader rehabilitation programmes.

Limb Activation

Joanette and Brouchon (1984) and Joanette, Brouchon, Gauthier and Samson (1986) observed that a patient showed significantly less neglect when using her left hand to point to targets than she did when using her right. Halligan and Marshall (1989) observed similar effects of hand use in the performance of cancellation and line bisection tests. This could be explained in a number of ways. Firstly, the patient's hand and arm may form a visual cue and either serve to attract attention to the left, or to re-contextualise the left of the task as being to the 'right' of something else. Secondly, the difficulty or novelty of using the left hand may induce a generally more alert state (the positive effects of such general alerting are discussed in the next section). Thirdly, making movements with the left hand may produce a general 'activating' effect on the impaired right hemisphere, assisting it in competing with the intact left hemisphere. Finally, Rizzolatti and Camarda (1987) have argued that spatial attention is intimately connected with the intention to perform motor actions. It is therefore possible that the location of the movement rather directly serves to enhance perceptual/attentional representations of that region.

In a series of single case and group studies, Robertson and colleagues examined some of these possibilities (Robertson & North, 1992; Robertson & North, 1993; Robertson & North, 1994; Robertson, North, & Geggie, 1992; Robertson, Tegnér, Goodrich, & Wilson, 1994). The results can be summarised as follows:

1. Movement of the left hand to the left of the body midline reduced perceptual neglect, whether or not that movement was visible to the patient.
2. Movement of the *right* hand to the *left* of midline did not produce a significant reduction in neglect compared with a no movement condition.
3. Movement of the left hand alone, but to the *right* side of the body midline did not produce a significant reduction in spatial neglect.
4. Simultaneous movement of both hands (whether both to the left of the body midline, both to the right of midline, or with each hand in its congruent location) abolished the benefits of the left hand moving in isolation. In

one study, spatial performance during bilateral movements was actually worse than in the no movement condition.

5. With different patients, the left 'limb activation' effect has been shown to work in the context of cancellation tasks performed in 'near space' (within reaching distance on the table top) and 'far space' (2.44 meters away; Robertson & North, 1993 – see Halligan & Marshall, 1991 for discussion on dissociations for neglect in near and far space), for reading tasks (Robertson & North, 1992; Robertson & North, 1993; Robertson & North, 1994), for a purely tactile exploratory task (Robertson et al., 1992), for walking trajectories (Robertson et al., 1994), and for covert shifts of attention (that is moving the focus of attention in space without accompanying eye or head movements; Mattingley, Robertson, & Driver, 1998).

6. In an initial study, Robertson and North (1993) found that passive movements of the left hand (i.e. when the experimenter moved the patient's fingers) did not produce a reduction in neglect – although in this case the right hand was simultaneously moving in order to perform the cancellation task. Subsequently, however, Frassinetti, Rossi and Ladavas (2001) have shown that passive abduction and adduction of the left arm can produce benefits.

The results strongly suggest that the benefits of moving the left hand cannot be adequately explained by a visual cueing argument. The possibility that the effect is mediated by generalised arousal caused by the novelty or difficulty of moving the left hand is also difficult to sustain, given the abolition of benefits in bi-manual movement conditions. The fact that neither movement of the left hand in right space, nor movement of the right hand in left space were sufficient to produce the effect suggests a) that it is neither a simple effect of the location of action facilitating attention to that region nor b) a simple effect of left hand movement 'activating' the right hemisphere. The hemispheric activation hypothesis may, however, be tenable if it is argued that a combination of the movement and the region of space in which that movement occurs is necessary to produce a strong enough effect.[2]

Whatever the precise mechanisms, the results suggest that encouraging use of the left limb to the left side of the body may be of value in rehabilitation. This has now been explored in a number of studies. One of the difficulties is that many neglect patients under-use their left limbs, despite residual function. To counter this, Robertson et al. (1992) developed an automatic cueing

---

[2]   Interestingly, although interactions between movement and spatial attention have not been found in healthy adults (Bonfiglioli, Duncan, Rorden, & Kennett, in press), they appear to be present in young children. Dobler et al. (2001a) found that asking six and seven year old children to make (hidden) hand movements immediately prior to judging pre-bisected lines exerted a significant influence over their subsequent perception. The direction of the influence was consistent with that seen in adult neglect.

device. The 'neglect alert device' consisted of a button, variable timer and a buzzer. Patients were asked to hold the button in their left hand and remember to press it as frequently as possible while performing other tasks. If the patients did not press the button for a particular interval (usually around 8 seconds) the buzzer would be activated, reminding the patients to continue these actions. In the first series of case studies, Robertson et al. (1992) demonstrated the effectiveness of the device in improving reading and cancellation task performance. The effects were persistent in at least one patient for at least three weeks following the end of formal training. Persistent effects have been found in subsequent studies using more ecological measures (Robertson, Hogg, & McMillan, 1998a; Wilson, Manly, Coyle, & Robertson, 2000). In accounting for this persistence, it has been suggested that a positive feedback loop may be established whereby greater awareness of left space leads in turn to increased spontaneous use of the left hand.

Although some apparently severe left-sided motor problems may have an attentional component, it remains true that many patients with neglect also suffer from dense hemiplegia or find left-sided movements painful or impossible. Such patients seem, therefore, unlikely candidates to benefit from limb activation effects. Recently, however, we have examined whether observing someone else's movements may produce benefits.

The term 'mirror neurons' has been coined to refer to populations of brain cells that are active both during the execution of movement and the observation of someone else making the same movement (Di Pellegrino, Fadiga, Fogassi, Gallesem, & Rizzolatti, 1992; Gallese, Fadiga, Fogassi, & Rizzolatti, 1996; Rizzolatti, Fadiga, Gallese, & Fogassi, 1996a). Such cells have been argued to play a role in motor learning by imitation and in understanding another's actions (a 'motor idea'; Fadiga, Fogassi, Gallese, & Rizzolatti, 2000; Iacoboni et al., 1999). In human functional imaging studies, that have almost invariably considered the effects of watching another making movements with the *right* hand, such populations have been detected in left inferior frontal gyrus (BA 45; Rizzolatti et al., 1996b; Grafton, Arbib, Fadiga, & Rizzolatti, 1996), left rostral parietal cortex (BA 40) and left supplementary motor area (Grafton et al., 1996). In a study examining observed movements of the mouth, right hand and right foot, the pattern of activations suggested a rather specific topographical distribution of these effects (Buccino et al., 2001). The question we (Manly, Woldt, George, & Warburton, in preparation) considered, therefore, was whether patients with neglect and left hemiplegia could benefit from a 'limb activation' effect simply through observing somebody else make movements with their left hand?

Given that patients must have numerous opportunities to observe other people moving, it may seem unlikely that additional observation of movements would have any effect. However, in many situations it might be rather unhelpful to have our motor system activated by any movements that happen to be going on around us (imagine the effect of being at the disco, for example) and attention may, therefore, be an important mediator for this process. It is certainly the case that existing studies of mirror neurons have implicitly focused the participant's attention on another's actions. As people with unilateral neglect will tend to have rather poor attention in general, a rather specific focus on another's activity may be necessary to see any potential effect.

We tested six patients with right hemisphere lesions and left unilateral neglect on a simple naming task. Four of the patients were unable to make intentional movements with their left hand or arm. In the test, the patients first watched a video clip of an actor making repeated grasping gestures with his left or right hand. As the clips continued in a box at the centre of a computer monitor, a spatially distributed array of twelve objects (pictures, letters etc) appeared around it. By asking the patients to name the objects, we were able to get an estimate of their perception of the spatial extent of the screen without requiring them to make any hand movements themselves. Presented in a random order, the three conditions showed the actor making movements with his left hand, his right hand or remaining still for an equal period of time. Compared with the stationery condition, both hand movements were associated with significantly improved naming performance. Observing the actor's left hand moving was, however, associated with significantly better performance than observing identical movements of the right hand. It should be noted that the actor's moving left hand appears towards the right side of the screen. Consequently this effect is unlikely to emerge as the result of a purely visual cueing effect. We are currently investigating how specific this effect is to biological movement by using an additional control in which a dot moves in the same location and frequency as the hand.

Increasing general arousal – behavioural and pharmacological effects

Many neuropsychological deficits are neither absolute (in the sense that a patient can show some residual capacity) nor entirely stable (in the sense that performance will vary from one time or context to another). Whilst these fluctuations may reflect random variation or 'noise' within the system, if it is possible to identify factors that are consistently associated with improved levels of performance, these may have value in rehabilitation. Neglect illustrates these characteristics extremely well. It is rare to work with a patient who has absolutely no ability to become aware of information to the left and, within individuals, the extent and severity of neglect can be extremely variable. As discussed, one factor that reliably modulates neglect in some patients is activity of the left limbs. Another appears to be patients' state of general alertness or 'readiness-to-respond'.

In addition to chronic spatial neglect, damage to the right hemisphere has long been known to produce disproportionate deficits in a cluster of abilities variously termed alerting, arousal, vigilance or sustained attention (De Renzi & Fagliono, 1965; Boller, Howes, & Patten, 1970; Heilman et al., 1978; Howes & Boller, 1975; Heilman & Van Den Abell, 1979; Wilkins, Shallice,

& McCarthy, 1987; Rueckert & Grafman, 1996). This neuropsychological association has now received support from the normal functional imaging literature (Pardo, Fox, & Raichle, 1991; Cohen & Semple, 1988; Cohen, Semple, Gross, King, & Nordahl, 1992; Lewin et al., 1996; Sturm et al., 1999). It would be expected, therefore, that many patients with neglect would also show these deficits.

In fact, evidence suggests that this association may be more specific. Robertson et al. (1997b) asked a large group of patients to perform a rather boring task in which they were asked to keep count of the number of tones heard within a particular interval. Although this task had previously been shown to be sensitive to right hemisphere lesions (Wilkins et al., 1987), Robertson et al. observed no difference in performance between neurological patients with left hemisphere damage, and patients with right hemisphere damage *who did not show neglect*. The group of patients with right hemisphere damage who *did* show neglect were, however, extremely poor at performing this simple, non-spatial, sustained attention test. Samuelsson et al. (1988), using a different reaction time paradigm, reached similar conclusions – namely that within groups with right hemisphere lesions, chronic neglect was disproportionately associated with non-spatial attention deficits.

Robertson, Mattingley, Rorden and Driver (1998b) investigated whether there may be a direct modulatory relationship between general alertness and spatial inattention to the left. A group of patients showing neglect were asked to perform the computerised spatial task of judging which of two lateralised stimuli had appeared first (so called 'prior entry' task; Stelmach & Herdman, 1991). Under normal circumstances, the patients' pathological bias predisposes them to see the right sided stimuli as appearing first (Rorden, Mattingley, Karnath, & Driver, 1996). In Robertson et al.'s study, however, when a loud tone was presented immediately before a trial, the patients' neglect was either significantly ameliorated, abolished or, in some cases even reversed. As the tone had no predictive value for whether the left or right target would appear first, the result was interpreted as a direct effect of transitory changes in alertness on spatial awareness. These results have recently been replicated in a case of a child with neglect of developmental origin (Dobler et al., 2001b).

Although this form of external alerting does not easily lend itself to long-term rehabilitation, particularly as the novelty of the tone may be important, other means of inducing more generally alert states have been explored. Robertson, Tegnér, Tham, Lo and Nimmo-Smith (1995) trained patients in a self-instructional procedure. In the training, the patients were asked to perform rather boring (although not particularly spatial) activities such as sorting cards or coins. Occasionally – and with the patients' prior consent – the therapist would create a loud, *inherently* alerting noise by slapping the table-top. When this occurred, the patients were instructed to say a phrase such as 'Pay Attention!', the idea being to associate this self-instruction with the sensation of increased alertness. As the training progressed, the patients were first instructed take over the generation of the alerting stimulus by wrapping on the table as they said 'Pay Attention!'. After being encouraged to use the verbal cue out-load while imagining the alerting stimulus, they were finally asked to simply imagine the stimulus and the instruction and to indicate to the therapist when they were doing this. Although compliance with this training is difficult to assess, the procedure nevertheless produced significant improvements in the non-spatial tone counting measure described above. Importantly, significant reductions in spatial neglect were observed coincident with this shift, despite the absence of any spatially specific training or instruction.

Given the apparently beneficial effects of increased arousal/alertness on spatial attention, and indeed the negative effects of sedative medication (Lazar et al., 2002), an alternative approach to behavioural training may be to use pharmacological stimulants. Fleet, Valenstein, Watson and Heilman (1987) administered bromocriptine to two patients. This was associated with improvements in some, but not all, neglect measures – improvements that reversed when the medication was withdrawn. Hurford, Stringer and Jann (1998) compared the effects of methylphenidate ('Ritalin') with bromocriptine. They report that, although methylphenidate produced benefits compared with the no-treatment condition, bromocriptine produced the stronger results. These preliminary studies suggest that medication may indeed have a role within rehabilitation for neglect, although larger fully controlled trials are required.

Summary of rehabilitation for neglect

It is clear that a number of very different approaches have produced significant reductions in unilateral spatial neglect. As well as helping patients, several of these techniques have also been useful in clarifying the underlying nature of the disorder, and raised important theoretical questions for further study. In terms of the clinical application of these techniques, there remain some important questions, including:

- Neglect is a heterogeneous condition and none of the techniques described here have been effective for *all* patients. Is it useful to treat neglect as homogeneous entity in terms of rehabilitation? Are there particular patterns of response associated with different manifestations of neglect, or different lesion locations, that can allow us to better target interventions?
- Are the effects of different interventions additive in some cases?
- To date, the effects of rehabilitation have generally been assessed on standardised tests given up to one month post-intervention. In addition to investigating the maintenance of these improvements over the longer term, results showing that neglect can 're-emerge' in apparently recovered patients under demanding conditions (Bartolomeo, 2000) – or when drowsy (Lazar et al., 2002) – means that generalisation to complex everyday activities requires careful evaluation.

- Given the links between neglect and non-spatial disorders, is reducing the spatial bias sufficient *in itself* to promote significantly improved outcomes? In other words, although spatial neglect may be the most salient symptom for some patients, is it their biggest problem?

The Rehabilitation of Non-Spatial Attention

Targeting functional goals

As discussed, deficits in non-spatial attention are among the most commonly reported problems following traumatic brain injury and stroke (e.g. Oddy et al., 1985; Brooks & McKinlay, 1987; Van Zomeren & Burg, 1985; Leclerk & Zimmermann, 2002; Conkey, 1938; Van Zomeren, 1981; Van Zomeren & Burg, 1985; Van Zomeren & Deelman, 1978; Ponsford & Kinsella, 1992; Robertson, Ward, Ridgeway, & Nimmo-Smith, 1996; Leclerk & Azouvi, 2002; Robertson, Manly, Andrade, Baddeley, & Yiend, 1997a; Rousseaux, Fimm, & Cantaglio, 2002). In comparison with unilateral neglect, specific rehabilitation for this cluster of disorders is at a very early stage. Although there is not the space here to do justice to the weighty topic of assessment,[3] it is worth re-emphasising some of the difficulties faced by clinicians in this respect. In assessing and treating unilateral neglect we are dealing with a problem that is strikingly different to the behaviour of healthy individuals and one that is relatively simple to operationally define (i.e. the left is worse than the right). While there are questions about generalisation of improvements, it is clearly the case that many measures used in neglect (e.g. finding and crossing out lines on a page) bear a reasonable resemblance to everyday difficulties faced by patients (e.g. finding and reaching for food on a plate). In contrast, non-spatial attention deficits are generally quantitatively rather than qualitatively different from normal capacity limitation. Given that they are likely to pervade most activities, they are difficult to assess in a manner that controls out other causes of poor performance (e.g. memory deficits, motor problems and so forth). The measures that allow some conceptual specificity are often so abstract and focused that it calls into question the extent to which they reflect everyday difficulties and whether, if they are the sole index of change, generalisation to complex activities has taken place.

One way out of this difficulty is to effectively ignore attention as a mediating variable and instead focus on functional goals. Wilson and Robertson (1992), for example, worked with a man who had suffered a head injury and who reported difficulty in 'keeping his mind' on what he was reading. They first established a baseline in which the patient used a counter to record when he felt his attention wandering from his book. At the outset of the treatment

---

[3]   Readers are directed towards books by Parasuraman (1998) and Leclerk and Zimmermann (2002) for an in-depth discussion of attention concepts and measurement. Useful sections on the clinical assessment of attention appear in Lezak (1995) and Crawford, Parker and McKinlay (1992).

phase, he began by reading for a very short period during which, according to the baseline data, a lapse was unlikely to occur. If this was the case, the duration of reading at the next session was increased by 10%. Over 160 sessions, the patient showed steady improvement and eventually reached his goal of reading without 'slips' for 5 minutes.

As many of the man's cognitive abilities (e.g. memory, general intelligence) were relatively intact – and he could read adequately for brief periods – it is reasonable to assume that there was strong attentional component to his difficulty. As reading duration was the sole outcome measure, however, whether or not the training improved his attention in a more general sense remains an open question in this case.

Alderman, Fry and Youngson (1995) highlight another case in which attention was thought to underlie the maintenance of difficulties in everyday life – in this example, very severe behavioural problems. SK was a young woman who suffered diffuse damage and focal lesions to the temporal lobes as the result of herpes simplex encephalitis. Three months after the injury, her behaviour at the rehabilitation centre was causing disruption to her own and others' programmes. In particular she was said to produce extremely loud comments about her own actions, the actions of others and their disabilities, and to do so in a near continuous manner. Initial behavioural treatment (in which SK was asked to give up a reward token each time the behaviour occurred) produced significant reductions in frequency but generalisation to a different context was disappointing. Hypothesising that SK may be rather unaware of her actions and therefore not ideally placed to reduce them, Alderman et al. then set out to train awareness. When walking with her therapist, SK was given a counter and asked to record each time she noticed herself making a verbal utterance. Comparison of her ratings with those of her therapist confirmed a vast disparity, with SK underestimating the frequency of her behaviour by approximately 90%. After a period during which she was prompted by the therapist to record instances as they occurred, SK was then given rewards conditional upon increasing the accuracy of her own monitoring. Only when this accuracy had improved to above 70% was any further attempt made to reduce the *frequency* of the behaviour – which was now successful. Again, it is unclear whether these improvements in self-monitoring and attention were specific to the verbal behaviour. The most important result, in terms of the likelihood of SK's returning to community living, however, was that the behaviour was reduced.

Training attention using abstract tasks

Personal computers provide a now relatively cheap and highly standardised method for attention training. Although such exercises in the field of memory have tended to produce improvements that are specific to the trained material rather than to the learning process in general (e.g. Glisky, Schacter, & Tulving, 1986a; Glisky, Schacter, & Tulving, 1986b) this may not be the case for other capacities.

In a randomised controlled study, Gray, Robertson, Pentland and Anderson (1992) offered 15 hours of computerised training to people with attentional problems resulting from a brain injury. The exercises included: a reaction time task with feedback on speed, a task requiring the identification of two identical digit strings from a briefly presented array of 4, a digit-symbol translation task, and a colour-word Stroop task. On completion of the training, the patients showed significant improvements on two untrained measures (the WAIS-R Picture Completion subtest and the Paced Auditory Serial Addition Task PASAT) relative to the control group who had received similar periods of recreational computing. When reassessed six months later, these improvements had been well maintained and indeed now extended to a wider range of measures. Generalisation to functional activities of everyday life was not examined in this study.

In light of the proposed functional separation between different forms of attention (sustained attention, selective attention and so forth), and suggestions in the literature that attention training effects might be rather specific, Sturm, Willmes, Orgass and Hartje (1997) set out to specifically test this hypothesis in a rehabilitation study. Thirty-eight patients with quantified attention deficits (mainly resulting from stroke) took part in the trial using the AIXTENT[4] computerised package. The package consisted of distinct modules, each designed to train a specific attention function. In one of the sustained attention module tasks, for example, patients watch several aircraft slowly flying across radar screen. Their task is to look out for abrupt changes in any of the aircraft's velocity or the transitory appearance of new objects on the screen, signalling detection by pressing a button. In contrast, the selective attention training tasks include a 'photo safari', a much more briskly paced activity in which the patients are asked to 'take photos' of some, but not all, objects that pop-up from a scenic background. The other training modules were for alertness and divided attention. The difficulty of the all the tasks was automatically and incrementally increased in response to adequate performance.

To evaluate the success and the specificity of the training, Sturm and colleagues administered the modules to each patient in a randomly selected *order*. They hypothesised that, if the training was indeed specific, improvements in sustained attention function should be greater following sustained attention training than, for example, selective attention training. Evaluation was made using repeated administrations of the computerised Test of Attentional Performance ('TAP'; Zimmermann, North, & Fimm, 1993) – a battery that allows separable assessment of different attentional components.

The hypothesis was broadly supported. Detection rates for targets in the untrained TAP vigilance task was significantly improved, for example, only after sustained attention training and not following training in selective or divided attention. Similarly, reaction times in the selective attention test

---

4   An English Language version of this package is under development.

were improved following selective attention training, but not after training of sustained attention. As might be expected, some crossover effects were also observed (divided attention performance being significantly enhanced following training in selective attention, for example). The results have now been substantially replicated in a multi-centre study in which each patient was exposed to only one of the training modules (Sturm et al., 2002a).

Supporting residual function

Variability is a central, if not definitive, feature of 'attention' deficits. The fact that performance on a task may, at one time, be adequate and, at another, quite deficient suggests that many of the basic components required for performance (e.g. vision, reading skill, motor responses) are present but for some reason are unreliably orchestrated to produce the desired results. As we saw with some interventions for neglect, if it is possible to identify factors that are consistently associated with better levels of performance, these may have value in rehabilitation.

Many of these 'interventions' will be of a type we all use in everyday life. These may include making sure the TV and radio are turned off before attempting an important activity or in planning regular breaks *before* concentration begins to flag. Given that patients may have limited insight into their deficits, or have trouble in spontaneously adjusting their behaviour to take account of deficits, it should not be assumed that these will be applied without assistance.

The extent to which poor performance on neuropsychological tests may be related to poor motivation or reluctance to expend 'mental effort' is often a tricky question, particularly on attention measures that are designed to be tedious and unrewarding. Of course, low motivation, or indifference to outcome, can itself be a consequence of brain injury (Stuss & Benson, 1983; Stuss & Benson, 1986), as well as resulting from patients becoming dispirited by repeated experience of failure, or from pre-morbid factors. It is certainly the case that 'motivating' instructions have been associated with improved performance relative to baseline on attentional measures (Blackburn, 1958; Shankweiler, 1959; Sturm et al., 2002b) and therefore by extension, may be effective in increasing attentional performance across a range of everyday tasks.

We (Manly, Hawkins, Evans, Woldt, & Robertson, 2002) have recently explored the (perhaps obvious) possibility that patients may be better able to usefully attend if they are reminded to do so. In order to mimic some of the complexities and competing demands of real-life tasks, we adapted Shallice and Burgess' (1991) Six Elements task. In this measure (the 'Hotel Test') the patients were provided with materials for 5 activities plausibly associated with running a hotel (sorting conference labels into alphabetical order, checking bills, proof-reading a tourist leaflet and sorting the coins from the charity collection). They were told that over the 15 minutes of the test they should try and sample each of the jobs but were warned that each task in isolation would take longer than the available 15 minutes to complete. As with the Six Elements, therefore, the test emphasised the patients' ability to keep track of this main goal and to flexibly shift between tasks when appropriate. Also in line with the earlier finding, 10 TBI patients performed significantly more poorly than IQ matched controls, the key error being to get caught up in one of the component tasks to the detriment of monitoring the overall goal. When however, the patients were exposed to randomly timed auditory 'beeps' – and having been instructed to use these as a reminder to 'think about what they were doing', their performance was not only significantly improved but was also no longer distinguishable from that of the control group. The results suggest that, at least in this group, the key reason for poor performance was a failure to maintain sufficient attention on the main goal rather than, for example, forgetting what that goal was. It also suggests that, if the *use* of residual capacities is supported by cueing, performance in quite complex functional activities may be improved.

Summary of rehabilitation for non-spatial attention
Although the rehabilitation of non-spatial attention is at an early stage (not least because theoretical development and assessment in this area are at an early stage) there are, nevertheless, optimistic signs. There is good evidence that functional difficulties in everyday life that seem to be partially determined by attention problems can be successfully retrained – although the extent to which this is possible will no doubt vary with the task.[5] There is also good evidence from a number of studies that repeated and progressive training, even on abstract computer tasks, can generalise to untrained measures. A clear direction for future work is to establish whether the functional goal based training approach produces more general improvements in attention function, and whether the abstract training produces benefits that generalise to functional real-life goals.

Acknowledgement

The writing of this chapter was supported by the UK Medical Research Council.

---

[5] There is of course abundant evidence that, with sufficient practice, many tasks that are initially attentionally demanding can come to be performed in a relatively 'automatic' fashion (Shiffrin & Schneider, 1977; Schneider, Dumais, & Shiffrin, 1984) – a feature that should not be overlooked in the rehabilitation of specific activities.

References

Alderman, N., Fry, R.K., & Youngson, H.A. (1995). Improvement in self-monitoring skills, reduction of behaviour disturbance and the dysexecutive syndrome: Comparison of response cost and a new programme of self-monitoring training. *Neuropsychological Rehabilitation, 5(3)*, 193-221.

Antonucci, G., Guariglia, C., Judica, A., Magnotti, L., Paoloucci, S., Pizzamiglio, L., & Zoccolotti, P. (1995). Effectiveness of neglect rehabilitation in a randomized group-study. *Journal of Clinical and Experimental Neuropsychology, 17*, 383-389.

Barrett, A.M., Crucian, G.P., Beversdorf, D.Q., & Heilman, K.M. (2001). Monocular patching may worsen sensory-attentional neglect: A case report. *Archives of Physical Medicine and Rehabilitation, 82(4)*, 516-518.

Bartolomeo, P. (2000). Inhibitory processes and spatial bias after right hemisphere damage. *Neuropsychological Rehabilitation, 10(5)*, 511-526.

Beis, J.M., Andre, J.M., Baumgarten, A., & Challier, B. (1999). Eye patching in unilateral spatial neglect: Efficacy of two methods. *Archives of Physical Medicine and Rehabilitation, 80*, 71-76.

Ben-Yishay, Y., Diller, L., Gerstman, L., & Haas, A. (1968). The relationship between impersistence, intellectual function and outcome of rehabilitation in patients with left hemiplegia. *Neurology, 18*, 852-861.

Bisiach, E., & Luzzatti, C. (1978). Unilateral neglect of representational space. *Cortex, 14*, 129-133.

Blackburn, H.J. (1958). Effects of motivating instructions on reaction time in cerebral disease. *Journal of abnormal and social psychology, 56*, 359-366.

Blanc-Garin, J. (1994). Patterns of recovery from hemiplegia following stroke. *Neuropsychological Rehabilitation, 4*, 359-385.

Boller, F., Howes, D., & Patten, D.H. (1970). A behavioural evaluation of brain scan results with neuropathalogical findings. *Lancet, 1*, 1143-1146.

Bonfiglioli, C., Duncan, J., Rorden, C., & Kennett, S. (in press). Action and perception: Evidence against converging selection processes. *Visual Cognition*.

Bradshaw, J.L., & Mattingley, J.B. (1995). *Clinical Neuropsychology: Behavioural and Brain Science*. San Diego: Academic Press.

Brain, R. (1941). Visual disorientation with special reference to lesions of the right hemisphere. *Brain, 64*, 244-272.

Broadbent, D.E. (1958). *Perception and Communication*. London: Pergamen Press.

Brooks, D.N., & McKinlay, W. (1987). Return to work within the first seven years of severe head injury. *Brain Injury, 1*, 5-15.

Buccino, G., Binkofski, F., Fink, G.R., Fadiga, L., Fogassi, L., Gallese, V., Seitz, R.J., Zilles, K., Rizzolatti, G., & Freund, H. (2001). Action observation activates premotor and parietal areas in a somatotopic manner: an fMRI study. *European Journal Of Neuroscience, 13(2)*, 400-404.

Butter, C., & Kirsch, N. (1992). Combined and separate effects of eye patching and visual stimulation on unilateral neglect following stroke. *Archives of Physical Medicine and Rehabilitation, 73*, 1133-1139.

Cappa, S.F., Sterzi, R., Vallar, G., & Bisiach, E. (1987). Remission of hemineglect and anosognosia during vestibular stimulation. *Neuropsychologia, 25*, 775-782.

Cherney, L.R., Halper, A.S., Kwasnica, C.M., Harvey, R.L., & Zhang, M. (2001). Recovery of functional status after right hemisphere stroke: Relationship with unilateral neglect. *Archives of Physical Medicine and Rehabilitation, 82(3)*, 322-328.

Chung, C.S., Caplan, L.R., Yamamoto, Y., Chang, H.M., Lee, S.J., Song, H.J., Lee, H.S., Shin, H.K., & Yoo, K.M. (2000). Striatocapsular haemorrhage. *Brain, 123*, 1580-1862.

Cohen, R.A., & Kaplan, R.F. (1993). Attention as a multicomponent process – neuropsychological validation. *Journal of Clinical and Experimental Neuropsychology, 15(3)*, 379.

Cohen, R.M., & Semple, W.E. (1988). Functional localization of sustained attention. *Neuropsychiatry, Neuropsychology and Behavioural Neurology, 1*, 3-20.

Cohen, R.M., Semple, W.E., Gross, M., King, A.C., & Nordahl, T.E. (1992). Metabolic brain pattern of sustained auditory discrimination. *Experimental Brain Research, 92(1)*, 165-172.

Conkey, R.C. (1938). Psychological changes associated with head injuries. *Archives of Psychology, 232*, 1-62.

Crawford, J., Parker, D.M., & McKinlay, L. (1992). *A handbook of neuropsychological assessment*. Hove: Laurence Earlbaum.

Damasio, A.R., Damasio, H., & Chui, H.C. (1980). Neglect following damage to frontal lobe or basal ganglia. Neuropsychologia, *18*, 123-132.

De Renzi, E., & Fagliono, P. (1965). The comparative efficiency of intelligence and vigilance tests in detecting hemispheric cerebral damage. *Cortex, 1*, 410-433.

de Seze, M., Wiart, L., Bon-Saint-Come, A., Debelleix, X., de Seze, M., Joseph, P.A., Mazaux, J.M., & Barat, M. (2001). Rehabilitation of postural disturbances of hemiplegic patients by using trunk control retraining during exploratory exercises. *Archives of Physical Medicine and Rehabilitation, 82(6)*, 793-800.

Denes, G., Semenza, C., Stoppa, E., & Lis, A. (1982). Unilateral spatial neglect and recovery from hemiplegia. A follow-up study. *Brain, 105*, 543-552.

Di Pellegrino, G., Fadiga, L., Fogassi, L., Gallesem, V., & Rizzolatti, G. (1992). Understanding Motor Events – A Neurophysiological Study. *Experimental Brain Research, 91(1)*, 176-180.

Diller, L., & Weinberg, J. (1977). Hemi-inattention in rehabilitation: The evolution of a rational rehabilitation program. In E.A. Weinstein & R.P. Friedland (Eds.), *Advances in Neurology, Vol. 10*. New York: Raven Press.

Dobler, V., Manly, T., Atkinson, J., Wilson, B.A., Ioannou, K., & Robertson, I.H. (2001a). Interaction of hand use and spatial selective attention in children. *Neuropsychologia, 39(10)*, 1055-1064.

Dobler, V., Manly, T., Robertson, I.H., Polichroniadis, M., Verity, C., Goodyer, I., & Wilson, B.A. (2001b). Modulation of hemispatial attention in a case of developmental unilateral neglect. *Neurocase, 7(185)*.

Driver, J., & Halligan, P.W. (1991). Can visual neglect operate in object-centred co-ordinates? An affirmative single-case study. *Cognitive Neuropsychology, 8*, 475-496.

Duhamel, J.-R., Colby, C.L., & Goldberg, M.E. (1992). The updating of the representation of visual space in parietal cortex by intended eye movements. *Science, 255*, 90-92.

Fadiga, L., Fogassi, L., Gallese, V., & Rizzolatti, G. (2000). Visuomotor neurons: ambiguity of the discharge or 'motor' perception? International *Journal of Psychophysiology, 35*, 165-177.

Farnè, A., Rossetti, Y., Tonolio, S., & Ladavas, E. (2002). Ameliorating neglect with prism adaptation: visuo-manual and visuo-verbal measures. *Neuropsychologia, 40*, 718-729.

Fleet, W.S., Valenstein, E., Watson, R.T., & Heilman, K.M. (1987). Dopamine agonist therapy for neglect in humans. *Neurology, 37*, 1765-1771.

Frassinetti, F., Angeli, V., Meneghello, F., Avanzi, S., & Ladavas, E. (2002). Long-lasting amelioration of visuospatial neglect by prism adaptation. *Brain, 125*, 608-623.

Frassinetti, F., Rossi, M., & Ladavas, E. (2001). Passive limb movements improve visual neglect. *Neuropsychologia, 39(7)*, 725-733.

Fullerton, J., McSherry, P., & Stout, M. (1986). Albert's Test: a neglected test of perceptual neglect. *Lancet* 22 Feb, 430-432.

Gallese, V., Fadiga, L., Fogassi, L., & Rizzolatti, G. (1996). Action recogniton in the premotor cortex. *Brain, 119,* 593.

Glisky, E.L., Schacter, D.L., & Tulving, E. (1986a). Computer learning by memory-impaired patients: acquisition and retention of complex knowledge. *Neuropsychologia, 24,* 313-328.

Glisky, E.L., Schacter, D.L., & Tulving, E. (1986b). Learning and retention of computer-related vocabulary in memory-impaired patients: method of vanishing cues. *Journal of Clinical and Experimental Neuropsychology, 8,* 292-312.

Grafton, S.T., Arbib, M.A., Fadiga, L., & Rizzolatti, G. (1996). Localization of grasp representations in humans by positron emission tomography 2. Observation compared with imagination. *Experimental Brain Research, 112(1),* 103-111.

Gray, J., & Robertson, I. (1989). Remediation of attentional difficulties following brain injury: three experimental single case studies. *Brain Injury, 3,* 163-170.

Gray, J.M., Robertson, I.H., Pentland, B., & Anderson, S.I. (1992). Microcomputer based cognitive rehabilitation for brain damage: a randomised group controlled trial. *Neuropsychological Rehabilitation, 2,* 97-116.

Halligan, P.W., & Marshall, J.C. (1989). Laterality of motor response in visuo-spatial neglect: a case study. *Neuropsychologia, 27,* 1301-1307.

Halligan, P.W., & Marshall, J.C. (1991). Left neglect for near but not far space in man. *Nature, 350,* 498-500.

Halligan, P.W., & Marshall, J.C. (1994a). Focal and global attention modulate the expression of visuo-spatial neglect: a case study. *Neuropsychologia, 32,* 13-21.

Halligan, P.W., & Marshall, J.C. (1994b). Right-sided cueing can ameliorate left neglect. *Neuropsychological Rehabilitation, 4,* 63-73.

Heide, W., & Kompf, D. (1997). Specific parietal lobe contribution to spatial constancy across saccades. In P. Thier & H.O. Karnath (Eds.), *Parietal lobe contributions to orientation in 3D space* (pp. 49-172). Heidelberg: Springer-Verlag.

Heilman, K.H., & Van Den Abell, T. (1979). Right hemisphere dominance for mediating cerebral activation. *Neuropsychologia, 17,* 315-321.

Heilman, K.M., Schwartz, H.D., & Watson, R.T. (1978). Hypoarousal in patients with the neglect syndrome and emotional indifference. *Neurology, 28,* 229-232.

Heilman, K.M., & Valenstein, E. (1979). Mechanisms underlying hemispatial neglect. *Annals of Neurology, 5,* 166-170.

Hier, D.B., Davis, K.R., Richardson, E.P., & Mohr, J.P. (1977). Hypertensive putaminal hemorrhage. *Annals of Neurology, 1,* 152-159.

Hier, D.B., Mondlock, J., & Caplan, L.R. (1983). Recovery of behavioural abnormalities after right hemisphere stroke. *Neurology, 33,* 345-350.

Howes, D., & Boller, F. (1975). Simple reaction time: Evidence for focal impairment from lesions of the right hemisphere. *Brain, 98,* 317-322.

Hurford, P., Stringer, A., & Jann, B. (1998). Neuropharmacologic treatment of hemineglect: A case report comparing bromocriptine and methylphenidate. *Archives of Physical Medicine and Rehabilitation, 79(3),* 346-349.

Iacoboni, M., Woods, R.P., Brass, M., Bekkering, H., Mazziotta, J.C., & Rizzolatti, G. (1999). Cortical Mechanisms of Human Imitation. *Science, 286,* 2526-2528.

Joanette, Y., & Brouchon, M. (1984). Visual allesthesia in manual pointing: some evidence for a sensori-motor cerebral organization. *Brain and Cognition, 3,*152-165.

Joanette, Y., Brouchon, M., Gauthier, L., & Samson, M. (1986). Pointing with left versus right hand in left visual field neglect. *Neuropsychologia, 24,* 391-396.

Karnath, H.O. (1994). Subjective body orientation in neglect and the interactive contribution of neck muscle proprioception and vestibular stimulation. *Brain, 117,* 1001-1012.

Karnath, H.O., Christ, K., & Hartje, W. (1993). Decrease of contralateral neglect by neck muscle vibration and spatial orientation of trunk midline. *Brain, 116,* 383-396.

Karnath, H.O., Ferber, S., & Himmelbach, M. (2001). Spatial awareness is a function of the temporal not the posterior parietal lobe. *Nature, 411*, 950-953.

Karnath, H.O., Schenkel, P., & Fischer, B. (1991). Trunk orientation as the determining factor of the 'contralateral' deficit in the neglect syndrome and as the physical anchor of the internal representation of body orientation in space. *B, 114*, 1997-2014.

Kumral, E., Evyapan, D., & Balkir, K. (1999). Acute caudate vascular lesions. *Stroke, 30*, 100-108.

Ladavas, R., Shallice, T., & Zanella, M.T. (1997). Preserved semantic access in neglect dyslexia. *Neuropsychologia, 35*, 257-70.

Lawson, I.R. (1962). Visual-spatial neglect in lesions of the right cerebral hemisphere: A study in recovery. *Neurology, 12*, 23-33.

Lazar, R., Fitzsimmons, B., Marshall, R., Berman, M., Bustillo, M., Young, W., Mohr, J., Shah, J., & Robinson, J. (2002). Reemergence of stroke deficits with midazolam challenge. *Stroke, 33(1)*, 283-285.

Leclerk, M., & Azouvi, P. (2002). Attention after traumatic brain injury. In M. Leclerk & P. Zimmermann (Eds.), *Applied Neuropsychology of Attention* (pp. 257-279). Hove: Psychology Press.

Leclerk, M., & Zimmermann, P. (2002). *Applied Neuropsychology of Attention.* Hove: Psychology Press.

Lewin, J.S., Friedman, L., Wu, D., Miller, D.A., Thompson, L.A., Klein, S.K., Wise, A.L., Hedera, P., Buckley, P., Meltzer, H., Friedland, R.P., & Duerk, J.L. (1996). Cortical localization of human sustained attention: Detection with functional MR using a visual vigilance paradigm. *Journal of Computer Assisted Tomography, 20(5)*, 695-701.

Lezak, M.D. (1995). *Neuropsychological Assessment (3rd ed.).* New York: Oxford University Press.

Mackworth, N.H. (1948). The breakdown of vigilance during prolonged visual search. *The Quarterly Journal of Experimental Psychology, 1(1)*, 6-21.

Manly, T., Hawkins, K., Evans, J.J., Woldt, K., & Robertson, I.H. (2002). Rehabilitation of Executive Function: Facilitation of effective goal management on complex tasks using periodic auditory alerts. *Neuropsychologia, 40(3)*, 271-281.

Mattingley, J.B. (in press). Visuomotor adaptation to optical prisms: a new cure for sptaial neglect? *Cortex*.

Mattingley, J.B., & Bradshaw, J.L. (1994). Can tactile neglect occur at an intra-limb level? Vibrotactile reaction times in patients with right hemisphere damage. *Behavioural Neurology, 7*, 67-77.

Mattingley, J.B., Driver, J., Beschin, N., & Robertson, I.H. (1997). Attentional competition between modalities: Extinction between touch and vision after right hemisphere damage. *Neuropsychologia, 35(6)*, 867-880.

Mattingley, J.B., Robertson, I.H., & Driver, J. (1998). Modulation of covert visual attention by hand movement: evidence from parietal extinction after right-hemisphere damage. *Neurocase, 4*, 245-253.

Mesulam, M.M. (1981). A cortical network for directed attention and unilateral neglect. *Annals of Neurology, 10*, 309-325.

Mirsky, A.F., Anthony, B.J., Duncan, C.C., Ahearn, M.B., & Kellam, S.G. (1991). Analysis of the elements of attention: A neuropsychological approach. *Neuropsychology Review, 2*, 109-145.

Oddy, M., Coughlan, T., Tyerman, A., & Jenkins, D. (1985). Social Adjustment after closd head injury: a further follow-up seven years after injury. *Journal of Neurology, Neurosurgury and Psychiatry, 48*, 564-568.

Ogden, J.A. (1985). Anterior-posterior interhemispheric differences in the loci of lesions producing visual hemineglect. *Brain and Cognition, 4*, 59-75.

Paolucci, S., Antonucci, G., Grasso, M., & Pizzamiglio, L. (2001a). The role of unilateral spatial neglect in rehabilitation of right brain-damaged ischemic stroke patients: A matched comparison. *Archives of Physical Medicine and Rehabilitation, 82(6)*, 743-749.

Paolucci, S., Grasso, M.G., Antonucci, G., Bragoni, M., Troisi, E., Morelli, D., Coiro, P., De Angelis, D., & Rizzi, F. (2001b). Mobility status after inpatient stroke rehabilitation: 1-year follow-up and prognostic factors. *Archives of Physical Medicine and Rehabilitation, 82(1)*, 2-8.

Parasuraman, R. (1998). *The Attentive Brain*. Massachusetts: MIT.

Pardo, J.V., Fox, P.T., & Raichle, M.E. (1991). Localization of a human system for sustained attention by positron emission tomography. *Nature, 349*, 61-64.

Pizzamiglio, L., Antonucci, G., Judica, A., Montenero, P., Rrazzano, C., & Zoccolotti, P. (1992). Cognitive rehabilitation of the hemineglect disorder in chronic-patients with unilateral right brain-damage. *Journal of Clinical and Experimental Neuropsychology, 14(6)*, 901-923.

Pizzamiglio, L., Frasca, R., Guariglia, C., Incoccia, C., & Antonucci, G. (1990). Effect of optokinetic stimulation in patients with visual neglect. *Cortex, 26*, 535-540.

Ponsford, J., & Kinsella, G. (1992). Attentional Deficits following closed-head injury. *Journal of Clinical and Experimental Neuropsychology, 14(5)*, 822-838.

Posner, M.I. (1993). Interaction of arousal and selection in the posterior attention network. In A. Baddeley & L. Weiskrantz (Eds.), *Attention: Selection, Awareness and Control* (pp. 390-405). Oxford: Clarendon Press.

Posner, M.I., & Petersen, S. E. (1990). The attention system of the human brain. *Annual Review of Neuroscience, 13*, 25-42.

Posner, M.I., & Walker, J.A. (1984). The Effects of Parietal Injury on Covert Orienting of Attention. *Journal of Neuroscience, 4*, 1863-1874.

Redding, G.M., & Wallace, B. (1997). *Adaptive Spatial Alignment*. Mahway, N.J.: Lawrence Earlbaum Associates.

Riddoch, M.J., & Humphreys, G.W. (1983). The effect of cueing on unilateral neglect. *Neuropsychologia, 21*, 589-599.

Rizzolatti, G., & Camarda, R. (1987). Neural circuits for spatial attention and unilateral neglect. In M. Jeannerod (Ed.), *Neurophysiological and Neuropsychological Aspects of Neglect*. Amsterdam: North Holland Press.

Rizzolatti, G., Fadiga, L., Gallese, V., & Fogassi, L. (1996a). Premotor cortex and the recognition of motor actions. *Cognitive Brain Research, 3*, 131-141.

Rizzolatti, G., Fadiga, L., Matelli, M., Bettinardi, V., Paulesu, E., Perani, D., & Fazio, F. (1996b). Localization of grasp representations in humans by PET .1. Observation versus execution. *Experimental Brain Research, 111(2)*, 246-252.

Robertson, I., Gray, J., & McKenzie, S. (1988). Microcomputer-based cognitive rehabilitation of visual neglect: three multiple-baseline single-case studies. *Brain Injury, 2*, 151-163.

Robertson, I.H., & Frasca, R. (1992). Attentional load and visual neglect. International *Journal of Neuroscience, 62*, 45-56.

Robertson, I.H., Hogg, K., & McMillan, T.M. (1998a). Rehabilitation of Unilateral Neglect: Improving Function by Contralesional Limb Activation. *Neuropsychological Rehabilitation, 8(1)*, 19-29.

Robertson, I.H., & Manly, T. (1999). Sustained Attention Deficits in Time and Space. In G.W. Humphreys, J. Duncan, & A.M. Treisman (Eds.), *Attention, space, and action: Studies in cognitive neuroscience*. Oxford: Oxford University Press.

Robertson, I.H., Manly, T., Andrade, J., Baddeley, B.T., & Yiend, J. (1997a). 'Oops!': Performance correlates of everyday attentional failures in traumatic brain injured and normal subjects. *Neuropsychologia, 35(6)*, 747-758.

Robertson, I.H., Manly, T., Beschin, N., Haeske-Dewick, H., Hömberg, V., Jehkonen, M., Pizzamiglio, L., Shiel, A., Weber, E., & Zimmerman, P. (1997b). Auditory Sustained Attention is a Marker of Unilateral Spatial Neglect. *Neuropsychologia, 35*, 1527-1532.

Robertson, I.H., Mattingley, J.M., Rorden, C., & Driver, J. (1998b). Phasic alerting of neglect patients overcomes their spatial deficit in visual awareness. *Nature, 395*, 169-172.

Robertson, I.H., & North, N. (1992). Spatio-motor cueing in unilateral neglect: the role of hemispace, hand and motor activation. *Neuropsychologia, 30*, 553-563.

Robertson, I.H., & North, N. (1993). Active and passive activation of left limbs: influence on visual and sensory neglect. *Neuropsychologia, 31*, 293-300.

Robertson, I.H., & North, N. (1994). One hand is better than two: motor extinction of left hand advantage in unilateral neglect. *Neuropsychologia, 32*, 1-11.

Robertson, I.H., North, N., & Geggie, C. (1992). Spatio-motor cueing in unilateral neglect: three single case studies of its therapeutic effectiveness. *Journal of Neurology, Neurosurgery and Psychiatry, 55*, 799-805.

Robertson, I.H., Ridgeway, V., Greenfield, E., & Parr, A. (1997c). Motor recovery after stroke depends on intact sustained attention: A two year follow-up study. *Neuropsychology, 11(2)*, 290-295.

Robertson, I.H., Tegnér, R., Goodrich, S.J., & Wilson, C. (1994). Walking trajectory and hand movements in unilateral left neglect: A vestibular hypothesis. *Neuropsychologia, 32(12)*, 1495-1502.

Robertson, I.H., Tegnér, R., Tham, K., Lo, A., & Nimmo-Smith, I. (1995). Sustained attention training for unilateral neglect: Theoretical and rehabilitation implications. *Journal of Clinical and Experimental Neuropsychology, 17*, 416-430.

Robertson, I.H., Ward, A., Ridgeway, V., & Nimmo-Smith, I. (1996). The structure of normal human attention: The Test of Everyday Attention. *Journal of the International Neuropsychological Society, 2*, 523-534.

Rode, G., Rossetti, Y., & Boisson, D. (1999). Improvement of mental imagery after prism exposure in neglect: a case study. *Behavioural Neurology, 11*, 251-258.

Rorden, C., Mattingley, J.B., Karnath, H., & Driver, J. (1996). Visual extinction and prior entry: Impaired perception of temporal order with intact motion perception after unilateral parietal damage. *Neuropsychologia, 35(4)*, 421-433.

Ross, F.L. (1992). The use of computers in occupational therapy in visual scanning training. *American Journal of Occupational Therapy, 46*, 314-322.

Rossetti, Y., Rode, G., Pisella, L., Farne, A., Li, L., Boisson, D., & Perenin, M.T. (1998). Prism adaptation to a rightward optical deviation rehabilitates left hemispatial neglect. *Nature, 395*, 166-169.

Rossetti, Y., Rode, G., Pisella, L., Farné, A., Ling, L., & Boisson, D. (1999). Sensorimotor plasticity and cognition: prism adaptation can affect various levels of space representation. In M. Grealy & J.A. Thomson (Eds.), *Studies in Perception and Action* (pp. 265-269). Hove, UK: Lawrence Erlbaum Associates.

Rousseaux, M., Fimm, B., & Cantaglio, A. (2002). Attention disorders in cerebro-vascular disease. In M. Leclerk & P. Zimmermann (Eds.), *Applied Neuropsychology of Attention* (pp. 280-304). Hove: Psychology Press.

Rubens, A.B. (1985). Caloric stimulation and unilateral visual neglect. *Neurology, 35*, 1019-1024.

Rueckert, L., & Grafman, J. (1996). Sustained attention deficits in patients with right frontal lesions. *Neuropsychologia, 34(10)*, 953-963.

Samuelsson, H., Hjelmquist, E., Jensen, C., Ekholm, S., & Blomstrand, C. (1988). Nonlateralized attentional deficits: An important component behind persisting visuospatial neglect? *Journal of Clinical and Experimental Psychology, 20(1)*, 73-88.

Samuelsson, H., Jensen, C., Ekholm, S., Naver, H., & Blomstrand, C. (1997). Anatomical and neurological correlates of acute and chronic visuospatial neglect following right hemisphere stroke. *Cortex, 33*, 271-85).

Schneider, W., Dumais, S.T., & Shiffrin, R.M. (1984). Automatic and Control Processing and Attention. In R. Parasuraman & D.R. Davies (Eds.), *Varieties of Attention* . Orlando: Academic Press.

Sea, M.C., Henderson, A., & Cermack, S.A. (1993). Patterns of visual spatial inattention and their functional significance in stroke patients. *Archives of Physical Medicine and Rehabilitation, 74*, 355-361.

Serfaty, C., Soroker, N., Glicksohn, J., Sepkuti, J., & Myslobodsky, M.S. (1995). Does monocular viewing improve target detection in hemispatial neglect? *Restorative Neurology and Neuroscience, 9*, 7-13.

Shallice, T., & Burgess, P. (1991). Deficit in strategy application following frontal lobe damage in man. *Brain, 114*, 727-741.

Shankweiler, D.P. (1959). Effects of success or failure instructions on reaction time in patients with brain damage. *Journal of Comparitive and Physiological Psychology, 52*, 546-549.

Shiffrin, R.M., & Schneider, W. (1977). Controlled and automatic human information processing: II. Perceptual learning, automatic attending, and a general theory. *Psychological Review, 84*, 127-190.

Sprague, J.M. (1966). Interaction of cortex and superior colliculus in mediation of visually guided behaviour in the cat. *Science, 153*, 1544-1547.

Stelmach, L.B., & Herdman, C.M. (1991). Directed attention and the detection of temporal order. *Journal of Experimental Psychology: Human Perception and Performance, 17*, 539-540.

Stone, S.P., Halligan, P.W., & Greenwood, R.J. (1993). The incidence of neglect phenomena and related disorders in patients with an acute right or left-hemisphere stroke. *Age and Ageing, 22(1)*, 46-52.

Stone, S.P., Patel, P., Greenwood, R.J., & Halligan, P.W. (1992). Measuring visual neglect in acute stroke and predicting its recovery: the visual neglect recovery index. *Journal of Neurology, Neurosurgery and Psychiatry, 55*, 431-436.

Stone, S.P., Wilson, B.A., Wroot, A., Halligan, P.W., Lange, L.S., Marshall, J.C., & Greenwood, R.J. (1991). The assessment of visuo-spatial neglet after acute stroke. *Journal of Neurology, Neurosurgery and Psychiatry, 54*, 345-350.

Sturm, W., Fimm, B., Cantagallo, A., Cremel, N., North, P., Passadori, A., Pizzamiglio, L., Rousseaux, M., Zimmermann, G., Deloche, G., & Leclerk, M. (2002a). Computerized training of specific attention deficits in stroke and traumatic brain injured patients: A multicentric efficacy study. In M. Leclerk & P. Zimmermann (Eds.), *Applied Neuropsychology of Attention* (pp. 257-279). Hove: Psychology Press.

Sturm, W., Fimm, B., Cantagallo, A., Cremel, N., North, P., Passadori, A., Pizzamiglio, L., Rousseaux, M., Zimmermann, P., Deloche, G., & Leclercq, M. (2002b). Computerised training of specific attention deficits in stroke and traumatic brain injured patients: a multicentric efficacy study. In M. Leclercq & P. Zimmermann (Eds.), *Applied Neuropsychology of Attention.* Hove: Psychology Press.

Sturm, W., Simone, A. d., Krause, B.J., Specht, K., Hesselmann, V., Radermacher, I., Herzog, H., Tellmann, L., Muller-Gartner, H.W., & Willmes, K. (1999). Functional anatomy of intrinsic alertness: evidence for a fronto-parietal-thalamic-brainstem network in the right hemisphere. *Neuropsychologia, 37(7)*, 797-805.

Sturm, W., Willmes, K., Orgass, B., & Hartje, W. (1997). Do specific attention deficits need specific training? *Neuropsychological Rehabilitation, 7(2)*, 81-103.

Stuss, D., & Benson, D.F. (1983). Neuropsychological studies of the frontal lobes. *Psychological Bulletin, 95*, 3-28.

Stuss, D.T., & Benson, D.F. (1986). *The Frontal Lobes.* New York: Raven Press.

Tilikete, C., Rode, G., Rossetti, Y., Pichon, J., Li, L., & Boisson, D. (2001). Prism adaptation to a rightward optical deviation improves postural imbalance in left-hemiparetic patients. *Current Biology, 11*, 524-528.

Vallar, G., & Perani, D. (1986). The anatomy of unilateral neglect after right-hemisphere stroke lesions: A clinical/CT scan correlation study in man. *Neuropsychologia, 24*, 609-622.

Van Zomeren, A.H. (1981). *Reaction Time and Attention after Closed Head Injury.* Lisse: Swets and Zeitlinger.

Van Zomeren, A.H., & Brouwer, W.B. (1992). Assessment of attention. In J. Crawford, D.M. Parker, & L. McKinlay (Eds.), *A Handbook of Neuropsychological Assessment* (pp. 241-266). Hove: Laurence Earlbaum.

Van Zomeren, A.H., & Burg, W.V. d. (1985). Residual complaints of patients two years after severe closed head injury. *Journal of Neurology, Neurosurgery and Psychiatry, 48,* 21-28.

Van Zomeren, A.H., & Deelman, B.G. (1978). Long-term recovery of visual reaction time after closed head injury. *Journal of Neurology, Neurosurgery and Psychiatry, 41,* 452-457.

Velasco, F., Velasco, M., Ogarrio, C., & Olvera, A. (1986). Neglect induced by thalamotomy in humans: a quantitative appraisal of the sensory and motor deficits. *Neurosurgery, 19,* 744-751.

Wagenaar, R.C., Wieringen, P.C.W.V., Netelenboss, J.B., Meijer, O.G., & Kuik, D.J. (1992). The transfer of scanning training effects in visual attention after stroke: five single case studies. *Disability Rehabilitation, 14,* 51-60.

Walker, R., Young, A.W., & Lincoln, N.B. (1996). Eye patching and rehabilitation in unilateral neglect. *Neuropsychological Rehabilitation, 6,* 219-231.

Webster, J., Jones, S., Blanton, P., Gross, R., Beissel, G., & Wofford, J. (1984). Visual scanning training with stroke patients. *Behaviour Therapy, 15,* 129-143.

Webster, J.S., McFarland, P.T., Rapport, L.J., Morrill, B., Roades, L.A., & Abadee, P. S. (2001). Computer-assisted training for improving wheelchair mobility in unilateral neglect patients. *Archives of Physical Medicine and Rehabilitation, 82(6),* 769-775.

Weinberg, J., Diller, L., Gordon, W., Gertsman, L., Lieberman, A., Lakin, O., Hodges, G., & Ezrachi, O. (1977). Visual scanning training effect on reading -related tasks in acquired right brain damage. *Archives of Physical Medicine and Rehabilitation, 58,* 479-486.

Weintraub, S., & Mesulam, M. (1987). Right cerebral dominance in spatial attention: further evidence based on ipsilateral neglect. *Archives of Neurology, 44,* 621-625.

Wilkins, A.J., Shallice, T., & McCarthy, R. (1987). Frontal lesions and sustained attention. *Neuropsychologia, 25,* 359-365.

Wilson, B., Cockburn, J., & Halligan, P. (1987). *The Behavioural Inattention Test.* Titchfield, Hampshire: Thames Valley.

Wilson, C., & Robertson, I.H. (1992). A home-based intervention for attentional slips during reading following head injury: a single case study. *Neuropsychological Rehabilitation, 2,* 193-205.

Wilson, F.C., Manly, T., Coyle, D., & Robertson, I.H. (2000). The effect of contralesional limb activation training and sustained attention training for self-care programmes in unilateral spatial neglect. *Restorative Neurology and Neuroscience, 16(1),* 1-4.

Zihl, J. (2000). *Rehabilitation of Visual Disorders following Brain Injury.* Hove: Psychology Press.

Zimmermann, P., North, P., & Fimm, B. (1993). Diagnosis of attentional deficits: Theoretical considerations and presentation of a test battery. In F. Stachowiak (Ed.), *Developments in the assessment and rehabilitation of brain damaged patients* . Tubingen: G Narr-Verlagg.

Chapter 4

REHABILITATION OF EXECUTIVE DEFICITS

Jonathan J. Evans

Oliver Zangwill Centre for Neuropsychological Rehabilitation, Ely MRC Cognition and Brain Sciences Unit, Cambridge, UK

Introduction

Deficits in executive functioning cause devastating social handicap after brain injury and therefore represent a major challenge for rehabilitation. The term 'executive functions' refers to a set of skills or processes required for effective problem-solving, planning and organisation, self-monitoring, initiation, error correction and behavioural regulation. Almost all theories of executive functioning have arisen from attempts to understand the role of the frontal lobes in cognition. Luria (1966) conceptualised the frontal lobes as being involved in problem solving, a process which includes the three phases of strategy selection, application of operations and evaluation of outcomes. Duncan (1986) described the role of the frontal lobes in terms of 'goal maintenance'. He argued that the frontal lobes are involved in identifying 'goals' or behavioural objectives and managing actions that will lead to the achievement of those goals. Duncan suggested that frontal lobe damage causes 'goal neglect', whereby the individual with a brain injury is able to identify what he or she needs to achieve and may be able to derive a plan, but during the course of the operation of the plan, the main goals may become neglected and actions no longer lead to achieving the goal. Whilst not completely random, behaviour is no longer goal-directed.

Baddeley and Wilson (1988) drew on the work of Rylander (1939) who described how individuals who suffer damage to the frontal lobes have impairments in attention (being easily distracted), have difficulties grasping the whole of a complicated state of affairs (an abstraction problem), and whilst they may be able to work along routine lines, they have difficulties in new situations. Baddeley (1986) coined the term dysexecutive syndrome as a replacement for the anatomically constrained term 'frontal lobe syndrome'. He suggested that one of the functions of the frontal lobes is that of the 'central executive' component of working memory.

Baddeley (1986) equated the concept of the central executive with that of the 'Supervisory Attention System' (S.A.S), described by Norman and Shallice (see Shallice, 1988). They discussed the control of action in terms of two levels of control; an automatic schema driven level (involving a non-conscious automatic control process referred to as contention scheduling) and the more conscious level referred to in terms of the S.A.S. This supervisory system was seen as responsible for, 'producing a response to novelty that is planned rather than one that is routine or impulsive' (Shallice, 1988, p. 345). More specifically the S.A.S. was described as being required in situations that involve; (1) planning or decision making; (2) error correction or troubleshooting; (3) responses that are not well learned or where they contain novel sequences of actions; (4) dangerous or technically difficult decisions; (5) situations that require the overcoming of a strong habitual response or resisting temptation.

Shallice and Burgess (1996) argued that the S.A.S. can be fractionated into a set of basic sub-components, or sub-processes and present evidence (based on neuropsychological dissociations and functional brain imaging), for the fractionation. They argue that responding appropriately to novelty requires three processes – (1) a process which results in the creation of a temporary new schema (since routine behaviour is governed by existing schema, novel behaviour will require the creation of a new schema), (2) a special purpose working memory that is required for the implementation of the temporary new schema and (3) a system that monitors, evaluates and accepts or rejects actions depending upon their success in solving the novel problem.

One source of evidence that the S.A.S. can be fractionated is that the sub-processes of S.A.S. dissociate. Patients with brain injury may have difficulty with one or more of the processes, whilst others remain intact. For example some patients appear to be aware that a problem exists, but may fail to identify more than one potential solution or make an adequate plan. Consequently the patient may respond to a problem with impulsive actions. Impulsivity is a relatively common consequence of brain injury, particularly where the frontal lobes have been involved. The individual appears to 'act without thinking', doing the first thing that comes to mind, failing to think of alternative solutions to a problem and failing to anticipate the consequences of the chosen action. In contrast, some patients are able to generate a plan, but plans are never translated into action. In each case the end result will be essentially the same in that the problem is not dealt with adequately, but for different reasons. Those reasons become important when considering the rehabilitation of these problems.

The Consequences of Executive Problems after Brain Injury

The consequences of frontal lobe damage were most dramatically illustrated in the most famous of all 'dysexecutive' patients, Phineas Gage (Macmillan, 2000). He lost part of his frontal lobes as a consequence of a tamping iron being accidentally blasted through his skull. Probably the most remarkable thing about Phineas Gage was that he survived at all. However, he developed a tendency to be disinhibited and had an inability to follow through with intended plans. He failed to keep his job and became socially inept. Similarly patient EVR described by Eslinger and Damasio (1985) who had a large orbito-frontal meningioma removed, was described as having an IQ of over 130 and the ability to perform well on a wide variety of cognitive tasks, even post-injury. Yet as a consequence of his injury, his life became disastrously disorganised. He had previously been a successful professional and a respected member of the community, but he ended up losing his job, going bankrupt, being divorced, subsequently marrying a prostitute and divorcing again. He was described as having immense difficulties in making simple decisions, such as where to go out to dinner or what toothpaste to buy. The three patients described by Shallice and Burgess (1991) were all similar to EVR in that they appeared to have a combination of adequate general intellectual ability, impaired executive ability and disastrously organised lives. Patient RP (Evans, Emslie, & Wilson, 1998) similarly showed adequate general intellectual and memory functioning but impaired attention and executive skills. As a consequence, RP was unable to translate intention into action, to plan ahead, and sustain attention whilst carrying out tasks. She was unable to work or effectively manage the household and required constant support and supervision from her husband who had to give up his job to care for her. Crepeau and Scherzer (1993) provide further evidence of the social handicap caused by dysexecutive syndrome. They describe the results of a meta-analytic study that showed that the presence of impairments in executive functioning was a key factor predicting whether or not individuals will return to work.

Rehabilitation of Executive Impairments

A key issue in rehabilitation is whether interventions should be aimed at treating the underlying impairment (i.e. restoring the lost function) or seek to provide clients with strategies that enable them to compensate for the impairment. As discussed below, the evidence that executive problems can be restored is not wholly convincing, whilst there is more evidence that mental strategies, or external aids can produce real benefits.

Re-training or restoring impaired executive functioning
Evidence that executive dysfunction can be returned to normal is slim, if not non-existent. Placebo controlled single-case studies of the drug Idazoxan

(Sahakian, Coull, & Hodges, 1994) in patients diagnosed with frontal lobe dementia are promising. However, it is not clear that frontal lobe dementia is a good model for non-progressive, single event brain damage. Nevertheless, this work clearly needs expanding so that the potential benefit of pharmacological interventions is adequately assessed. Further work must also address the extent to which improvement of performance on specific tests of planning, such as those used in studies to date, generalises to everyday problem solving.

Retraining approaches to rehabilitation make the assumption that practicing a particular cognitive function through tasks and exercises will enable that function to return, in a more or less normal fashion. Von Cramon, Matthes-von Cramon and Mai (1991) and von Cramon and Matthes-von Cramon (1992) describe a group based training programme described as 'problem-solving therapy', which is seen as a retraining approach. Von Cramon and colleagues note that the broad aim of problem-solving therapy is to provide patients 'with techniques enabling them to reduce the complexity of a multi stage problem by breaking it down into more manageable portions. A slowed down, controlled and step wise processing of a given problem, should replace the unsystematic and often rash approach these patients spontaneously prefer' (1991, p. 46). The therapy approach adopts a problem-solving framework which draws on the work of d'Zurilla and Goldfried (1971). The specific aims of the therapy are to enhance the patients' ability to perform each of the separate stages of problem-solving, through practice on tasks that are designed to exercise the skills required for each of the separate stages. These stages include (a) identifying and analysing problems; (b) separating information relevant to a problem solution from unimportant and irrelevant data; (c) recognising the relationship between different relevant items of information and if appropriate combining them; (d) producing ideas/solutions; (e) using different mental representations (e.g. verbal, visual, abstract patterns such as flow charts) in order to solve a problem; and (f) monitoring solution implementation and evaluate solutions.

Exercises for working on the ability to separate information relevant to a problem from unimportant or irrelevant data include practice at formulating 'wanted' small ads and telegrams, where the need for only including relevant information is at a premium. Practice at generating ideas is gained from tasks such as completing unfinished stories, for and against discussions of current affairs and practice brainstorming sessions. Patients are encouraged to monitor solution implementation via the use of work books, and group activities where a patient is asked to be a co-therapist during a game (e.g. Mastermind), drawing other players' attention to mistakes, irregularities and unnecessary moves. Therapy runs for a period of about six weeks with an average of 25 sessions. Each group involves four to six clients who initially work independently, but as soon as possible two clients work together on an assignment, with the division of labour being clearly explained. Finally, task orientated groups are established in which each individual in the group takes on the responsibility for finding the solution to the part of a project, (e.g. organising a visit to a museum in the city centre).

Von Cramon et al. (1991) compared a group of patients who received problem-solving therapy (n = 20), with a group of patients who received a control 'Memory Therapy' Group (n = 17). The control group allowed for the possibility that clients might benefit from general advice and group activity, rather than specifically from the tasks aimed at exercising executive skills. They showed that patients who underwent problem-solving therapy showed some improvement in tests of general intelligence and problem solving (Tower of Hanoi) compared with controls. Von Cramon and colleagues demonstrated some generalisation of problem-solving skills to untrained test tasks but there was no evidence of generalisation to everyday situations. Evidence for the latter is hard to obtain because of measurement difficulties but it is clearly important that some evidence is obtained of generalisation to situations outside of formal test sessions. Von Cramon and colleagues also noted that a small number of patients actually deteriorated on tests. They hypothesised that this was due to an increased awareness of the complexity of problems on the part of the patient, leading to confusion about how to respond. By contrast, such patients had a pre-treatment propensity towards premature or ill-considered actions, some of which would have been correct by chance.

Internal strategies

A number of interventions aimed at helping clients with attention and executive difficulties might be considered as 'internal' strategies. Typically this means that the individual is using a mental routine or self-instructional technique of some sort.

Cicerone and Wood (1987) provide a good example of the use of the self-instructional technique in a 20 year old man with a severe head injury. He was described as functioning relatively independently, but impulsively interrupted conversations and generally appeared not to think before he did something. They used the Tower of London Test as a training task, asking the client to state each move he was about to make while attempting to solve the problem and then to state the move while he performed it. In stage two the patient was asked to repeat the first stage except to whisper rather than speak aloud. Finally in the third stage he was asked to 'talk to himself', (i.e. to think through what he was doing). This approach was successful in improving performance on the trained task, but more importantly, there was generalisation to two other untrained tasks. In addition, with some generalisation training, there were improvements in general social behaviour, rated by independent raters. The main change brought about by this simple self-instructional technique was that it helped the patient to slow his approach to the task in hand and, in effect, develop a habit of thinking through his actions rather than responding impulsively.

Von Cramon and Matthes-von Cramon (1995) provide an example of an internalised check list routinely applied to compensate for executive deficits. They describe GL, a 33-year-old Physician who had a traumatic brain injury at the age of 24, resulting in bilateral frontal lobe damage. Despite the injury, GL passed his medical exams post injury (though after several failures). He was described as having 'drifted' through several jobs in neurosurgery, pathology and the pharmaceutical industry. His problems were characterised as involving a lack of overview and being dependent upon meticulous instructions. He was unable to benefit from feedback, spending too much time on routine activities and being unable to adapt himself to the requirements of novel or changing situations. In the study, a protected work trial was established in a hospital pathology lab and he was provided with prototypical reports on autopsy. It was noted that he tended to jump to conclusions about diagnosis and he was therefore taught a set of rules/guidelines for the systematic process of diagnosis. These rules were initially provided in the form of a written checklist, which, over time, GL learned and was able to apply without the need to refer to the checklist. GL improved his ability to diagnose correctly and to write reports. However, there was no generalisation to a novel planning task.

Another approach is to teach a more general strategy that can be applied in a variety of situations. Levine et al. (2000) described the use of a Goal Management Training (GMT) technique in two studies. Study 1 evaluated the technique with a group of head-injured patients on paper-and-pencil tasks. The second study described the use of this technique with one post-encephalitic patient seeking to improve her meal preparation abilities. The GMT technique was derived from Duncan's (1986) concept of 'goal neglect'. The principle is that patients with frontal lobe damage fail to generate goal (or sub-goal) lists of how to solve problems (and achieve goals), and/or may fail to monitor progress towards achieving sub- or main goals. The training has 5 stages, which are first defined for the patient, and include (1) Stop and think what I am doing, (2) Define the main task, (3) List the steps required, (4) Learn the steps, (5) Whilst implementing the steps, check that I am on track, or doing what I intended to do. After each stage is introduced, illustrative examples from the patient's own life are used as well as mock examples. In the first study, the GMT was applied in a single one-hour session, with testing on several target tasks undertaken afterwards. Levine et al showed improved performance on three paper and pencil tasks, but generalisation to everyday life was not examined. Study 2 addressed the question of application of GMT in a more practical task. Patient KF suffered from a meningo-encephalitic illness, which resulted in some general intellectual decline, attentional, memory and executive functioning deficits. A particular problem for KF was meal preparation, with four specific areas of difficulty; failure to assemble the necessary ingredients, misinterpretation of written instructions, repeated checking of instructions and sequencing/omission errors. The measure used to evaluate the efficacy of GMT was the number of problem behaviours evident during meal preparation tasks (as well as performance on the paper and pencil tasks used in Study 1). GMT was applied over two sessions, and was adapted so that tasks relating to meal preparation and involving the various stages of GMT were created. The results of the study were that KF showed a significant reduction in errors in meal preparation stages over the course of the intervention. Although baseline data were collected that indicated the problem with meal preparation was clearly evident and this improved post-training, the lack of control variable information means that spontaneous recovery cannot be ruled out, especially given that she was only 5 months post-illness at the time of the study. Nevertheless, the study does raise the possibility that GMT may be a useful technique (especially considering the apparent efficacy based on a relatively small amount of training time).

Evans (2001) describes a group approach, adapted from the von Cramon group described above and from the Goal Management Training of Robertson (1996; See also Levine et al. 2000) described in more detail below. The Attention and Problem Solving group is one component of a holistic rehabilitation programme. The first few sessions of the group (which runs twice a week for 8–10 weeks) primarily address attentional difficulties, and the later sessions are used to introduce a problem-solving framework to the clients. This framework is presented as a paper-based checklist of the stages of problem solving. The stages are illustrated in Figure 1. An accompanying template is also provided that can be used to proceed through the stages using a written format, but clients are encouraged, through practice at using the framework with the template, to internalise the framework so that in time the use of the framework becomes more automatic. No formal evaluation of this group has yet been undertaken, but the successful use of this framework by one client, David, is described later.

Fasotti, Kovacs, Eling and Brouwer (2000) developed a compensatory strategy training that they call Time Pressure Management. The aim was to teach brain-injured patients a technique to help compensate for slow information processing. The strategy consisted of a general self-instruction ('Give myself enough time to do the task') followed by four specific steps; (1) Ask yourself if two or more things for which there is not enough time must be done at the same time? If yes, go to step 2, if not, do the task, (2) Make a short plan of which things can be done before the actual task begins, (3) Make an emergency plan describing what to do in case of overwhelming time pressure, (4) Use the plan and emergency plan regularly, monitor performance during the task. This simple approach is essentially focused on teaching patients to be more planful and more consciously aware of their performance, with a particular emphasis on helping patients to become better managers of their environment. Fasotti et al. showed that use of the strategy helped patients improve performance on a practice task, though once again no evidence for generalisation to everyday life was provided.

Shallice and Burgess's (1996) model of the problem solving processes associated with the functioning of the supervisory attentional system highlights the importance of the retrieval from memory of past experience. When faced with a novel task or problem, the strategy of recalling incidents of tackling

Goal Management (Problem Solving) Framework

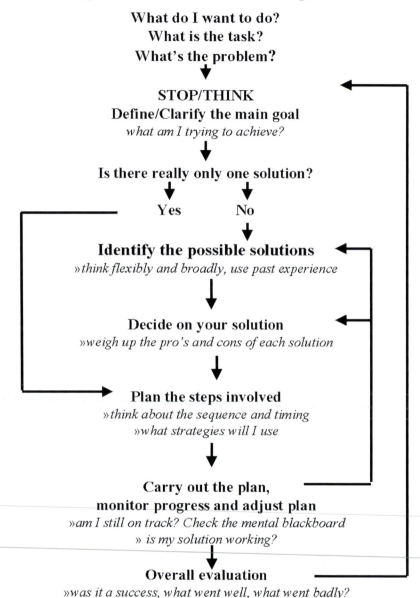

What do I want to do?
What is the task?
What's the problem?

STOP/THINK
Define/Clarify the main goal
what am I trying to achieve?

Is there really only one solution?

Yes   No

Identify the possible solutions
»think flexibly and broadly, use past experience

Decide on your solution
»weigh up the pro's and cons of each solution

Plan the steps involved
»think about the sequence and timing
»what strategies will I use

Carry out the plan,
monitor progress and adjust plan
»am I still on track? Check the mental blackboard
» is my solution working?

Overall evaluation
»was it a success, what went well, what went badly?

OLIVER ZANGWILL CENTRE FOR NEUROPSYCHOLOGICAL REHABILITATION

Fig. 1. The Goal Management Framework used to aid clients develop a systematic approach to problem solving and goal management.

similar problems in the past may help in the present situation. Dritschel, Kogan, Burton, Burton and Goddard (1998) demonstrated that people with head injury often fail to refer to previous experiences in solving practical planning tasks, such as describing how they would book a holiday, get a new job or find a new place to live. Hewitt, Evans and Dritschel (2000) hypothesised that if patients were given a brief training relating to the retrieval of autobiographical memories, they would improve in their ability to plan practical tasks. The training took the form of an illustration of the value of recalling specific autobiographical experiences from the past in practical problem-solving, a cue-card to prompt specific memory retrieval and practice at doing this in order to plan how to tackle a particular task. The performance of two groups of subjects was compared, one receiving the training and the other not. The results showed that the training group improved significantly more than the no-training group in terms of the number of specific memories recalled, the number of steps and the overall effectiveness of the plan produced in relation to a set of eight hypothetical practical demands (e.g. how would you organise a surprise birthday party, how would you find a new house). Incorporating some form of training relating to retrieval of specific autobiographical memories may be helpful in a problem-solving training programme.

External strategies

The most common strategy in the rehabilitation of memory problems is to teach the use of external aids, such as checklists, diaries or electronic organisers. Such aids are also useful for people who have planning and organisational problems. For some individuals, the process of writing things down seems to be the critical step in that it prevents a more impulsive style of responding to situations. For others, the process of writing things down makes the process of generating possible solutions and weighing up the pros and cons of those solutions more manageable. For individuals with significant working memory or speed of information processing deficits, it may be difficult to use the framework 'in mind', and an external written approach may be more helpful.

Poor sequencing of tasks is a possible consequence of executive disorder and in some cases checklists prove to be useful. The case of GL, the doctor who improved his performance in writing pathology reports was described above. He used a checklist approach, but was able to internalise the checklist so that the task, even though complex, became essentially routine. Burke, Zencius, Wesolowiski and Doubleday (1991) describe six case studies where checklists were used in order to help clients develop and carry out plans. For example, the case of a 38 year old man who had problems with sequencing steps in a task, such as planing timber in the wood shop. Using a multiple baseline across tasks procedure, it was demonstrated that introduction of checklists improved performance, which was maintained even after the checklists were withdrawn. This suggests that the client had learned a task routine. However, significantly, the client was also better at a task for which the checklist had not been introduced. The authors concluded that he was able to spontaneously generalise the use of a structured approach to the new situation. What was perhaps critical was the fact that the structured checklist approach was introduced not just for one task, but across a range of tasks in a systematic fashion, encouraging the client to learn both specific tasks and a general approach to new situations.

One specific form of executive deficit is an impairment in the ability to initiate action. In this case, checklists may be useful, but may rely too heavily on the patient initiating the checking of the list and following through on actions. An aid that is more effective at prompting action is required. One such aid that appears to have this function is NeuroPage. This system was developed by Hersh and Treadgold (1994) and has been demonstrated to be effective for people with memory and executive impairment (Wilson, Evans, Emslie, & Malinek, 1997; Wilson, Emslie, Quirk, & Evans, 2000). The system utilises radio paging technology and involves the patient wearing an alphanumeric pager. Reminders of things to do are entered onto a central computer using NeuroPage software. This automatically sends out the message via a modem to a paging company, which then sends out the message to the patient's pager, which bleeps and delivers a text message. NeuroPage was used with Patient RP (Evans, Emslie, & Wilson, 1998), who suffered a cerebro-vascular accident as a result of a ruptured aneurysm. Her main problem was that she had difficulty translating intention into action. She was also distractible and had difficulty completing tasks. Despite adequate memory and intelligence, RP's combination of executive and attentional deficits had a significant impact on her day to day life. Although she could accurately say what she had to do, she had to be prompted to do many things, such as take her medication, or water her plants. She was highly distractible. When she did manage to set off to do a task, she was frequently distracted by something else along the way and failed to return to the original task. She therefore took a huge amount of time to get things done. She also found it difficult to be organised and planful enough to cook a family meal. A study of RP's performance in carrying out a range of day to day tasks, using an ABAB single case experimental design, showed that NeuroPage was highly effective in helping RP to complete tasks she needed to do on time. This significantly reduced the stress on her husband. Evans et al. noted that there appeared to be two important aspects to the success of the paging system. The first was the presentation of an external text message that appeared to be important for RP and prompted behaviour in a way that an internal intention to act failed to do. This is consistent with Luria's view of the frontal lobes being involved in the control of behaviour by inner speech. The second aspect was the bleeping of the pager that provided an arousal boost to facilitate RP's initiation of tasks and help her sustain attention during the course of task completion. One issue in the use of alerting devices is the possibility that the individual will habituate to the sound and it will lose its alerting effect. This is a danger if alerts are being used very frequently and so highlights the importance of managing the frequency so that it retains its alerting capacity.

Manly, Hawkins, Evans and Robertson (2002) also examined the impact of external alerting. Performance of patients who had suffered traumatic brain injury on a multi-element task was tested under two conditions. The task used, the Hotel Test, is similar in format to the Modified Six Elements Test (Wilson et al., 1996). It involves the patient completing 6 different tasks, including a prospective remembering task, that are presented as tasks that might be given to an assistant hotel manager (e.g. making up bills, arranging conference delegate cards, looking up phone numbers, sorting charity box coins, proof reading a leaflet and pushing a button to open a door). Like the Six Elements Test, not everything from all of the tasks can be completed in the 15 minutes allocated. Two parallel versions were used in the two experimental conditions. In one condition, an external alert (a tone on an audio tape) was presented at random, relatively infrequent intervals. In the other condition no tone was presented. The study used a counterbalanced, crossover design. The results showed that participants performed more effectively during the bleeped condition, than the control condition. It was argued that the alerting tones improved the link between a well represented goal and current behaviour. The tones did not specifically prompt task switching, but rather seemed to improve the ability to maintain the overall task goal actively in mind, and hence switch tasks more flexibly.

For some people, particularly those with very severe executive impairments or with a combination of executive and other difficulties, the provision of external aids might not be effective and it is necessary to consider changing some aspect of their physical or social environment. Work with family, friends and colleagues is one form of environmental modification approach. Helping relatives and carers to understand the nature of executive difficulties can help to minimise negative responses to problems arising from a dysexecutive syndrome. For example one of the most difficult things for families to appreciate is that an initiation difficulty is not laziness. Another is that the person may remember some things and not others due to attentional problems rather than not bothering to remember. Education can have an important role in helping families both to understand, and modify their own behaviour in relation to clients (for a case example see O'Brien, Prigatano and Pittman 1988). A combination of difficulties can sometimes result in problem behaviour such as aggressive or stereotyped behaviour, each of which may prevent the client from participating in other rehabilitation activities and cause significant disruption for family, friends and carers. In this situation, it is often necessary to provide a highly structured environment with the opportunity for very frequent feedback in order to help clients to shape and modify their behaviour. The work of Alderman and colleagues (Alderman & Burgess, 1990; Alderman & Ward, 1991; Alderman & Burgess, 1994; Alderman, this volume) illustrates the use of behaviour modification techniques, originally developed in the context of work with people with complex patterns of neurobehavioural disability, which are relevant in the context of the combination of memory and executive impairments in this client group.

The rehabilitation interventions described here provide a range of treatment options for people with various forms of executive dysfunction. However, most people referred for rehabilitation do not have just one area of cognitive impairment. Hence for any one individual there is typically a need for a range of interventions to be used. Furthermore, a comprehensive rehabilitation programme will aim to help the individual client to identify strategies for compensating for, or coping with, cognitive impairments, and also support the client in the application of those strategies in practical, personally relevant situations. The following case example illustrates this process in the context of a neuropsychological rehabilitation programme.

Case Example: David

At the age of 34, David suffered a cerebro-vascular accident, resulting in a right internal capsule infarct. He was a Chemical Engineer. Following an acute hospital admission, and then a period of inpatient rehabilitation, he returned home some four months post-injury. He had been unable to return to work, and had been medically retired. Eleven months post-injury David was referred to an intensive inter-disciplinary outpatient neuropsychological rehabilitation programme (Wilson et al., 2000). The main problems reported included;
- mental tiredness
- difficulty doing more than one thing at once
- difficulty sustaining his concentration (either being very easily distracted or totally focused and locked into something)
- bumping into things on the left
- poor sense of the passage of time
- difficulty thinking ahead or organising things
- difficulty initiating things (intends to do things, but doesn't do them)

Neuropsychological assessment revealed generally satisfactory verbal and non-verbal reasoning and memory skills. There was some evidence of persisting neglect, though only typically manifested in visually crowded and dynamic environments. There was however evidence of very significant problems with attention, affecting tests of visual selective, divided and sustained attention, such as those in the Test of Everyday Attention (Robertson, Ward, Ridgeway, & Nimmo-Smith, 1994). He also demonstrated difficulties on tests of planning and strategy application, such as the Key Search and Zoo Map tasks in the Behavioural Assessment of the Dysexecutive Syndrome (Wilson, Alderman, Burgess, Emslie, & Evans, 1996). On a practical test of planning and preparing an unfamiliar meal, he completed the task, but nevertheless showed evidence of difficulties with attention (failing to notice an item he was searching for) and with problem solving (e.g. in response to being unable to locate an item, and to noticing that an ingredient was not cooking fast enough). One of his hobbies was painting miniature military figures, which he had enjoyed doing while listening to the radio. However, since his injury he had found it impossible to do these two tasks at the same time, and having become dispirited with his performance on the painting task following several attempts, had stopped painting. He was frustrated with his situation, and lacked confidence in himself. This also impacted on his relationship with his wife. David's lack of initiative and low confidence meant that the relationship with his wife lacked reciprocity.

In conjunction David, the clinical team constructed a set of rehabilitation programme goals. These were:

1. David will demonstrate an accurate understanding of the consequences of his brain injury consistent with his two week detailed assessment report.
2. David will report an accurate understanding of the effect of his injury on his relationship with his wife and have identified strategies that he could use to manage his relationship more effectively.
3. David will demonstrate effective use of problem solving strategies in social and functional situations as rated by himself, his wife and the clinical team.
4. David will demonstrate effective use of attention strategies in social and functional situations as rated by himself, his wife and the clinical team.
5. David will manage negative automatic thoughts in a range of family, social and leisure situations and rate himself as confident in specified situations.
6. David will plan his weekly schedule independently and complete 80% of activities successfully and without reporting excessive fatigue.
7. David will take responsibility for household budgeting and stay within an agreed monthly budget.
8. David will be engaged in a voluntary work trial and have a personal development plan.
9. David will be engaged in a physical leisure activity on a twice-weekly basis.

The goals reflect four key processes involved in neuropsychological rehabilitation – (1) developing insight/awareness, (2) managing mood and psychological adjustment, (3) developing compensatory strategies for cognitive impairments, (4) applying strategies in functional, 'real life' situations. These processes are dependent upon each other in order to progress. As part of his programme, David attended an Understanding Brain Injury Group, as well as working with his Individual Programme Coordinator to develop a personal report of his own brain injury, the consequences and the strategies he uses to compensate for his cognitive difficulties. In David's case, the two main areas of cognitive impairment were attention and executive functioning. He attended the group described earlier, and worked with a psychologist to develop personally relevant strategies. Two approaches were taken to attentional problems. One was to use specific strategies to compensate for deficits and the other was to train performance on specific tasks in order to reduce the attentional load of these tasks. To compensate for difficulties with sustained attention, David learned to manage his environment better, to reduce distractions. A functional example was when having friends to visit selecting appropriate (e.g. quiet, ambient) music. He also developed a mental routine of checking his attention and where necessary re-focusing his attention to the task in hand. In order to develop this routine initially he used an alarm clock that he set for 15 minute intervals. A good example of where cognitive and mood management strategies overlapped was when watching films. Pre-injury one of his great pleasures was watching a film together with his wife. However, post-injury it had become a struggle. He would find that after 20 minutes or so, he would start to find it hard to concentrate. He would then engage in a mental battle with himself, in effect trying to 'force himself' to stay with the film. But this battle in itself was a distraction and made it harder, so that he nearly always gave up watching, but felt bad. The approach used here was to use the mental check after 15 minutes to ask himself, 'Am I still concentrating? If not do I want to re-focus my attention or take a break?' He also used video recorded films more so that he could break and return to a film if he wanted. However, what he found in general was that by giving himself permission to take a break, he more often than not actually chose to simply re-focus his attention. For some activities, he was aware that he was prone to getting 'locked into' the task. This happened most often if playing computer games. Here the problem seemed to be related to a dual-tasking problem, whereby he could not monitor peripheral stimuli and hence the passage of time effectively. In these situations he relied on using an external alarm (on an electronic organiser).

Two of the specific situations that David identified were difficult as a result of dual tasking problems were playing badminton and painting his miniature figures. When playing Badminton he found it difficult to play a shot and move to the next point in anticipation of the return shot. He also found it difficult to play and keep track of the score. Both of these he had done with ease before the injury. In this case it was hypothesised that the physical process of playing a shot was now taking more cognitive resources (it was not as automatic as it had been and required more conscious attention). The solution here was rather straightforward. David was simply encouraged to focus on the process of playing the shots and to practice regularly, to re-establish his skill level in the physical task. Then as his physical performance improved, he was able to gradually introduce the tasks of trying to think more about anticipating shots and also keeping the score. A similar approach was taken to returning to painting his figures. He began by doing short periods in very quiet environments, and building up the physical skills. Then very gradually, classical music was introduced, then music with lyrics and then talk based radio programmes.

With regard to problem solving or goal management, there were several areas of difficulty. Although some difficulty with planning had been identified in the standard assessments, there was evidence in most practical situations that he could identify solutions to problems. However he lacked confidence in his ability and also had major difficulties with initiation of intended actions. David was therefore trained in the use of the goal management or problem solving framework, which was practiced with hypothetical problems and then personally relevant problems that arose during the course of the programme. David reported that he found the structured approach of the framework (which he could do mentally, rather than needing to write down) useful. It appeared that the formality of the process helped him to develop confidence that the solutions he derived were likely to be reasonable. He demonstrated use of the framework in coping with problems such as losing his electronic organiser, finding that some accommodation did not have his booking and was full, and in planning a weekend away with his wife. To compensate for his difficulties with task initiation, a self-instructional approach was adopted. David used a phrase that he said to himself, which was, 'Just Do It!' This seemed to provide a sufficient attentional 'kick', that David was able to follow through on a greatly increased number of tasks. Once again a key issue was the role of mood factors in exacerbating the effect of the cognitive impairment. Armed with the strategies, the tools for coping, his confidence increased, and this in turn was a significant factor in itself in facilitating the initiation of actions.

In conjunction with the development of strategies, David was also focused on the functional goals, but of course as he developed confidence in the application of strategies so he was able to apply them in a range of situations. He commenced a voluntary work placement in a Heritage Trust. He developed a planning system using his electronic organiser to schedule activities with more appropriate pacing. He took on the family budgeting role. He engaged in just one physical leisure activity per week. His increased level of confidence in problem solving and initiation meant that he felt he was less dependent upon his wife, which enabled him to engage in a more adult, equal relationship with her.

In summary, David presented with relatively circumscribed deficits in attention and executive deficits, which had a dramatic effect on his day today functioning. In terms of Shallice and Burgess's (1996) model of the supervisory attentional system, David's main impairments could be thought of being in relation to the implementation of plans and monitoring of attention and action. This knowledge lead to the development of strategies focused on improving initiation (e.g. the 'Just Do It!' strategy) and monitoring (e.g. the mental checking routine). He had less difficulty with actual planning, though lacked confidence in this, and then use of the problem-solving framework seemed to be helpful in the development of his confidence in this respect. Not all clients in rehabilitation are as successful as David. Many have even more complex combinations of problems and less insight/awareness. Nevertheless cases such as David's highlight how effective the rehabilitation process can be under the right circumstances, and the importance of the integrated mood and cognitive management approaches in a context of practical, functional and personally relevant activities.

Summary and Conclusions

Dysexecutive problems represent a major challenge for rehabilitation, and yet have received rather little attention, at least in the rehabilitation literature. A comprehensive tool-kit of techniques for such problems does not yet exist. This must be in part due to the lack of theoretical consistency with regard to the nature of executive functions and the problems that form the dysexecutive syndrome. Theoretical developments, partly driven by localisation evidence from functional imaging studies. are heading towards fractionation of concepts such as the Supervisory Attentional System or the Central Executive. A fractionated system means that specific problems may occur in isolation and that sophisticated rehabilitation should be able to target impaired systems. Whether such systems can be 'restored or retrained' remains to be addressed further, with pharmacological treatments and stem cell implantation techniques offering some hope for the future. There is some evidence that re-training approaches focused on teaching people problem-solving skills can be effective and have practical benefits. Furthermore, evidence is accumulating slowly that a range of specific compensatory techniques can be effective. Some techniques or strategies might be described as impairment-focused and general (e.g. NeuroPage for alerting, or self-instructional training for reducing impulsivity), where others are highly specific to a particular functional task or situation (e.g. the use of a checklist for task completion). For most individuals some combination of both approaches may be beneficial, though insight levels may be a major factor in deciding what approach to use. For those with poor (treatment-resistant) insight, who will have difficulties spontaneously using general strategies, then task specific approaches are likely to be more effective, though of course severe insight difficulties will make even these approaches problematic. It seems likely that these techniques will be most effective when applied in the context of a comprehensive, inter-disciplinary neuropsychological rehabilitation programme.

References

Alderman, N. & Burgess, P.W. (1990). Integrating cognition and behaviour: A pragmatic approach to brain injury rehabilitation. In R. Wood and I. Fussey (Eds.), *Cognitive Rehabilitation in Perspective*. Basingstoke: Taylor and Francis Ltd., pp. 204-228.

Alderman, N. & Ward, A. (1991). Behavioural treatment of the dysexecutive syndrome: Reduction of repetitive speech using response cost and cognitive overlearning. *Neuropsychological Rehabilitation, 1*, 65-80.

Alderman, N. & Burgess, P. (1994). A comparison of treatment methods for behaviour disorder following herpes simplex encephalitis. *Neuropsychological Rehabilitation, 4*, 31-48.

Baddeley, A.D. (1986). *Working Memory*. Oxford: OUP.

Baddeley, A.D. & Wilson, B.A. (1988). Frontal amnesia and the dysexecutive syndrome. *Brain and Cognition, 7*, 212-230.

Burke, W.H., Zencius, A.H., Wesolowski, M.D. & Doubleday, F. (1991). Improving executive function disorders in brain injured clients. *Brain Injury, 5*, 241-252.

Cicerone, K.D. & Wood, J.C. (1987). Planning disorder after closed head injury: A case study. *Archives of Physical Medicine and Rehabilitation, 68*, 111-115.

von Cramon, D., Matthes-von Cramon, G. & Mai, N. (1991). Problem-solving deficits in brain injured patients: A therapeutic approach. *Neuropsychological Rehabilitation, 1*, 45-64.

von Cramon, D. & Matthes-von Cramon, G. (1992). Reflections on the treatment of brain injured patients suffering from problem-solving disorders. *Neuropsychological Rehabilitation, 2*, 207-230.

von Cramon, D. & Matthes-von Cramon, G. (1995) Back to work with a chronic dysexecutive syndrome. *Neuropsychological Rehabilitation, 4*, 399-417.

Crepeau, F. & Scherzer, P. (1993). Predictors and Indicators of Work status after Traumatic Brain Injury: A Meta Analysis. *Neuropsychological Rehabilitation, 3*, (1), 5-35.

Dritschel, B.H. Kogan, L., Burton, A., Burton, E., & Goddard, L. (1998). Everyday planning difficulites following brain injury: a role for autobiographical memory. *Brain Injury, 12*, 875-886.

Duncan, J. (1986). Disorganisation of behaviour after frontal lobe damage. *Cognitive Neuropsychology, 3*, 271-290.

Eslinger, P.J. & Damasio, A.R. (1985). Severe disturbance of higher cognition after bilateral frontal lobe ablation: patient EVR. *Neurology, Cleveland, 35*, 1731-1741.

Evans, J.J., Emslie, H., & Wilson, B.A. (1998). External cueing systems in the rehabilitation of executive impairments of action. *Journal of the International Neuropsychological Society, 4*, 399-408.

Evans (2001). Rehabilitation of the dysexecutive syndrome. In R.L.I. Wood, & T. McMillan, (Eds.), *Neurobehavioural Disability and Social Handicap*. Hove: Psychology Press.

Fasotti, L., Kovacs, F., Eling, P.A.T.M., & Brouwer, W.H. (2000). Time pressure management as a compensatory strategy training after closed head injury. *Neuropsychological Rehabilitation, 10*, 47-65.

Hersh, N. & Treadgold, L. (1994). Prosthetic memory and cueing for survivors of traumatic brain injury. *Unpublished report obtainable from Interactive Proactive Mnemonic Systems*, 6657 Camelia Drive, San Jose, California.

Hewitt, J., Evans, J.J., & Dritchel, B. (2000). Improving planning skills in people with traumatic brain injury through the use of an autobiographical episodic memory cueing procedure. Paper presented at the Autumn Meeting of the British Neuropsychological Society, 23 November, Nottingham, UK.

Levine, B., Robertson, I.H., Clare, L., Carter, G., Hong, J., Wilson, B.A., Duncan, J., & Stuss, D.T. (2000). Rehabilitation of executive functioning: An experimental-clinical validation of Goal Management Training. *Journal of the International Neuropsychological Society, 6*, 299-312.

Luria, A.R. (1966). *Higher Cortical Functions in Man*. New York: Basic Books.

Macmillan. M. (2000). *An Odd Kind of Fame: Stories of Phineas Gage*. London: MIT Press

Manly, T., Hawkins, K., Evans, J.J., & Robertson, I.H. (2002). Rehabilitation of executive function: facilitation of effective goal management on complex tasks using periodic auditory alerts. *Neuropsychologia, 40*, 271-281.

O'Brian, K.P., Prigatano, G.P., & Pittman, H.W. (1988). Neurobehavioural education of a patient and spouse following right frontal oligodendroglioma excision. *Neuropsychology, 2*, 145-159.

Robertson, I.H. (1996). *Goal Management Training: A Clinical Manual*. Cambridge: PsyConsult.

Robertson, I.H. (1999). The rehabilitation of attention. In D.T. Stuss, G. Winocur, & I.H. Robertson, (Eds.), *Cognitive Rehabilitation* (pp. 302-313). Cambridge: CUP.

Robertson, I.H., Ward, T., Ridgeway, V., & Nimmo-Smith, I. (1994). *The Test of Everyday Attention*. Flempton: Thames Valley Test Company.

Rylander, G. (1939). *Personality Changes After Operations on the Frontal Lobes. Acta Psychiatrica et Neurologica* Supplementum XX. Copenhagen: Ejnar Munksgaard.

Sahakian, B.J., Coull, J.J., & Hodges, J.R. (1994). Selective enhancement of executive function in a patient with dementia of the frontal lobe type. *Journal of Neurology, Neurosurgery and Psychiatry, 57*, 120-121.

Shallice, T. (1988). *From Neuropsychology to Mental Structure*. Cambridge: Cambridge University Press.

Shallice, T. & Burgess, P. (1991). Deficits in strategy application following frontal lobe damage in man. *Brain, 144*, 727-741.

Shallice, T. & Burgess, P. (1996). The domain of the supervisory process and temporal organisation of behaviour. *Philosphical Transactions: Biological Sciences, 351*, 1405-1412.

Wilson, B.A., Alderman, N., Burgess, P. Emslie, H., & Evans, J.J. (1996). *The Behavioural Assessment of the Dysexecutive Syndrome*. Flempton: Thames Valley Test Company.

Wilson, B.A., Emslie, H., Quirk, K. & Evans, J.J. (2001). Reducing everyday memory and planning problems by means of a paging system: a randomised control crossover study. *Journal of Neurosurgery, Neurology and Psychiatry, 70*, 477-482.

Wilson, B.A., Evans, J.J., Emslie, H., & Malinek, V. (1997). Evaluation of NeuroPage: A new memory aid. *Journal of Neurology, Neurosurgery and Psychiatry, 63*, 113-115.

Wilson, B.A., Evans, J.J., Brentnall, S., Bremner, S., Keohane, C., & Williams, W.H. (2000). The Oliver Zangwill Centre for Neuropsychological Rehabilitation: A partnership between health care and rehabilitation research. In A.-L. Christensen & B.P. Uzzell (eds.), *International Handbook of Neuropsychological Rehabilitation* (pp. 231-246). New York: Kluwer Academic/Plenum Publishers.

van Zomeren, A.H. & Brouwer, W.H. (1994) *Clinical Neuropsychological Assessment of Attention*. New York: OUP.

d'Zurilla, T.J. & Goldfried, M.R. (1971). Problem-solving and behaviour modification. *Journal of Abnormal Psychology, 78*, 107-126.

Chapter 5

REHABILITATION OF MEMORY DEFICITS

Barbara A. Wilson

MRC Cognition and Brain Sciences Unit, Cambridge, and
The Oliver Zangwill Centre, Ely, UK

Introduction

Memory difficulties are one of the commonest cognitive problems arising from injury to the brain and, consequently, form a large part of cognitive rehabilitation. Unlike the study of memory itself, or the interest shown in memory performance, there has been until quite recently, little scientific enquiry into the remediation or amelioration of memory problems after brain injury. Neither has there been much effort until the past few years in relating theory to the practical experiences of memory impaired people or vice versa. Although considerate effort has gone into pharmacological research in the attempt to find a drug to improve or halt memory decline, this is beyond the scope of this chapter. The interested reader is referred to Curran and Weingartner (2002) This chapter highlights successful approaches to memory rehabilitation that have developed over the past two decades, it discusses guidelines that have been established in memory rehabilitation as a result of theoretical investigations of amnesia. Reference is made to the role of theory in those cases where theory has influenced the clinical management of memory problems. The four major approaches within memory rehabilitation involve (1) environmental adaptations, (2) new technology, (3) new learning, and (4) holistic approaches incorporating emotional, social, behavioural and cognitive aspects of memory deficits. A discussion of these approaches is provided together with an example of a young man receiving a holistic programme for his memory difficulties.

Theoretical Influences on Memory Rehabilitation

It is probably true to say that the main theoretical influences on neuropsychology and neuropsychological rehabilitation have come from (a) the study of neuropsychology itself; (b) cognitive (neuro)psychology, which provides us with theoretical models to help explain phenomena and predict patterns of behaviour; and (c) behavioural psychology, which has provided us with a number of intervention strategies that can be modified or adapted for use with people with brain injury (see Wilson, 1999 for further discussion).

Behavioural psychology has also provided strategies to help us assess everyday manifestations of neuropsychological impairments, analyse problems and evaluate the efficacy of treatments. One branch of behavioural psychology in particular, learning theory, has been important in helping neuropsychologists improve learning in people with brain injury (Baddeley & Wilson, 1994).

There are, of course, numerous other sources that have affected the development of neuropsychology and neuropsychological rehabilitation. These include neurology, psychiatry, gerontology, occupational therapy, linguistics, ergonomics, information technology and others. All of them serve to emphasise the fact that neuropsychology and neuropsychological rehabilitation are areas requiring a broad theoretical base – or, perhaps one should say, several theoretical bases (Wilson, 1997)

It is apt, I think, to point out there that it is simply not sufficient for cognitive psychologists to suggest that neuropsychological rehabilitation should be driven by theories solely from their own subdiscipline. The danger of following one model or theoretical approach too closely, without considering other possible influential sources, is that we might become too confined and constrained. (Wilson, 2002). Take, for example, the concomitant difficulties that are often associated with memory impairment such as anxiety, fear and depression. These problems need to be addressed as part of memory rehabilitation (see Chapter 7 in this volume). Here models of emotion, such as Beck's influential model of emotional disorders (Beck, 1976; 1996) are playing an increasingly important role in the rehabilitation of people with memory disorders. Prigatano (2000) believes that dealing with the emotional effects of brain injury is essential to rehabilitation success. Social factors and individual personality need to be taken into account when designing rehabilitation. Pre- and post morbid life styles will also be influential in determining the nature of treatment.

It is not always clear to what extent the problems are cognitive or emotional in origin. Howieson and Lezak (1995) for example, describe a patient who was referred for help because he 'forgot' to go to bed at night. Those responsible for the referral saw the patient's difficulties as being connected with memory failure when in fact the nocturnal activity and agitation were emotional in origin. In contrast, relatives of a patient with amnesia following head injury may believe that memory failure is due to emotional trauma caused by the accident. The main point here is that rehabilitation needs to draw on a number of theoretical fields and models to deal with the wide ranging and complex problems faced by survivors of brain injury (Wilson, 2002).

Ways of Understanding Memory

Although there are several models of memory functioning and not all are uniformly accepted, the following is taken primarily from three influential models of memory namely the Working Memory Model (Baddeley & Hitch, 1974), the systems model of long term memory and associated brain structures (Squire & Knowlton, 1995) and the model of Markowitsch (1998).

Length of storage
The Working Memory model of Baddeley and Hitch (1974) subdivides memory into three main types depending both on time-based and conceptual differences. The first system, *sensory memory*, is a brief and rather literal trace that results from a visual, auditory or other sensory event, probably lasting no longer than a quarter of a second. This is the system we use to make sense of moving pictures (visual sensory memory) or language (auditory sensory memory). Most people with damage to this system would present with perceptual or language disorders and we would not normally think of them as having memory problems.

The second system, *working memory*, is considered to have two main components or functions. The first of these is *short-term* or *immediate* memory and lasts for several seconds. This period of time can be extended to several minutes if the person is rehearsing or concentrating on the particular information. Unlike sensory memory, information in working memory has already undergone substantial cognitive analysis, so it is typically represented in meaningful chunks such as words or numbers. We use this system when looking up a new telephone number and holding on to it long enough to dial.

The second component of working memory is a *central executive* that can be conceived of as an organiser, controller or allocator of resources. This component enables us to both to drive a car and talk to our passenger at the same time. Sufficient resources are allocated to each of these tasks, and if a demanding or unusual situation occurs on the road we stop talking while all our resources are required to deal with the unexpected situation.

The third system in the Baddeley and Hitch (1974) model is *long-term memory*, which encodes information in a reasonably robust form and can last for decades. Although there are differences in memory for things that happened 10 minutes ago and things that happened 10 years ago, the differences are less clear-cut than those between the sensory (quarter of a second) and immediate (few seconds) memory systems. All the systems described so far are connected with *retrospective memory*, that is remembering information or events that have already occurred. Frequently, however, we want to remember to do something in the future, such as take our medicine, water the plants, or make a telephone call. The system activated for remembering to do something is known as *prospective memory*. It is significant that many of the complaints of memory impaired people refer to failures in prospective memory.

Type of information to be remembered

In 1972 Tulving (1972) produced an influential paper distinguishing two types of memory: semantic and episodic. *Semantic memory* is memory for our knowledge about the world, for example, remembering that Brussels is the capital of Belgium, or that a squirrel has a bushy tail. Semantic memory is also concerned with our knowledge of social customs, the meanings of words, the colours and textures of objects, and how things smell. Most memory impaired patients do not forget this kind of information, although they may have difficulty adding to their store of semantic knowledge. Amnesic patients are often unable, for example, to learn new words that enter the vocabulary after their neurological insult.

Episodic memory, on the other hand, represents what most of us would think of as memory in that it refers to a specific episode that has been experienced and can be recalled. Thus, remembering what television programme you watched last night, when you last had your hair cut or what you read a few minutes ago, are all examples of episodic memory. This system is frequently damaged in people with organic memory impairment and episodic memory deficits are perhaps the most noticeable characteristic of the amnesic syndrome.

A third system that operates differently from either semantic or episodic memory is *procedural memory*, the system used for learning skills such as swimming or typing. People get better with practice and can demonstrate the skill even though they may not remember how they learned to ride swim or type. JC, a young amnesic patient of mine, successfully learned to type even though he had no conscious recollection of learning. In his words, 'Practical skills developed without me being aware of how this came about. I could do things without being able to explain how.' Procedural memory is typically normal or nearly normal in amnesic patients.

The stages involved in remembering

Typically there are three stages involved in remembering: *encoding, storage*, and *retrieval*. Encoding refers to the registration stage, or getting the information into memory. Storage refers to the maintenance of information in the memory store, and retrieval refers to the stage of extracting or recalling the information when it is required. After a neurological insult to the brain, each of these stages can be affected.

Suggestions as to how to improve encoding, storage and retrieval include:

- Simplifying the information you give to a memory impaired person.
- Reducing the amount of information supplied at any one time.
- Ensuring there is minimal distraction.
- Making sure the information is understood – by asking the person to repeat it in his/her own words.
- Encouraging the person to link or associate information with material that is already known.
- Trying to ensure processing at a deeper level – by encouraging the person to ask questions.
- Using the 'little and often' rule i.e. it is better to work for a few minutes several times a day or during a session than to work for the same amount of time in one chunk.
- Making sure learning occurs in different contexts to avoid context specificity and enhance generalisation.

Recall and recognition

Recall and recognition are two of the main ways we remember information. Recall involves actively finding the information to be remembered. In some situations, however, we do not need to recall the information but to recognise it. Most of us at some time have been unable to tell someone how to find a particular street, but can nevertheless take ourselves there with no trouble. Most memory impaired people find recall harder than recognition, although both systems are usually affected. Some people might have difficulty with both verbal and visual information while others might have problems in only one of these modalities.

Explicit and implicit memory

In many situations we need to consciously recall information we have received. For example, if I asked someone where they spent last Christmas, and they could tell me, they would be using *explicit memory*, i.e. consciously recalling the desired information. If, on the other hand, I asked someone when and where they learned to swim, and the steps by which they gained expertise, they would probably find this difficult. They could demonstrate how to swim, that is they could have *implicit memory* of this skill, they would remember how to do it even if they were unable to explain it with any great ease or remember when and how they learned the skill. Like procedural memory, implicit memory is usually intact or relatively intact in people with organic memory impairment.

Retrograde and anterograde memory

One of the questions frequently asked by relatives of memory impaired people is, 'Why can s/he remember what happened several years ago, but not what happened yesterday?' The short answer is that old memories are stored differently in the brain from new memories. Although information acquired before a neurological insult may be forgotten, this is usually for a specific time period ranging from a few minutes for some head-injured people to several decades for some people with Korsakoff's syndrome or herpes simplex encephalitis. Memory loss dating from before the insult is known as *retrograde amnesia* (RA). RA is usually less of a problem and less handicapping for the memory impaired person than *anterograde amnesia*, which refers to memory difficulties dating from the time of the neurological insult (although see Kapur, 1993, for a review of RA).

It should be noted here that these are not mutually exclusive systems. Instead they are simply different ways of considering the breakdown of memory. For example, procedural memory is a subcategory of implicit memory; explicit memory covers both episodic and semantic memory and anterograde amnesia represents an impairment in the ability to add to semantic memory as well as an impairment in episodic memory. Thus competing terms are often used for similar concepts.

Strategies for Memory Rehabilitation

Environmental adaptations
The most that we might be able to do for a patient with widespread cognitive impairments is change or adapt the environment in some way in order to reduce the load on the patient's memory. An example of this is given by Harris (1980)when he describes a geriatric unit in the USA with a high rate of incontinence until somebody painted all the lavatory doors a distinctive colour. The rate of incontinence decreased, presumably because more people could remember that the lavatories were behind the distinctly coloured doors.

Similar approaches can be used in a variety of settings. Signposts, for example, can be placed strategically around the hospital or home. Doors can be labelled so that patients know which is the dining room, which is the bedroom and so forth. The patient's bed itself can be labelled. As well as providing signposts and labels, therapists should make sure that (a) the printing is large enough to be legible to those with failing eyesight, (b) the labels/signs are placed in prominent positions, (c) the labels are discriminable against their backgrounds, and (d) the terminology used is familiar to the patient. Further examples of environmental adaptation can be found in Wilson (1995) and Wilson and Evans (2000).

Compensating for memory deficits
Compensation is one of the major tools for enabling people with brain injury to cope in everyday life. Wilson and Watson (1996) described a framework for understanding compensatory behaviour in people with organic memory impairment. Wilson (2000) went on to use this framework to consider compensation for other cognitive deficits. The framework was developed from one proposed by Bäckman and Dixon (1992) and further modified by Dixon and Bäckman (1999). The framework distinguishes four steps in the evolu-

tion of compensatory behaviour, namely origins, mechanisms, forms and consequences.

The origins of compensatory behaviour take place when there is either (1) a decrease in a given skill without an accompanying decrease in environmental demands, or (2) an increase in environmental demands without an accompanying increase in the skills required for successful performance.

Mechanisms are ways in which a match between everyday demands and skill deficits is achieved. One way is to offset the mismatch by an increase in time and effort; a second way is to use a substitute skill; and a third way is to adapt or adjust to the new situation by relaxing the criteria of success or by changing expectations.

Forms of compensatory behaviour refer to the manner and extent to which compensatory behaviour differs from the behaviour of a normal person in a similar situation. These forms may involve the same behaviour a normal person would use with more time and effort expended; or they may involve substitute skills and these may be ones normal people use but only infrequently; or they may be entirely new behaviours not used by the general population. Consequences of compensatory behaviour may be functional and adaptive, and reduce the mismatch between environmental demand and skill, or they may be maladaptive and fail to reduce the mismatch.

Wilson and Watson (1996) considered how Bäckman and Dixon's framework might apply to people with memory impairments. Although much of the framework was useful it was insufficient to account for all the successes and failures in learning to compensate demonstrated by people with organic memory impairment. For example, Bäckman and Dixon (1992) consider severity of impairment affects the extent to which compensation occurs and suggest compensatory behaviour follows a U-shaped curve whereby people with very mild or very severe deficits will not compensate whereas those with moderate deficits will. They provide examples of normal elderly adults who compensate better than young adults who do not need to compensate, and Alzheimer patients who do not have the wherewithal to compensate. Wilson and Watson (1996) regarded this as only partially true and cite the example of severely amnesic people who can compensate despite very severe problems provided they have few additional cognitive deficits.

Two recent studies consider factors that predict good use of compensations (Evans, Wilson, Needham, & Brentnall, in press; Wilson & Watson, 1996). The main predictors appear to be age (younger people compensate better), severity of impairment (very severely impaired people compensate less well), specificity of deficit (those with specific memory problems compensate better than those with more widespread cognitive impairments) and premorbid use of strategies (those using compensation aids pre-morbidly appear to do better).

External aids and new technology
Most people without memory impairments make frequent use of external aids. A follow-up study of 45 memory impaired people (Wilson, 1991b)

showed more aids are likely to be used 5-10 years after the end of formal rehabilitation than during rehabilitation. A recent study (Evans et al., in press) interviewed 101 brain injured people and their families to find out what strategies were used to compensate for memory impairments and how effective were the compensations. The variables that best predicted use of memory aids were current age, time since injury, the number of aids used premorbidly and good attentional skills.

Few people in the Wilson (1991a) and the Evans et al. (in press) studies were using technological aids such as electronic organisers despite increasing use of technology in society as a whole. Nevertheless the growth in technology has benefited memory rehabilitation in several ways and this benefit is likely to increase in the future. 'Smart' houses, for example, employ computers and videos to monitor and control the living environments of people with dementia. The aim of people developing and using this technology is to increase independence and activity and to improve the quality of life for confused elderly people. If successful for this population, there is no reason why 'smart' houses cannot be adopted for other people with cognitive impairments.

Two 'smart' houses are up and running in Norway (Graeme Slaven, personal communication) addressing problems such as falls, disorientation, inadequate meals, poor hygiene, emergencies and limited home management. With the rapid development of technology, it is possible that 'smart' houses will become more important in the next decade or so, and would seem a fruitful area for psychologists, engineers, architects and computer programmers to join forces to design and evaluate new environments. Another recent and exciting tool in memory rehabilitation is NeuroPage®, developed for use with brain injured memory impaired people. NeuroPage® is a simple and portable paging system designed in California by the engineer father of a head injured son working together with a neuropsychologist (Hersch & Treadgold, 1994) NeuroPage® uses a computer linked by modem and telephone to a paging company. The scheduling of reminders or cues for each individual is entered into the computer and, from then on, no further human interfacing is necessary. On the appropriate day and time NeuroPage® automatically transmits the reminder information to the paging company who transmits the message to the individual's pager.

The system avoids most of the problems faced by memory impaired people when they try to use a compensatory aid or strategy. Employing aids or strategies involves memory, so the very people who need them most have the greatest difficulty using them. They forget to use them, may be unable to program them, may use them unsystematically and may be embarrassed by them. In contrast, NeuroPage® can be controlled by one rather large button, easy to press even for those with motor difficulties. It is highly portable, it has an audible or vibratory alarm depending on the preference of the user, it has an accompanying explanatory message and is, to many people's minds, prestigious.

In a pilot study (Wilson, Evans, Emslie, & Malinek, 1997), NeuroPage® was evaluated with 15 brain injured people whose memory difficulties followed head injury, stroke or tumour. Using an ABA design whereby the first A phase was the baseline period, B the treatment and the second A phase the post-treatment baseline, we demonstrated that all 15 participants benefited significantly from NeuroPage®. The average number of problems tackled for the group as a whole was 3.86 with a range of 1–7 and a mode of 4. Typical reminders included 'take your medication', 'feed the dog/cat', 'pack your things for college/work', and 'check your diary'.

For the group as a whole, the mean percentage success for completing tasks in the first baseline period was 37.08, while in the treatment phase this rose to 85.56. Using an Odds Ratio Test (Everitt, 1995), which takes into account different underlying success rates for each target and calculates an average improvement factor, it was found that each participant showed a significant improvement. There were, however, wide individual differences, with some subjects changing from 0% success in the baseline period to over 90% success in the treatment period through to those with more modest changes such as 6.67% in the baseline stage to 22.93% in the treatment stage.

There were also wide variations between subjects in the post-treatment baseline phase. The mean success of the group as a whole was 74.46%, i.e. better than in the first baseline phase. The Odds Ratio Test indicated that 11 of the 15 participants were significantly better than in the baseline phase and 4 were not. The implications here are that some participants 'learn' to do what is expected during treatment, i.e. they learn to take their medication, feed the dog and pack their school bag, while other people will always require reminders to carry out tasks.

Two single case studies with NeuroPage® showed how the system can enhance independence in people with memory and/or planning problems (Evans, Emslie, & Wilson, 1998; Wilson, Emslie, Quirk, & Evans, 1999). Finally, a recently completed study of 143 people using a randomised control crossover design replicated the findings of the pilot study and showed that NeuroPage® significantly reduces the everyday problems of brain injured people with memory and planning difficulties (Wilson, Emslie, Quirk, & Evans, 2001).

In addition to NeuroPage®, recent work with pocket-computer memory aids shows that it is possible for people with memory deficits to learn to use two different types of pocket-computer (a touchscreen and a keyboard machine). There were individual preferences for one or other machine although high users tended to prefer the keyboard pocket-computer, while less frequent users made more entries with the touchscreen pocket-computer. The authors felt this demonstrated the need for rehabilitation staff to distinguish ability to use a machine from willingness to use a machine (Wright et al., 2001).

For further discussion of the use of computers and other technological equipment in memory rehabilitation, the reader is referred to Glisky (1995) and Kapur (1995). External aids appear to work through capitalising on residual episodic memory unlike errorless learning described below which is probably more dependent on implicit memory.

New learning

Useful as external aids new technology and environmental adaptations may be, they are rarely sufficient on their own. Memory impaired people need to learn some new information on some occasions. People's names, for example, can be written down in a notebook but in normal social interaction we need to greet people by name (at least every now and again). Referring to a notebook to retrieve the name would impair natural communication. Although learning names is difficult for many people and particularly so for those with organic memory impairment, a number of studies have shown that it is possible to teach names to amnesic people using strategies to improve learning. Wilson (1987) evaluated the strategy of visual imagery to teach names and demonstrated that it is virtually always superior to rote repetition. Thoene and Glisky (1995) also found that visual imagery was superior to other methods for teaching people's names to amnesic patients. More recently, Clare, Wilson, Breen, and Hodges (1999) were able to teach a 74-year-old man in the early stages of Alzheimer's disease the names of his colleagues at a social club. A combination of strategies was used including finding a distinctive feature of the face together with backward chaining and expanding rehearsal. A follow up study showed that much of this information was maintained two years after the end of treatment (Clare, Wilson, Carter, Hodges, & Adams, 2001).

Another principle, from experimental investigations into memory that can help brain injured people to learn more efficiently, is the principle of distributed practice. If learning trials are spaced or distributed, this leads to faster learning than massed practice whereby the same amount of information or practice is presented in one chunk (Baddeley & Longman, 1978; Lorge, 1930). In similar vein, Landauer and Bjork (1978) found that learning was improved if the information to be retained was tested over gradually increasing intervals. Such expanded rehearsal (otherwise known as spaced retrieval) is now a widely used procedure in helping people with memory and learning difficulties (see Camp, 2001, for a fuller discussion).

Some strategies from the field of study techniques (e.g Robinson, 1970) and learning disability (e.g.Yule & Carr, 1987), have been applied in neuropsychological rehabilitation (Wilson, 1991a) and work continues in ways to improve learning. One series of potentially important studies in recent years has involved errorless learning.

Errorless learning has for many years been used to teach new skills to people with learning disabilities (Cullen, 1976; Jones & Eayrs, 1992; Sidman & Stoddard, 1967) but until quite recently the principle has not been employed to any great extent with neurologically impaired adults. As the name implies, errorless learning involves learning without errors or mistakes. Most people can learn or benefit from their errors because they remember their mistakes and, therefore, avoid making the same mistake repeatedly.

People without episodic memory, however, cannot remember their mistakes so fail to correct them. Furthermore, the very fact of engaging in a behaviour may strengthen or reinforce that behaviour. Consequently, for someone with a severe memory impairment, it makes sense to ensure that any behaviour which is going to be reinforced is correct rather than incorrect.

Work on errorless learning in memory impaired adults was not only influenced by the earlier studies from the field of learning disability, but also by studies of implicit learning from the field of cognitive neuropsychology. There have been numerous studies showing that amnesic patients can learn some things normally or nearly normally even though they may have no conscious recollection of learning anything at all (Baddeley, 1990; Brooks & Baddeley, 1976; Graf & Schacter, 1985; Glisky & Schacter, 1987, 1989). Glisky and Schacter (1987, 1989) tried to use the implicit learning abilities of amnesic subjects to teach them computer technology. Although some success was achieved, this was at the expense of considerable time and effort. This and other attempts to build on the relatively intact skills of memory impaired people has, on the whole, been disappointing. One reason for failures and anomalies could be that implicit learning is poor at eliminating errors. Error elimination is a function of explicit not implicit memory. Consequently, if subjects are forced to rely on implicit memory (as amnesic subjects are), trial-and-error learning becomes a slow and laborious process.

Baddeley and Wilson (1994) published the first study demonstrating that amnesic patients learn better when they are prevented from making mistakes during the learning process. This was a theoretical study in which a stem completion task was used to teach severely memory impaired patients lists of words. Each of the 16 amnesic patients in the study showed better learning when they were prevented from making mistakes (i.e., prevented from guessing) than when they were forced to guess (i.e., forced to make mistakes). Since then, several single case studies have been carried out with memory impaired patients comparing errorful and errorless learning for teaching practical, everyday, information (Wilson, Baddeley, Evans, & Shiel, 1994). In the majority of cases, errorless learning proved to be superior to trial-and-error learning. Squires, Hunkin, and Parkin (1996) Wilson and Evans (1996) and Evans et al. (2000) report further studies.

Results from recent work (Evans et al., 2000) involving ten errorless learning experiments, suggest that tasks and situations which depend on implicit memory (such as stem completion tasks or retrieving a name from a first letter cue) are more likely to benefit from errorless learning methods than tasks which require explicit recall of new situations. Nevertheless, Wilson et al. (1994) demonstrated new explicit learning in a memory impaired head injured patient. Clare et al. (1999) also demonstrated explicit learning in a man with Alzheimer's disease. The Evans et al.(2000) studies found that the more severely amnesic patients benefited to a greater extent from errorless learning methods than those who are less severely impaired, although this may only apply when the interval between learning and recall is relatively short. One of the implications from this finding is that errorless learning should be combined with expanding rehearsal to enhance its effectiveness. Recent work in Cambridge suggests that errorless learning works primarily by capitalising on implicit memory rather than strengthening impaired episodic memory.

Holistic Approaches to Memory Rehabilitation

Wilson (1997) suggests there are currently four main approaches to cognitive rehabilitation, namely cognitive retraining through exercises or stimulation; strategies derived from theoretical models from cognitive neuropsychology; strategies derived from a combination of methodologies and techniques particularly neuropsychology, cognitive psychology and behavioural psychology; and holistic approaches that address cognitive, social and emotional sequelae of brain injury. Although each of these approaches has strengths and weaknesses, the holistic approach might be the best in terms of improving independence, employability and quality of life for people with non-progressive brain damage (Cope, 1994; Mehlbye & Larsen, 1994; Prigatano et al., 1994; Rattok et al., 1992).

Holistic programmes offer both group and individual therapy to increase the brain injured person's understanding of his or her problems, to improve insight, to help develop compensatory strategies for cognitive deficits and to consider work or other meaningful activities the brain injured person can engage in. It is important to address emotional issues because people with cognitive deficits become more distressed as they become more aware of their difficulties. Thus distress can interfere with new learning and adjustment just as it does for people without brain damage.

An example of a holistic rehabilitation programme for a man with cognitive, social and emotional difficulties is provided by Wilson, Evans and Williams (in press). They describe Carl, a young man who sustained a severe head injury in a road traffic accident when he was 21 years of age. He was in coma for 4 months and in Post Traumatic Amnesia for 2–3 months. Of average intellectual ability, Carl had some deficits of attention and fluency. He had a retrograde amnesia of several years and could remember little of his earlier life except that he was a fan of Manchester United Football Club. Despite a good immediate memory, his anterograde memory was poor, he forgot conversations, could not remember what he had been doing or was about to do. He became socially withdrawn, refused to go out because he could not remember what he had said or what others had said to him. He also became obsessive about checking things, for example, whether he had locked the door and whether he had his wallet, keys and mobile telephone with him.

During his rehabilitation programme Carl received individual and group therapy to deal with his varied problems. He attended the 'Understanding Brain Injury' group to improve insight into his strengths and weaknesses. This group meets daily, has an educational focus that teaches people about the brain and the consequences of brain injury. Clients are encouraged to take notes, learn from the handouts provided, review their progress and develop and share understanding of their own injuries. In the Memory Group, Carl was encouraged to use a filofax for daily planning, a voice organiser to record conversations and an electronic organiser to alert him (by means of an alarm and message printed on the screen) to carry out activities such as telephoning a friend or taking exercise. He also attended a group for Stress Management. Here Carl was taught (a) breathing exercises and (b) how to identify hierarchies to work through to enable him to participate in social occasions, community activities and physical exercise.

In the Attention Group, he was helped to attend more efficiently and to 'burn-in' images so that he would not need to check and re-check. He also received vocational counselling, individual psychological support and individual memory sessions to back up the group sessions.

After 4 months in the rehabilitation programme, Carl started on a college course, he was socialising with friends and going to clubs or pubs 2–3 times a week, he was independent in the local and wider community, his checking and tidying rituals were considerably reduced and he expressed greater confidence in himself in the use of strategies to manage his memory and engage in activities. Carl commented 'I have got my life back'.

Summary and Conclusions

Memory should be regarded as a multifunctional cognitive system that can be understood in a number of ways. We can consider the length of time information is stored, the type of information stored, the stages involved in remembering, whether information is recalled or recognised, whether implicit or explicit information is required, or whether memories date from before or after the neurological insult.

Most memory impaired people have difficulty learning and remembering new information; they have a normal, or nearly normal, immediate memory span, but have problems remembering after a delay or distraction, and they usually have a period of retrograde amnesia that may range from minutes to decades.

Although restoration of memory functioning is unlikely to occur in the majority of people whose memory impairments follow neurological insult, there is, nevertheless, much that can be done to reduce the impact of disabling and handicapping memory problems and foster understanding of the issues involved. These include: dealing with emotional sequelae such as anxiety and depression, which are often associated with organic memory impairment;

environmental modifications that can enable very severely impaired people to cope in their daily lives despite lack of adequate memory functioning; teaching people how to use external memory aids to help them compensate for their memory difficulties; and the employment of errorless learning principles to improve the learning ability of memory impaired people.

References

Bäckman, L., & Dixon, R.A. (1992). Psychological compensation: A theoretical framework. *Psychological Bulletin, 112*, 259-283.

Baddeley, A.D. (1990). *Human memory: Theory and practice*. London: Lawrence Erlbaum Associates.

Baddeley, A.D., & Hitch, G. (1974). Working memory. In G.H. Bower (Ed.), *The psychology of learning and motivation, Vol. 8*, (pp. 47-89). New York: Academic Press.

Baddeley, A.D., & Longman, D.J.A. (1978). The influence of length and frequency on training sessions on the rate of learning to type. *Ergonomics, 21*, 627-635.

Baddeley, A.D., & Wilson, B.A. (1994). When implicit learning fails: Amnesia and the problem of error elimination. *Neuropsychologia, 32*, 53-68.

Beck, A.T. (1976). *Cognitive therapy and emotional disorders*. New York: International Universities Press.

Beck, A.T. (1996). Beyond belief: A theory of modes, personality, and psychopathology. In P.M. Salkovskis (Ed.), *Frontiers of cognitive therapy* (pp. 1-25). New York: The Guilford Press.

Brooks, D.N., & Baddeley, A.D. (1976). What can amnesic patients learn? *Neuropsychologia, 14*, 111-122.

Camp, C.J. (2001). From efficacy to effectiveness to diffusion: Making the transitions in dementia intervention research. *Neuropsychological Rehabilitation, 11*, 495-517.

Clare, L., Wilson, B.A., Breen, E.K., & Hodges, J.R. (1999). Errorless learning of face-name associations in early Alzheimer's disease. *Neurocase, 5*, 37-46.

Clare, L., Wilson, B.A., Carter, G., Hodges, J.R., & Adams, M. (2001). Long-term maintenance of treatment gains following a cognitive rehabilitation intervention in early dementia of Alzheimer type: A single case study. *Neuropsychological Rehabilitation, 11*, 477-494.

Cope, N. (1994). Traumatic brain injury rehabilitation outcome studies in the United States. In A.-L. Christensen & B.P. Uzzell (Eds.), *Brain injury and neuropsychological rehabilitation: International perspectives* (pp. 201-220). Hillsdale, NJ: Lawrence Erlbaum Associates.

Cullen, C.N. (1976, 25th March 1976). Errorless learning with the retarded. *Nursing Times*, 45-47.

Curran, V., & Weingartner, H. (2002). The Psychopharmacology of Memory. In A.D. Baddeley, M. Kopelman, & B.A. Wilson (Eds.), *Handbook of Memory Disorders* (Second ed., pp. 123-141). Chichester: Wiley & Sons.

Dixon, R.A., & Bäckman, L. (1999). Principles of compensation in cognitive neurorehabilitation. In D. T. Stuss, G. Winocur, & I.H. Robertson (Eds.), *Cognitive neurorehabilitation: A comprehensive approach* (pp. 59-72). New York, NY: Cambridge University Press.

Evans, J.J., Emslie, H., & Wilson, B.A. (1998). External cueing systems in the rehabilitation of executive impairments of action. *Journal of the International Neuropsychological Society, 4*, 399-408.

Evans, J.J., Wilson, B.A., Needham, P., & Brentnall, S. (in press). Who makes good use of memory-aids: Results of a survey of 100 people with acquired brain injury. *Journal of the International Neuropsychological Society.*

Evans, J.J., Wilson, B.A., Schuri, U., Andrade, J., Baddeley, A., Bruna, O., Canavan, T., Della Sala, S., Green, R., Laaksonen, R., Lorenzi, L., & Taussik, I. (2000). A comparison of 'errorless' and 'trial-and-error' learning methods for teaching individuals with acquired memory deficits. *Neuropsychological Rehabilitation, 10*, 67-101.

Everitt, B. (1995). *Cambridge dictionary of statistics in the medical sciences.* Cambridge: Cambridge University Press.

Glisky, E.L. (1995). Computers in memory rehabilitation. In A.D. Baddeley & B.A. Wilson & F.N. Watts (Eds.), *Handbook of memory disorders* (pp. 557-575). Chichester: John Wiley.

Glisky, E.L., & Schacter, D.L. (1987). Acquisition of domain-specific knowledge in organic amnesia: Training for computer-related work. *Neuropsychologia, 25*, 893-906.

Glisky, E.L., & Schacter, D.L. (1989). Extending the limits of complex learning in organic amnesia: Computer training in a vocational domain. *Neuropsychologia, 27*, 107-120.

Graf, P., & Schacter, D.L. (1985). Implicit and explicit memory for new associations in normal and amnesic subjects. *Journal of Experimental Psychology: Learning, Memory and Cognition, 11*, 501-518.

Harris, J.E. (1980). We have ways of helping you remember. *Concord: The Journal of the British Association of Service to the Elderly, 17*, 21-27.

Hersch, N., & Treadgold, L. (1994). NeuroPage: The rehabilitation of memory dysfunction by prosthetic memory and cueing. *NeuroRehabilitation, 4*, 187-197.

Howieson, D.B., & Lezak, M.D. (1995). Separating memory from other cognitive problems. In A.D. Baddeley, B.A. Wilson, & F.N. Watts (Eds.), *Handbook of memory disorders* (pp. 411-426). Chichester: John Wiley.

Jones, R.S.P., & Eayrs, C.B. (1992). The use of errorless learning procedures in teaching people with a learning disability. *Mental Handicap Research, 5*, 304-312.

Kapur, N. (1993). Focal retrograde amnesia in neurological disease: A critical review. *Cortex, 29*, 217-234.

Kapur, N. (1995). Memory aids in the rehabilitation of memory disordered patients. In A.D. Baddeley, B.A. Wilson, & F.N. Watts (Eds.), *Handbook of memory disorders* (pp. 533-556). Chichester: John Wiley.

Landauer, T.K., & Bjork, R.A. (1978). Optimum rehearsal patterns and name learning. In M.M. Gruneberg, P.E. Morris, & R.N. Sykes (Eds.), *Practical aspects of memory* (pp. 625-632). London: Academic Press.

Lorge, I. (1930). *Influence of regularly interpolated time intervals upon subsequent learning*: Quoted in H.H. Johnson & R.L. Solso (1971) An introduction to experimental design in psychology: A case approach. New York: Harper & Row.

Markowitsch, H.J. (1998). Cognitive neuroscience of memory. *Neurocase, 4*, 429-435.

Mehlbye, J., & Larsen, A. (1994). Social and economic consequences of brain damage in Denmark. In A.-L. Christensen & B.P. Uzzell (Eds.), *Brain injury and neuropsychological rehabilitation: International perspectives* (pp. 257-267). Hillsdale, NJ: Lawrence Erlbaum Associates.

Prigatano, G.P. (2000). Rehabilitation for traumatic brain injury. *The Journal of the American Medical Association, 284*, 1783.

Prigatano, G.P., Klonoff, P.S., O'Brien, K.P., Altman, I.M., Amin, K., Chiapello, D., Shepherd, J., Cunningham, M., & Mora, M. (1994). Productivity after neuropsychologically oriented milieu rehabilitation. *Journal of Head Trauma Rehabilitation, 9*, 91-102.

Rattok, J., Ben-Yishay, Y., Ezrachi, O., Lakin, P., Piasetsky, E., Ross, B., Silver, S., Vakil, E., Zide, E., & Diller, L. (1992). Outcome of different treatment mixes in a multidimensional neuropsychological rehabilitation programme. *Neuropsychology, 6,* 395-416.

Robinson, F.P. (1970). *Effective study.* New York: Harper and Row.

Sidman, M., & Stoddard, L.T. (1967). The effectiveness of fading in programming simultaneous form discrimination for retarded children. *Journal of Experimental Analysis of Behavior, 10,* 3-15.

Squire, L., & Knowlton, B. (1995). Memory, hippocampus and brain systems. In M. Gazzaniga (Ed.), *The Cognitive Neurosciences.* Boston: MIT Press.

Squires, E.J., Hunkin, N.M., & Parkin, A.J. (1996). Memory notebook training in a case of severe amnesia: Generalising from paired associate learning to real life. *Neuropsychological Rehabilitation, 6,* 55-65.

Thoene, A.I.T., & Glisky, E.L. (1995). Learning of name-face associations in memory impaired patients: A comparison of different training procedures. *Journal of the International Neuropsychological Society, 1,* 29-38.

Tulving, E. (1972). Episodic and semantic memory. In E. Tulving & W. Donaldson (Eds.), *Organization of memory* (pp. 381-403). New York: Academic Press.

Wilson, B.A. (1987). *Rehabilitation of memory.* New York: Guilford Press.

Wilson, B.A. (1991a). Behaviour therapy in the treatment of neurologically impaired adults. In P.R. Martin (Ed.), *Handbook of behavior therapy and psychological science: An integrative approach* (pp. 227-252). New York: Pergamon Press.

Wilson, B.A. (1991b). Long term prognosis of patients with severe memory disorders. *Neuropsychological Rehabilitation, 1,* 117-134.

Wilson, B.A. (1995). Memory rehabilitation: Compensating for memory problems. In R.A. Dixon & L. Bäckman (Eds.), *Compensating for psychological deficits and declines: Managing losses and promoting gains* (pp. 171-190). Mahwah, NJ: Lawrence Erlbaum Associates.

Wilson, B.A. (1997). Cognitive rehabilitation: How it is and how it might be. *Journal of the International Neuropsychological Society, 3,* 487-496.

Wilson, B.A. (1999). *Case studies in neuropsychological rehabilitation.* New York: Oxford University Press.

Wilson, B.A. (2000). Compensating for cognitive deficits following brain injury. *Neuropsychology Review, 10,* 233-243.

Wilson, B.A. (2002). Towards a comprehensive model of cognitive rehabilitation. *Neuropsychological Rehabilitation, 12,* 97-110.

Wilson, B.A., Baddeley, A.D., Evans, J.J., & Shiel, A. (1994). Errorless learning in the rehabilitation of memory impaired people. *Neuropsychological Rehabilitation, 4,* 307-326.

Wilson, B.A., Emslie, H., Quirk, K., & Evans, J. (1999). George: Learning to live independently with NeuroPage®. *Rehabilitation Psychology, 44,* 284-296.

Wilson, B.A., Emslie, H.C., Quirk, K., & Evans, J.J. (2001). Reducing everyday memory and planning problems by means of a paging system: A randomised control crossover study. *Journal of Neurology, Neurosurgery and Psychiatry, 70,* 477-482.

Wilson, B.A., & Evans, J.J. (1996). Error free learning in the rehabilitation of individuals with memory impairments. *Journal of Head Trauma Rehabilitation, 11,* 54-64.

Wilson, B.A., & Evans, J.J. (2000). Practical management of memory problems. In G.E. Berrios & J.R. Hodges (Eds.), *Memory disorders in psychiatric practice* (pp. 291-310). Cambridge: Cambridge University Press.

Wilson, B.A., Evans, J.J., Emslie, H., & Malinek, V. (1997). Evaluation of Neuro-Page: A new memory aid. *Journal of Neurology, Neurosurgery and Psychiatry, 63,* 113-115.

Wilson, B.A., Evans, J.J., & Williams, H. (in press). Memory problems. In A.D. Tyerman (Ed.), *Rehabilitation after traumatic brain injury: A psychological approach.* Leicester: The British Psychological Society.

Wilson, B.A., & Watson, P.C. (1996). A practical framework for understanding compensatory behaviour in people with organic memory impairment. *Memory, 4,* 465-486.

Wright, P., Rogers, N., Hall, C., Wilson, B. A., Evans, J.J., Emslie, H., & Bartram, C. (2001). Comparison of pocket-computer aids for people with brain injury. *Brain Injury, 15,* 787-800.

Yule, W., & Carr, J. (Eds.). (1987). *Behaviour modification for people with mental handicaps* (2nd ed.). London: Croom Helm.

Chapter 6

REHABILITATION OF LANGUAGE DISORDERS

Anastasia M. Raymer[1,2] and
Lynn M. Maher[2,3,4]

[1]Dept. of Early Childhood, Speech-Language Pathology, &
Special Education,
Old Dominion University, Norfolk, Virginia
[2]Dept. of Veterans Affairs Brain Rehabilitation Research
Center, Gainesville, Florida
[3]Dept of Physical Medicine and Rehabilitation, Baylor College
of Medicine, Houston, Texas
[4]Dept. of Veterans Affairs Center for Healthy Aging with Disabilities, Houston, Texas

Language functions are mediated by the left cerebral hemisphere in the majority of right- and left-handed individuals (Benson & Ardila, 1996). Individuals with neurologic disorders, such as stroke, trauma, tumor, and degenerative conditions, that damage left cortical and subcortical regions may incur verbal and written language impairments. Aphasia is an impairment in the comprehension and production of verbal language caused by acquired brain damage (Damasio, 1992). The language disturbance may affect grammatical (word order and word endings), lexical (word selection), semantic (word meaning), and phonological (speech sounds) aspects of language. Acquired alexia and agraphia are impairments of reading and writing that frequently co-occur with aphasia, as orthographic functions, which draw upon some of the same symbolic language mechanisms used in verbal language, are mediated by the left hemisphere as well. The right cerebral hemisphere contributes to additional aspects of communication abilities, including processing of discourse, figurative language (e.g., idioms, humor), and prosody (Myers, 1999). Therefore right hemisphere damage can lead to subtle impairments of communication as well.

Rehabilitation specialists, including speech-language pathologists and neuropsychologists, concern themselves with the treatment of language and communication difficulties encountered by individuals with aphasia and related communication disorders. In this chapter, we will restrict our discussion to the impairments of verbal language typically observed in individuals with left hemisphere damage. In the first section, we will describe theoretical approaches to the classification and interpretation of language disorders. We will then provide an overview of the rehabilitation approaches used to address impairments of verbal language functions, restrictions to communication activities posed by the language impairments, and environmental facilitators or barriers to communication, an orientation consistent with the Classification of Functioning, Disability, and Health (World Health Organization, 2001).

Theoretical Approaches to Language Disorders

Researchers have devised a number of approaches to classification and interpretation of the language impairments that arise following brain damage. The earliest neurologic syndrome approaches utilized a brain ablation paradigm to correlate behavioral impairment with specific anatomical brain regions. This approach eventually gave way to cognitive neuropsychological theories which elaborated on the structures and processes involved in language processing. More recently, researchers have described distributed neural network models for analysis of language and aphasia. The approaches provide different contributions to our understanding of aphasia and have implications for clinical approaches to language assessment and treatment.

Syndrome Classifications for Language Disorders

Broca in the 1860s is usually credited with recognizing that loss of spoken language is associated with lesions of the left inferior frontal cortex. Wernicke and Lichtheim (cited in Caplan, 1993) later extended notions of language impairment and developed a model in which 'centers' for different auditory, motor, and conceptual components of language processing are localized and interconnected in the left hemisphere. On the basis of their model, they distinguished different syndromes of aphasia that may occur following brain damage. A number of aphasia syndrome classification schemes have been proposed since that time (Benson & Ardila, 1996). Although each system incorporates somewhat different terminology, the patterns of language breakdown are similar to those originally described by Wernicke and Lichtheim.

Table 1. Aphasia Syndromes (+ intact; – impaired).

Aphasia Syndrome	Fluency	Repetition	Auditory Comprehension	Naming
Broca's	nonfluent	–	+*	–
Transcortical Motor	nonfluent	+	+*	–/+
Global	nonfluent	–	–	–
Mixed Transcortical	nonfluent	+	–	–
Wernicke's	fluent	–	–	–
Transcortical Sensory	fluent	+	–	–/+
Conduction	fluent	–	+*	–
Anomic	fluent	+	+	–

*may have difficulty understanding grammatically complex sentences

To classify the aphasias, we must consider language functioning in four key areas: auditory comprehension, repetition, fluency of verbal expression, and confrontation naming (Table 1). Aphasia assessment batteries (e.g., Boston Diagnostic Aphasia Examination, Goodglass, Kaplan, & Barresi, 2001; Western Aphasia Battery, Kertesz, 1982) typically include subtests to evaluate language functions across these four language domains. Additional assessment tools are available to assess functioning for specific language processes such as confrontation naming (e.g., Boston Naming Test, Kaplan, Goodglass, & Weintraub, 2001) or auditory comprehension (e.g., Revised Token Test, McNeil, & Prescott, 1978).

Fluency of verbal expression warrants specific description as this dimension of language processing often poses a challenge in clinical aphasiology. Fluency in this context refers to the ease with which an individual produces fully elaborated conversational sentences, in distinct contrast to verbal fluency for single words as measured in a controlled oral word association test (Borkowski, Benton, & Spreen, 1967). At least five different aspects of verbal expression contribute to verbal fluency (Greenwald, Nadeau, & Rothi, 2000). Amount of verbal output, grammatical, articulatory, and prosodic integrity of the utterances, and ability to initiate and elaborate utterances all coalesce to provide fluent verbal expression. A serious disturbance of any one or more of these aspects of verbal expression may render the clinical impression of nonfluent verbal production. Fluent verbal expression, while adequate in overall amount as well as articulatory and prosodic flow of utterances, can be undermined in the accuracy of the lexical, phonological, and grammatical content of utterances such that verbal expression is unclear and difficult to understand. In general, nonfluent aphasias occur as a consequence of lesions affecting left pre-rolandic regions, and fluent aphasias occur following lesions involving left post-rolandic structures and sparing pre-rolandic regions.

Nonfluent Aphasias

Four general patterns of nonfluent aphasia can be observed. In individuals with *Broca's aphasia*, both verbal expression and repetition are nonfluent and *agrammatic* due to omissions of grammatical words (e.g., auxiliaries, articles) and word endings (e.g., plurals, verb tense). Their prosody may be flattened and they may have difficulty initiating and sequencing articulatory movements, sometimes referred to as *apraxia of speech* (Kearns, 1997). Individuals with Broca's aphasia may have *asyntactic* comprehension leading to difficulty understanding grammatically complex sentences (e.g., passives). Word retrieval is impaired, especially for verbs (e.g., Damasio & Tranel, 1993; Zingeser & Berndt, 1990). Broca's aphasia is associated with large left frontal-subcortical lesions (Damasio & Damasio, 1989; Kreisler et al., 2000).

In *transcortical motor aphasia* (TCMA), verbal expression is rendered nonfluent due to lack of dynamic verbal initiation, and poor ability to elaborate utterances (Rothi, 1997). Preserved repetition sometimes leads to *echolalia* in utterances. Word retrieval in picture naming may be intact, or disrupted by perseverations in naming (Benson & Ardila, 1996). Auditory comprehension may be impaired for grammatically-complex sentences. TCMA has been described acutely with left hemisphere lesions of the mesial frontal cortex (supplementary motor area), dorsolateral frontal cortex, or thalamus (Alexander, Benson, & Stuss, 1989; Kreisler et al., 2000).

In *global aphasia*, patients are severely nonfluent, with verbal output limited to *automatisms* (e.g., cursing, I don't know) and *stereotypies* (repeated use of a nonmeaningful word) which at times are spoken with meaningful intonation (Goodglass et al., 2001). Repetition, word retrieval and auditory comprehension are severely impaired. Global aphasia is typically associated with extensive left pre- and post-rolandic damage (Damasio & Damasio, 1989; Kertesz, 1979) and persists when lesions extend into Wernicke's area and anterior periventricular white matter (Naeser, Gaddie, Palumbo, & Stiassny-Eder, 1990; Naeser, Palumbo, Helm-Estabrooks, Stiassny-Eder, & Albert, 1989).

Mixed transcortical aphasia is the counterpart to global aphasia in which repetition is relatively spared, whereas all other language domains are severely impaired. This infrequent syndrome occurs with damage to left anterior and posterior cortical watershed regions that preserve left perisylvian cortex (Rothi, 1997).

Fluent Aphasias

Likewise, four fluent aphasia syndromes have been described. *Wernicke's aphasia* is characterized by fluent verbal expression in which there is a press to speak or *logorrhea*. Spontaneous verbalizations, repetition, and spoken naming are disrupted by paraphasias and neologisms. Auditory comprehension is severely undermined. Yet it is possible for some patients to have fairly preserved comprehension and seem anosognosic or unaware of their unintelligible verbal output (Maher, Rothi, & Heilman, 1994; Marshall, Robson, Pring, & Chiat, 1998). Wernicke's aphasia is associated with lesions affecting the posterior portion of the left superior temporal gyrus (Damasio & Damasio, 1989; Kreisler et al., 2000).

In *transcortical sensory aphasia* (TSA), although repetition abilities are intact, fluent verbal expression and naming are marked by numerous paraphasias (Rothi, 1997). Lesions affect the left angular gyrus (e.g., Alexander, Hiltbrunner, & Fischer, 1989), thus TSA may be associated with Gerstmann syndrome.

Conduction aphasia is a form of fluent aphasia in which there is inordinate difficulty with repetition relative to other language abilities (Kohn, 1992). Phonemic paraphasias are common in verbal tasks, and patients often exhibit *conduit d'approche*, successive attempts to self-correct their mispronunciations. Individuals with conduction aphasia may display asyntactic comprehension (Heilman & Scholes, 1976). The lesions associated with conduction aphasia tend to involve the left supramarginal gyrus, insula, and underlying white matter (Damasio & Damasio, 1989; Anderson et al., 1999).

Anomia or word retrieval difficulty is common across aphasia syndromes. Some individuals, however, tend to present with anomia as an isolated symptom, or *anomic aphasia* (Goodglass & Wingfield, 1997). Word retrieval errors in conversation or picture naming tasks may include circumlocutions, semantic paraphasias, or response omissions. Nouns may be more affected than verbs (Zingeser & Berndt, 1990). Anomic aphasia may occur acutely with lesions in the left temporo-occipital junction or thalamus (e.g., Foundas, Daniels, & Vasterling, 1998; Raymer et al., 1997).

The aphasia syndrome approach has advocates who propose that syndrome classification schemes provide a common nomenclature to discuss patients and to generally represent patterns of language breakdown (Heilman & Rothi, 1987). Kreisler et al. (2000) confirmed the importance of the classical anatomical regions in the determination of aphasic symptoms, at least in the acute stage. However, there are a number of limitations to the aphasia syndrome approach. Some estimate that as few as 40% of subjects can be consistently classified into one of the aphasia syndromes (Goodglass et al., 2001). Variations across individuals in location and extent of left hemisphere lesions leads to disparities in the presentation of language symptoms across individuals with putatively similar aphasia syndromes. The lesion approach cannot account for distant effects of the lesion *(diaschisis)* in acute aphasia or compensatory mechanisms that may be operative in chronic aphasia. Finally, aphasia syndrome presentation does not necessarily indicate decisions to be made for language rehabilitation, which are guided more by the constellation of aphasic symptoms than by the overall syndrome classification. Out of the need to decipher some of the differences in language impairments across patients with aphasia, other approaches to description of language disorders have been developed.

Cognitive Neuropsychological Approaches to Language Disorders

The cognitive neuropsychological (CN) approach represents a melding of interests in cognitive psychology and neuropsychology. The goal of cognitive psychologists is to elucidate the functional architecture (representations and processes) involved in various cognitive activities, including language. Cognitive neuropsychologists study impairments of cognitive functions following brain damage, providing a converging source of evidence for the functional architecture of cognitive systems (Coltheart, 2001; Hillis, 2001). The models of language developed in the CN approach are considerably more elaborated than the Wernicke-Lichtheim model. One depiction of the language system is represented in Figure 1 where we have integrated mechanisms involved in lexical and sentence processing into one basic model of language. Details of the model are the subject of continuous inquiry, but generally, this simplified version of the language system is schematized as a set of stored representations (knowledge) and processes (procedures) that implement those representations in the comprehension and production of words and sentences. Independent orthographic and phonologic mechanisms store representations and accomplish processes involved in language functioning across modalities of input (e.g., spoken or written words, viewed objects) and modes of response output (e.g., writing, speech).

Acquired brain damage that disrupts functioning of a language structure or process can result in predictable constellations of symptoms across all language tasks that implement the impaired mechanism. Of course, brain damage often affects multiple language mechanisms, leading to a clinical challenge to disentangle the sources of dysfunction associated with an individual's pattern of disordered language. A clinical assessment battery that is available to guide assessment of language functions from the CN perspective is the Psycholinguistic Assessment of Language Processing Abilities (PALPA)(Kay, Lesser, & Coltheart, 1992).

It would be a lengthy deliberation to describe all the patterns of language breakdown that could be envisioned with disruption of the complex model of language proposed in Figure 1. (For recent reviews see Raymer & Rothi, 2001; Mitchum & Berndt, 2001; Beeson & Hillis, 2001). For the sake of this discussion, we will give some general patterns that will be observed with breakdown at various stages in the language system. Modality specific recognition impairments are likely to follow disruption of early auditory or visual analysis as well as the input lexicons. Intact performance would be observed in tasks requiring recognition through alternative input modalities and production of language responses that are not instigated by the impaired input modality. For example, impairment of either auditory analysis or the

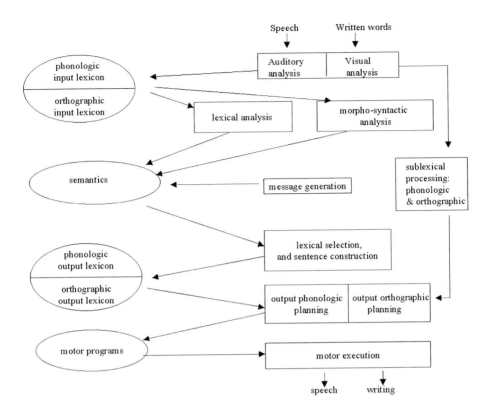

Fig. 1. Model of Language Comprehension and Production (after Caplan, 1993) with representations in ovals and processes in squares.

phonologic input lexicon would disrupt performance in all tasks requiring implementation of either of those early stages of language processing, including auditory comprehension, repetition, writing to dictation, and naming to spoken definitions. Performance for tasks using written and object input would be intact, however.

Likewise, mode-specific production impairments could be evident with dysfunction of either orthographic or phonologic output lexicons or output planning. So, for example, impairment of the orthographic output lexicon would lead to difficulty when spelling to dictation or to picture confrontation, or in spontaneous writing tasks. Performance for verbal tasks would be unaffected in oral picture naming, oral reading, and spontaneous conversation.

Semantic system dysfunction would be associated with impairment in all tasks that require processing of the meaning of words and sentences, including auditory and reading comprehension, picture naming, and spontaneous oral and written generation of words and sentences. However, the ability to repeat spoken messages, copy written material, and read aloud and spell to dictation words with regular spelling-to-sound correspondences (e.g., lake, chin) may still be accomplished with sublexical processes that allow for translation of phonologic and orthographic information.

Morpho-syntactic processes are independent for input and output processing. Therefore, a production impairment related to sentence construction processes would lead to difficulty in sentence generation spontaneously, to picture description, or in story retelling. Auditory and reading comprehension for sentences may be preserved as input morpho-syntactic analysis processes are intact.

The clinician applying the CN approach will analyze patterns of impaired and retained performance across language tasks to develop an understanding of the levels of language dysfunction that are responsible for impaired language performance (Hillis, 2001). In turn, information garnered about stages of language dysfunction may allow the clinician to target language treatment in theoretically motivated directions to either restore language functions or to circumvent impaired functions and use compensatory means to communicate. That is, a CN analysis will orient the clinician to *what* language behavior is impaired, but not *how* to address that dysfunction. This type of detailed CN assessment can be time-consuming, however, and there are limitations to this approach as well. In particular, the language components represented in the models are likely under-specified. The clinical utility of the CN analysis has been called into question by reports indicating that language deficits that arise from dysfunction of different language mechanisms may be modified by the same language intervention, and individuals with similar language deficits may not respond in similar ways to treatments (Hillis, 1993). Finally, this approach fails to take into account other cognitive capacities that may affect performance such as attention or memory (Crosson, 2000a, 2000b). Some of these concerns have led to the generation of distributed network models of language processing.

Neural Network Models

According to Mesulam (2000), the neuroanatomic substrates of cognitive domains take the form of large-scale distributed neural networks that contain interconnected cortical and subcortical nodes. Each major node of a network participates in multiple intersecting networks. In this way a single lesion may disrupt functioning in multiple networks, and a specific cognitive domain may be impacted by a variety of lesions. Support for this approach is found in connectionist or parallel distributed models (PDP) of language and related behaviors and impairments. Sophisticated computational simulations of language learning and language impairment have been adapted for orthographic, phonological, lexical, and syntactic processing (e.g., Plaut, 1996; Martin, Dell, Saffran, & Schwartz, 1994.)

Nadeau (2000; Nadeau & Rothi, 2001) reviewed some of the key features of neural network models that have implications for language functions and disorders. He noted that a distinction in neural network models, as compared to cognitive neuropsychological models, is that knowledge is represented in the strengths of the connections among the nodes of the network array. Processing in the array is massively parallel in that many nodes activate or inhibit other nodes in the array as a signal is propagated through the network. That is, processing derives from the activity of the nodes, and not from separate mechanisms as is implied in CN language models. Nadeau also indicated that disruption of neural network models by brain lesions leads to graceful degradation of functioning within the network. This property of neural models is consistent with the tendency for many errors in aphasia comprehension and production to be closely related, either semantically or phonologically, to the target language interpretation. It is not until there is major degradation in the network that severe language dysfunction will arise.

The application of neural network models to the study of aphasia and its treatment is still in its infancy, and at present these network models suffer from a lack of physiologic constraint (Price, 2000). However, the ability of distributed network models to account for connections across cognitive domains and to address the neural processes that might underlie these behaviors suggests they may have a significant impact in the future.

Treatment of Language Disorders

The clinician analyzes a patient's pattern of language dysfunction to develop an appropriate plan for management of the consequences of aphasia in keeping with the prognosis for recovery (Benson & Ardila, 1996). Although aphasia is likely to persist, some recovery is anticipated. In general, a positive prognosis may be expected when the aphasia results from a recovering neurological disease, is in the first 6-12 months of recovery, and results from a lesion that is smaller, spares subcortical white matter, and is unilateral. Psychosocial factors such as age, gender, premorbid abilities, handedness, emotional state, and family support contribute to aphasia recovery but have a less potent impact (Benson & Ardila, 1996).

For most individuals, treatment may be beneficial for helping them to improve their language and communication abilities beyond the levels that would be anticipated from spontaneous recovery alone (Robey, 1998; Wertz et al., 1986). However, the exact approach taken for an individual with aphasia will depend on a number of medical, philosophical, and psychosocial factors. Foremost is the patient's constellation of language dysfunctions. Treatment methods have been devised to address impairment of auditory comprehension and verbal expression. Within each modality, treatment methods vary depending upon level of breakdown at single-word semantic and phonological stages of processing versus sentence-level morpho-syntactic processing.

WHO Classification of Language Interventions

In addition to classifying language treatments according to modalities of language dysfunction, intervention strategies can be distinguished in a format consistent with the WHO (2001) International Classification of Functioning, Disability, and Health (ICF). In the most recent iteration of the WHO model, there are three distinct categories of influences on the ability of a person to successfully perform physical activities: body structure/function, activities and participation, and environmental factors. In the category of body structure/function are included the mental functions for language and other higher cognitive functions. When these mental functions are disrupted by acquired neurologic disease, cognitive disorders such as aphasia, dyslexia, and dygraphia may be observed. Some treatment approaches that address the disability posed by disruption of language functions are aimed at restoring or restitution of specific language functions. Other approaches circumvent impaired functions and engage alternative cognitive mechanisms to assist in reorganizing or vicariatively improving language functions (Rothi, 1995; Wilson, 1997, 1999) (Table 2).

A second category of influences on disability relates to activities and participation in life situations (WHO, 2001). Because of the loss of language and cognitive functions, the individual may experience restrictions and limitations

Table 2.   Approaches to treatment of specific language functions in aphasia.

Word retrieval treatments
      Cueing Hierarchies
      Semantic Comprehension Treatment
      Semantic Feature Analysis Training
      Phonological Comprehension Treatment
      Voluntary Control of Involuntary Utterances
      Verbal + Gestural Facilitation

Treatments for sentence production deficits
      Sentence Production Program for Aphasia
      Linguistic-Specific Training
      Melodic Intonation Therapy
      Mapping Therapy

Table 3: Approaches to enhance communication activities and participation:

Implement alternative modes of expression:
      Pantomime and Gestural codes (Amer-Ind, American Sign Language)
      Facial expression and emotional prosody
      Writing and drawing
Promoting Aphasics' Communicative Effectiveness
Group Therapy

in their ability to use language to communicate, accomplish many daily life activities, interact with other persons, or participate in educational, employment, civic and other social opportunities. Some treatment approaches for individuals with language disorders are devised to improve general use of strategies and compensatory measures to enhance communication as an activity that allows for participation in communication interchanges (Table 3).

A third category in the WHO (2001) classification includes analysis of the environmental factors that either facilitate or provide a barrier to the use of language functions. Some approaches to aphasia treatment are geared at modifying aspects of the environment to remove barriers or to facilitate the language and communication environment (Table 4). In this realm we include treatment approaches that involve support systems as well as products such as technological and pharmacologic interventions.

Treatments for Specific Language Functions

Auditory comprehension
Restitutive treatment for lexical processing is based on the premise that systematic auditory stimulation will facilitate recovery from aphasia (Duffy, 1994; Schuell, Jenkins, & Jimenez-Pabon, 1964). Auditory stimulation training incorporates repeated practice with auditory-verbal tasks such as answering questions, manipulating objects, and pointing to command. Clinicians manipulate characteristics of the words (e.g., familiarity, semantic category, emotionality), the paralinguistic aspects of the auditory-verbal signal (e.g., rate, pauses, intonation), and task conditions (e.g., number of response choices, length of auditory input, redundancy and repetitions) to systematically increase the level of difficulty of auditory processing over time. Positive results of auditory stimulation training have been reported in single case studies (see Jacobs, 2001, for a review) and as part of group studies of aphasia therapy (Wertz et al., 1981, 1986). Computerized training programs are particularly amenable to auditory stimulation practice (Aftonomos, Appelbaum, & Steele, 1999; Katz, 2000).

In contrast to general auditory comprehension training, cognitive neuropsychological training studies address specific phonologic or semantic dysfunctions underlying impaired auditory comprehension in some individuals (Grayson, Hilton, & Franklin, 1997; Morris, Franklin, Ellis, Turner, & Bailey, 1996). In this type of auditory lexical training, patients participate in tasks that target either phonologic (sound and syllable discriminations, and matching spoken words to pictures or written words with similar sounds), or semantic (yes/no question verification regarding semantic attributes of words, and matching spoken words to corresponding picture amid semantically-related foils, or matching spoken words to associated pictures or written words), aspects of lexical processing, depending on the source of auditory comprehension impairment in a given individual. Directed semantic or phonologic training may lead to improved auditory comprehension abilities in some individuals (Grayson et al., 1997; Morris et al., 1996).

Restitutive sentence comprehension treatments often incorporate a linguistic approach to sentence training (e.g., Haendiges, Berndt, & Mitchum, 1997; Jacobs & Thompson, 2000). For example, in Mapping Therapy, which incorporates the visual modality in training (e.g., Jones, 1986; Byng, 1988), patients are taught to understand syntactically complex reversible sentences by translating from grammatical word order (e.g., subject noun, verb, object noun) to the semantic roles (e.g., agent, action, object) played by words in the sentence. In sentences such as passive structures (e.g., The girl was called by the boy), there is not a direct mapping between grammatical word order and semantic roles, leading to comprehension difficulties for some individuals with aphasia. Repeated practice with syntactically complex sentences may lead to improved comprehension abilities (see Fink, 2001, for a recent review).

Other treatment methods attempt to circumvent auditory comprehension impairments by summoning alternative visual input modalities to reorganize comprehension abilities for spoken words. For example, lip-reading (Shindo, Kaga, & Tanaka, 1991), word reading (Hough, 1993), and systematic gesture processing as in Visual Action Therapy (Helm-Estabrooks & Albert, 1991) have led to improved auditory word comprehension skills in some patients with aphasia.

Word retrieval

Individuals with both fluent and nonfluent forms of aphasia present with difficulties in word retrieval tasks. Because of the common occurrence of word retrieval impairments in aphasia, many techniques have been investigated to remediate this problem (Helm-Estabrooks, 1997). One of the most common approaches is the use of cueing hierarchies in the context of picture naming tasks. When a patient fails to name a picture, the clinician systematically provides cues that have more and more potent influence to assist the individual in retrieving the intended word. Cues such as sentence completions (e.g., You stir coffee with a ...), initial phonemes (e.g., 'sp'), rhyming words (It sounds like moon.), or imitation (say 'spoon') may assist the individual to retrieve intended words. With practice over time, word retrieval skills may be facilitated or the individual may learn to self-cue (see Patterson, 2001, for a recent review).

Recent investigations have examined restitutive techniques influenced by cognitive neuropsychological models that delineate semantic and phonological stages in word retrieval (Hillis, 1998; Raymer & Rothi, 2001). Some naming treatment studies target semantic stages of lexical processing in that the patient is required to act upon the meanings of target words. For example, pairing word comprehension tasks and word production may improve word retrieval abilities (e.g., Drew & Thompson, 1999; Marshall, Pound, White-Thompson, & Pring, 1990; Nickels & Best, 1996). In semantic feature analysis (SFA) training, patients view a grid that cues them to systematically activate the semantic attributes of a target word (e.g., category, function, location), ultimately leading to production of the target word (e.g., Boyle, 2001; Boyle & Coelho, 1995; Lowell, Beeson, & Holland, 1995).

Other restitutive treatments focus on the phonological stage of word retrieval. Patients practice word production as they think about how words sound, how many syllables are in the words, initial phonemes, and rhyming words. They rehearse the words during picture naming, reading, or repetition activities (e.g., Hillis, 1993; Miceli, Amitrano, Capasso, & Caramazza, 1996; Raymer, Thompson, Jacobs, & leGrand, 1993). However, studies that have contrasted word retrieval treatments within subjects suggest that semantic treatment may have a more powerful influence than phonological treatment (Ennis et al., 2000; Howard, Patterson, Franklin, Orchard-Lisle, & Morton, 1985; Raymer & Ellsworth, 2002).

Some patients with severe aphasia and pronounced word retrieval impairments may require specialized methods to improve word production. One technique useful for some patients rendered nonverbal by aphasia is Voluntary Control of Involuntary Utterances (VCIU; Helm-Estabrooks & Albert, 1991). VCIU is based on Luria's (1970) concept of intrasystemic reorganization as clinicians train patients to gain volitional control over any retained automatically-spoken utterances, and then to modify those responses into other similar words. Systematic practice moving from automatic to volitional production of words in meaningful contexts may lead to an expanded vocabulary in some individuals.

In addition to restorative treatments, a number of reorganization treatments have been described to promote use of strategies to vicariatively mediate word retrieval, circumventing impaired lexical mechanisms. One method that has been explored as an alternative means to mediate word retrieval is the use of gestural pantomimes. Consistent with Luria's (1970) notion of intersystemic reorganization, patients are trained to combine pantomimes with spoken words to facilitate word retrieval (e.g., Pashek, 1997, 1998; Raymer & Thompson, 1991). Crosson and colleagues (Crosson, 2000a; Richards, Singletary, Rothi, Koehler, & Crosson, 2002) have reported the benefits of nonsymbolic (nonmeaningful) limb movements for word retrieval training as well. Advantages of the use of nonsymbolic limb movements in training are that they can be implemented with all types of words, regardless of the meaning, and that they are less vulnerable to disruption by limb apraxia (Maher & Ochipa, 1997). On the other hand, a benefit of pantomime training is that even when word retrieval abilities do not improve, general communication abilities often are enhanced through the use of pantomimes.

Sentence production
Some individuals with aphasia, particularly those with nonfluent forms of aphasia, need training that focuses on improving the use of fluent, grammatical sentences. As in sentence comprehension treatments, the premise

of some restitutive sentence production treatments is to practice producing
sentences that vary systematically from less complex to more complex grammatical structures. As patients experience production difficulty, clinicians
model and expand target sentences, and patients then rehearse sentences to
facilitate correct production. The methods vary in the context used for sentence practice, including story completion activities (e.g., Helm-Estabrooks
& Nicholas, 1999), picture description (Haendigas et al., 1997; Kearns,
1985), or sentence reading (e.g., Thompson, 2001). With repeated practice
over time, some patients improve use of complete, grammatical sentences.
Contrary to methods often used in training hierarchies, Thompson, Ballard,
and Shapiro (1998) have reported that practice with grammatically more
complex sentence types (e.g., object relative clauses) can generalize to less
complex sentence structures (e.g., who-questions) in some individuals with
aphasia.

A reorganization approach to sentence production treatment is Melodic
Intonation Therapy, a treatment designed to invoke the right hemisphere's
intonational capacity to support sentence production (Sparks, 2001). In this
systematic program, patients produce sentences while tapping rhythmically
and using highly intoned, sing-song patterns. Over time the melody is reduced
to a more natural prosodic pattern and the tapping discontinues. The method
has been deemed effective for improving sentence production, particularly
in patients with Broca's aphasia (Therapeutics and Technology Assessment
Subcommittee of the American Academy of Neurology [AAN], 1994; see
also Martin, Kubitz, & Maher, 2001). Evidence for the neural reorganization
invoked by MIT was provided by Belin and colleagues (1996) who reported
that patients showed increased left frontal activation and right posterior deac-
tivation following participation in MIT, contrary to what might be predicted
following melodic training, and suggesting that rhythmic tapping may be a
critical element of the MIT procedure.

The possibility that tapping may be more important than intonation in
the MIT protocol was explored by Boucher, Garcia, Fleurant, and Paradis
(2001). They found that rhythmic tapping was more effective than intonation
for improving sentence production in two individuals with nonfluent aphasia. Raymer, Rowland, Haley, and Crosson (2002) implemented a training
procedure in which their patient made alternating tapping movements of the
left hand in left space to improve sentence production in an individual with
transcortical motor aphasia.

Finally, some interest has been placed on a treatment approach for
verbal expression patterned after research in physical therapy advocating
constrained use of compensatory measures and forced use of impaired motor
systems (Taub, Uswatte, & Pidikiti, 1999). Pulvermuller and colleagues
(2001) applied the principle of constrained language use during intervention
in which patients were required to respond only with verbal responses, word
or sentence, during intensive (3 hours/day for 2 weeks) language enrichment
activities that took place in small groups. No nonverbal communication

strategies were accepted. Clinicians used shaping and modeling to expand the verbal repertoire of patients across sessions. This intensive forced use of language led to significant improvements in language functions (auditory comprehension and naming) as compared to a comparable amount of traditional impairment-oriented treatment provided on a less intensive schedule.

Treatments for Communication Activities and Participation

Some approaches to aphasia treatment, sometimes termed 'functional' treatments, target the overall limitations that aphasia poses for a patient's general communication activities (Aten, 1994). These types of treatments encourage individuals to incorporate any strategies, verbal and nonverbal, to improve communication with conversational partners. Surprisingly, many patients with aphasia do not naturally attempt to use alternative means to communicate and need direct instruction and practice to improve their abilities in this area. Patients are often instructed to use writing or drawing to convey ideas (Rao, 1995). They are encouraged to use intonation or facial expressions to express emotions. Some severely impaired patients need to establish a system of body signals to indicate yes and no (head nods, thumbs up). Clinicians frequently encourage patients to use symbolic gestures or pantomimes, such as Amer-Ind (Skelly, 1979) to enhance communication.

Promoting Aphasics' Communicative Effectiveness (PACE) is a training technique that uses the functional approach as the clinician and patient participate in a communication barrier activity (Davis & Wilcox, 1981). The patient has to provide any verbal or nonverbal cues possible to convey to the clinician an item depicted on a picture card. The client/clinician interchange in PACE emphasizes use of all communication channels in a natural communicative context.

An efficient setting in which to apply functional language strategies is in the context of group aphasia therapy (Elman, 1999; Marshall, 1999). In group aphasia treatment, a small number of individuals with aphasia interact in language activities designed to promote conversation and use of communication strategies. Activities center around daily living activities, current events, hobbies, and other interests. Participation in group aphasia treatment emphasizing use of functional communication strategies has been reported to lead to significant improvements on some language and communication measures (Elman & Bernstein-Ellis, 1999).

Facilitating the Communication Environment

A number of intervention strategies exist that influence the communication 'environment' for individuals with acquired language disorders. Environmental treatments are designed to facilitate language and communication abilities using external sources which can include pharmacologic interventions and technological devices as well as support provided by communication partners. In addition, some environmental modifications can be construed as means to remove barriers to successful communication.

Pharmacologic intervention in aphasia

Language impairments result from disruption of neurobiological substrates of language functions. Thus clinicians have explored pharmacologic methods to maximize plasticity and recovery in the impaired neurologic system leading to improvements in language functions. The premise of this type of intervention is that drugs are necessary to replace neurotransmitters that are undermined following brain lesion (Shisler, Baylis, & Frank, 2000). Although there is some degree of skepticism in the treatment literature (Small, 1994, 2000), some studies have reported that pharmacologic interventions may enhance recovery from aphasia.

Because frontal lobe regions depend on dopaminergic input for proficient functioning, the dopaminergic agonist bromocriptine has been administered to a number of patients with nonfluent aphasia following left frontal lesions. Studies have documented improvements in verbal fluency measures, particularly in the reduction of pausing and improved word retrieval, in selected patients (e.g., Albert, Bachman, Morgan, & Helm-Estabrooks, 1988; Gold, Van Dam, & Silliman, 2000; Gupta, Mlcoch, Scolaro, & Moritz, 1995; Raymer et al., 2001). Other studies with bromocriptine, including one double-blind, placebo-controlled investigation, reported no significant benefits on language measures (MacLennan, Nicholas, Morley, & Brookshire, 1991; Sabe et al., 1995).

Cholinergic input seems to play a critical role in left hemisphere temporal and thalamic functioning, leading some investigators to explore treatments with cholinergic drugs for aphasia. Administration of cholinergic agents physostigmine (Jacobs et al., 1996) and bifemelane (Tanaka, Miyazaki, & Albert, 1997) has been associated with improved word retrieval skills in patients with fluent aphasia. Likewise, treatment with donepezil resulted in to improved verbal fluency in one patient with nonfluent aphasia (Hughes, Jacobs, & Heilman, 2000).

Finally, some studies have explored the role that norepinephrine may play in increasing cortical excitability during recovery from neurologic damage. Treatment with the noradrenergic agonist dextroamphetamine has been associated with improved aphasia recovery in one double-blind placebo controlled investigation (Walker-Batson et al., 1991, 2001). The effect may relate at least in part to behavioral treatment paired with the drug administration, however (McNeil et al., 1997).

Clinicians are particularly interested in the potential that pharmacologic intervention may play in promoting recovery from aphasia and other cognitive, sensory, and motor impairments. Unfortunately, some studies have conflated pharmacologic and behavioral interventions and it is not clear as to the relative contributions of these two distinct aspects of treatment.

Technological aids to communication

Some individuals with profound impairments of verbal expression in aphasia may need to implement some type of external aid to express personal needs and ideas. Simple paper and pencil can allow some patients to draw or write messages. More often, clinicians develop inexpensive low-tech picture pointing boards or notebooks to help patients communicate by pointing to pictures or words. Software programs are available to design personalized devices with icons that are pertinent to an individual's needs and interests.

Other individuals are interested in exploring high-tech options to improve communication abilities. Specialized augmentative and alternative communication (AAC) devices or computers outfitted with appropriate hardware and software allow some patients to express themselves using spelling, mouse clicks, or touch screens. Unfortunately, some patients with aphasia may have difficulty manipulating some AAC systems as fairly sophisticated language capability is necessary to successfully operate some of these devices (Hux, Beukelman, & Garrett, 1994). Nevertheless, some researchers have been successful in training patients with severe aphasia to use computer-assisted communication programs (e.g., Weinrich, Boser, & McCall, 1999; Weinrich, Shelton, Cox, & McCall, 1997).

Communication support systems

Finally, an area that addresses means to both facilitate and reduce barriers to effective communication is intervention aimed at the conversational partners of individuals with aphasia. Lyon (1997) has advocated moving communication partners into the treatment room to improve communication in the aphasia dyad through counseling and training on the use of productive strategies to enhance communication and reduce frustration. Interactions can be videotaped and analyzed for sources of breakdown and other potentially more effective communication options can be explored (Boles, 1998). A number of strategies that can be implemented by communication partners are provided in Table 4. Some options are designed to enhance the auditory comprehension of individuals with aphasia, whereas others as meant to promote resolution of breakdown emanating from the speaker with aphasia. Kagan, Black, Duchan, Simmons-Mackie, and Square (2001) have documented that conversational partners can be trained to use a variety of conversational support and repair strategies that may not naturally be used by untrained individuals during communication exchanges with individuals with aphasia.

Table 4.   Partner strategies to facilitate or reduce barriers in the aphasic communication dyad.

To facilitate auditory comprehension
        Gain eye contact and speak directly to the individual.
        Use short, grammatically simple sentences.
        Speak at a slower rate while maintaining a natural prosody.
        Do not speak louder.
        Repeat sentences and then revise the utterance is necessary .
        Talk about familiar topics.
        Signal when the topic changes.
        Embellish messages with alternative communication channels.
        (writing, drawing, gestures, facial expression)

To facilitate verbal expression of the speaker with aphasia
        Gently provide missing words or multiple choice options.
        Encourage circumlocution and use of nonverbal channel to communicate
        messages.
        Reiterate messages so speaker can confirm messages were understood as
        intended.
        Encourage speaker to disregard simple errors when intent of messages is
        not disrupted.
        Write down ideas when breakdown occurs and return to them later.

Efficacy of Aphasia Treatment

The optimal methods for exploring treatment efficacy are in randomized controlled trials or in meta-analyses (Therapeutics and Technology Assessment
Subcommittee of AAN, 1994). Other types of treatment research designs,
which often fail to implement subject randomization, are less favored.
Developing appropriate research studies to establish the efficacy of aphasia
treatment is a challenging endeavor (Holland & Wertz, 1988). Group studies
are undermined by the heterogeneity of the language impairments observed
across individuals with aphasia. An effective treatment for one form of aphasia or one individual with aphasia may not be effective for another, thereby
reducing the aggregate effect of an aphasia treatment. A number of subject
selection characteristics must be controlled. Nevertheless, a number of investigators have examined the efficacy of aphasia treatment using a variety of
experimental designs with positive outcomes.

    Holland, Fromm, DeRuyter, and Stein (1996) reviewed more than 200
aphasia treatment studies in the English literature. These included 20 group
studies with more than 60 subjects with aphasia. They concluded that the
effects of aphasia treatment for individuals with a single hemisphere stroke
significantly surpass the effects of spontaneous recovery alone, particularly
if individuals receive 3 hours of treatment per week for at least 5 months.
Moreover, three different meta-analyses examining 45 (Whurr, Lorch, &
Nye, 1992), 21 (Robey, 1994), and 55 (Robey, 1998) different aphasia

treatment studies have corroborated the view that treatment leads to greater language improvements than does spontaneous recovery alone.

The majority of aphasia treatment studies have implemented single subject experimental treatment designs (SSDs), time series designs that are well-suited to address the heterogeneous factors involved in aphasia treatment (McReynolds & Thompson, 1986). Meta-analyses of treatment effect sizes reported in SSDs have indicated that, despite the fact that most experimental subjects were in chronic stages of aphasia, large effect sizes have been reported with a variety of aphasia treatments (Robey, Schultz, Crawford, & Sinner, 1999; Robey, McCallum, & Francois, 1999).

Summary

The language system is a complex and interactive mechanism involving representations and processes for phonologic, semantic, and morpho-syntactic aspects of language. When impaired through acquired brain damage, particularly affecting the left cerebral hemisphere, an array of language impairments may arise. Clinicians implement a variety of treatment options when providing intervention to patients with language impairments.

Some language function-oriented treatment methods are restorative in nature, attempting to re-activate language representations and processes as in normal language functioning. Others are intended to reorganize language functions by engaging alternative cognitive systems to mediate language functions. Other types of interventions address the reduction in communication activities and life participation posed by language impairment, circumventing language impairments and capitalizing upon retained communication functions. Finally, some interventions are aimed at modifying external factors in the environment to either facilitate or reduce barriers to language and communication. These have included newer types of pharmacologic interventions to increase brain plasticity and recovery of language functioning. Attempts to demonstrate the efficacy of language interventions have shown large treatment effect sizes beyond what would be expected from spontaneous recovery alone.

Clinicians are continuing research efforts to devise novel methods of behavioral and/or pharmacologic intervention. Newer methods to assess the effectiveness and outcomes of treatment will allow for a distinction between statistical and clinical significance of our treatment research findings. Technological advances are allowing for an examination of the neurobiologic bases of treatment effects. The future of treatment research is likely to be very prosperous, and our patients with language impairments are likely to benefit in substantial ways in the years ahead.

Acknowledgments

Preparation of this chapter was supported in part by grants from NIH-NIDCD to the University of Florida (P50 DC03888-01A1) (subcontracts to Old Dominion University and Baylor College of Medicine) and the Department of Veterans Affairs Rehabilitation Research & Development Service to the Brain Rehabilitation Research Center, Gainesville, Florida, and the Center for Healthy Aging with Disabilities, Houston, Texas.

References

Aftonomos, L.B., Appelbaum, J.S., & Steele, R.D. (1999). Improving outcomes for persons with aphasia in advanced community-based treatment programs. *Stroke, 30,* 1370-1379.

Albert, M.L., Bachman, D.L., Morgan, A., & Helm-Estabrooks, N. (1988). Pharmacotherapy for aphasia. *Neurology, 38,* 877-879.

Alexander, M.P., Benson, D.F., & Stuss, D.T. (1989). Frontal lobes and language. *Brain and Language, 37,* 656-691.

Alexander, M.P., Hiltbrunner, B., & Fischer, R.S. (1989). Distributed anatomy of transcortical sensory aphasia. *Archives of Neurology, 46,* 885-892.

Anderson, J.M., Gilmore, R., Roper, S., Crosson, B., Bauer, R.M., Nadeau, S., et al., (1999). Conduction aphasia and the arcuate fasciculus: A reexamination of the Wernicke-Geschwind model. *Brain and Language, 70,* 1-12.

Aten, J.L. (1994). Functional communication treatment. In R. Chapey (Ed.), *Language intervention strategies in adult aphasia, 3rd ed.* (pp. 292-303). Baltimore: Williams & Wilkins.

Beeson, P.M., & Hillis, A.E. (2001). Comprehension and production of written words. In R. Chapey (Ed.), *Language intervention strategies in aphasia and related neurogenic communication disorders, 4th ed.* (pp. 572-604). Philadelphia: Lippincott Williams & Wilkins.

Belin, P., Van Eeckhout, P.H., Zilbovicius, M, Remy, P., Francois, C., Guillaume, S., et al., (1996). Recovery from nonfluent aphasia after melodic intonation therapy: A PET study. *Neurology, 47,* 1504-1511.

Benson, D.F., & Ardila, A. (1996). *Aphasia: A clinical perspective.* New York: Oxford University Press.

Boles, L. (1998). Conversational discourse analysis as a method for evaluating progress in aphasia: a case report. *Journal of Communication Disorders, 31,* 261-273.

Borkowski, J.G., Benton, A.L., & Spreen, O. (1967). Word fluency and brain damage. *Neuropsychologia, 5,* 135-140.

Boucher, V., Garcia, L.J., Fleurant, J., & Paradis, J. (2001). Variable efficacy of rhythm and tone in melody-based interventions: implications for the assumption of a right-hemisphere facilitation in non-fluent aphasia. *Aphasiology, 15,* 131-149.

Boyle, M. (2001). Semantic feature analysis: The evidence for treating lexical impairments in aphasia. *ASHA Division 2: Neurophysiology & Neurogenic Communication Disorders, 11 (2),* 23-28.

Boyle, M., & Coelho, C.A. (1995). Application of semantic feature analysis as a treatment for aphasic dysnomia. *American Journal of Speech-Language Pathology, 4,* 94-98.

Byng, S. (1988). Sentence processing deficits: Theory and therapy. *Cognitive Neuropsychology, 5,* 629-676.

Caplan D. (1993). *Language: Structure, processing, and disorders*. Cambridge, MA: MIT Press.

Coltheart, M. (2001). Assumptions and methods in cognitive neuropsychology. In B. Rapp (Ed.), *The handbook of cognitive neuropsychology* (pp. 3-21).

Crosson B. (2000a). Systems that support language processes: attention. In S.E. Nadeau, L.J.G. Rothi, & B. Crosson (Eds.), *Aphasia and language: Theory to practice* (pp. 372-397). New York: Guilford Press.

Crosson, B. (2000b). Systems that support language processes: verbal working memory. In S.E. Nadeau, L.J.G. Rothi, & B. Crosson (Eds.), *Aphasia and language: Theory to practice* (pp. 399-418). New York: Guilford Press.

Damasio, A.R. (1992). Aphasia. *New England Journal of Medicine, 326,* 531-539.

Damasio, H., & Damasio, A.R. (1989). *Lesion analysis in neuropsychology.* New York: Oxford University Press.

Damasio, A.R., & Tranel, D. (1993). Nouns and verbs are retrieved with differently distributed neural systems. *Proceedings of the National Academy of Sciences, USA, 90,* 4957-4960.

Davis, G., & Wilcox, M. (1981). Incorporating parameters of natural conversation in aphasia treatment. In R. Chapey (Ed.), *Language intervention strategies in adult aphasia* (pp. 169-194). Baltimore: Williams & Wilkins.

Drew, R.L., & Thompson, C.K. (1999). Model-based semantic treatment for naming deficits in aphasia. *Journal of Speech, Language, and Hearing Research, 42,* 972-989.

Duffy, J.R. (1994). Schuell's stimulation approach to rehabilitation. In R. Chapey (Ed.), *Language intervention strategies in adult aphasia, 3rd ed.,* (pp. 146-174). Baltimore: Williams & Wilkins.

Elman, R.J. (1999). *Group treatment of neurogenic communication disorders.* Woburn, MA: Butterworth-Heinemann.

Elman, R.J., & Bernstein-Ellis, E. (1999). The efficacy of group communication treatment in adults with chronic aphasia. *Journal of Speech, Language and Hearing Research, 42,* 411-419.

Ennis, M.R., Raymer, A.M., Burks, D.W., Heilman, K.M., Nadeau, S., & Rothi, L.J.G. (2000). Contrasting treatments for phonological anomia: unexpected findings [Abstract]. *Journal of the International Neuropsychological Society, 6,* 240.

Fink, R.B. (2001). Mapping treatment: an approach to treating sentence level impairments in agrammatism. *ASHA Division 2: Neurophysiology & Neurogenic Communication Disorders, 11 (3),* 14-23.

Fink, R.B., Schwartz, M.F., & Myers, J.L. (1998). Investigations of the sentence-query approach to mapping therapy. *Brain and Language, 65,* 203-207.

Foundas, A.L., Daniels, S.K., & Vasterling, J.J. (1998). Anomia: Case studies with lesion localization. *Neurocase, 4,* 35-43.

Gold, M., VanDam, D., & Silliman, E.R. (2000). An open-label trial of bromocriptine in nonfluent aphasia: a qualitative analysis of word storage and retrieval. *Brain and Language, 74,* 141-156.

Goodglass, H., Kaplan, E., & Barresi, B. (2001). *The assessment of aphasia and related disorders* (3rd ed.). Baltimore: Lippincott Williams & Wilkins.

Goodglass, H., & Wingfield, A. (Eds.).(1997). *Anomia: Neuroanatomical and cognitive correlates.* San Diego, CA: Academic Press.

Grayson, E., Hilton, R., & Franklin, S. (1997). Early intervention in a case of jargon aphasia: efficacy of language comprehension therapy. *European Journal of Disorders of Communication, 32,* 257-276.

Greenwald, M.L., Nadeau, S.E., & Rothi, L.J.G. (2000). Fluency. In S.E. Nadeau, L.J.G. Rothi, & B. Crosson (Eds.), *Aphasia and language: Theory to practice* (pp. 31-39). New York: Guilford Press.

Gupta, S.R., Mlcoch, A.G., Scolaro, C., & Moritz, T. (1995). Bromocriptine treatment of nonfluent aphasia. *Neurology, 45,* 2170-2173.

Haendiges, A.N., Berndt, R.S., & Mitchum, C.C. (1997). Assessing the elements contributing to a 'mapping' deficit: A targeted treatment study. *Brain and Language, 52,* 276-302.

Heilman, K.M., & Rothi, L.J.G. (1987). Aphasia: Syndrome subtypes. *Current Neurology, 71,* 277-294.

Heilman, K.M., & Scholes, R.J. (1976). The nature of comprehension errors in Broca's, conduction and Wernicke's aphasics. *Cortex, 12,* 258-265.

Helm-Estabrooks, N. (1997). Treatment of aphasic naming problems. In H. Goodglass & A. Wingfield (Eds.), *Anomia: Neuroanatomical and cognitive correlates* (pp. 189-202). San Diego, CA: Academic Press.

Helm-Estabrooks, N., & Albert, M.L. (1991). *Manual of aphasia therapy.* Austin, TX: Pro-Ed.

Helm-Estabrooks, N., & Nicholas, M. (1999). *Sentence production program for aphasia.* Austin, TX: Pro-Ed.

Hillis, A.E. (1993). The role of models of language processing in rehabilitation of language impairments. *Aphasiology, 7,* 5-26.

Hillis, A.E. (1998). Treatment of naming disorders: New issues regarding old therapies. *Journal of the International Neuropsychological Society, 4,* 648-660.

Hillis, A.E. (2001). Cognitive neuropsychological approaches to rehabilitation of language disorders: Introduction. In R. Chapey (Ed.), *Language intervention strategies in aphasia and related neurogenic communication disorders, 4th ed.* (pp. 513-523). Philadelphia: Lippincott Williams & Wilkins.

Holland, A.L., Fromm, D.S., DeRuyter, F., & Stein, M. (1996). Treatment efficacy: Aphasia. *Journal of Speech and Hearing Research, 39,* S27-S36.

Holland, A.L., & Wertz, R.T. (1988). Measuring aphasia treatment effects: Large-group, small-group, and single-subject studies. In F. Plum (Ed.), *Language, communication and the brain* (pp. 267-273). New York: Raven Press.

Hough, M. (1993). Treatment of Wernicke's aphasia with jargon: A case study. *Journal of Communication Disorders, 26,* 101-111.

Howard, D., Patterson, K., Franklin, S., Orchard-Lisle, V., & Morton J. (1985). Treatment of word retrieval deficits in aphasia. *Brain, 108,* 817-829.

Hughes, J.D., Jacobs, D.H., & Heilman, K.M. (2000). Neuropharmacology and linguistic neuroplasticity. *Brain and Language, 71,* 96-101.

Hux, K., Beukelman, D.R., & Garrett, K.L. (1994). Augmentative and alternative communication for persons with aphasia. In R. Chapey (Ed.), *Language intervention strategies in adult aphasia, 3rd ed.* (pp. 338-357). Baltimore: Williams & Wilkins.

Jacobs, B.J. (2001). Treatment of lexical comprehension impairments in aphasia. *ASHA Division 2: Neurophysiology & Neurogenic Communication Disorders, 11 (2),* 4-11.

Jacobs, B.J., & Thompson, C.K. (2000). Cross-modal generalization effects of training noncanonical sentence comprehension and production in agrammatic aphasia. *Journal of Speech, Language, and Hearing Research, 43,* 5-20.

Jacobs, D.H., Shuren, J., Gold, M., Adair, J.C., Bowers, D., Williamson, D.J.G., & Heilman, K.M. (1996). Physostigmine pharmacotherapy for anomia. *Neurocase, 2,* 83-91.

Jones, E.V. (1986). Building the foundations for sentence production in a non-fluent aphasic. *British Journal of Disorders of Communication, 21,* 63-82.

Kagan, A., Black, S.E., Duchan, J.F., Simmons-Mackie, N., & Square, P. (2001). Training volunteers as conversation partners using 'supported conversation for adults with aphasia' (SCA): A controlled trial. *Journal of Speech, Language, and Hearing Research, 44,* 624-638.

Kaplan, E., Goodglass, H., & Weintraub, S. (2001). *Boston naming test* (2nd ed.). Philadelphia: Lippincott Williams & Wilkins.

Katz, R.C. (1994). Computer applications in aphasia treatment. In R. Chapey (Ed.), *Language intervention strategies in adult aphasia, 3rd ed.* (pp. 322-337). Baltimore: Williams & Wilkins.

Kay, J., Lesser, R., & Coltheart, M. (1992). *PALPA: Psycholinguistic assessments of language processing in aphasia.* Hove, UK: Erlbaum.

Kearns, K.P. (1997). Broca's aphasia. In L.L. LaPointe (Ed.), *Aphasia and related neurogenic language disorders* (pp. 1-40). New York: Thieme.

Kearns, K.P. (1985). Response elaboration training for patient initiated utterances. In R.H. Brookshire (Ed.), *Clinical aphasiology* (pp. 196-204). Minneapolis: BRK Publishers.

Kertesz, A. (1979). *Aphasia and associated disorders.* Orlando: Grune & Stratton.

Kertesz, A. (1982). *Western aphasia battery.* Orlando: Grune & Stratton.

Kohn, S. (Ed.). (1992), *Conduction aphasia.* Hillsdale, NJ: Erlbaum.

Kreisler, A., Godefroy, O., Delmaire, C., Debachy, B., Leclercq, M., Pruvo, J.P., & Leys, D. (2000). The anatomy of aphasia revisited. *Neurology, 54,*1117-1122.

Lowell, S., Beeson, P.M., & Holland, A.L. (1995). The efficacy of a semantic cueing procedure on naming performance of adults with aphasia. *American Journal of Speech-Language Pathology, 4,* 109-114.

Luria, A.R. (1970). *Traumatic aphasia.* The Hague: Mouton.

Lyon, J. (1997). Volunteers and partners: Moving intervention outside the treatment room. In B. Shadden & M.A. Toner (Eds.), *Aging and communication* (pp. 299-323). Austin, TX: Pro-Ed.

MacLennan, D.L., Nicholas, L.E., Morley, G.K., & Brookshire, R.H. (1991). The effects of bromocriptine on speech and language function in a man with transcortical motor aphasia. In T.E. Prescott (Ed.), *Clinical aphasiology, Vol. 20* (pp. 145-155). Austin, TX: Pro-Ed.

Maher, L.M., & Ochipa, C. (1997). Management and treatment of limb apraxia. In L.J.G. Rothi & K.M. Heilman (Eds.), *Apraxia: The neuropsychology of action* (pp. 75-91). Hove, UK: Psychology Press.

Maher, L.M., Rothi, L.J., & Heilman, K.M. (1994). Lack of error awareness in an aphasic patient with relatively preserved auditory comprehension. *Brain and Language, 46,* 402-418.

Maher, L.M., Singletary, F., Swearengin, J.A., Moore, A.B., Wierenga, C.E., Crosson, B., Clayton, M.C., Butler, L.V., Kendall, D., & Rothi, L.J.G. (2002). An errorless learning approach to sentence generation in aphasia [Abstract]. *Journal of the International Neuropsychological Society, 8,* 177.

Marshall, J., Pound, C., White-Thomson, M., & Pring, T. (1990). The use of picture/word matching tasks to assist word retrieval in aphasic patients. *Aphasiology, 4,* 167-184.

Marshall, J., Robson, J., Pring, T., & Chiat, S. (1998). Why does monitoring fail in jargon aphasia? Comprehension, judgment and therapy evidence. *Brain and Language, 63,* 79-107.

Marshall, R.C. (1999). *Introduction to group treatment for aphasia: Design and management.* Woburn, MA: Butterworth-Heinemann.

Martin, N., Dell, G.S., Saffran, E.M., & Schwartz, M.F. (1994). Origins of paraphasias in deep dysphasia: testing the consequences of a decay impairment to an interactive spreading activation model of lexical retrieval. *Brain and Language, 47,* 609-660.

Martin, V.C., Kubitz, K.R., & Maher, L.M. (2001). Melodic intonation therapy. *ASHA Division 2: Neurophysiology & Neurogenic Communication Disorders, 11 (3),* 33-37.

McNeil, M.R., Doyle, P.J., Spencer, K.A., Goda, A., Flores, D., & Small, S.L. (1997). A double-blind, placebo-controlled study of pharmacological and behavioural treatment of lexical-semantic deficits in aphasia. *Aphasiology, 11,* 385-400.

McNeil, M., & Prescott, T. (1978). *Revised token test*. Austin, TX: Pro-Ed.

Mesulam, M.-M. (2000). *Principles of behavioral and cognitive neurology*. New York: Oxford University Press.

McReynolds, L.V., & Thompson, C.K. (1986). Flexibility of single-subject experimental designs: Part I: Review of the basics of single-subject designs. *Journal of Speech and Hearing Disorders, 51,* 194-203.

Mitchum, C.C., & Berndt, R.S. (2001). Cognitive neuropsychological approaches to diagnosing and treating language disorders: Production and comprehension of sentences. In R. Chapey (Ed.), *Language intervention strategies in aphasia and related neurogenic communication disorders, 4th ed.* (pp. 551-571). Philadelphia: Lippincott Williams & Wilkins.

Morris, J., Franklin, S., Ellis, A.W., Turner, J.E., & Bailey, P.J. (1996). Remediating a speech perception deficit in an aphasic patient. *Aphasiology, 10,* 137-158.

Myers, P.S. (1999). *Right hemisphere damage*. San Diego: Singular Publishing.

Nadeau, S.E. (2000). Connectionist models and language. In S.E. Nadeau, L.J.G. Rothi, & B. Crosson (Eds.), *Aphasia and language: Theory to practice* (pp. 299-347). New York: Guilford Press.

Nadeau, S.E. & Rothi, L.J.G. (2001). Rehabilitation of subcortical aphasia. In R. Chapey (Ed.), *Language intervention strategies in aphasia and related neurogenic communication disorders, 4th ed.* (pp. 457-471).

Nadeau, S.E., Rothi, L.J.G., & Crosson, B. (Eds.). (2000). *Aphasia and language: Theory to practice*. New York: Guilford Press.

Naeser, M.A., Gaddie, A., Palumbo, C.L., & Stiassny-Eder, D. (1990). Late recovery of auditory comprehension in global aphasia. Improved recovery observed with subcortical temporal isthmus lesion vs Wernicke's cortical area lesion. *Archives of Neurology, 47,* 425-432.

Naeser, M.A., Palumbo, C.L., Helm-Estabrooks, N., Stiassny-Eder, D., & Albert, M.L. (1989). Severe nonfluency in aphasia. Role of the medial subcallosal fasciculus and other white matter pathways in recovery of spontaneous speech. *Brain, 112,* 1-38.

Nickels, L., & Best, W. (1996). Therapy for naming disorders (Part II): Specifics, surprises, and suggestions. *Aphasiology, 10,* 109-136.

Pashek, G.V. (1997). A case study of gesturally cued naming in aphasia: Dominant versus nondominant hand training. *Journal of Communication Disorders, 30,* 349-366.

Pashek, G.V. (1998). Gestural facilitation of noun and verb retrieval in aphasia: A case study. *Brain and Language, 65,* 177-180.

Patterson, J.P. (2001). The effectiveness of cueing hierarchies as a treatment for word retrieval impairment. *ASHA Division 2: Neurophysiology & Neurogenic Communication Disorders, 11* (2), 11-18.

Plaut, D.C. (1996). Relearning after damage in connectionist networks: toward a theory of rehabilitation. *Brain and Language, 52,* 25-82.

Price, C. (2000). Functional imaging studies of aphasia. In J.C. Mazziotta, A.W. Toga & R.S.J. Frackowiak (Eds.) *Brain mapping: The disorders* (pp. 181-200). San Diego: Academic Press.

Pulvermuller, F., Neininger, B., Elbert, T., Mohr, B., Rockstroh, B., Koebbel, P., & Taub, E. (2001). Constraint-induced therapy of chronic aphasia after stroke. *Stroke, 32,* 1621-1626.

Rao, P.R. (1995). Drawing and gesture as communication options in a person with severe aphasia. *Topics in Stroke Rehabilitation, 2,* 49-56.

Raymer, A.M., Bandy, D., Schwartz, R.L., Adair, J.C., Williamson, D.J.G., Rothi, L.J.G., & Heilman, K.M. (2001). Effects of bromocriptine in a patient with crossed aphasia. *Archives of Physical Medicine and Rehabilitation,82,* 139-144.

Raymer, A.M., & Ellsworth, T.A. (2002). Contrasting treatments for verb retrieval impairment in aphasia: a case study. *Aphasiology, 16,* 1031-1045.

Raymer, A.M., Foundas, A.L., Maher, L.M., Greenwald, M.L., Rothi, L.J.G. & Heilman, K.M. (1997). Cognitive neuropsychological analysis and neuroanatomic correlates in a case of acute anomia. *Brain and Language, 58,* 137-156.

Raymer, A.M., & Rothi, L.J.G. (2001). Cognitive approaches to impairments of word comprehension and production. In R. Chapey (Ed.), *Language intervention strategies in aphasia and related neurogenic communication disorders, 4th ed.* (pp. 524-550). Philadelphia: Lippincott Williams & Wilkins.

Raymer, A.M., Rowland, L., Haley, M., & Crosson, B. (2002). Nonsymbolic movement training to improve sentence generation in transcortical motor aphasia: A case study. *Aphasiology, 16,* 493-506.

Raymer, A.M., & Thompson, C.K. (1991). Effects of verbal plus gestural treatment in a patient with aphasia and severe apraxia of speech. In T.E. Prescott (Ed.), *Clinical aphasiology, Volume 12* (pp. 285-297). Austin, TX: Pro-Ed.

Raymer, A,M,, Thompson, C.K., Jacobs, B., & leGrand, H.R. (1993). Phonologic treatment of naming deficits in aphasia: Model-based generalization analysis. *Aphasiology, 7,* 27-53.

Richards, K., Singletary, F., Rothi, L.J.G., Koehler, S., & Crosson, B. (2002). Activation of intentional mechanisms through utilization of nonsymbolic movements in aphasia rehabilitation. *Journal of Rehabilitation Research and Development, 39,* 445-454.

Robey, R.R. (1994). The efficacy of treatment for aphasic persons: A meta-analysis. *Brain and Language, 47,* 582-608.

Robey, R.R. (1998). A meta-analysis of clinical outcomes in the treatment of aphasia. *Journal of Speech, Language, and Hearing Research, 41,* 172-187.

Robey, R.R., McCallum, A.F., & Francois, L.K. (1999, June). A meta-analysis of single-subject research on treatments for aphasia. Presentation at the Clinical Aphasiology Conference, Key West, FL.

Robey, R.R., Schultz, M.C., Crawford, A.B., & Sinner, C.A. (1999). Single-subject clinical-outcome research: Designs, data, effect sizes, and analyses. *Aphasiology, 13,* 445-473.

Rosen, H.J., Peterson, S.E., Linenweber, M.R., Snyder, A.Z., White, D.A., Chapman, L., et al. (2000). Neural correlates of recovery from aphasia after brain damage to left inferior frontal cortex. *Neurology, 55,* 1883-1894.

Rothi, L.J.G. (1995). Behavioral compensation in the case of treatment of acquired language disorders resulting from brain damage. In R.A. Dixon & L. Mackman (Eds.), *Compensating for psychological deficits and declines: Managing losses and promoting gains* (pp. 219-230). Mahwah, NJ: Erlbaum.

Rothi, L.J.G. (1997). Transcortical motor, sensory, and mixed aphasias. In L.L. LaPointe (Ed.), *Aphasia and related neurogenic language disorders, 2nd ed.* (p. 91-110). New York: Thieme.

Sabe, L., Salvarezza, F., Garcia Cuerva, A., Leiguarda, R., & Starkstein, S. (1995). A randomized, double-blind, placebo-controlled study of bromocriptine in nonfluent aphasia. *Neurology, 45,* 2272-2274.

Schuell, H., Jenkins, J.J., & Jimenez-Pabon, E. (1964). *Aphasia in adults.* New York: Harper & Row.

Shindo, M., Kaga, K., & Tanaka, Y. (1991). Speech discrimination and lip reading in patients with word deafness or auditory agnosia. *Brain and Language, 40,* 153-161.

Shisler, R.J., Baylis, G.S., & Frank, E.M. (2001). Pharmacological approaches to the treatment and prevention of aphasia. *Aphasiology, 14,* 1163-1186.

Skelly, M. (1979). *Amer-Ind gestural code based on universal American Indian hand talk.* New York: Elsevier.

Small, S.L. (1994) Pharmacotherapy of aphasia: A critical review. *Stroke, 25,* 1282-1289.

Small, S.L. (2000). The future of aphasia treatment. *Brain and Language, 71,* 227-232.

Sparks, R.W. (2001). Melodic intonation therapy. In R. Chapey (Ed.), *Language intervention strategies in aphasia and related neurogenic communication disorders* (pp. 703-717). Philadelphia: Lippincott Williams & Wilkins.

Tanaka, Y., Miyazaki, M., & Albert, M.L. (1997). Effects of increased cholingergic activity on naming in aphasia. *Lancet, 350,* 116-117.

Taub, E., Uswatte, G., Pidikiti, R. (1999). Constraint-induced movement therapy: a new family of techniques with broad application to physical rehabilitation-a clinical review. *Journal of Rehabilitation Research & Development, 36,* 237-251.

Therapeutics and Technology Assessment Subcommittee of the American Academy of Neurology (1994). Assessment: Melodic intonation therapy. *Neurology, 44,* 566-568.

Thompson, C.K. (2001). Treatment of underlying forms: A linguistic specific approach for sentence production deficits in agrammatic aphasia. In R. Chapey (Ed.), *Language intervention strategies in aphasia and related neurogenic communication disorders, 4th ed.* (pp. 605-628). Philadelphia: Lippincott Williams & Wilkins.

Thompson, C.K., Ballard, K.J., & Shapiro, L.P. (1998). The role of syntactic complexity in training wh-movement structures in agrammatic aphasia: Optimal order for promoting generalization. *Journal of the International Neuropsychological Society, 4,* 661-674.

Walker-Batson, D., Curtis, S., Natarajan, R., Ford, J., Dronkers, N., Salmeron, E., Lai, J., Unwin, D.H. (2001). A double-blind, placebo-controlled study of the use of amphetamine in the treatment of aphasia. *Stroke, 32,* 2093-2098.

Weinrich, M., Boser, K.I., & McCall, D. (1999). Representation of linguistic rules in the brain: Evidence from training an aphasic patient to produce past tense verb morphology. *Brain and Language, 70,* 144-158.

Weinrich, M., Shelton, J.R., Cox, D.M., & McCall, D. (1997). Remediating production of tense morphology improves verb retrieval in chronic aphasia. *Brain and Language, 58,* 23-45.

Wertz, R.T., Collins, M.J., Weiss, D., Kurtzke, J.F., Friden, T., Brookshire, R.H., et al. (1981). Veterans administration cooperative study on aphasia: A comparison of individual and group treatment. *Journal of Speech and Hearing Research, 24,* 580-594.

Wertz, R.T., Weiss, D.G., Aten, J.L., Brookshire, R.H., Garcia-Bunuel, L., Holland, A.L., et al. (1986). Comparison of clinic, home and deferred language treatment for aphasia. *Archives of Neurology, 43,* 653-658.

Whurr, R., Lorch, M.P., & Nye, C. (1992). A meta-analysis of studies carried out between 1946 and 1988 concerned with the efficacy of speech and language therapy treatment for aphasic patients. *European Journal of Disorders of Communication, 27,* 1-17.

Wilson, B.A. (1997). Cognitive rehabilitation: how it is and how it might be. *Journal of the International Neuropsychological Society, 3,* 487-496.

Wilson, B.A. (1999). *Case studies in neuropsychological rehabilitation.* Oxford: Oxford University Press.

World Health Organization (WHO). (2001, May). International classification of functioning, disability and health. Available: www.who.int/classification/icf.

Zingeser, L.B., & Berndt, R.S. (1990). Retrieval of nouns and verbs in agrammatism and anomia. *Brain and Language, 39,* 14-32.

Chapter 7

NEURO-REHABILITATION AND COGNITIVE BEHAVIOUR THERAPY FOR EMOTIONAL DISORDERS IN ACQUIRED BRAIN INJURY

W. Huw Williams

University of Exeter, UK

Introduction

Survivors of Acquired Brain Injury (ABI) are at particular risk of developing mood disorders. Negative psychological reactions to neurological trauma may be caused by a complex interaction of a host of factors. The task of assessment is made even more difficult because survivors often have difficulties in reporting their own emotions accurately. Although challenging, rehabilitation of emotional disorders is acknowledged as one of the key areas for development in neurological services. In this chapter we provide an overview of the assessment and rehabilitation of emotional and mood disorders following ABI in post-acute settings. Individual cases are described, based on work conducted within cognitive rehabilitation programmes augmented with cognitive behaviour therapy.

Rehabilitation and Emotion

In 'holistic' rehabilitation survivors are encouraged to become 'insightful' and to 'take on' an active role in their own rehabilitation. Mclellan (1997) for example, noted that rehabilitation is a 'shared process between survivor and staff [in which the survivor] is to choose the destination and the route taken, but also do most of the work' (p.1). In Cognitive Rehabilitation staff attempt to engage their clients in ways that enable them to develop awareness, and acceptance, of their cognitive deficits so as to develop strategies to compensate for them (Wilson, 1997). The balancing act of engaging a person to develop insight and self-determination, yet take on board deficits and potential obstacles to plan for, is challenging, and the process of rehabilitation may well be emotionally charged. During the process of coming to understand, accept, and cope with a memory problem that perhaps threatens return to work, a survivor may grieve the loss of their skills and be anxious about the future (see Prigatano, 1986). Indeed, Wilson (2001) recently described rehabilitation as both a science and an art in the demands that it places on staff. Done without creativity and flexibility, it can appear to 'force' insight, which is not only an un-productive strategy, but is also alienating and dis-empowering for the person. In contrast, enabling a person to recognise the need to check the evidence for applying a memory strategy might lead to some possible alliances. In rehabilitation, then, the person needs to be engaged in, and guided through, a process of exploration and discovery. The gains, it is hoped, would be continued engagement with a service until meaningful goals, which are self-sustaining, self-actualising and rewarding (such as being in a job that is manageable and that one likes), are achieved. However it might also mean achieving a 'good enough' degree of insight for acceptance of on-going support, that can mitigate against a fall off in emotional well-being and further denudation of social roles.

Rehabilitation staff not only attend to general emotional issues in rehabilitation, but also work with, and through, the emotional crises of survivors and families. Referrals to outpatient and outreach programmes are not often on the basis of a circumscribed neurological issue or goal, but are usually due to lack of insight, development of mood problems, chemical dependency, or threatened (or actual) family disintegration (see Harris, 1997). A recent large-scale population-based study by Teasdale and Engberg (2001) revealed that approximately 3–4% of those who suffered Traumatic Brain Injury (TBI) later committed suicide. Consequently there have been calls for more comprehensive guidance, and indeed services, to be developed, for the assessment and management of mood disorders in brain injury (Lewis, 2001).

Mood Disorders in ABI Groups

There have been various attempts to detail the types and frequency of mood disorders following ABI. The majority of research has been conducted in

Traumatic Brain Injury (TBI). There has been much variability between studies in terms of the measures used, perspectives taken (client and/or significant other) and timescale of assessment. From the existing evidence, there is much to indicate that mood disturbance of various forms is very common following ABI. The seminal work of Brooks, Campsie, Symington, Beattie, and McKinley (1987), revealed how the emotional and behavioural consequences of brain injury were more common and distressing for carers than purely cognitive problems. More recently, Bowen, Neumann, Conner, Tennant and Chamberlain (1998), using the Wimbledon Self-report Scale for Mood Disorders, found a 38% rate of 'caseness' for mood disorders in 77 survivors 6 months after injury. Hibbard, Uysal, Kepler, Bogdany and Silver (1998) investigated patterns of mood disorders in TBI with the Structured Clinical Interview for DSM-IV. They found that the most frequent diagnoses were major depression and specific anxiety disorders, and that co-morbidity was high, with 44% of individuals having two or more diagnoses.

A complicating factor for the general assessment of mood disorders in ABI is that there is a lack of appropriate measures of psychiatric/mental health status for TBI groups. Measures in use have usually been developed for other, non-brain injured groups, and may lack validity when used with ABI groups (see Bowen et al., 1998; Williams, Evans, & Wilson, 1999). Moreover, it important to note that TBI leads to complex forms of emotional disturbance, often associated with dysexecutive and amnestic syndromes. Therefore, it is more likely that a person with TBI would suffer a syndrome of neurological-emotional reactions than a singular form of emotional disturbance (Berrios, personal communication). Sometimes the neurological factors are more prominent, and at other times the emotional reaction is more prominent. Due to these issues, false positives and false negative findings on psychiatric or mood measures may be common in ABI practice. Reliance, then, on 'routine' screening measures, is particularly problematic in ABI, and, as such, care needs to be taken to conduct assessment from different perspectives (the client's, the partner's, and/or significant others') with a range of techniques (interviews, cognitive tests, mood measures, behavioural checklists and observation). From such assessments it may become possible to understand how a mood disorder may represent elements of a person's overall neuro-behavioural syndrome. In terms of rehabilitation, a clinical formulation of elements that contribute to a mood disorder can inform areas for intervention, such as the symptoms a survivor is most troubled by and/or for which goals may be set.

Depression

Depression can be viewed as a persistent state of low self-esteem, sadness and hopelessness (about the world, future and self). It has been suggested that depression may become more prevalent in TBI groups over time, given successive losses and difficulties establishing control over life post-injury (Brooks et al., 1987). The grief literature, emphasising losses experienced, and difficulties in 'moving' through to stages of resolution, is particularly helpful in understanding depression. The coping literature provides key themes relating to the notion of learned helplessness, which may become an entrenched state for the survivor (discussed below). Studies of depression and TBI have 'consistently shown a strong association regardless of instruments or procedures used' (Satz, Forney, Zaucha, Asarnow, Light et al., 1998, p. 538). Using the Beck Depression Inventory (Beck, Ward, & Mendelson, 1961), Garske and Thomas (1992) found that, of 47 TBI survivors, 55% had clinical symptoms of mild to severe depression. Kreutzer, Seel and Gourley (2000) investigated depression following TBI using standardized diagnostic criteria (DSM-IV) in 722 outpatients with brain injury. They found that 42% of patients with brain injury met DSM-IV criteria for diagnosis of major depressive disorder. In addition, they noted that fatigue, frustration, and poor concentration were the most commonly cited manifestations of depression. Research into risk factors for depression is limited. Ownsworth and Oei (1998), in a general review, suggested that the following factors made TBI survivors particularly susceptible to depression: pre-existing psychiatric disturbance; sustained injury involving the left anterior region of the brain; significant impairment of self-awareness; and unrealistic expectations of resuming pre-injury social roles and experiencing failure doing so. However, it should be noted that impairments in self-awareness has been shown to be a protective factor for mood disorders (see Williams, Evans, Needham, & Wilson (2002)). Indeed, it may well be that as survivors become more aware – over time and by rehabilitation – of the implications of the injuries for their life goal and social roles that they may suffer emotional distress (see discussion in Fleminger, Oliver, Williams, & Evans, (in press)). For example, Godfrey et al. (1993) noted that the presentation of emotional dysfunction (i.e. depression, anxiety and poor self-esteem) coincided with improved insight of behavioural, cognitive and social impairments in closed head injury (CHI) patients.

A major difficulty in assessing depression following brain injury is that apparent depressive symptoms – such as irritability, frustration, fatigue, poor concentration and apathy – may occur as a direct result of brain damage rather than due to depression. Indeed, Fleminger et al. (in press) noted that, given the paucity of studies making direct comparisons of the rates of symptom endorsement between the differing clinical groups (depressed, depressed and brain injured and brain injured) it is difficult to confirm the symptoms that specifically characterise depression following brain injury. Aloia, Long and Allen (1995) compared the symptom profiles of depression in head injured patients and non-head injured patients. The findings suggested that the picture of depression in head-injury was similar to that in non-head-injury. However, Kreutzer, Seel, and Gourley (2001) in a review of the literature, noted that the symptoms irritability, lack of interest, moving slowly, fatigue and forgetfulness as being more common after brain injury regardless of depression. Moreover, apathy, or loss of motivation, is frequently observed among brain-injured patients and is often associated with depression. It may be helpful to note that Marin (1990, 1991) draws a distinction between apathy as a symptom of depression and 'true' apathy which 'describes only those patients whose lack of motivation is not attributable to a diminished level of consciousness, an intellectual deficit or emotional distress' (p. 22).

Suicide is, as we have noted above, disturbingly common after TBI. Depression is a major (but not only) risk factor for suicide. Harris and Barraclough (1997) undertook a meta-analysis of suicide following various medical and psychiatric conditions. They calculated Standardized mortality ratios (SMRs) for each disorder by comparing the sums of their observed and expected values. For both civilian and war brain injuries they calculated that risk of suicide after brain injury was raised over 3 fold from that expected in the general population (for further discussion see Fleminger et al. (in press)). The presence of depression in the context of a neurological injury presents a volatile set of conditions for assessment and management of suicidality. Indeed, in the general psychiatric literature, a history of head injury is regarded as a risk factor for suicide in depression (Mann, Waternaux, Haas & Malone, 1999). Teasdale and Engberg (2001) noted that risk factors for suicide in their study of TBI included female gender, being aged between 21-60, and having a co-diagnosis of substance misuse. In general, the following issues may need to be addressed in suicidality in ABI: lack of planning and problem solving for 'getting out' of depressed mood; poor memory that affects ability to cope with problematic situations; emotional lability and/or dis-inhibition and impulsiveness that might increase the risk of acting without considering the consequences of actions; poor emotional expression, leading to depressed state going un-noticed; and perseveration over negative material, leading to a spiral of negative thinking (see Klonoff & Lage, 1995; Tate, Simpson, Flanagan & Coffey, 1997 for risk factors, assessment, and recommendations for management of suicide).

Anxiety disorders

There are a range of anxiety disorders, such as generalised anxiety disorder (GAD), phobias, panic disorder, obsessive compulsive disorder (OCD) and post-traumatic stress disorder (PtSD). As a group, anxiety disorders are the most commonly diagnosed mental health disorder in general mental health settings. They are suspected to be common after brain injury, although possibly under-diagnosed due to difficulties in identifying symptoms in the context of other issues (see Scheutzow & Wiercisiewski, 1999). For many, anxiety may be associated with the adjustment process to the brain injury and may, for example, be focused on feeling out of control and insecure over their future and social roles.

GAD has been reported, and is often associated with depression (see Jorge, Robinson, Starkstein, & Arndt, 1993). OCD was considered rare in brain injured groups, although there is increasing evidence of it occuring (see Lishman, 1998). OCD is characterised by symptoms of either recurrent intrusive thoughts and/or compulsive repetitive behaviours. It tends to present in the context of an affective disorder with symptoms of tension, rumination, self-doubt, indecision and compulsive preoccupation. McKeown (1984) found 3 of a sample of 25 survivors of mild brain injury, and a further individual from a twin study, to have severe OCD. There was an absence of any pre-morbid features in 3 of the 4 cases. Berthier, Kulisevsky, Gironell and Lopez (2001) reported a study of 10 people with TBI who had OCD. They noted that the patterns of OCD symptoms (such as a high frequency of obsessions regarding contamination, somatic symptoms, need for symmetry, and compulsions such as cleaning and checking) were relatively well specified.

Scheutznow and Wiercisiewski (1999) described the case of a TBI survivor assessed as having a panic disorder who presented with clear anxiety symptoms, with avoidance of activities due to a fear of suffering a heart attack. Phobic reactions are infrequently reported in the literature, although, clinically, patients are often found to have stress responses in reaction to particular stimuli. Such reactions might be best understood within the literature on PtSD. Recent studies have shown that PtSD is a relatively common mood disorder for survivors of mild and severe brain injury (Bryant, 2001; Bryant, Marossezesky, Crooks, Baguley, & Gurka, 2000; Hickling, Gillen, Blanchard, Buckley, & Taylor, 1998; McMillan, 1996; Ohry, Rattock, & Solomon, 1996; Williams, Evans, Wilson, & Needham, in press (a)). Bryant et al. (2000) found that 27% of 96 survivors of mild and severe TBI had PtSD. In a study of a representative community sample of 66 severe TBI survivors, 18% were shown to have moderate to severe PtSD symptoms (Williams et al., in press (a)). PtSD is characterised by intrusive experiences, hyper-vigilance, anxiety, fear and avoidance of activities. If left untreated it may severely limit a person's ability to function. PtSD and TBI were previously considered to be mutually exclusive, as it was thought that the survivor's lack of memory of the event negated the possibility of vivid intrusive cognitions and avoidance behaviours (Sbordone & Leiter, 1995). However, survivors have been shown to have 'islands of memory' of their trauma, such as being stuck in a car wreckage, or of later, secondary experiences, which could fuel intrusive ruminations (McMillan, 1996). Others have been traumatised by confabulated memories of the traumatic event (see King, 1996). Cases have also been documented of people with no memory of the event having traumatic re-experiences and avoidance behaviours following exposure to environments similar to their trauma (see McNeil & Greenwood, 1996). It has been suggested that if an event is unexpected, but has the biological significance of a life threat, then it may be stored in memory despite disruption to areas of the brain that store declarative memories (Markowitsch, 1998). Indeed, such theoretical mechanisms in TBI are consistent with fear-conditioning hypotheses for PtSD which hold that traumatic experiences can be processed independently of higher cortical functions (Brewin, Dalgleish, & Joseph, 1996; Bryant, 2001). Indeed, the nature of the event, for example, 'coming out of the blue' and beyond any perceived control by the person, giving a heightened sense of threat to self, has been shown to be associated with the presence and severity of PtSD symptoms (see Williams, Williams & Ghadiali, 1998; Williams, Evans, Wilson, & Needham, in press (b)).

Principal Agents and Contributory Factors for Mood Disorders in TBI

There are a host of factors that contribute to the development of mood disorders. Recent developments in this area have lead to the argument that a bio-psycho-social account is needed for understanding psychosocial outcome in TBI (see Macmillan, Martelli, Hart, & Zasler, 2002). Principal factors include the following: the nature and severity of the neurological injury; the pre-injury history of the survivor; the survivor's adjustment and coping systems; the type and nature of the event suffered; and the presence of additional stresses. In addition, the forms of support available and the length of time elapsed since the injury need to be considered.

Neurological factors

The brain is the system that contains, creates and controls our reactions to the world. Injuries of any form may lead to emotional disturbance. As described above, some injuries may be more destructive to one's emotional integrity than others. An understanding of the breakdown in neurological functions is crucial for the understanding and management of any form of emotional disorder following brain injury. Two main forms of neurological deficits may lead to emotional dysfunction: composite (those involving a number of systems working together to produce functional behaviours) and specific (more circumscribed deficits of parts of a module). Of the composite problems, the most common (and crucial) is the dysexecutive syndrome, frequently seen in injuries to the frontal areas. Indeed, this disorder is particularly problematic for emotional functioning as executive systems are critical for 'handling' cognitive acts that modulate emotional processing. One crucial 'composite' result of effective executive functioning is having insight and awareness of one's circumstances and status. 'Specific' neurological deficits may lead to circumscribed forms of impaired emotional processing, including: motivation problems arising from injuries to the cingulate gyrus; inability to process others' emotional expression, associated with injuries to the amygdala; and inability to respond appropriately in situations that should be of concern, due to lesions of the ventromedial prefrontal cortex. An assessment of emotion therefore requires a consideration of neurological and neuropsychological profiles such that relevant causal agents are identified for rehabilitation. It is not within the scope of this chapter to consider such disorders in detail. Lishman (1998) provides a comprehensive overview of the assessment and management of neurologically-based emotional disorders. Eames (2001) provides insights into differentiating symptoms associated with neurological injury and psychiatric disorders. Judd (1999) gives a lucid account of neuropsychothera-peutic approaches for such problems in community settings.

Pre-injury history

In terms of predicting outcome in TBI, particularly emotional status, there is an aphorism that holds that, 'It is not only the kind of injury that matters, but the kind of head' (Symonds, 1937, p. 1092). Research on pre-injury char-acteristics and psychosocial outcome has focused on two main areas. Firstly, the presence of positive personality traits that might enhance psychosocial outcome (such as determination, resourcefulness and stability) and secondly, the absence of such positive elements, which may be reflected in difficult pre-morbid psychosocial histories, and could put people at risk of adverse outcomes (see Tate, 1998). The general position that a set of pre-injury per-sonality characteristics is a major determinant on outcome was summarised as follows: 'In most cases after severe head injury, the personality and behav-ioural changes that occurred 'tend either to be an exaggeration of previous traits or to occur in patients that might have been expected to develop mental disorder without having had their brains damaged' (Brooks, 1984, p. 139, in Lishman, 1998, p. 174). Whilst acknowledging that there may be some likelihood of such effects, Lishman (1998) notes that, 'it has proved difficult to specify what special aspects of [premorbid] personality are important' (p. 174). He added that the evidence for personality types being associated with particular outcomes is 'impressionistic and hampered by lack of opportunity for objective assessments before the injury occurred' (p. 174).

It is, however, well established that gender and age are pre-injury risk factors. TBI occurs most frequently in the 18-25 year-old age group, with males outnumbering females by a ratio of at least 2:1 (Tate, 1998). Within this group, it is possible that anti-social and/or risk taking characteristics might contribute towards risk of injury, and might be associated with poorer longer-term outcome. However, it is also very likely that such characteristics would be transient rather than permanent characteristics of the person. As Tate (1998) noted: young men may 'frequently tend to be nonconformist, risk takers, immature, have difficulty with authority and so forth simply by virtue of their life stage' (p. 8).

Premorbid social maladjustment (PSM) indices, such as educational achievement, work history and 'nervous illness' were described in a seminal paper by Symonds and Russell (1943). It had been generally held that people with poor PSM profiles were overly represented in samples of TBI survivors. More recent research has revealed more complex interactions than had been assumed between pre-injury status and psychosocial wellbeing. Tate (1998) investigated pre-injury delinquency, conviction and substance dependency in a study with 100 head injured survivors. She found that 11 had evidence of such PSM characteristics. Furthermore she found that PSM was not predictive of psychosocial functioning 6 months post-trauma. In a further study, using the Eysenck Personality Questionnaire-Revised (including scales measuring psychoticism, tough-mindedness, addiction, and criminality), Tate found that it was possible to identify a sub-group of participants with elevated scores for dispositional traits, but that such traits were not associated with psychosocial outcome. She found that post-traumatic amnesia (PTA) length was the only correlate of poorer outcome.

There is, however, some evidence of an association between pre-injury factors and mental health outcome both direct, and by implication. In Bowen et al.'s (1998) study, it was found that pre-morbid occupational status was associated with the development of mood disorders following injury. Deb, Lyons and Koutzoukis (1999) found that pre-injury factors such as lower social class and lower educational achievement were associated with psychiatric caseness according to the Clinical Interview Schedule-Revised. Dunlop, Udvarhelyi, Stedem, O'Connor, Isaacs et al. (1991) that found that a prior history of alcohol misuse was associated with poorer outcome. More recently, Macmillan, Martelli, Hart and Zasler (2002) found that pre-injury psychiatric status and drug use history were predictive of poorer outcome in terms of return to work.

It is likely then, that there may well be particular patterns of pre-injury characteristics that exert an influence on how the person copes with their injuries and their aftermath. It may well be that the type of head is important, but the type of resources and opportunities the person had, and has, must also be considered.

Grief, coping and adjustment

Survivors of TBI have been noted to become depressed, withdrawn and anxious as a reaction to the disruption caused to their lives, their losses, and the chronic frustration associated with their acquired disabilities (Rosenthal & Bond, 1990). There has been increased interest in understanding why some survivors are protected from, and others more vulnerable to, developing such reactions. Grief models, and more recently, models of stress and coping, have been adopted to conceptualise responses to injury. The stress-coping models, which are in part evolved from grief models, and also cognitive behavioural theory, are purported to be comprehensive bio-psycho-social frameworks for understanding the complex interaction of pre-injury, injury and post-injury factors on mood and behaviour.

Grief models provide a framework for understanding how survivors might understand their losses and come to understand and cope with them (see Jackson, 1988). In general, reactions to loss may involve initial stages of shock and denial, then stages of anger and depression, leading through to adjustment and reintegration. An important aspect of such models is that there is not necessarily a progression through all stages of grief, as it is possible to have different combinations of each form of emotion at the same time, with one or other possibly being more salient. TBI leads to a particularly complicated form of grief because emotional denial (if it occurs) may well follow actual lack of awareness – anosognosia. Furthermore, the person may have lost the very skills and opportunities for reinvestment in life, for example, when poor memory skills undermine the ability to work. Moreover, losses may also be cumulative and ongoing for survivors. In the early stages, the person may be experiencing a loss of function (cognitive or physical), but they may subsequently start to experience other losses, perhaps relating to work, and/or a partner. It is not surprising that a pervasive sense of grief may occur in the context of a disintegrated sense of self. As one client noted, 'I live in the ruins of my old self'. Individual differences in emotional reaction to loss might then be understood in terms of a person's 'stage' of grieving, tasks of grieving, and awareness.

Stress-coping theories of adaptation have as their key theme the interaction of pre-injury coping styles and stress caused by the demands and conflicts of the aftermath of the neurological event (see Kendall & Terry, 1996). An individual's adjustment may be influenced by successive efforts to master the demands and conflicts triggered by their trauma with, over time, adaptive or un-helpful coping styles being developed. Such conceptualisations are argued to be consistent with the general stress and coping literature (Folkman, Lazarus, Dunkel-Schetter et al., (1986) and the literature on coping in physical illness (Moos & Schaefer, 1984). Moos and Schaefer, for example, described three key coping skills in the context of physical illness: appraisal-focused coping – finding a pattern of meaning in a crisis; problem-focused coping – seeking to confront the 'reality' by constructing a more satisfactory situation; and emotion-focused coping – focusing on managing emotional reactions. The adoption of particular styles of coping may be related to the development of mood disorder and general psychosocial outcome.

Moore and Stambrooke (1992, 1995) examined how long-term outcome may be mediated by coping styles. They followed up 131 survivors of TBI and found two main clusters of 'coping' styles related to outcome. They reported that one group tended to have an external locus of control, and used an indiscriminate variety of all styles of coping and tended to have poor psychosocial outcome (with reports such as, 'I'd do anything to stop the pain...Life stopped...I'm being punished'). The second group tended to have a mainly problem-solving approach, and good outcomes ('it was a terrible day...I appreciate life and family more... take a day at a time'). In a similar vein, Malia, Powell and Torode (1995) reported a study in which 74 ABI survivors were shown to be less likely to have good psychosocial outcomes if their coping styles were avoidant, emotion-focused or 'wishful'. More recently, Finset and Andersson (2000) investigated coping styles of 70 ABI survivors and a non-injured control group. They reported that the ABI group tended to have a less differentiated coping style than the controls. They also found two main dimensions to coping responses in the ABI group – approach and avoidance. A lack of active-approach coping responses was associated with apathy, and avoidant coping was associated with depression. They suggested that apathy was related to sub-cortical and right hemisphere lesions. Unfortunately, it was not possible to control for dysexecutive problems contributing to the un-planful coping responses described in these studies. What is important in the context of rehabilitation, then, is that styles of coping might not necessarily represent 'static' pre-injury dispositions, and need to be understood in the contest of the survivor's neurological profile, and general post-injury psychological reactions.

Trauma of the event

As described above, it has become more widely accepted that the event leading to a brain injury can be emotionally traumatic. Many survivors of traumatic events have great difficulty in developing adaptive ways of coping with changes in their lives and their emotional trauma, and typically become isolated and withdrawn (Brewin, 1984). Within the context of a 'stress and coping' model described above, it can be argued that some survivors may have had a combination of factors that have enabled them to adjust to changes in their lives caused by their trauma. However, their adjustment might also be influenced by having suffered emotional trauma during the event itself. There is evidence in non-TBI groups that some survivors have greater risk of developing PtSD under less severe trauma conditions than others. However, under severe trauma conditions both 'at risk' and 'not at risk' groups appear equally likely to develop the disorder. In a recent study Williams et al. (in press, a) found that pre-injury factors (such as educational achievement and occupational status) did not predict the development of PtSD. However, attribution to others for the event was associated with the development of symptoms, whilst poor insight was a protective factor in the development of symptoms.

Additional issues & stresses

It is beyond the scope of this chapter to cover the myriad sources of stress for ABI survivors. However, it is important to note some additional critical issues for assessment and management of mood disorders. Firstly, many survivors may suffer relationship problems, with breakdown of partnership and/or changes in family roles (see Kendall & Terry, 1996). In many cases of ABI there may be physical disabilities causing additional stress. Survivors may often have problems with pain, particularly headache, and in TBI, pain due to orthopaedic injuries (see Andary, Crewe, Anzel, Haines, Kulkarni et al., 1997), which may be associated with the maintenance of emotional distress, such as PtSD symptoms (see Bryant, Marosszezecky, Crooks, Baguley, Gurka, & Joseph, 1999). Symptoms of sleep disorder are also very frequent, and may exacerbate problems in cognition and affect (Cohen, Oksenberg, Snir, & Stern, 1994). Furthermore, as has been noted above, misuse of alcohol and/or drugs may become significant problems for survivors, either as an exacerbation of a pre-injury condition, and/or a maladaptive coping strategy (see Kreutzer, Witol, & Marwitz, 1997).

Neurorehabilitation and Emotion

In this section there will be a consideration of the neuro-rehabilitative input required for the management of mood disorders in ABI groups. However, it is important to note that psychopharmacological interventions are often used in combination with other modalities, such as CBT.

Pharmacological intervention and considerations

Reviews of recent psychopharmacology for depression and anxiety in ABI are available (see Fleminger et al. (in press) and Williams, Evans, & Fleminger (in press) respectively). In general, there appears to be evidence for the efficacy of anti-depressant medication after stroke in treating depression (see Turner-Stokes & Hassan (2002)) and there is anecdotal evidence to support the use of SSRIs in brain injury (Sloan, Brown, & Pentland, 1992). Unfortunately, there do not appear to be any RCT evaluations of antidepressant efficacy for depression after traumatic brain injury (see Fleminger et al. (in press)). There is an indication that depression following brain injury may be more difficult to treat than when in isolation. For example, a controlled comparison study by Dinan and Mobayed (1992) found that patients who were depressed following head injury appeared to respond less well to amitriptyline that depressed patients without a head injury. Fleminger et al. (in press) noted that 'neuropsychiatrists would recommend starting with an SSRI, partly because these drugs probably have less effect on reducing seizure threshold particularly when compared with tricyclic antidepressants'.

Psychological treatments are considered to be the mainstay of the management of anxiety in those with a brain injury – as those without brain injury (see Lishman, 1998). With severe symptoms, or symptoms that do not respond to psychological treatment, a pharmacological strategy may be suggested. Antidepressants with sedative properties may be valuable in some patients with anxiety, and may also help the insomnia which is often present (Williams et al., in press). Zafonte, Cullen, and Lexell, (2002) provide a review of the mechanisms, efficacy, and side effects of serotonin agents in traumatic brain injury for the treatment of depression, and for panic disorder, obsessive-compulsive disorders, agitation, sleep disorders, and motor dysfunction. Williams et al. (in press) noted that Benzodiazepines should be avoided in those with chronic symptoms or in those with evidence of substance abuse, also that the potential side effects of the anxiolytics appear to dictate which drug is chosen. Indeed, caution must be exercised in general with the use of psychotropic medication with brain injured groups. First, such medications might exacerbate the symptoms of the brain injury. For example, psychotropics may produce derealisation – a common symptom after brain injury, therefore such survivors are particularly vulnerable to this side effect. Second, because of the cognitive problems experienced by such survivors many may have difficulty in maintaining appropriate management of a pharmacological regime.

Case Illustrations of Cognitive Rehabilitation and Cognitive Behaviour Therapy (CBT):
The following cases are provided to illustrate how cognitive rehabilitation and CBT may be integrated for the management of mood disorders in ABI. Two individuals were treated at a centre for cognitive rehabilitation. In both cases there was a diagnosed mood disorder (OCD and PtSD), and co-morbidity with other disorders (depression, and depression with alcohol misuse respectively), in the context of general neuropsychological deficits.

General cognitive rehabilitation programme
The assessment process consisted of neuropsychological evaluation, multi-disciplinary therapy assessments interviews, clinical psychology and neuropsychiatric evaluations, administration of mood and behaviour inventories, and self and observer ratings of cognitive, mood and behavioural symptoms over a two week period (for further details see Williams, Evans, & Wilson, 1999). Mood and psychiatric assessments followed DSM-IV guidelines for diagnoses of psychiatric disorders (American Psychiatric Association, 1994). The rehabilitation programme consisted of five components: (1) goal setting procedures; (2) coordinating therapists for facilitating survivor's understanding of intervention and goals; (3) intervention on awareness of impairments and emotional reactions; (4) therapeutic group milieu for encouraging awareness and acceptance and use of strategies; and (5) supported social re-integration for follow-through of strategy use in home or work settings.

For each survivor, the individualised programmes contained an intensive rehabilitation phase followed by a community re-integration phase (attending the centre on 1–2 days per week, for example). Family members, partners and/or friends of the participant were invited to attend a support group to facilitate their understanding of the participant and to derive mutual emotional support. In cognitive groups survivors were encouraged to develop their understanding of their brain injury and its consequences, and how to manage and compensate for cognitive problems, for example, in a memory group.

CBT and rehabilitation
In the programme, clients were provided with individual and group sessions designed from a CBT perspective. CBT has been shown to be highly effective for the management of a range of mood disorders in the general mental health groups (see Roth & Fonaghy, 1996). Importantly, CBT has at its centre, a Socratic, metacognitive process of guided discovery that enables a person to share in an examination of their cognitive, emotional and behavioural experiences. CBT provides systematic means for addressing such issues as: negative automatic thoughts; negative cognitive schemas; unhelpful behaviour profiles; social engagement and, importantly, hope. CBT is advocated as particularly suited for people with ABI as it contains systems for managing generalisability of 'therapeutic work' from the treatment session (diaries and workbooks etc.)

and promotes social and emotional control skills learning (Ponsford et al., 1995; Williams & Jones, 1997). Moreover, cognitive rehabilitation and CBT both have an emphasis on enabling survivors to gain skills, record progress, challenge pessimism and promote self-efficacy. CBT appears particularly well-suited for integration with cognitive rehabilitation as it provides systems and strategies for structuring interventions for people with cognitive disabilities (Ponsford, 1995; Manchester & Woods, 2001; Williams & Jones, 1997).

Case Illustration; OCD and Depression

CBT for OCD includes behavioural exposure, response prevention and management of negative intrusive thoughts. CBT has shown to be effective, in general, and in prevention of relapse (Roth & Fonagy, 1996). Davey and Tallis (1994) described additional features to a CBT treatments, inlcuding attentional strategies for managing self-doubt.

History
DC was a security system officer at the time of injury. He had suffered a TBI in an RTA (coma of 4 weeks, PTA of 2-3 months). He also suffered ortho-paedic injuries. He was seen two years post-injury. His family had become concerned over his withdrawn state, lack of purpose, and low mood. He had a dense retrograde amnesia and a poor anterograde memory. He exhibited a range of compulsive behaviours, involving tidying, and checking. He did not have any premorbid psychological or psychiatric history of note.

Neuropsychological status and mood state
DC's pre-injury and current IQ, and processing speed were in the average range. His attentional skills and memory were impaired. He noted that he did not 'trust' himself to remember activities, of which there were few. He had a limited daily routine. He often 'tidied up', and on rare trips from the house, checked that the cooker was off and that the doors were locked, up to 20 times. He socialised with difficulty, 'checking himself' for personal pos-sessions 'constantly'. He believed himself to be 'a mess' and therefore socially unacceptable. He also had fears over harming his legs if he engaged in any activities. His scores on the Hospital Anxiety and Depression Scale (HADS, Zigmond & Snaith, 1983) were in the moderate and mild ranges for anxiety and depression, respectively. However, in interview, he was assessed as being at risk of suicidal depression in the longer term.

Formulation
DC had a dense amnesic disorder with attentional difficulties consequent upon his TBI. His immediate visual recall was a particular strength. OCD symptoms appeared to be related to the following: (1) cognitive disorders triggering self-doubt and rumination with checking as an overcompensation

for poor memory; (2) checking and tidying, providing a means of controlling aspects of his immediate environment and sense of safety in the absence of other, more meaningful, activities; (3) behaviours being negatively reinforced by avoidance (the behaviour 'saved' him from social demands); (4) distorted self-image being maintained, and exacerbated, by avoidance of activities, with core beliefs being highly negative and leading to negative automatic thoughts; (5) health fears contributing to general avoidance behavioural pattern; (6) problems being maintained and exacerbated by a lack of opportunity for developing adaptive responses.

General intervention

DC was provided with support for developing an external memory system which included: filofax for long term memory; voice organiser for supporting delayed memory; and electronic organiser for prospective memory/reminding. He was also supported in developing stress management skills, including: relaxation skills; management of negative automatic thoughts (NATs); and attentional skills for 'burning in' what he had 'just done'. A graded exposure programme was developed based on his least to most worrisome situations in 3 domains: social-leisure; community-mobility; and physical activities. Over a period of 8 months, DC was provided with a programme that progressed from developing basic emotional and cognitive control skills through to integrating their use in functional situations. He was provided with specific clinical psychology input to develop his integrated use of such skills, with interdisciplinary input across all areas of his hierarchies.

Specific interventions

For socialising, DC had a hierarchy that included the following situations, and associated negative automatic thoughts: calling a friend ('they're only putting up with me...anyway, I'll forget what we talked about'); going to a pub, and staying for 40 minutes ('I'll repeat myself...I'll look a mess') and going to a club ('I'll get pushed and hurt my legs'). Over the course of intervention, DC became skilled at using relaxation to prepare for situations and answer NATs, and became engaged in activities. For example, for making a call, he had a plan of using breathing exercises and getting a note-pad for questions to ask and noting responses. On 'checking the evidence' for 'being a nuisance' to friends, he found that, when reviewing his mood diary on his organiser, he had examples of friends asking his advice, joking, and making joint plans.

For socialising and community mobility, DC initially needed to develop his skills for leaving the house. This included 'over-attending' to indications that the door was locked (when closing the door, he was instructed to listen to the click, and the serrated key making a scraping sound when coming out of the lock). He also practised making a visual image of where things were before leaving the house, so he could 'recreate' the image later ('I left the phone on the tabletop, picture it, don't worry'). When socialising he used his voice-corder to note any future plans (where to meet later, for example), and relaxation skills if needed. Regarding his physical health worries, he was supported in identifying and managing catastrophic NATs.

Outcome

DC reported increased confidence in integrating such skills to achieve his goals. At discharge from the programme he had made progress in all areas, socialising regularly, travelling independently, and being engaged in a range of physical activities. His scores on anxiety and depression ratings were reduced to the non-clinical range. He noted: 'I've had my life back...I spent all the time since the accident at home watching TV..afraid that if I do something I'd look foolish... [I'm now with friends or] making new friends...using strategies...that was confusing for a while but over time you get used to the new habits, and what technique to use where and when, and you get to trust it...and [you] get confident...[but] you've got to watch for that vicious cycle, of withdrawal.' DC had maintained his progress at a 6 months review.

Case illustration: PtSD, alcohol misuse and depression

CBT is widely accepted as a treatment for PtSD and includes a combination of exposure therapy, stress inoculation training and cognitive therapy (Rothbaum, Meadows, Resick, & Foy, 2000). McMillan (1991) described the successful use of a behavioural approach for managing intrusive and avoidant symptoms in the case of a survivor of severe head injury who had complete amnesia for the event. McNeil and Greenwood (1996) described a CBT package with a survivor of severe brain injury from a road traffic accident (RTA). It was found that treating the PtSD symptoms lead to changes in behaviour, which had been originally thought to have been un-modifiable due to organic 'personality changes'.

History

KE was seen 2.5 years following a TBI in a RTA. His girlfriend, a passenger, died in the accident. He had a coma of 1–2 days and a post-traumatic amnesia of up to a week. He suffered multiple skull fractures, and facial and orthopaedic injuries. He lost his job as a sales person and had had two unsuccessful returns to work. He had started a new relationship, which was under threat due to anger outbursts.

Assessment

KE's verbal and visuo-spatial reasoning skills were largely intact although he had mild executive problems and a reduction in processing speed. His memory and attentional skills were poor. His cognitive difficulties were compounded by mild diplopia. There was no prior history of psychiatric disturbance or substance abuse. He reported that he could recollect an island of memory for the trauma event: '[I was] coming around for a short period...[I] felt I was dying...I remember...I was in the car. Smoke ...there was blood...I couldn't see...couldn't breathe...I reached for my girlfriend, she was lying there...[passenger seat]...she was dead.'. He reported nightmares every night and frequent flashbacks during the day. He admitted alcohol misuse to cope with his problems, especially for aiding sleep. On the Impact of Events Scale (IES) (Horowitz, Wilner, & Alvarez, 1979) his score was in the severe range. On the HADS, his score for anxiety was in the severe range, and depression in the moderate range.

Formulation

KE had executive, memory and attentional difficulties. He was noted to have severe PtSD, including intrusive re-experiences, avoidance behaviours and emotional blunting. PtSD symptoms were contributed to by survivor guilt and a grief reaction. He had mild generalised anxiety and mild to moderate depression, and a moderate alcohol dependency. He had moderate insight into his mood disturbance. His symptoms were maintained in the absence of opportunities to develop adaptive responses. Without appropriate support, he was assessed as being at risk of continuing to experience PtSD symptoms and to develop more severe depression in the long term.

General intervention

KE attended the programme to pursue goals related to managing his anger, alcohol, and PtSD symptoms, and for developing occupational opportunities. Through cognitive groups KE identified and later demonstrated the use of systems and strategies for managing his planning, memory and attentional difficulties. For example, he used a palm-top computer to plan and monitor activities at home, such as undertaking basic DIY tasks. This was particularly helpful for providing him with reminders to stop working and take breaks and spend time with his step-children. In mood groups KE developed his awareness of factors that influenced his mood from a CBT perspective. He was also supported in developing coping skills, such as relaxation strategies, 'thought catching' and evidence checking. He also received twice-weekly individual CBT sessions with a clinical psychologist focusing on identifying immediate triggers and background mediators for his mood and developing his coping skills. Using the palm-top computer he was supported in recording the following: alcohol intake; sleep pattern and problems; arguments, including antecedents, behaviour and consequences; and nightmares or flashbacks. He received individual and group input regarding alcohol misuse and anger management techniques.

Specific interventions

As KE became reliable in recording his emotional status he progressed to achieving specific input on his PtSD symptoms, with goals including addressing his monitoring and management of intrusive re-experiences. For example, he received individual sessions in which he was asked to describe current trauma re-experiences in increasingly more detail whilst being prompted to use relaxation strategies. On one occasion he had reported (from notes on his palm top) being distressed after watching a television police drama involving a car chase. He had become breathless and agitated. Whilst recounting the episode in a session, he recounted his 'island of memory' from the trauma event, and noted how the steering wheel had trapped him. With guidance to use relaxation techniques to 'stay in the present', he continued to explore the memory to become increasingly exposed to it. In later group sessions he reported being more able to process the event without the expected surge of anxiety. KE was also supported in identifying a part-time work placement (in a Do-It-Yourself (DIY) store). He was encouraged to develop a paced, planful approach to managing the demands of this work placement, and counselled to maintain a part-time role.

Outcome

At discharge, KE had achieved goals regarding his emotional status and work. He managed his anger, alcohol, and PtSD symptoms consistently. For example, he had nightmares occasionally rather than nightly, and could use relaxation strategies for aiding sleep, which meant he drank less alcohol, and was more able to function during the day. He was also holding down a part-time job in a DIY store. His score for depression was reduced from the clinical to non-clinical range, although his anxiety score remained somewhat elevated. His scores on the IES were reduced from the severe to the moderate range. These gains were maintained at a 6-month review, and his alcohol intake had continued to reduce (down by 50% to 'safe' levels). However, as suggested by his IES scores, he continued to have some trauma-related nightmares and intrusive thoughts. He noted that he did not misuse alcohol to avoid such intrusions, and felt much more able to control PtSD symptoms. KE was referred on to case management services locally.

Conclusions

Neurological trauma can lead to many forms of emotional distress and survivors frequently develop mood disorders. Recent advances in cognitive rehabilitation, in combination with developments in CBT, have yielded the possibility of systems and strategies for managing cognitive and emotional disorders for many ABI survivors. It must be emphasised that the assessment and management of mood disorders in ABI is complicated by a host of factors, and needs to be comprehensive in order to arrive at realisable goals. However, given the mental health risks of survivors of ABI, services need to be developed which provide screening for mental health issues such that more detailed management plans, including in-depth assessments, can be conducted. With such developments, more people may have access to services that could protect, and even promote, their social and psychological well being.

References

Aloia, M.S., Long, C.J., & Allen, J.B. (1995). Depression among the head-injured and non-head-injured: a discriminant analysis. *Brain Injury, 9(6)*, 575-583.

American Psychiatric Association (1994). *Diagnostic and Statistical Manual – IV.* American Psychiatric Association, Washington.

Andary, M.T., Crewe, N., Anzel, S.K., Haines, P., Kulkarni, M.R., Stanton, D.F., Thompson, A. & Yosef, M. (1997). Traumatic brain injury/chronic pain syndrome: A case comparison study. *Clinical Journal of Pain, 13*, 244-250.

Beck, A.T., Ward C.H., & Mendelson, M. (1961). An inventory for measuring depression. *Archives of General Psychiatry, 4*, 561-571.

Berthier, M., Kulisevsky, J., Gironell, A. & Lopez, O.L. (2001). Obsessive-compulsive disorder and traumatic brain injury: Behavioural, cognitive and neuroimaging findings. *Neuropsychiatry, Neuropsychology & Behavioral Neurology, 14*, 23-31.

Bowen, A., Neumann, V., Conners, M., Tennant, A., & Chamberlain, M.A. (1998). Mood disorders following traumatic brain injury: Identifying the extent of the problem and the people at risk. *Brain Injury, 12*, 177-190.

Brewin, C. (1984). Attributions for industrial accidents: Their relationship to rehabilitation outcome. *Journal of Social & Clinical Psychology, 2*, 156-164.

Brewin, C.R., Dalgleish, T., & Joseph, S. (1996). A dual representation theory of posttraumatic stress disorder. *Psychological Review, 103*, 670-686.

Brooks, N., Campsie, L., Symington, C., Beattie, A. & McKinley, W. (1987). The effects of severe head injury on patient and relative within seven years of injury. *Journal of Head Injury Rehabilitation, 2*, 1-13.

Bryant, R.A. (2001). Posttraumatic stress disorder and traumatic brain injury: Can they co-exist? *Clinical Psychology Review, 21*, 931-948.

Bryant, R.A., Marossezesky, J.E., Crooks, J., Baguley, I. & Gurka, J. (2000). Coping style and post-traumatic stress disorder following severe traumatic brain injury, *Brain Injury, 14*, 175-180.

Bryant, R.A., Marosszezecky, J.E., Crooks, J., Baguley, I.G., Gurka, J.A. & Joseph, A. (1999). Interaction of posttraumatic stress disorder and chronic pain following traumatic brain injury. *Journal of Head Injury Rehabilitation, 14*, 588-594.

Cohen, M., Oksenberg, A., Snir, D., & Stern, M.J. (1994). Temporally related changes in sleep complaints in traumatic brain injured patients. *Journal of Neurology, Neurosurgery and Psychiatry, 55*, 313-315.

Coughlan, A.K., & Storey, P. (1988). The Wimbledon Self-Report Scale: Emotional and mood appraisal. *Clinical Rehabilitation, 2*, 207-213.

Deb, S., Lyons, I. & Koutzoukis, C (1999). Neurobehavioural symptoms one year after a head injury. *British Journal of Psychiatry, 174*, 360-365.

Davey, G.L & Tallis, F. (1994). New Worrying: perspectives on theory, assessment, and treatment. New York: Wiley.

Dinan, T.G., & Mobayed, M. (1992). Treatment resistance of depression after head injury: a preliminary study of amitriptyline response. *Acta Psychiatrica Scandinavica, 85(4)*, 292-294.

Dunlop, T.W., Udvarhelyi, G.B., Stedem, A.F.A, O'Connor, J.M.C., Isaacs, M.L., Puig, J.G. & Mather, J.H (1991). Comparison of patients with and without emotional/behavioral deterioration during the first year after traumatic brain injury. *Journal of Neuropsychiatry and Clinical Neurosciences, 3*, 150-156.

Eames, P. (2001). Distinguishing the neuropsychiatric, psychiatric, and psychological consequences of acquired brain injury. In R.L.L. Woods & T.M. McMillan (Eds.), *Neurobehavioural Disability & Social Handicap Following Traumatic Brain Injury.* Hove: Psychology Press.

Finset, A. & Andersson, S. (2000). Coping strategies in patients with acquired brain-injury: Relationships between coping, apathy, depression and lesion location. *Brain Injury, 14*, 887-905.

Fleminger, S., Oliver, D., Williams, W.H., & Evans J.J. (in press). The Neuropsychiatry of Depression after Brain Injury. Special issue of *Neuropsychological Rehabilitation*.

Folkman, S., Lazarus, R.S., Dunkel-Schetter, C. et al. (1986). The dynamics of stressful encounters: Cognitive appraisal, coping, and encounter outcomes. *Journal of Personality & Social Psychology, 50*, 992-1003.

Garske G.G. & Thomas, K.R. (1992). Self-reported self-esteem and depression: Indexes of psychosocial adjustment following severe traumatic brain injury. *Rehabilitation Counselling Bulletin, 36*, 44-52.

Harris, D.P. (1997). Outcome measures and a program evaluation model for postacute brain injury rehabilitation. *Journal of Outcomes Measurement, 1*, 23-30.

Harris, E.C., Barraclough, B. (1997) Suicide as an outcome for mental disorders: A meta-analyis. *British Journal of Psychiatry, 170*, 205-228.

Hickling, E.J., Gillen, R., Blanchard, E.B., et al., (1998). Traumatic brain injury and posttraumatic stress disorder: a preliminary investigation of neuropsychological test results in PTSD secondary to motor vehicle accidents. *Brain Injury, 12(4)*, 265-274.

Hibbard, M.R., Uysal, S., Keple, K., Bogdany, J. & Silver, J. (1998). Axis I psychopathology in individuals with traumatic brain injury. *Journal of Head Trauma Rehabilitation, 13*, 24-39.

Horowitz, M., Wilner, N. & Alvarez, W. (1979). Impact of events scale: A measure of subjective stress. *Psychosomatic Medicine, 41*, 209-218.

Jackson, H. (1988). Brain, cognition and grief. *Aphasiology, 2*, 89-92.

Jorge, R.E., Robinson, R.G., Starkstein, S.E. & Arndt, S.V. (1993). Depression and anxiety following traumatic brain injury. *Journal of Neuropsychiatry & Clinical Neurosciences, 5*, 369-374.

Judd, T. (1999). Neuropsychotherapy & community integration: Brain illness, emotions & behaviour. In A.E. Puente & C.P. Reynolds (Eds), *Critical Issues in Neuropsychology*. London: Kluwer Academic.

Kendall, E & Terry D.J. (1996). Psychosocial adjustment following closed head injury: A model for understanding individual differences and predicting outcome. *Neuropsychological Rehabilitation, 6*, 101-132.

King, N.S. (1997). Posttraumatic stress disorder and head injury as a dual diagnosis: Islands of memory as a mechanism. *Journal of Neurology, Neurosurgery & Psychiatry, 62 (1)*, 82-84.

Klonoff, P. & Lage, G.A. (1995). Suicide in patients with traumatic brain injury: Risk and prevention. *Journal of Head Trauma Rehabilitation, 10*, 16-24.

Kreutzer, J.S., Seel, R.T. & Gourley, E. (2001). The prevalence and symptoms of depression after traumatic brain injury: A comprehensive examination. *Brain Injury, 15*, 563-576.

Kreutzer, J.S., Witol, A. & Marwitz, J.H. (1997). Alcohol and drug use among young persons with traumatic brain injury. In E.D. Bigler, E. Clark, et al. (Eds.),*Childhood Head Injury: Diagnosis, Assessment & Intervention*. Austin: Pro-ed.

Lewis, G. (2001). Mental health after head injury. *Journal of Neurology, Neurosurgery & Psychiatry, 71*, 431.

Lishman, W. (1998). *Organic Psychiatry (3rd ed.)*. Oxford: Blackwell Science.

Macmillan, P.J., Martelli, M.F., Hart, R.P. & Zasler, N.D. (2002). Pre-injury status and adaptation following traumatic brain injury. Brain Injury, *16*, 41-49.

Malia, K., Powell, T. & Torode, M. (1995). Coping and psychosocial function after brain injury. *Brain Injury, 9*, 607-618.

Manchester, D. & Woods, R.L.L. (2001). Applying cognitive therapy in neurobehavioural rehabilitation. In R.L.L. Woods & T. M. McMillan (Eds), *Neurobehavioural Disability & Social Handicap Following Traumatic Brain Injury*. Hove: Psychology Press.

Mann, J.J., Waternaux, C., Haas, G.L. & Malone, K.M. (1999). Toward a clinical model of suicidal behaviour in psychiatric patients. *American Journal of Psychiatry, 156*, 181-189.

Markowitsch, H.J. (1998). Cognitive Neuroscience of Memory, *Neurocase, 4*, 429-435.

Marin, R.S. (1990). Differential diagnosis and classification of apathy. *American Journal of Psychiatry, 147(1)*, 22-30.

Marin, R.S. (1991). Apathy: a neuropsychiatric syndrome. *Journal of Neuropsychiatry & Clinical Neurosciences, 3(3)*, 243-54.

McKeown, J., McGuffin, P. & Robinson, P. (1984). Obsessive-compulsive neurosis following head injury. A report of four cases. *British Journal of Psychiatry, 144*, 190-192.

McMillan, T.M. (1996). Post-traumatic stress disorder following minor and severe closed head injury: 10 single cases. *Brain Injury, 10*, 749-758.

McNeil, J. & Greenwood, R. (1996). Can PTSD occur without amnesia for the precipitating event? *Cognitive Neuropsychiatry, 1*, 239-246.

McLellan, D.L. (1997). Introduction to Rehabilitation. In B.A. Wilson & D.L. McLellan (Eds.) *Rehabilitation Studies Handbook* (pp. 1-21). Cambridge: University Press.

Moore, A.D. & Stambrook, M. (1995a). Cognitive moderators of outcome following traumatic brain injury: A conceptual model and implications for rehabilitation. *Brain Injury, 9*, 109-130.

Moore A.D. & Stambrook, M. (1992 b): Coping strategies and locus of control following traumatic brain injury: A cluster analytic approach. *Brain Injury, 6*, 89-94.

Moos, R. & Schaefer, J.A. (1984). The crisis of physical illness: An overview and conceptual approach. In Moos, R. (Ed.), *Coping with Physical Illness: New directions*. New York: Plenum Press.

Oddy, M. & McMillan, T.M. (2001). Future directions: Brain injury services in 2010. In R.L.L. Woods & T.M. McMillan (Eds.), *Neurobehavioural Disability & Social Handicap Following Traumatic Brain Injury*. Hove: Psychology Press.

Ohry, A., Rattock J., & Solomon, Z. (1996). Post-traumatic stress disorder in brain injury patients, *Brain Injury, 10*, 687-695.

Ownsworth, T.L. & Oei,T. (1998). Depression after traumatic brain injury: Conceptualization and treatment considerations. *Brain Injury, 12*, 735-751.

Ponsford, J., Sloan, S., & Snow, P. (1995). *Traumatic Brain Injury: Rehabilitation for everyday adaptive living*. Psychology Press, Hove.

Prigatano, G.P. (1986). *Neuropsychological Rehabilitation After Brain Injury*. Baltimore:John Hopkins University.

Prigatano, G.P., Fordyce, D.J., Ziener, H.K., Roueche, J.R., Pepping, M. & Wood, B.D. (1984). Neuropsychological rehabilitation and closed head injury in young adults. *Journal of Neurology, Neurosurgery and Psychiatry, 9*, 91-102.

Rosenthal, M., & Bond, M.R. (1990). Behavioural and psychiatric sequelae. In M. Rosenthal, E.R. Griffith, M.R. Bond, & J.D. Miller (Eds.), *Rehabilitation of the Adult and Child with Traumatic Brain Injury, 2nd ed.* (pp. 179-192). Philadelphia: F.A. Davis.

Roth A.D., Fonagy P. (1996). *What works for whom? A critical review of psychotherapy research*. New York, Guilford Press.

Rothbaum, B.D., Meadows, E.A., Resick, P. & Foy, D.W. (2000). Cognitive behavior therapy: Guidelines for treatment of PTSD. *Journal of Traumatic Stress, 13*, 558-562.

Satz, P., Forney, D.L., Zaucha, K., Asarnow, R.B., Light, R., McCleary, C., Levin, H., Kelly, D., Bergsneider, M., Hovda, D., Martin, N., Namerow, N. & Becker, D. (1998). Depression, cognition, and functional correlates of recovery outcome after traumatic brain injury. *Brain Injury,12,* 537-553.

Sbordone, R.J. & Leiter, J.C. (1995). Mild traumatic brain injury does not produce posttraumatic stress disorder. *Brain Injury, 9,* 405-412.

Scheutzow, M.H. & Wiercisiewski, D.R. (1999). Panic disorder in a patient with traumatic brain injury: A case report and discussion. *Brain Injury, 13,* 705-714.

Sloan, R.W., Brown, K.W., & Pentland, B. (1992). Fluoxetine as a treatment of emotional lability after brain injury. *Brain Injury, 6,* 315-319.

Symonds, C.P. (1937). Mental disorder following head injury. *Proceedings of_the Royal Society of Medicine, 30,* 1081-1094.

Symonds, C.P. & Russell, W.R. (1943). Accidental head injuries. Prognosis in service patients. *Lancet,* ic, 7-10.

Tate, R. (1998). 'It is not only the kind of injury that matters, but the kind of head': The contribution of premorbid psychosocial factors to rehabilitation outcomes after severe traumatic brain injury. *Neuropsychological Rehabilitation, 8,* 1-18.

Tate, R., Simpson, G., Flanagan, S. & Coffey, M. (1997). Completed suicide after traumatic brain injury. *Journal of Head Trauma Rehabilitation, 12,* 16-28.

Teasdale, T. & Engberg A.W. (2001). Suicide after traumatic brain injury: a population study. *Journal of Neurology, Neurosurgery and Psychiatry, 71,* 436-440.

Turner-Stokes, L., & Hassan, N. (2002). Depression after stroke: a review of the evidence base to inform the development of an integrated care pathway. Part 2: Treatment alternatives, *Clinical Rehabilitation, 16(3),* pp. 248-260.

Williams, W.H, Evans, J.J., & Fleminger, S. (in press). Neurorehabilitation and Cognitive Behaviour Therapy of Anxiety Disorders after Brain Injury: An overview and a Case Illustration of Obsessive Compulsive Disorder. Special Issue, *Neuropsychological Rehabilitation.*

Williams, W.H., Evans, J.J., Needham, P. & Wilson, B.A. (2002). Neurological,cognitive and attributional predictors of posttraumatic stress symptoms after traumatic brain injury. *Journal of Traumatic Stress, 15,* 397-401.

Williams, W.H., Evans, J.J. & Wilson, B.A. (1999). Outcome measures for survivors of acquired brain injury in day and outpatient neurorehabilitation programmes. *Neuropsychological Rehabilitation, 9,* 421-436.

Williams, W.H., Evans, J.J., Wilson, B.A., & Needham, P. (in press). Prevalence of post-traumatic stress disorder symptoms after severe traumatic brain injury in a representative community sample. *Brain. Injury*

Williams, W.H. & Jones, R.S. (1997). Teaching cognitive self-regulation of independence and emotion control skills. In D. Dagnan, K. Loumidis, & BizaKroeze (Eds.), *Cognitive Therapy for People with Learning Disabilities.* London: Routledge.

Williams, W.H., Williams, J.M.G., & Ghadiali, E.J. (1998). Autobiographical memory in traumatic brain injury: Neuropsychological and mood predictors of recall. *Neuropsychological Rehabilitation, 8,* 43-60.

Wilson, B.A. (1989). Models of cognitive rehabilitation. In P. Eames & R. Wood (Eds.), *Models of Brain Rehabilitation* (pp. 117-141). London: Chapman & Hall.

Wilson, B.A. (1997). Cognitive rehabilitation: How it is and how it might be. *Journal of the International Neuropsychological Society, 3,* 487-496.

Wilson, B.A. (2001). Cognitive Rehabilitation: Science or Art. Paper presented at the *British Psychological Society Conference,* Glasgow.

Zafonte, R.D, Cullen, N., & Lexell, J. (2002) Serotonin agents in the treatment of acquired brain injury. *Journal-of-Head-Trauma-Rehabilitation, 17(4),* 322-334.

Zigmound A.S., Snaith R.P. (1983). The Hospital Anxiety and Depression Scale. *Acta Psychiatrica Scandinavica, 67,* 361-370.

Chapter 8

ENHANCING OUTCOMES AFTER TRAUMATIC BRAIN INJURY: A SOCIAL REHABILITATION APPROACH

Robyn L Tate[1], Barbara Strettles [2], Thelma Osoteo[2]

[1] Rehabilitation Studies Unit, Department of Medicine, University of Sydney and Royal Rehabilitation Centre Sydney, Australia
[2] Brain Injury Rehabilitation Unit, Liverpool Hospital, Sydney, Australia

'Adults with disabilities and their families want the same things other people do – a place to live, a job, an education, recreation, friendships and family life.'
Racino & Williams (1994, p. 39)

Concepts and principles

Social functioning after traumatic brain injury (TBI) can be conceptualised from at least two perspectives. Firstly, disturbance in social functioning as an *impairment*, directly caused by the TBI. These executive impairments that straddle the domains of cognition and behaviour frequently arise as a result of frontal systems dysfunction. Included are difficulties with social skills (Godfrey & Shum, 2000; Marsh, 1999), pragmatic communication (McDonald,

Togher, & Code, 1999; McGann & Werven, 1995), social problem solving (Levine, van Horn, & Curtis, 1993; Kendall, Shum, Halson, Bunning, & The, 1997), and behavioural controls (Alderman, Fry, & Youngson, 1995; Medd & Tate, 2000; Wood, 1987). An alternative perspective conceptualises disturbance in social functioning after TBI as *disablement,* affecting three broad domains in particular: occupational activities, interpersonal relationships, and independent living skills. It is not only impairments in executive functioning that may cause disablement in social functioning – any type of motor-sensory or neuropsychological impairment may also adversely affect social functioning; for instance, hemiparesis restricting a person's ability to play sport, amnesia limiting a person's capacity to engage in and remember conversations, thereby impacting on their capacity to maintain interpersonal relationships and so forth.

This volume contains a number of chapters that are relevant to the first perspective of social functioning, impairments, (see in particular Chapter 4 on executive deficits and Chapter 9 on behaviour and conduct disorders). Rehabilitation of impairments in social aspects of executive functions is becoming more widely discussed and incorporated into rehabilitation programs (see above chapters and also Grattan & Ghahramanlou, 2002; Sohlberg & Mateer, 2001). In order to avoid repetition, the present chapter focuses on the second perspective: social functioning as disablement after TBI, much of which also applies to acquired brain injury in general. We present our rehabilitation approach to maximising a person's social functioning after TBI and provide an overview of our clinical practice.

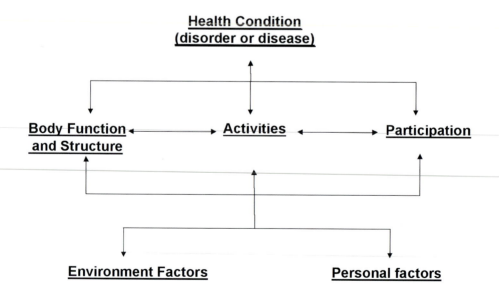

Fig. 1. International Classification of Function.

There is not a direct correspondence between impairments and their effects upon social functioning. The International Classification of Functioning (ICF, WHO, 2001) provides a helpful framework to understand the complex set of factors contributing to social functioning after TBI and other health conditions. The ICF differs in significant ways from the original model, the International Classification of Impairments, Disabilities and Handicaps (ICIDH, WHO, 1980), including: (1) the use of neutral terminology (Activity replaces Disability; Participation replaces Handicap), (2) use of the term Disablement in a generic sense, without specific demarcation between limitations in Activity and restriction in Participation, and (3) the introduction of Contextual Factors (both environmental and personal) which may exert a facilitating effect or cause barriers to participation (see Fig. 1).

Figure 2 illustrates the way in which the ICF is interactive and different outcomes may be achieved depending on various configurations in impairments, disablement and contextual factors. Impairments caused by TBI (whether neuropsychological e.g., memory impairment, or motor-sensory e.g., dysarthria) may cause limitation in activities (e.g., at the general level, work) and restriction in the person's capacity to participate in everyday life situations (e.g., at the specific level, unable to do their job as a receptionist). Contextual factors will influence the outcome, however: an understanding employer may alter the work duties so that they are compatible with the person's impairments (e.g., changing reception work for clerical duties).

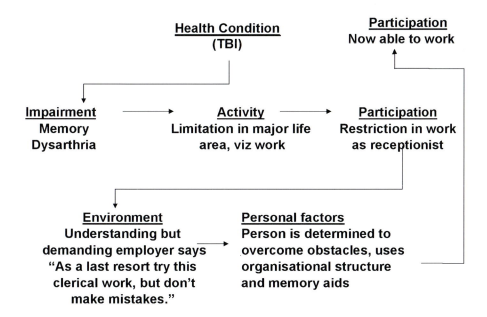

Fig. 2. International Classification of Functioning: Contextual factors.

Moreover, the individual's personal qualities in terms of, for example, their level of drive and determination to be employed may result in them using organisational strategies and memory aids as part of their work practice to compensate for their memory impairment, thereby reducing or even eliminating disablement in the work and employment domain.

The ICF has many comparable features to other models of adjustment after TBI described in the literature. Thirty years ago Lishman (1973) drew a distinction between direct effects of the injury (in WHO terms, impairments and disabilities) and indirect effects of the injury (in WHO terms, contextual variables). Recent work (e.g., Godfrey, Knight, & Partridge, 1996; Kendall & Terry, 1996; Moore, & Stambrook, 1995) has seen more refined analyses of the way in which outcome and adjustment are influenced by impairments, disabilities, and contextual variables (personal and environmental resources), collectively termed antecedents. An important contribution of this research describes the way in which the impact of the antecedent variables on outcome and adjustment is mediated by the individual's cognitive appraisals of the situation and particular coping strategies.

Thus, for the purposes of the present chapter, 'social' refers to the effects of impairments on the person's daily activities and participation in everyday life, as mediated by contextual and other factors. Thence, social rehabilitation refers to procedures used to maximise resumption of social aspects of participation in daily activities, particularly for independent living, interpersonal relationships, work and leisure activities. This perspective of disablement in social functioning has considerable overlap with the literature on community integration. The aforementioned three broad domains (occupational activities, interpersonal relationships, and independent living) are those we used in our earlier work examining psychosocial outcomes after TBI (Tate, Lulham, Broe, Strettles, & Pfaff, 1989) and later in developing a measuring instrument of psychosocial reintegration (Tate, Hodgkinson, Veerabangsa, & Maggiotto, 1999; Tate, Pfaff, Veerabangsa, & Hodgkinson, in submission). Subsequent to our initial report, other researchers have independently affirmed the relevance of these three areas of social functioning for the TBI group (McColl, Carlson, Johnston et al., 1998; Willer, Rosenthal, Kreutzer, Gordon, & Rempel, 1993).

In the opinion of Ylvisaker and Feeney (Feeney, Ylvisaker, Rosen, & Greene, 2001; Ylvisaker & Feeney, 1998, 2000), traditional rehabilitation models use a hierarchical treatment approach: first addressing neurologically-based impairments; then, if difficulties persist, activity limitation; and finally participation restriction. Their clinical practice reverses the hierarchy so that the first line of attack is to increase participation (in ICIDH terminology, reduce handicap). They enumerate a number of principles or 'critical intervention themes', summarised in Table 1, which guide their rehabilitation practice, and they argue for rehabilitation that is contextualised, collaborative, and person-focused. Their approach arises from their experience with individuals who frequently exhibit challenging behaviours (generally premor-

Table 1. Critical intervention themes.

Adapted from Ylvisaker and Feeney (2000)	
Context	The context of delivery of rehabilitation needs to involve personally meaningful themes, activities, settings and interactions.
Everyday routines and everyday people	Appropriately structured everyday activities provide the best context. People relevant to the life of the person with TBI (eg. family, work supervisors) should be involved in their rehabilitation
Apprenticeship training and collaboration	Information and skill is acquired *during* task completion. Supports and mediation are provided initially, then systematically withdrawn at appropriate times. Professional staff work in collaboration with clients to achieve goals.
Reconstructing a sense of self	Impairments and the associated activity limitation and participation restriction necessitate that the individual restructures their sense of self and have successful experiences associated with their new identity.

bid, which are then compounded by impairments from the TBI). It addresses the aforementioned multifactorial contributions to adjustment, and thereby provides a helpful model for clinical practice after discharge from inpatient rehabilitation.

It is well known that TBI spans the gamut from the most minor of injuries to those of extreme severity, in which a person can be unresponsive for many months. Our work focuses largely on those with severe injuries, with durations of posttraumatic amnesia (PTA) usually in excess of one week. Yet the nature and degree of impairments and levels of recovery, as measured by scales such as the Glasgow Outcome Scale (GOS, Jennett & Bond, 1975; Jennett, Snoek, Bond, & Brooks, 1981), show extreme individual variability. Confusion has often arisen in distinguishing between severity of the initial injury and severity of outcome, but it is far from the case that a person with a severe injury necessarily has severe impairments or severe disability. Although there is a significant correlation between severity of injury and degree of recovery, levels of outcome of individuals with severe injuries span the ranges of GOS categories. For example, at an average of six years posttrauma, our consecutive series of 100 severely injured rehabilitation admissions (mean duration of PTA 11.6 weeks, with PTA in excess of one month in 74%) comprised 49 individuals with Good Recovery, 27 with Moderate Disability, 17 with Severe Disability, none were in the Persistent Vegetative State and seven had died (Tate et al., 1989). It thus follows that goals of social rehabilitation will be very much dependent upon, in the first instance, the nature and degree of disablement.

Within this constraint, the philosophical tenet that guides our rehabilitation service is that all individuals are entitled to work or have alternative meaningful occupational activity, be part of a social network, and live in their own home in the community. Also implied, is that they have access to community resources and activities, in the form of transport. It is helpful to put these principles in the context of those other clinicians have described to empower people with disability from TBI, as summarised in Table 2. At a more specific level, Durgin (2000) provides a thought-provoking analysis of strategies to combat traditional, over-restrictive practices, as well as those to permit considered and reasonable risk-taking to enable the person's return to community living.

Table 2. Principles guiding community integration after TBI.

Racino and Williams (1994)	Willer and Corrigan (1994)
1. People using the services and their families know themselves best	1. No two individuals with acquired brain injury are alike
2. Services must promote self-sufficiency and community membership	2. Skills are more likely to generalize when taught in the environment where they are to be used
3. Services should be functional and take place in relevant environments	3. Environments are easier to change than people
4. People using services should have the option to hire, manage, and fire their own staff	4. Community integration should be holistic
5. All people with TBI have a place to participate and contribute in the community	5. Life is a place-and-train venture
6. Support resources includes 'natural' supports, community supports, and personal assistance services	6. Natural supports last longer than professionals
7. People should live in generic, affordable, and accessible housing within communities and neighbourhoods	7. Interventions must not do more harm than good
8. The provision of support services should be separated from the selection of a place to live	8. The service system presents many of the barriers to community integration
9. Medical services should only be provided for medical issues	9. Respect for the individual is paramount
10. Hope is an essential fuel for the future	10. Needs of individuals last a lifetime; so should their resources

Social Rehabilitation in Practice: the Liverpool Hospital Approach

a) Structure of the service

The following overview of our clinical practice draws upon the infrastructure provided by a government-funded, regionally-based, specialist TBI rehabilitation service located at Liverpool Hospital in Sydney, Australia. This service, originally established at Lidcombe Hospital in the 1970s (inpatient unit in 1976 and community service in 1979), has been described elsewhere (Broe, Lulham, Strettles, Tate, Walsh, & Ross, 1982). Since 1989, the Liverpool service has been one of the 13 participating units in the New South Wales Brain Injury Rehabilitation Program – a state-wide program initiated as a partnership between the Department of Health and the Motor Accidents Authority of New South Wales.

As shown in Table 3, selection criteria to the service are few and liberal: age, place of residence, and having sustained a TBI. The admission criteria are occasionally waived in exceptional circumstances. For example, young people from the region with other types of acquired brain injury, most commonly hypoxia or stroke, are admitted if there are no other suitable services to meet their needs, such as dealing with confusion and agitation in a mobile patient

Table 3. Liverpool hospital brain injury rehabilitation service.

Admission criteria:
- Age at injury 16-60 years
- Resident in geographical catchment area (South Western and Southern Sydney Area Health Services – population approx. 1.1 million)
- Sustained traumatic brain injury

Clinical service components:
- 16-bed inpatient unit
- 4-bed transitional living unit located in the community
- 4-bed respite cottage located in the community (Camden House)
- multi-disciplinary inpatient team
- multi-disciplinary community team
- *Head-2-Work* program located in the community in an industrial factory

Staffing levels for community team (16.7 full-time equivalents):
- 0.6 team leader
- 5 case managers
- 1 clinical psychologist
- 1.6 medical rehabilitation specialists
- 1.5 neuropsychologists
- 2 occupational therapists
- 1 physiotherapist
- 1 recreation officer
- 1 speech pathologist
- 2 social workers

during the post-acute stages. In its current configuration, the rehabilitation service has a number of components, with the community team drawing heavily upon the transitional living unit (TLU), respite cottage, and *Head-2-Work* program. This integrated service allows for a continuum of care from the time of inpatient admission.

The focus of the present chapter on social rehabilitation describes services provided by the community team, after the person has been discharged from inpatient rehabilitation. This service has not arisen because it is a cheaper option than inpatient rehabilitation, as appears to be driving the agenda of some programs described from North America, but rather the service exists because many people are discharged from inpatient rehabilitation with continuing limitations and restrictions in everyday living that call for continued therapy and provision of services.

b) Cornerstones of the service

There are four essential clinical features of the community service. It is nonselective, and the rehabilitation programs are needs-driven, community-based, and largely individually-focused.

(1) Individuals are unselected

The underlying philosophy of the service is one of equity of access to rehabilitation. Thus, it is nonselective and all individuals are accepted who meet the previously described very liberal admission criteria. People are not rejected on the basis of the nature or severity of impairments, nor their psychosocial and economic backgrounds. Consequently, individuals are often admitted who are difficult to work with and who may not have favourable prognoses: those with challenging behaviours, problems with awareness, current substance usage, history of and/or current psychiatric symptomatology, criminal histories, previous unemployment, as well as those who do not have private health or other type of insurance or compensation.

(2) Needs-driven rehabilitation

There are three aspects to a needs-driven rehabilitation service. Firstly, all eligible people are admitted to the service who have needs, irrespective of the time posttrauma. One implication of this is that the number of people involved in the service at any one time is large. During the calendar year 2000, 467 individuals received services from the community team (Tate, Strettles, & Osoteo, in submission). The workload for the 17 staff in the team is thus intense, with 8,046 occasions of service provided during 2000. Secondly, it is recognised that no single profession has the requisite skills and expertise to address the diverse range of needs presented by people with TBI and their families. Thus, a multidisciplinary team is necessary to effect social rehabilitation and maximal community reintegration.

Finally, a needs-driven approach means that there is no designated timeframe for an individual's involvement in a program. Essentially, an individual and/or family can be a member of the service while-ever that person has needs that the service can meet. Thus when some goals are met (e.g., accommodation in the community), others goals can be set which build upon previous ones (e.g., being able to travel independently by public transport). Furthermore, as circumstances change new issues arise that are addressed, as the following example illustrates:

In 1987, at age 45, Bill sustained a minor brain injury, but subsequently deteriorated and at two days posttrauma was in status epilepticus. Left temporo-parietal subdural haematomata were repeatedly evacuated, both before and after insertion of a ventriculo-peritoneal shunt. In 1988, after 12 months inpatient rehabilitation, he was discharged to the care of his parents and referred to the community team. Although independent in basic self-care activities, Bill was not otherwise inde-pendent, largely because of his neuropsychological deficits (memory disorder, cognitive rigidity, perseveration and marked inertia). The community team continues involvement in Bill's case at the time of writing. Over this 14-year period, there have been 119 occasions of service from the community team. These were not evenly spread across the years, but rather waxed and waned – there have been years when Bill has been discharged from the service, but re-referral occurs when specific issues arise, such as the death of his mother in 1998 and father's subsequent illness. At that point, respite care was made available, he was re-assessed in the TLU for independent living, accommodation options and community activities were explored, with input from the case manager, occupational therapist and social worker.

Thus a second philosophical tenet is the commitment to provision of services throughout the person's life, based on the recognition that needs and circum-stances change over time. In our experience, rehabilitation after TBI is not usually a discrete 'repair and fix' job; rather, for many people it is a lifelong process of adaptation.

(3) Community-based therapy programs

When rehabilitation is community-based, there is the opportunity for it to be conducted in context. Clinicians have often pointed to the importance of contextually-based therapies (Cervelli, 1990; Hayden, Moreault, LeBlanc, & Plenger, 2000; Sloan, Balicki, & Winkler, 1996; Ylvisaker & Feeney, 2000). Opportunities for social rehabilitation in inpatient settings are often fairly contrived and artificial, and hence social rehabilitation is best conducted in the community after the patient has been discharged from inpatient rehabili-tation. Moreover, during inpatient rehabilitation the energies of the patient and family are usually focused on recovery of more basic functions – mobil-ity, communication, cognition and activities of daily living. It is generally the case that they are not emotionally ready to tackle the social consequences of TBI until around the time of discharge. The risk is, however, that once the patient is discharged from inpatient rehabilitation, social rehabilitation is not conducted at all. This is because the focus of many outreach teams is on the coordination and liaison component of case management, in which the person is referred to other services as required, rather than the provision of those services within the team. The Liverpool approach is distinctive in that case managers work in partnership with therapists. The advantage is that the individual receives a holistic, coordinated, integrated and planned service. The people and their families become well known to team members, who are then in a position to address current needs and anticipate future ones.

A central aspect of the rehabilitation program is networking with other government and non-government agencies and working in tandem with generic services provided in the community. Frequently, there are barriers to accessing generic services because, in Australia at least, these focus on older persons or those with disabilities from other causes that make such services unsuitable for the group with TBI. Closely related, is the fact that staff members involved in generic services generally do not understand issues pertaining to acquired brain injury. This applies both to accessing services to enhance community living (e.g., housing support, recreational options), as well as getting assistance in times of crisis, such as suicidality. Recommended practice in the latter domain is for specialist brain injury services to work together with generic mental health and other services (Kuipers & Lancaster, 2000; Tate, Simpson, Flanagan, & Coffey, 1998). By providing services within the team we can support people while they are accessing services to optimise the chances of success, as Bill's previous example demonstrates:

When Bill's mother died and his father's health was failing, the goal of independent housing was explored. Following a four-week assessment in the TLU, the case manager sought the social worker's involvement, who met with Bill and made application to the Department of Housing. This was not restricted to completing the forms and paperwork, but rather involved a counselling approach to help Bill become more aware of the issues involved in independent living, and assist him to generate his own solutions to potential problems. The social worker attended meetings between Bill and the Department of Housing to ensure correct information was given and that Bill was not disadvantaged by staff not understanding his disabilities and his inability to follow through the process. Because of the social worker's advocacy role, she became an important support person for Bill at this time. The occupational therapist's involvement initially focused intensively on household management, particularly the development of strategies for financial management and budgeting for bills, which had arisen from his independent living assessment as an area of special difficulty.

(4) Individually-focused rehabilitation

An individually-focused approach allows for establishing an active rehabilitation program, driven by goal planning, which is specific to the individual's unique constellation of impairments, functional limitations and restrictions, environmental circumstances, and personal characteristics. The individually-focused approach does not imply that the person is treated in isolation, nor that he or she is a passive entity who has therapeutic procedures *applied* to him or her. Rather, the rehabilitation process is tri-level involving the person, their family and their culture/community. The therapist or case manager acts as a facilitator, with the ultimate aim being to gradually withdraw supports during a transition phase so that the person becomes more independent. A hierarchical approach is adopted which guides the plan of action:

- first provide information,
- then provide the means (depending on the issues and the person's level of disablement, this may range from assisting with transport, making funds available, establishing environmental structures or using verbal prompts),
- and deal with issues that interfere with independent functioning,
- to ultimately enhance the individual's independence with the aim of the person generating their own outcomes with staff facilitating the process.

The level of disablement is important and for a proportion of the group with severe disability the rehabilitation program may be confined to the first three steps because their cognitive limitations mean that the best they can achieve will be access to services, and it may not be possible for them to generate their own outcomes. The goal for other clients with less disability is to optimise their independence, as shown in the following example:

Mick, a 25-year old jockey who lived in the country, fell from a horse in 1999 and was admitted to a local regional hospital. His initial Glasgow Coma Scale (GCS, Teasdale & Jennett, 1974) score was 15, but he was transferred to (another) Sydney hospital for neurosurgical management of a right frontal haemorrhage. Duration of PTA was 10 days. Mick's progress and functional recovery was good, and he was discharged home where he lived with his cousin, with referral to the regional brain injury rehabilitation outreach team. By 13 months posttrauma, Mick's family were concerned that he seemed to have difficulties coping and he moved to Sydney to live with his parents. The regional brain injury team referred him to our service. The assessments identified a constellation of problems: speech and language impairments, memory, planning and organising difficulties and depression mainly because he was unable to return to his former job. Therapies and strategy training with the speech pathologist, neuropsychologist and clinical psychologist were successful and the occupational therapist and case manager addressed vocational options. Mick was initially assessed and retrained at the unit's *Head-2-Work* program, and subsequently enrolled in an animal attendant course at a local community education college. Requirements of the course involved a workplace component and Mick was referred to *BreakThru*, a community supported work program. They arranged a job at Wattle Tree Farm, a local tourist attraction with bush animals, and provided job coaching and support. Mick's program with the community team spanned a 14-month period, and he was discharged from the service in April 2001, at that point still working at Wattle Tree Farm.

c) Clinical pathways

The clinical pathway of the service is described in Figure 3. Individuals are referred to the service either directly from the inpatient unit or the community, the latter including referrals from other services (such as general practitioners, solicitors, health services) and self/family referral. Referral to any part or stage of the service is possible, and is independent of whether, where or when they received other services related to their brain injury. Persons who are accepted to the service may be new admissions, or previous members of the service who were discharged but have been re-referred, usually because new issues have arisen with which they require assistance.

All persons accepted by the service attend a clinic, run by rehabilitation physicians four times during the week. The purpose of the clinic is not only for medical reasons, but also to identify pertinent issues via a psychosocial interview. New referrals are discussed at the weekly case conference, from

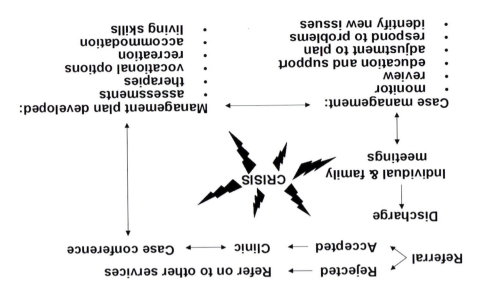

Fig. 3. Clinical pathway of Brain Injury Rehabilitation Unit.

which a management plan is developed. The management plan may include referral to staff of the community team for other services, which are both centre-based and provided in the home or community. Goal planning is conducted with each individual by various team members, along the lines of the process described by McMillan and Sparkes (1999).

The rehabilitation process is dynamic and involves initial fine-tuning and adjustment of the goals and rehabilitation plan to suit the individual/family needs. Adaptations to the management plan may occur for a variety of reasons, common ones being family dynamics and cultural expectations of the client and family, as the following example shows:

> Omar was a 28 year-old man of Middle Eastern background who sustained severe cognitive and physical disabilities as a result of a car accident in 1998. Following extensive inpatient rehabilitation, he remained severely disabled and was admitted to the TLU, specifically to increase his independence in personal care. Upon discharge home to his family he was able to manage personal care, requiring only minimal supervision. But these gains were soon eroded because the family insisted on doing everything for him, and this was Omar's expectation also. In their culture, a 'sick' person is cared for, and allowing such a person to do activities that are difficult for them is not the way a loved one should be treated (see Simpson, Mohr, & Redman, 2000). After negotiation, the family allowed a roster of paid carers to be involved in supervising and monitoring Omar's personal care, thereby implementing the discharge plan of maintaining his level of independence in personal care. Introduction of the carers was not without its difficulties, however, because the family did not understand their role – the family perceived that the carers, in merely 'watching' Omar, were not busy enough to earn their salary and so extra duties, such as housework, were requested. This necessitated the case manager negotiating a structure for the carers and educating the family about the carers' role, that Omar was not 'sick', and the importance of him doing things for himself.

The community case conference, combined with case management, mainly serves as the reporting mechanism for program monitoring, review and adjustment. As such, the case conference does not include the person or family, although we acknowledge that some clinicians advocate the active involvement of the individual and family in case conferences. Kneipp (1995) describes this process in detail, but she recognises that it is time consuming: team meetings are usually held monthly and the report described one three-hour meeting for a single individual, held in his or her own home. Our constraint is one of sheer numbers, with an annual caseload of around 500 individuals and their families.

Case management is integral to the organisation and coordination of the person's program, but additionally case managers are also the front-line people who frequently provide education and support to the individual and family, assess and respond to problems, resolve conflicts, and identify new issues as they arise. Hence, they work with the people in a very personal way, and there is nothing that the service will not do, literally adopting the 'whatever it takes' (Willer & Corrigan, 1994) philosophy or 'what can we do to make this happen?' (DePompei, Frye, DuFore, & Hunt, 2001, p. 236). Regular meetings with the person and family, as well as other service providers, are held with relevant community team members. At these meetings progress is reviewed and new goals, including discharge, are discussed. As Figure 3 shows, the process is not unidirectional, but rather is interactive and recursive. Moreover, in some instances the process can stop along the way, and intensity of involvement can also vary, until all issues are solved, goals are achieved and no further goals are identified, at which point discharge is an option. However, if goals are continuing or new goals are identified and new plans developed, then the individual will remain in the system. Crisis management is an important part of the service and will cut across established plans and programs. The following example shows the typical range of issues seen by the community team and methods of management:

Lee, aged 24, sustained severe TBI and other injuries (soft tissue and loss of vision in her left eye) as a result of a motor vehicle accident in 1998. She had migrated to Australia from South East Asia 10 years previously with her husband, 13-year old sister, and parents, and had been working in a retail factory for the previous two years. Initial GCS score was 8, duration of PTA was 58 days, and she required craniotomy to evacuate right extradural and subdural haematomata. On admission to the rehabilitation unit at 7 weeks posttrauma, she was agitated and percutaneous endoscopic gastrostomy (PEG) and tracheostomy tubes were in situ. Lee received a range of therapies and by the time of discharge at 4 months posttrauma, she was independently mobile, independent in self-care and cooking activities, but continued to have language impairments (word finding and keeping on track in conversations). The consequences of her continued neuropsychological deficits (in particular, impulsivity, slow processing speed, cognitive rigidity and limited attentional, new learning and planning skills) had been difficult to handle during inpatient rehabilitation, had not significantly responded to intervention, and additionally caused family friction during weekend leave.

Following discharge from inpatient rehabilitation, the community team took over Lee's management and continued rehabilitation: an attendant carer was arranged to allay concerns about Lee being by herself all day; the physiotherapist organised a home-based program to improve fitness and treatment of pain for the soft tissue injury; the occupational therapist continued working on independent living skills in the community and, along with the Royal Blind Society, the effects of Lee's visual impairments, and she attended a group-therapy program targeting social skills; the speech pathologist continued work on Lee's communication skills, and introduced memory retraining strategies; the recreation officer organised a structured weekly program because she was not yet ready to commence work retraining; the clinical psychologist targeted Lee's emotional and temper control problems; and the social worker provided support and strategies to the family to assist them to deal with her cognitive and behavioural changes. The overall program was coordinated and monitored by the case manager via home visits with the family, at first on a frequent basis, and then as the situation stabilised, less intensively.

Just on one year posttrauma, after eight months with the community team and three sets of rehabilitation plans later, Lee's situation was much improved. She was engaging in an Asian speaking social program, was fully independent in activities of daily living, with strategies in place for budgeting. She was still involved with the clinical psychologist, but was able to control her temper and anger in most situations. At this point in time she became depressed and therapy incorporated this focus. Social work involvement with the family increased due to family conflicts and Lee's husband's difficulty in adjusting to the situation. Respite at the Camden House was organised. The subsequent two years have focused on relationship issues between Lee and her husband. Lee's neuropsychological disabilities particularly impact upon her capacity to share intimacy and sexual relations. There are constant high levels of stress and unhappiness, but neither Lee nor her husband are prepared to end their marriage, and at the time of writing the clinical psychologist, social worker and case manager remain closely involved with Lee and her husband.

d) Specific components of the service

The components of the service addressing social rehabilitation as defined (viz. occupational activities, interpersonal relationships and independent living) are described in Table 4.

(1) Occupational activities

The occupational area is probably the most straightforward of the three social domains to effect changes, largely because of the range of options currently available. The review of Malec and Basford (1996) demonstrates the wide range of return to work rates, 0-79% in the 17 programs they reviewed. One reason for the variability is sample differences, particularly with respect to severity of injury and disability – samples with large proportions of people with less severe injuries or disabilities have better outcomes. For instance, Prigatano, Klonoff, O'Brien et al. (1994) reported 62.9% were working (full or part-time) on average at 3.5 years posttrauma, but 32% of their sample

Table 4. Specific pathways: Issues identified from the clinic or elsewhere.

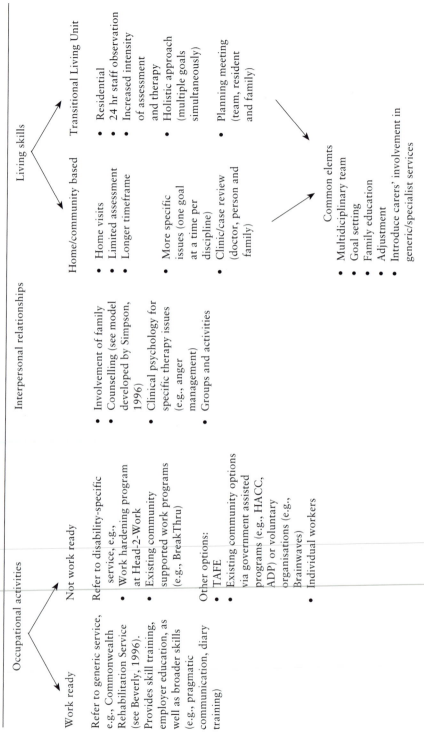

Occupational activities

Work ready

Refer to generic service, e.g., Commonwealth Rehabilitation Service (see Beverly, 1996). Provides skill training, employer education, as well as broader skills (e.g., pragmatic communication, diary training)

Not work ready

Refer to disability-specific service, e.g.,
• Work hardening program at Head-2-Work
• Existing community supported work programs (e.g., BreakThru)

Other options:
• TAFE
• Existing community options via government assisted programs (e.g., HACC, ADP) or voluntary organisations (e.g., Brainwaves)
• Individual workers

Interpersonal relationships

• Involvement of family
• Counselling (see model developed by Simpson, 1996)
• Clinical psychology for specific therapy issues (e.g., anger management)
• Groups and activities

Living skills

Home/community based

• Home visits
• Limited assessment
• Longer timeframe

• More specific issues (one goal at a time per discipline)
• Clinic/case review (doctor, person and family)

Transitional Living Unit

• Residential
• 24 hr staff observation
• Increased intensity of assessment and therapy
• Holistic approach (multiple goals simultaneously)
• Planning meeting (team, resident and family)

Common elemts
• Multidiciplinary team
• Goal setting
• Family education
• Adjustment
• Introduce carers' involvement in generic/specialist services

had an injury of only moderate or mild severity, with GCS scores greater than 8. Similarly, 48% of the sample of Malec, Smigielski, DePompolo and Thompson (1993) were in competitive work at one year after program completion, but selection criteria excluded those who were not independent in mobility, continence, communication, memory, and safety. By contrast, rates in unselected series of people with very severe injuries, such as our own, tend to be low (22% in full-time employment at, on average, six years posttrauma, Tate et al., 1989). This figure is comparable to those reported by other groups: 23% at one year reported by Harrison-Felix, Newton, Hall and Kreutzer (1996); 25% at seven years reported by Brooks, McKinlay, Symington and Beattie (1987); 38% at 2-5 years posttrauma found by Fleming, Tooth, Hassell and Chan (1999); 38% at four years found by Sander, Kreutzer, Rosenthal, Delmonico and Young (1996). More alarming, however, is that a large proportion do not work and have no alternative occupational activity in lieu of work (39% in our series).

In Australia, vocational rehabilitation services are either generic or disability specific. The main generic service is provided by a government-funded organisation, the Commonwealth Rehabilitation Service, with 170 sites throughout the country (Beverley, 1996). All persons with disability (physical, psychiatric, sensory and/or cognitive) of any aetiology are eligible and the service has a number of specialist acquired brain injury teams. A range of services is provided: workplace assessment, training and intervention; employer and co-worker education; developing job seeking plans for those who do not have a job to return to or who have not yet started work, as well as broader skills training including pragmatic communication (cf. Carlson & Buckwall, 1993), diary use in the workplace, counselling for psychological adjustment, fitness training to improve conditioning for job requirements, school and study interventions and so forth.

For those who are not yet ready to return to work or where the work re-entry process is likely to be protracted, a number of pre-work options are available through disability-specific programs, such as the rehabilitation unit's *Head-2-Work* program, a government (Workcover) accredited program of assessment and training which is located in an industrial factory, or community supported work programs for people with disability, including mental health, such as *BreakThru*. The latter service adopts a supported work philosophy, with job coaching and on-the-job support similar to other programs reported in the literature (Buffington & Malec, 1997; Kowalske, Plenger, Lusby, & Hayden, 2000; Kreutzer, Wehman, Norton, & Stonnington, 1988; Stapleton, Parente, & Bennett, 1989; Wehman, Kreutzer, West et al., 1990).

Avocational options are explored with the community team's recreation officer, using external agencies: study skills programs offered through community education colleges (Technical and Further Education, TAFE) or government assisted programs (Home and Community Care, HACC; Headway Adult Development Program, ADP). The recreation officer also promotes involvement of people who may be socially isolated by getting such people together and engaging in activities that are peer interactive, for example through the Brainwaves group, all with the aim of assisting individuals to manage their own leisure better. One exciting development is Potential Unlimited, a nine-month program developed by Thomas (1999) in conjunction with Outward Bound Australia, as a means to increase self-esteem and quality of life after TBI. The Headway ADP, an initiative the Brain Injury Unit launched in 1982, is probably the closest equivalent to the clubhouse model described by Jacobs (1997). It is now one of six community access programs in our state, offering both centre-based and community activities (as well as access plans from the home if the individual resides in the geographical area), and has participants involved in its management. Like the clubhouse model, there is no set timeframe for involvement, membership is open to all people irrespective of degree of disability or time posttrauma, and costs are low ($AUD100 per year or pro rata for those without insurance, but even then the fee is often waived if necessary). The main focus of the ADP is on community participation and access, but the program does not have the day-to-day member direction of the clubhouse model, or the structure of their various units (e.g., communication, kitchen, maintenance).

(2) Interpersonal relationships

Difficulties with interpersonal relationships are extremely common after TBI. Indeed, the impact of TBI upon family relationships can be dramatic and results in high levels of marital breakdown in rehabilitation samples – 55% in our series at six years posttrauma (Tate et al., 1989), 40% reported by Oddy, Coughlan, Tyerman and Jenkins (1985) at seven years, 49% over a 5–8 year period reported by Wood and Yurdakul (1997), 78% in Thomsen's (1984) group at 10–15 years posttrauma, and so forth. Detailed and specific interviewing of spouses reveals the 'severe problems' many of them have in their marital relationships (Gosling & Oddy, 1999). Interpersonal difficulties affect friendships, and social isolation is a frequent legacy of TBI as old friendships fall away and are not replaced by new ones (see review by Rowlands, 2000). Emotional distress after TBI has been consistently documented (see Chapter 7 of this volume), with high proportions showing symptoms indicative of depression, anxiety, anger, fatigue and mood disturbance, ranging from 44–60% in the sample of Perlesz, Kinsella and Crowe (2000), and slightly lower levels in their primary carers (35–49%).

A number of books on rehabilitation of acquired brain injury include chapters addressing interpersonal relationships, from perspectives of both personal adjustment to the effects of the injury, as well as altered interpersonal interactions that may arise from cognitive and behavioural impairments (see for example, Ponsford, Sloan, & Snow, 1995; Prigatano, 1999; Sohlberg & Mateer, 2001). The selection of methods (cognitive-behaviour therapy, solution-focused therapy, psychotherapy, narrative therapy, family therapy) will be dictated largely by the needs and cognitive limitations of the client.

Simpson (1996) has described a model of counselling adjustment that is drawn upon in the Liverpool service, which involves four components:

- understanding the nature of the injury and its sequelae,
- restructuring lifestyles and learning to adapt to changes in occupational activity, interpersonal relationships and living skills, described as 'learning through living',
- reintegrating identity in order to synthesise the premorbid sense of self with posttrauma changes that often involve a devalued identity, and
- acceptance that the future is hopeful, albeit not necessarily as it would have been had the injury not occurred.

The process of reintegrating identity, or 'reconstructing identity' to use Ylvisaker and Feeney's (2000) phrase, is far from easy. They use strategies, such as metaphor to effect positive change in the person's concept of self, e.g., eschewing 'self-as-victim' and developing 'self-as-master' models. They describe this model in a number of case studies: 'Jason willingly worked at developing scripts, strategies, systems of support and explicit rules of self-direction that he then practiced in his everyday interactions and activities.' (p. 21). At a more general level, rehabilitation interventions to address social isolation include very practical initiatives, such as Circles of Support (Wertheimer, 1995; Willer, Allen, Anthony, & Cowlan, 1993), whereas participation in occupational activities (e.g., Brainwaves, Headway ADP, clubhouse) also has an indirect effect on reducing social isolation.

(3) Independent living
It is not only disability in basic activities of daily living (i.e., personal care) and mobility that create barriers to people living independently after TBI, but it is also problems with instrumental activities of daily living (e.g., skills in shopping, use of transport, financial management) which are often due to impairments in executive functions. Difficulties with basic activities of daily living affect only the minority, in the order of 10% of rehabilitation samples (Ponsford, Olver, & Curran, 1995; Tate et al., 1989), whereas problems with instrumental activities are much more common: for example, Ponsford et al. report that 34% were not independent in community activities such as shopping, and 35% showed restriction in use of transport.

There are two components to our approach to independent living. Much of the work is home and community-based. Using home visits, programs are established and reviewed, specialised equipment is trialled, paid carers are inducted into the family situation, and families are educated and helped to adjust to changed circumstances. The second component uses the TLU as a resource for (usually a four-week) assessment and training period when an out-of-home program is more useful. A range of circumstances may point to the latter alternative: e.g., family dynamics precluding proper assessment, intensity of therapy required, complex situations involving behavioural regulation (e.g., not only *can* they do tasks, but also *do* they do them?), social interactions (e.g., attitudes and abilities when living in a shared household) and so forth. At the completion of the living skills program, either home-based or at the TLU, there is discussion of living options based on the outcomes of the assessment and training information as well as available supports, to enable people to make choices and decisions about where they want to live and with whom.

The main frustration, however, is the lack of suitable, community-based, long-term accommodation options, particularly for those people with significant disability (any of physical, cognitive or behavioural). For people from this group it is not only a matter of *locating* such accommodation, it is also the process of *maintaining* the person in that situation by providing whatever care and supports are necessary. These range from personal care through to budgeting skills, through to being able to get along with neighbours.

This chapter and its case illustrations show the types of strategies our team uses to continue supporting individuals to enable them to live in the community. In our experience, it is easier working with people from the outset of their injury, but even when people are admitted to the service many years posttrauma, it can still be possible to provide them with the necessary therapies and skills to enable them to live in the community, as shown by Bell and Tallman (1995) in their own program. They reported on five cases who were transferred directly from acute neurosurgical wards to long-term nursing homes. Following initial rehabilitation, which commenced at least 12 months posttrauma (and for two people more than nine years posttrauma), these individuals who were slow-to-recover were able to achieve significant gains and move out into the community. Similarly, in Gray and Burnham's (2000) sample of 306 patients who were slow to recover and did not commence rehabilitation until, on average, one year posttrauma, 86% was discharged to the community after, on average, one year of inpatient rehabilitation. See also McColl, Davies, Carlson and colleagues (1999) for a detailed, qualitative analysis of factors contributing to difficulties and success in community living in four people who made a transition from 24-hour supervised living.

Yet, independent living is more than simply *living* in the community. As Johnston and Lewis (1991) note, degree of supervision is an important consideration: 'although nominally 'in the community' the burden of such placement approximates that of institutional care' (p. 153). In their sample (n = 82), 24 people (29.3%) participating in their community re-entry program were already living in the community but required 24-hour supervision. At one year after program completion, this number decreased to five people (6.1%) who required such supervision. Moreover, Wood, McCrea, Wood and Merriman (1999) make the further comment that in their group of persons with serious neurobehavioural disability, a proportion of whom lived in the family home prior to rehabilitation, one criterion of success of the program was returning people to the family without the tension and disharmony that characterised the pre-rehabilitation situation.

Profile of a 12-month Cohort

A further issue relevant to this chapter pertains to evidence for the efficacy of the interventions and services delivered. While recognising this imperative, there are challenges in its implementation in systems such as the rehabilitation service provided by the community team. Our program is moving towards more targeted evaluations of the service, but specific, prospectively collected evaluative data are not currently available. The standard approach to program evaluation cannot be readily applied because the service is not a discrete program of intervention, but rather is an intricate and diverse network of services, extended over a protracted timeframe if necessary. Thus our philosophical approach, organisational structure and configuration of therapies/services for our very heterogenous group of clients, does not easily lend itself to measuring 'outcomes', as that term is traditionally used. Sometimes a successful outcome will refer to *maintaining* a person's level of independence, as the case of Omar demonstrated. Other times it will be *providing supports* to a person to enable him or her to continue living in the community, as Bill's case illustrated. As all the case illustrations in this chapter showed, however, the team does deal with identified needs and issues of the individual clients, and so in the absence of specific program evaluation data, we are able to examine some descriptive data documenting service delivery.

Earlier in this chapter we made reference to the survey we conducted of the 467 clients receiving services from the community team during the calendar year 2000 (Tate, Strettles & Osoteo, in submission). From this large group we extracted a computer-generated random sample of 50 clients and conducted a detailed file search on this subgroup. Table 5 provides descriptive data comparing the random sample and remaining 417 clients served during the year 2000; there were no statistically significant differences on any of the variables. By the end of the year 2000, median time posttrauma for the group was 24.5 months range 2.3 months to 36.0 years posttrauma: half the group (n = 26, 52%) was more than two years posttrauma, 15 (30%) were between 12 and 24 months posttrauma, with the remainder (n = 9, 18%) less than 12 months posttrauma. In spite of injury severity (76% of the random sample had duration of PTA of one week or more, and 30% greater than one month), 27 clients (54%) were classified as Good Recovery (all lower level) on the GOS, 14 (28.0%) as Moderate Disability (eight upper level; six lower level), and nine (18.0%) as Severe Disability (five upper level; four lower level).

As may be expected from the levels of disability experienced by the clients, the effects of the injury impacted dramatically upon their lives. Table 6 compares the premorbid and posttrauma status of the group. Premorbidly, four clients (8%) were unemployed, but posttrauma this escalated to 72%, a figure comparable with our other consecutive series described earlier in this chapter (Tate et al., 1989). Posttrauma return to work was closely linked to GOS category: with a single exception, the 11 people in competitive employment posttrauma were from the Good Recovery group. The occupational

Table 5.   Demographic and injury variables of 467 clients receiving services from the
            community team during 2000.

	Random sample (n = 50)	Remaining clients (n = 417)
	Median (Range)	Median (Range)
Age	33.5 (15-69)	34.85 (15-78)
Duration of PTA (days)	20.0 (1-183)	21.0 (0-183)
Number of occasions of service during 2000	9.0 (1-106)	8.0 (1-167)
	n (%)	n (%)
Sex		
Male	40 (80.0)	336 (80.6)
Female	10 (20.0)	81 (19.4)
Cause of injury:		
Road traffic accident	20 (40.0	224 (53.7)
Fall	14 (26.0)	91 (21.8)
Assault	10 (20.0)	52 (12.5)
Other	6 (12.0)	50 (12.0)

status for three of these 11 clients was skilled, and for the remainder was
unskilled. Moreover, whereas 12 clients were students at the time of their
injuries, there were only three students posttrauma, and each of these was
in the Good Recovery group. There was not a lot of change in marital status
(no change for 84%), or living situation (no change for 76%), but these gross
indices do not reflect differences that may well have occurred in the quality
of interpersonal relationships (e.g., marital unhappiness and stress, cf. Case
Lee) and living situation (e.g., caring for very disabled people in the family
home, cf. Case Omar).

Figure 4 shows the admission and discharge details of the random sample
during the course of the year 2000. It clearly demonstrates the long-term and
ongoing nature of the clients' involvement with the community team. At the
commencement of the year, 32 clients (64%) were already in the service; the
earliest admission to the community team for this group receiving services
during 2000, occurred in February 1992. Twenty-eight of these 32 clients
were still active members of the service at the end of the year, and four were
discharged during the course of the year. The other 18 clients (36%) entered
the service at some point during the year 2000, and 16 clients from this group
were still receiving services at the end of the year. Thus only two clients (4%)
were admitted to and discharged from the Community Service during the year

Table 6. Change in circumstances in the random sample (n = 50).

	Work			Marital status			Living arrangements	
	Pre n (%)	Post n (%)		Pre n (%)	Post n (%)		Pre n (%)	Post n (%)
Full Time*	26 (52%)	4 (8%)	Single	25 (50%)	28 (56%)	Parental home	23 (46%)	22 (44%)
Part Time*	6 (12%)	7 (14%)	Married/ de facto	18 (36%)	16 (32%)	Own home	19 (38%)	23 (46%)
Unemployed	4 (8%)	36 (72%)	Separated	7 (14%)	6 (12%)	Rent	8 (16%)	4 (8%)
Student	12 (24%)	3 (6%)				Group home	0	1 (2%)
Other	2 (4%)							

* Work status for those in competitive employment:
Premorbid: Professional/managerial (n = 4), Clerical (n = 2), Skilled (n = 10), Unskilled/semiskilled (n = 16); Posttrauma: Skilled (n = 3), Unskilled (n = 8).

2000. In all, there were three times as many admissions to the service (n = 18) than discharges from it (n = 6) during the course of the year in the random sample, which is a typical pattern to that of other years, and indicates the growth of the service over time.

From our file search we identified 11 types of issues representing social rehabilitation as described in this chapter. In keeping with the distinction drawn by McMillan and Sparkes (1999), many of the issues would be classified as staff action plans, rather than being client goals per se. The types of issues with active involvement from the team that were dealt with in the random sample during the course of the year, along with their 'outcomes' or action status, are displayed in Table 7. We classified the 11 types of issues within three domains, representing social rehabilitation as described in this chapter: occupational activity (work, study, recreation/leisure), interpersonal relationships (both intrapersonal for adjustment/mood, as well as behaviour/ social skills and family/friends issues), and living skills (including accommodation, transport, financial/legal, mobility/fitness/self-care, cognitive strategy training).

On average, clients received 17.2 occasions of service (median = 9.0, range 1-106) during the course of the year, and 2.4 (median = 3.0, range 0-6) social rehabilitation type issues were addressed. As anticipated, those clients remaining with the service over time had more severe injuries, as measured

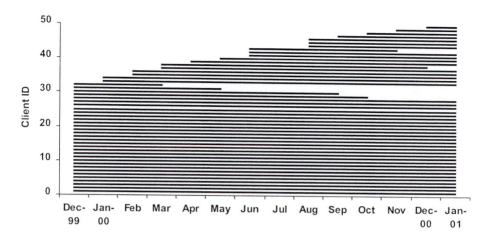

Fig. 4. Admissions to and discharges from the service during the year 2000.

Table 7.   Social rehabilitation type issues addressed with clients from the random sample.

	Number of clients with issues addressed during the year 2000	Percent of issues with action completed
	n (%)	
Occupational Activity	22 (44.0)	
Work	15 (30.0	100.0
Study	3 (6.0)	100.0
Recreation/leisure	5 (10.0)*	100.0
Interpersonal Relationships	27 (54.0)	
Psychological adjustment/mood	13 (26.0)	92.3
Behaviour/social skills	12 (24.0)	91.7
Family/friends	15 (30.0)	100.0
Living Skills	33 (66.0)	100.0
Accommodation	9 (18.0)	100.0
Transport	11 (22.0)	100.0
Financial/legal	8 (16.0)	100.0
Mobility/fitness/self care	17 (34.0)	100.0
Cognitive strategies	14 (28.0)	100.0

* Note: This figure is lower than usual because the staff position of Recreational Officer remained vacant during 2000.

by duration of PTA ($r = 0.69$, $p < 0.001$) and greater disability on the GOS (Good Recovery versus Moderate/Severe Disability, $r_{pb} = 0.32$, $p < 0.03$). Also as expected, the total occasions of service was associated with greater disability ($r_{pb} = 0.35$, $p < 0.02$), but not with chronicity ($r = 0.14$). There were, however, no associations between frequency of social rehabilitation type issues and injury severity ($r = 0.06$), degree of disability ($r_{pb} = 0.18$), or length of time since injury ($r = 0.01$).

Twenty-two clients (44%) had issues that were addressed in the occupational domain, 27 clients (52%) in the relationship area, and 33 clients (66%) in the living skills domain. In virtually all instances some resolution of the issue occurred during that year. This does not necessarily imply that an independent outcome occurred, such as return to work or independent living in the community. Moreover, although a specific issue was successfully dealt with, the client may not have been discharged from the service (cf. Fig. 4), because other issues may arise, as the case of Lee demonstrated. The following illustrations show the types of issues and action taken. In the occupational activities area, work issues, for example, were addressed with 15 clients, most of whom (n = 9) were in the Good Recovery group, and most (n = 9) were also less than 18 months posttrauma (seven of these nine were also in the Good Recovery group). In four clients, the work issues were fairly straight-forward, involving referral and limited liaison with vocational programs (*Head-2-Work* and the Commonwealth Rehabilitation Service). Three clients had specific difficulties (loss of job due to the client's errors, inability to cope with the workload, and memory impairments), which required targeted interventions in the workplace for the last two cases, each of which resulted in successful outcomes. The remaining eight clients with work issues required intensive monitoring, liaison and support, such as Brian, a 24 year-old skilled worker, who was injured seven months previously and admitted to the community team at 5.5 months posttrauma. He received 16 occasions of service relating to work issues over a four-month period. The nature of the contact with Brian was to develop a rehabilitation plan for him resuming work, then altering his work duties as a consequence of a seizure, and implementing strategies for him to combat his fatigue, physical intolerance, agitation, and organisational difficulties.

In the relationships domain, adjustment issues, for example, were addressed with 13 clients (seven of whom were classified as Moderate/Severe Disability), and included ongoing management of anxiety and/or depression in each client. Therapy was usually undertaken by the clinical psychologist, in association with the case manager, and often included the consultant psychiatrist. Not infrequently, issues needed to be worked through using an interpreter; 48% of the sample was from a non-English speaking background. It was not unusual for the management of adjustment and emotional issues to occur in the context of multiple problem areas, such as in the case of Tim, a 49-year old unemployed married man, who was almost four years posttrauma and was classified as Moderate Disability (upper level). His anxiety issues needed to be managed in the context of other social factors including impulsivity and anger management problems, family conflict, social isolation, changes in sleep and appetite, excessive alcohol use, and noncompliance with medication.

With reference to living skills, the accommodation area, for example, was an issue for nine clients, all of whom were classified as either Moderate or Severe Disability. Three clients required arrangements for a period of respite and for an additional two clients their situations were more complicated requiring respite while other interventions were implemented (restructuring of mortgage payments and applying for funds to improve inappropriate housing). For another client the accommodation issue pertained to building extensions to the existing house that necessitated discussions with the Office of the Protective Commission to release funds for this purpose. For three clients, challenging behaviours were jeopardising existing accommodation arrangements requiring liaison with the family and local Mental Health team.

In summary, these descriptive data provide a snapshot of the community team caseload in the random sample, representing some 10% of the workload in a typical year. At a general level, there is initial support for the efficacy of continued rehabilitation in the community from other programs run over shorter timeframes than our own. Seventeen of the 28 treatment studies reviewed by Hall and Cope (1995) focused on rehabilitation provided in the community, either day treatment or residential programs. Yet, while all studies reported improved posttreatment functioning on various outcome measures, commonly including health status measures such as independence and employment, only two of the studies used a matched control group (Fryer & Haffey, 1987; Prigatano, Fordyce, Zeiner, Roueche, Pepping, & Wood, 1984). The remaining investigations compared pre-intervention and postintervention measures in a single group of treated individuals. Moreover, as High, Boake and Lehmkuhl (1995, p. 23) remind us 'it is not enough to show that rehabilitation is effective; one must also be able to justify the effectiveness and expense of the individual components.'

Subsequent to the Hall and Cope (1995) review, a number of other treatment studies addressing rehabilitation for TBI in a community setting have appeared in the literature using stronger research designs, including Willer, Button and Rempel (1999) who conducted a case-controlled study comparing community-based residential treatment and home-based rehabilitation, and Powell, Heslin and Greenwood (2002) who conducted a randomised controlled trial comparing a goal-planned, individualised program at home (or other community setting) with written information regarding available services in the community. This methodologically superior study provides the strongest evidence to date to enable critical analysis of the relative strengths and weaknesses of interventions. Although there was no test of the specific components of their treatment package, the pattern of results provides some indication for future research directions. Of interest, improvements in general functioning did not occur, but rather were specific to activities of daily living (Barthel index) and some aspects of psychological well-being.

It is clear that the current pressing need is to use strong methodological designs and focus attention on evaluating specific components of programs that tap into the socialising and productive employment domains, the very essence of social rehabilitation. A new focus in the continued development of our service is strengthening the evaluative component, using specific projects. One relevant study currently in progress examines family education about living with a person with TBI, incorporating evidenced-based learning principles, as well as evaluating efficacy. Findings from this study will enable analysis of the way in which training and education are conducted and provide a basis to incorporate the results into our work practices. At the broader level, the Liverpool service, as part of the state-wide Brain Injury Rehabilitation Program, is in the process of obtaining consensus on standards of outcome measures at various times posttrauma that will be entered onto a statewide database. This will not only yield systematic documentation of progress at an individual level, but also enable service planning and development at a socio-political level.

The Broader Perspective

In summary, our approach to social rehabilitation, described within the context of a community rehabilitation team in this chapter, aims to enhance outcomes by increasing independence and self-determination, particularly in relation to occupational activities, interpersonal relationships and independent living. In so doing, we make a distinction between 'rehabilitation' and 'maintenance'. Because of the potentially large number of individuals served by community or outreach TBI teams, the focus can often be 'maintenance' – i.e., case management, liaison, addressing practical issues and crisis management. In our view, community teams also have the opportunity to include an active rehabilitation component, including isolated bursts of therapies (e.g., a finite number of sessions for anger management), as well as providing opportunities for individuals to 'get better' (i.e., 'cope better', 'feel better', 'act better'), not merely 'keep busy'. The essence of our approach is based on identifying issues, and then dissecting, what for the individual and family, can often appear to be huge, complex, insurmountable problems into manageable portions and thence into specific goals that can be addressed.

This approach has similarities to some elements of a number of other programs described in the literature (see the case management role as described in DePompei et al., 2001 and La Marche, Reed, Rich et al., 1995; and the interdisciplinary approach in Pace, Schlund, Hazard-Haupt et al., 1999), but in overall terms our program is unlike others reported in the literature. In particular, our model differs from other (predominantly neuropsychological) therapies that are conducted in an outpatient setting (see, for example, programs described in Christensen & Uzzell, 2000). In one sense, such programs are an extension of inpatient programs in that the clients come to a centre and participate in timetabled sessions addressing multiple potential impairment areas – communication, social skills, memory, attention, problem solving and so forth. Usually these types of programs are run over a set number of sessions, such as a three or six-month package, with some, such as New York-based Rusk Institute program (Daniels-Zide & Ben-Yishay, 2000), having fixed entry and exit dates.

Within the framework we adopt, there is also the argument to be made that social rehabilitation after TBI must to go beyond the clinical focus of the individual/family in order to encompass a broader socio-political perspective to effect social change. To this end, the Liverpool system has a fifth essential component that was not described in the foregoing, namely non-clinical services. One focus of activity of the non-clinical services that pertains to social rehabilitation is the development of information kits for consumers and professionals. Those currently available address information needs (Strettles, Simpson, & Mead, 1995), living skills (Shepherd & Strettles, 1999), sexuality (Simpson, 1999), and suicidality (Simpson, 2002). Submissions and consultations to government and non-government organisations are another way to address gaps in clinical services and improve quality. Submissions have been made on public housing, criminal justice, respite accommodation, and long-term care needs. Listing of submissions, research activities and other information about the service is available through their web site (www.swsahs.nsw.gov.au/biru).

In conclusion, this chapter has described our conceptual framework for social rehabilitation after TBI and provided an overview of our clinical practice. The distinctive features of the service are a commitment to ongoing and long-term involvement while-ever there are needs, along with a multidisciplinary team approach in which case managers work in partnership with therapists. For reasons previously outlined, we believe that rehabilitation to address social disablement in the areas of occupational activity, interpersonal relationships and independent living is best conducted in the community. The community-based component of our TBI service has evolved over more than 20 years and in its present configuration is a resource-intensive program. This, however, is largely a function of the volume (around 500 clients and their families per annum), rather than being an inherent requirement of the program, and hence does not impose a limitation to the implementation of the program in other services where the caseload is a fraction of our own. The clinical and nonclinical components of our service are dynamic and continue to evolve and develop to assist in realising our vision for better health, good health care and achieving the maximum quality of life for the person, their family and community.

References

Alderman, N., Fry, R.K., & Youngson, H.A. (1995). Improvement of self-monitoring skills, reduction of behavioiur disturbance and the dysexecutive syndrome of self-monitoring training. *Neuropsychological Rehabilitation, 5(3),* 193-221.

Bell, K.R., & Tallman, C.A. (1995). Community re-entry of long-term institutionalised brain-injured persons. *Brain Injury, 9(3)*, 315-320.

Beverley, K. (1996). The cutting edge – ABI vocational rehabilitation in the workplace: A NSW perspective. In J. Ponsford, P. Snow & V. Anderson (Eds.). *International perspectives in traumatic brain injury. Proceedings of the 5th Conference of the International Association for the Study of Traumatic Brain Injury and 20th Conference of the Australian Society for the Study of Brain Impairment* (pp. 367-372). Bowen Hills, Qld: Australian Academic Press.

Broe, G.A., Lulham, J.M., Strettles, B., Tate, R.L., Walsh, C.A., & Ross, G. (1982). The concept of head injury rehabilitation. In G.A. Broe and R.L. Tate (Eds.). *Brain Impairment. Proceedings of the 5th Annual Brain Impairment Conference* (pp. 59-68). Sydney: The Postgraduate Committee in Medicine of the University of Sydney.

Brooks, N., McKinlay, W., Symington, C., Beattie, A., & Campsie, L. (1987). Return to work within the first seven years of severe head injury. *Brain Injury, 1(1)*, 5-19.

Buffington, A.L.H., & Malec, J.F. (1997). The vocational rehabilitation continuum: Maximising outcomes through bridging the gap from hospital to community-based services. *Journal of Head Trauma Rehabilitation, 12(5)*, 1-13.

Carlson, H.B., & Buckwald, M.B.W. (1993). Vocational Communication Group treatment in an outpatient head injury facility. *Brain Injury, 7(2)*, 183-187.

Christensen, A.-L. & Uzzell, B.P. (Eds.). (2000). *International handbook of neuropsychological rehabilitation*. New York: Kluwer.

Cope, D.N., Cole, J.R., Hall, K.M., & Barkan, H. (1991). Brain injury: analysis of outcome in a post-acute rehabilitation system. Part 1: General analysis. *Brain Injury, 5*, 111-125.

Cervelli, L. (1990). Re-entry into the community systems of posthospital care. In: M. Rosenthal, E.R. Griffith, M.R. Bond, & J.D. Miller. (Eds.). *Rehabilitation of the adult and child with traumatic brain injury* (pp. 463-475). Philadelphia: FA Davis Co. 2nd ed.

Daniels-Zide, E., & Ben-Yishay, Y. (2000). Therapeutic milieu day program. In A.-L. Christensen & B.P. Uzzell (Eds.). *International handbook of neuropsychological rehabilitation*. (pp. 183-193). New York: Kluwer.

DePompei, R., Frye, D., DuFore, M., & Hunt, P. (2001). Traumatic Brain Injury Collaborative planning group: A protocol for community intervention. *Journal of Head Trauma Rehabilitation, 16(3)*, 217-237.

Durgin, C.J. (2000). Increasing community participation after brain injury: Strategies for identifying and reducing risks. *Journal of Head Trauma Rehabilitation, 15(6)*, 1195-1207.

Feeney, T.J., Ylvisaker, M., Rosen, B.H., & Greene, P. (2001). Community supports for individuals with challenging behavior after brain injury: An analysis of the New York State Behavioral Resource Project. *Journal of Head Trauma Rehabilitation, 16(1)*, 61-75.

Fleming, J., Tooth, L., Hassell, M., & Chan, W. (1999). Prediction of community integration and vocational outcome 2-5 years after traumatic brain injury rehabilitation in Australia. *Brain Injury, 13 (6)*, 417-431.

Fryer, I.J., & Haffey, W.J. (1987). Cognitive rehabilitation and community readaptation: outcomes from two program models. *Journal of Head Trauma Rehabilitation, 2(3)*, 51-63.

Godfrey, H.P.D., Knight, R.G., & Partridge, F.M. (1996). Emotional adjustment following traumatic brain injury: A stress-appraisal-coping formulation. *Journal of Head Trauma Rehabilitation, 11(6)*, 29-40.

Godfrey, H.P.D., & Shum, D. (2000). Executive functioning and the application of social skills following traumatic brain injury. *Aphasiology, 14(4)*, 433-444.

Grattan, L., & Ghahramanlou, M. (2002). The rehabilitation of neurologically-based social disorders. In: P. Eslinger (Ed.). *Neuropsychological interventions: Clinical research and practice.* (pp. 266-293). New York: Guildford.

Gosling, J., & Oddy, M. (1999). Rearranged marriages: marital relationships after head injury. *Brain Injury, 13(10),* 785-796.

Gray, D.S., & Burnham, R.S. (2000). Preliminary outcome analysis of a long-term rehabilitation program for severe acquired brain injury. *Archives of Physical Medicine and Rehabilitation, 81,* 1447-1456.

Hall, K.M., & Cope, D.N. (1995). The benefit of rehabilitation in traumatic brain injury: A literature review. *Brain Injury, 10(1),* 1-13.

Harrison-Felix, C., Newton, C.N., Hall, K.M., & Kreutzer, J.S. (1996). Descriptive findings from the traumatic brain injury model systems national data base. *Journal of Head Trauma Rehabilitation, 11(5),* 1-14.

Hayden, M.E., Moreault, A-M., LeBlanc, J., & Plenger, P. (2000). Reducing level of handicap in traumatic brain injury. An environmentally based model of treatment. *Journal of Head Trauma Rehabilitation, 15(4),* 1000-1021.

High, W.M., Boake, C., & Lehmkuhl, L.D. (1995). Critical analysis of studies evaluating the effectiveness of rehabilitation after traumatic brain injury. *Journal of Head Trauma Rehabilitation, 10(1),* 14-26.

Jacobs, H.E. (1997). The Clubhouse: Addressing work-related behavioural challenges through a supportive social community. *Journal of Head Trauma Rehabilitation, 12(5),* 14-27.

Jennett, B., & Bond, M.R. (1975). Assessment of outcome after severe brain damage. A practical scale. *Lancet, i,* 480-484.

Jennett, B., Snoek, J., Bond, M.R., & Brooks, N. (1981). Disability after severe head injury. *Journal of Neurology, Neurosurgery, and Psychiatry, 44,* 285-293.

Johnston, M.V., & Lewis, F.D. (1991). Outcomes of community re-entry programmes for brain injury survivors. Part 1: Independent living and productive activities. *Brain Injury, 5,* 141-154.

Kendall, E. & Terry, D.J. (1996). Psychosocial adjustment following closed head injury: A model for understanding individual differences and predicting outcome. *Neuropsychological Rehabilitation, 6(2),* 101-132.

Kendall, E., Shum, D., Halson, D., Bunning, S., & The, M. (1997). The assessment of social problem solving ability following traumatic brain injury. *Journal of Head Trauma Rehabilitation, 12,* 68-78.

Kneipp, S. (1995). A model for team meetings in non-residential community integrated programs. *Journal of Head Trauma Rehabilitation, 10(6),* 50-59.

Kowalske, K., Plenger, P.M., Lusby, B., & Hayden, M.E. (2000). Vocational reentry following TBI: An enablement model. *Journal of Head Trauma Rehabilitation, 15(4),* 989-999.

Kreutzer, J., Wehman, P., Morton, M., & Stonnington, H. (1988). Supported employment and compensatory strategies for enhancing vocational outcome following traumatic brain injury. *Brain Injury, 2,* 205-223.

Kuipers, P., & Lancaster, A. (2000). Developing a suicide prevention strategy based on the perspectives of people with brain injuries. *Journal of Head Trauma Rehabilitation, 15,* 1275-1284.

La Marche, J.A., Reed, L.K., Rich, M.A., Cash, A.W., Lucas, L.H. & Boll, T.J. (1995). The interactive community-based model of vocational rehabilitation. *Journal of Head Trauma Rehabilitation, 10(4),* 81-89.

Levine, M.J., van Horn, K.R., & Curtis, A.B. (1993). Developing models of social cognition in assessing psychosocial adjustments in head injury. *Brain Injury, 7(2),* 153-167.

Lishman, W.A. (1973). The psychiatric sequelae of head injury: A review. *Psychological Medicine, 3,* 304-318.

Malec, J.F., & Basford, J.S. (1996). Postacute brain injury rehabilitation. *Archives of Physical Medicine and Rehabilitation, 77*, 198-207.

Malec, J.F., Smigielski, J.S., DePompolo, R.W., & Thompson, J.M. (1993). Outcome evaluation and prediction in a comprehensive-integrated post-acute outpatient brain injury rehabilitation programme. *Brain Injury, 7*, 15-29.

Marsh, N.V. (1999). Social skill deficits following traumatic brain injury: Assessment and treatment. In: S. McDonald, L. Togher, & C. Code (Eds.). (1999). *Communication disorders following traumatic brain injury* (pp. 175-210). Hove, UK: Psychology Press.

McColl, M.A., Carlson, P., Johnston, J., Minnes, P., Shue, K., Davies, D., & Karlovits, T. (1998). The definition of community integration: perspectives of people with brain injuries. *Brain Injury, 12(1)*, 15-30.

McDonald, S., Togher, L., & Code, C. (Eds.). (1999). *Communication disorders following traumatic brain injury*. Hove, UK: Psychology Press.

McGann, W., & Werven, G. (1995). Social competence and head injury: a new emphasis. *Brain Injury, 9(1)*, 93-102.

McMillan, T.M., & Sparkes, C. (1999). Goal planning and neurorehabilitation: The Wolfson Neurorehabilitation Centre Approach. *Neuropsychological Rehabilitation, 9(3/4)*, 241-251.

Medd, J., & Tate, R.L. (2000). Evaluation of an anger management therapy programme following acquired brain injury: A preliminary study. *Neuropsychological Rehabilitation, 10(2)*, 185-201.

Moore, A.D., & Stambrook, M. (1995). Cognitive moderators of outcome following traumatic brain injury: A conceptual model and implications for rehabilitation. *Brain Injury, 9*, 109-130.

Oddy, M., Coughlan, T., Tyerman, A. & Jenkins, D. (1985). Social adjustment after closed head injury: a further follow-up seven years after injury. *Journal of Neurology, Neurosurgery, and Psychiatry, 48*, 564-568.

Pace, G.M., Schlund, M.W., Hazard-Haupt, T., Christensen, J.R., Lashno, M., McIver, J., Peterson, K., & Morgan, K.A. (1999). Characteristics and outcomes of a home and community-based neurorehabilitation programme. *Brain Injury, 13*, 535-546.

Perlesz, A., Kinsella, G., & Crowe, S. (2000). Psychological distress and family satisfaction following traumatic brain injury: Injured individuals and their primary, secondary and tertiary carers. *Journal of Head Trauma Rehabilitation, 15(3)*, 909-929.

Ponsford, J.L., Olver, J.H., & Curran, C. (1995). A profile of outcome: 2 years after traumatic brain injury. *Brain Injury, 9(1)*, 1-10.

Ponsford, J., Sloan, S., & Snow, P. (1995). *Traumatic brain injury: Rehabilitation for everyday adaptive living*. Hove, UK: Lawrence Erlbaum.

Powell, J., Heslin, J., & Greenwood, R. (2002). Community based rehabilitation after severe traumatic brain injury: a randomised controlled trial. *Journal of Neurology, Neurosurgery, and Psychiatry, 72*, 193-202.

Prigatano, G.P. (1999). *Principles of neuropsychological rehabilitation*. New York: Oxford University Press.

Prigatano, G.P., Fordyce, D.J., Zeiner, H.K., Roueche, J.R., Pepping, M., & Wood. B.C. (1984). Neuropsychological rehabilitation after closed head injury in young adults. *Journal of Neurology, Neurosurgery, and Psychiatry, 47*, 505-513.

Prigatano, G.P., Klonoff, P.S., O'Brien, K.P., Altman, I.M., Amin, K., Chiapello, D., Shepherd, J., Cunningham, M., & Mora, M. (1994). Productivity after neuropsychologically oriented milieu rehabilitation. *Journal of Head Trauma Rehabilitation, 9(1)*, 91-102.

Racino, J.A., & Williams, J.M. (1994). Living in the community: An examination of the philosophical and practical aspects. *Journal of Head Trauma Rehabilitation, 9(2)*, 35-48.

Rowlands, A. (2000). Understanding social support and friendship: Implications for intervention after acquired brain injury. *Brain Impairment, 1(2),* 151-164.

Sander, A., Kreutzer, J.S., Rosenthal, M., Delmonico, R., & Young, M.E. (1996). A multicentre longitudinal investigation of return to work and community following traumatic brain injury. *Journal of Head Trauma Rehabilitation, 11(5),* 70-84.

Shepherd, B., & Strettles, B. (1999). *Getting it all together. A kit for daily living when you have a brain injury.* Sydney: Brain Injury Rehabilitation Unit, South Western Sydney Area Health Service and Motor Accidents Authority.

Simpson, G.K. (1996). A model of adjustment counselling after traumatic brain injury. In J. Ponsford, P. Snow & V. Anderson (Eds.). *International perspectives in traumatic brain injury.* Proceedings of the 5th Conference of the International Association for the Study of Traumatic Brain Injury and 20th Conference of the Australian Society for the Study of Brain Impairment (pp. 403-406). Bowen Hills, Qld: Australian Academic Press.

Simpson, G.K. (1999). *You and me. An education program about sex and sexuality after traumatic brain injury.* Sydney: Brain Injury Rehabilitation Unit, South Western Sydney Area Health Service.

Simpson, G.K. (2002). *Suicide prevention after traumatic brain injury. A resource manual.* Sydney: Brain Injury Rehabilitation Unit, South Western Sydney Area Health Service.

Simpson, G.K., Mohr, R., & Redman, A. (2000). Cultural variations in the understanding of brain injury and brain injury rehabilitation. *Brain Injury, 14,* 125-140.

Sloan, S., Balicki, S., & Winkler, D. (1996). Community reintegration of people with traumatic brain injuries: Keys to success. In J. Ponsford, P. Snow & V. Anderson (Eds.). *International perspectives in traumatic brain injury.* Proceedings of the 5th Conference of the International Association for the Study of Traumatic Brain Injury and 20th Conference of the Australian Society for the Study of Brain Impairment (pp. 346-349). Bowen Hills, Qld: Australian Academic Press.

Sohlberg, M.M., & Mateer, C.A. (2001). *Cognitive rehabilitation. An integrative neuropsychological approach.* New York: Guildford.

Stapleton, M., Parente, R., & Bennett, P. (1989). Job coaching traumatically brain injured individuals: lessons learned. *Cognitive Rehabilitation, 7,* 18-21.

Strettles, B., Simpson, G.K., & Mead, D. (1995). *Head injury information kit.* Canberra: Department of Health, Housing and Community Services.

Tate, R.L., Hodgkinson, A.E., Veerabangsa, A., & Maggiotto, S. (1999). Measuring psychosocial recovery after traumatic brain injury: Psychometric properties of a new scale. *Journal of Head Trauma Rehabilitation, 14(6),* 543-557.

Tate, R.L., Lulham, J.M., Broe, G.A., Strettles, B., & Pfaff, A. (1989). Psychosocial outcome for the survivors of severe blunt head injury: The results from a consecutive series of 100 patients. *Journal of Neurology, Neurosurgery, and Psychiatry, 52,* 1128-1134.

Tate, R.L., Pfaff, A., Veerabangsa, A., & Hodgkinson A. (in submission). *Measuring psychosocial recovery after brain injury: Change versus competency.*

Tate, R.L., Simpson, G.K., Flanagan, S., & Coffey, M. (1997). Completed suicide after traumatic brain injury. *Journal of Head Trauma Rehabilitation, 12(6),* 16-28.

Tate, R.L., Strettles, B., & Osoteo, T. (in submission). *Patterns of service usage in community rehabilitation after acquired brain injury.*

Teasdale, G., & Jennett, B. (1974). Assessment of coma and impaired consciousness. *Lancet ii,* 81-84.

Thomas, M. (1999, October). *Potential Unlimited: Evaluation of a pilot programme.* Paper presented at the 4th Annual Research Forum of the NSW Brain Injury Rehabilitation Program, Sydney.

Thomsen, I.V. (1984). Late outcome of very severe blunt head trauma: a 10-15 year second follow-up. *Journal of Neurology, Neurosurgery, and Psychiatry, 47,* 260-268.

Wehman, P., Kruetzer, J., West, M., Sherron, P., Zasler, N., Groah, C., Stonnington, H.H., Burns, C., & Sale, P. (1990). Return to work for people with traumatic brain injury: a supported employment approach. *Archives of Physical Medicine and Rehabilitation, 71,* 1047-1052.

Wertheimer, A. (1995). *Circles of support: Building inclusive communities.* Bristol: Circles Network UK.

Willer, B.S., Allen, K., Anthony, J., & Cowlan, G. (1993). *Circles of support for individuals with acquired brain injury.* Buffalo: Rehabilitation Research and Training Center on Community Integration of Persons with Traumatic Brain Injury.

Willer, B., Button, J., & Rempel, R. (1999). Residential and home-based postacute rehabilitation of individuals with traumatic brain injury: a case control study. *Archives of Physical Medicine and Rehabilitation, 80,* 399-406.

Willer, B., & Corrigan, J.D. (1994). Whatever It Takes: a model for community-based services. *Brain Injury, 8,* 647-659.

Willer, B., Rosenthal, M., Kreutzer, J.S., Gordon, W.A., & Rempel, R. (1993). Assessment of community integration following rehabilitation for traumatic brain injury. *Journal of Head Trauma Rehabilitation, 8,* 75-87.

Wood, R.Ll. (1987). *Brain injury rehabilitation. A neurobehavioural approach.* London: Croom Helm.

Wood, R.Ll, Yurdakul, L.K. (1997). Change in relationship status following traumatic brain injury. *Brain Injury, 11(7),* 491-502.

World Health Organisation (WHO). (1980). ICIDH. *International classification of impairments, disabilities and handicaps.* Geneva: World Health Organisation.

World Health Organisation (WHO). (2001). ICF. *International classification of functioning, disability and health.* Geneva: World Health Organisation.

Ylvisaker, M., & Feeney, T. (1998). *Collaborative brain injury intervention. Positive everyday routines.* San Diego: Singular Publishing Group.

Ylvisaker, M., & Feeney, T. (2000). Reconstruction of identity after brain injury. *Brain Impairment, 1(1),* 12-28.

Chapter 9

REHABILITATION OF BEHAVIOUR DISORDERS

Nick Alderman

Kemsley Division, St Andrew's Hospital, Northampton, UK

Introduction

The presence of behaviour disorders amongst people who have sustained some form of neurological insult, particularly traumatic brain injury (TBI), has been well documented. Whilst confusion and agitation observed during the acute stage of recovery resolves in the majority of cases, a wide range of behavioural problems may emerge with the resolution of consciousness. These are varied, ranging from passivity to aggression, whilst others mimic symptoms characteristic of psychiatric disorders. Whilst behaviour disorders are not atypical following TBI, a reasonable expectation is that these will resolve with time. Unfortunately, studies, which have investigated long-term outcome, paint a picture that is contrary to this belief. Instead, the worrying trend is not only that behaviour disorders persist, but that they also become more severe (for example, see Brooks, McKinlay, Symington, Beattie, & Campsie, 1987; Johnson & Balleny, 1996). The number of TBI cases with severe, persistent behavioural problems is small (estimated as 0.3 per 100,000 per annum by Greenwood & McMillan [1993]). However, tenfold this figure are thought to retain persistent behaviour disorders which, although less severe, nevertheless serve to handicap everyday functioning (Johnson & Balleny, 1996). Not surprisingly, behaviour disorders constitute a considerable source of stress within families (McKinlay, Brooks, Bond, Martinage, & Marshall, 1981; Oddy, Coughlan, Tyerman, & Jenkins, 1985); in addition, neurological patients who are behaviour disordered are unpopular and tend to be avoided by rehabilitation professionals (Miller & Cruzat, 1981). An immediate consequence of this is that people in need of rehabilitation are excluded from such programmes. A longer term corollary may be that once discharged to the care of their families, persistent behaviour disorder renders management of such people at home untenable, and as a direct consequence they gravitate to placements that are clearly inappropriate for their needs, such as psychogeriatric, learning disability and long-stay secure psychiatric units, as well as prison (Eames & Wood, 1985a).

The range and type of behaviour disorders observed amongst neurological patients is extensive. However, some are more characteristic. For example, Wood (2001) refers to problems of labile mood, impulse control and personality change that are often associated with TBI, amongst a wider constellation of cognitive and behaviour symptoms that he collectively labels 'Neurobehavioral Disability'. Development of aggression has been especially highlighted (for example, see Miller, 1994) because of the impact this has on families and its poor prognosis regarding success in rehabilitation (Burke, Wesolowski, & Lane, 1988).

When does behaviour become a disorder?

There is little doubt that behaviour which is clearly harmful to the environment, and which places either the perpetrator or others around them at risk, can be more easily labelled as 'problematic' or a 'disorder'. People whose behaviour falls beyond the cultural and social limits of what is acceptable within their community may be highlighted (often by the judicial system) and identified as being likely recipients of treatment whose purpose is to reduce social handicap. A tendency has grown in clinical circles in recent years to label such disorders 'challenging behaviour', especially in the literature pertaining to learning disability. For example, in the UK Emerson, Barrett, Bell, Cummings, McCool, Toogood and Mansell (1987) defined challenging behaviour as that which jeopardises the safety of the person exhibiting them, or limits access to ordinary community facilities. Alderman (2001) embraced this view and argued that many of the post-acute behaviour disorders observed amongst neurological patients fall under the umbrella of 'challenging behaviour'. Alderman argued that behaviours should fall within this definition if they served to deny a person access to neurological rehabilitation services, as well as community facilities. In this way, disorders of initiation and passivity which characterise some forms of brain injury, and even the general coarsening of social behaviour which is often typical of TBI patients, are also classed as 'challenging' as their effect can be just as disabling as aggression if they function to exclude people from services of which they are in need.

Aetiology of Behaviour Disorders

There are many possible causes that drive behaviour disorders that are the sequelae of neurological insult. Identifying these, as they apply to the individual patient, is an ideal to be pursued if effective treatment is to be delivered. Unfortunately, this process is thwart with difficulty. One reason is that there are many different neurological conditions, each with their own distinctive neuropathology: behaviour disorders that characterise each condition will vary because of differences in the location and extent of the structural damage incurred. However, behavioural problems observed in people with similar neurological conditions may vary further because such patients do not constitute a homogenous group. This point was made by Mateer and Ruff (1990) who pointed out that no two brains are damaged in exactly the same way; consequently, not only are there differences regarding neuropathology, but also the probability that underlying cognitive systems are disrupted in identical ways is low. For example, Colthart (1991) estimated that the naming system could be impaired in up to 16,383 separate ways. Another set of factors that contributes to lack of homogeneity concerns other sequelae arising from insult. These may be extensive and include cognitive, emotional, physical and functional impairments, as well as overt behavioural problems. Wilson (1991) argued people rarely have just one or two specific problems arising from brain injury: instead, they routinely present with a combination of these difficulties, which are rarely identical.

The point is that whilst within specific diagnostic groups (for example, stroke and TBI) the location and extent of the neuropathology will initially dictate types of behaviour disorder, these will be subjected to a wide array of secondary influences which modify, sometimes considerably, how they are eventually manifested. The range of variables which influence development of behaviour disorders is considerable, but includes cognitive deficits, reactive disorders, denial and poor awareness, post-injury learning, poor frustration-tolerance, environmental factors, and exacerbation of pre-morbid traits. Space does not permit extensive elaboration of these here (see Alderman, submitted): however, the influence on behaviour of some of these will be illustrated through discussion of case material later in this chapter. Thus, behaviour disorders will invariably be the product of complex interaction between many factors. Seeking to find a single cause is probably not only conceptually too simplistic, but is fraught by methodological problems attributable to poor homogeneity.

A note on the 'Frontal Lobe Syndrome'

A little will now be said about the Frontal Lobe Syndrome simply because behaviourally disturbed neurological patients, particularly those who have sustained TBI, continue to be almost routinely ascribed this label. There is little doubt that this area of the brain has received most attention regarding cerebral correlates of behaviour disorder. An extensive breadth of anecdotal social and other changes observed after damage (actual and assumed) to the frontal lobes is evident in the literature. The case of Phineas Gage (see Kimble, 1963) remains one of the earliest and most striking examples of behaviour and personality changes which followed a penetrating injury of the brain which resulted in a large bilateral lesion of the ventromedial prefrontal cortex.

The range of symptoms historically attributed to frontal lobe syndrome is exhibited through a wide range of difficulties in everyday life. These may include problems with abstract reasoning, making decisions and showing good judgement; difficulties in maintaining attention; inappropriate social behaviour; difficulties in devising and following plans and with situations involving some forms of memory, for example, remembering to carry out intended actions at a future time (for review, see Levin, Eisenberg, & Benton, 1991; Stuss & Benson, 1986; Shallice, 1988).

However, whilst 'frontal lobe syndrome' implies the presence of a consistent pattern of behaviour disorder and other difficulties with a single cause, this is plainly not the case. Examination of patients with known frontal lobe damage demonstrates the presence of not just one, but a variety of different clusters of behaviour disorder, personality abnormality and functional problems. In addition, disorders attributed to frontal lobe damage are often found in the absence of frontal lobe pathology, or cannot be specifically attributed to them alone in the case of generalised, diffuse damage (Stuss & Benson, 1984; Bigler, 1990). Instead, recent advances in functional imaging have helped to emphasise how different brain areas work together as a system in the performance of all but the very simplest of tasks, a finding which questions the integrity of the concept of the frontal lobe syndrome. Indeed, Baddeley (1986) and Baddeley and Wilson (1988), have argued that it is a mistake to try and account for those functional changes attributed to this syndrome on the basis of localisation alone. These authors remind us that deficits associated with damage to other brain structures are not classified according to location, but instead by function. Baddeley and Wilson argue that a functional definition should be sought regarding types of deficit that arise following damage to the frontal lobes and the myriad of rich connections they have with posterior structures: hence their proposal of the term 'dysexecutive syndrome'.

A further advantage of this reconceptualisation of the frontal lobe syndrome to that of the dysexecutive syndrome, is to reduce the emphasis on attempting to ascribe deficits to specific brain sites, whilst highlighting that it is problems with function that should form the basis of most clinical activity, particularly when conducted within a rehabilitation environment. The focus on observable phenomena has led to the development of cognitive models that have attempted to account for behavioural manifestations of the underlying organic damage, irrespective of the site of injury. The models proposed by Shallice (1982) and Baddeley (1986) have achieved the greatest prominence, and have endeavoured to explain the presence of a range of functional problems through impairment of attentional control mechanisms. These models have proven very useful to clinicians in conceptualising the cause of some types of behaviour disorder, and have driven the development of a range of successful treatment programmes (for example see, Burgess & Alderman, 1990; Alderman, 1996; Alderman, Fry, & Youngson, 1995). An example of how the concept of the dysexecutive syndrome and cognitive models can be applied to the rehabilitation of behaviour problems will be presented later in this chapter.

Burgess, Alderman, Evans, Emslie and Wilson (1998) demonstrated that behaviours symptomatic of the dysexecutive syndrome are prevalent amongst people with acquired neurological damage. However, they also found evidence that it is a mistake to conceptualise the dysexecutive syndrome as a single clinical condition. Burgess and colleagues showed instead it fractionates at the level of behaviour into at least five discernible sub-syndromes or components. These were *inhibition* (behaviours arising through difficulties with response suppression), *intentionality* (those attributable to altered insight and the creation and maintenance of goal-related action), *executive memory* (behaviours resulting through impairment of those memory processes directly involved in executive function, for example confabulation), *positive affect* (those consistent with emotional and personality changes seen in people with dysexecutive problems, including aggression and euphoria) and lastly *negative affect* (emotional and personality changes that include shallowing of affect and increased apathy).

This work confirms that it is just as erroneous to simplify the dysexecutive syndrome to the level of a single unitary disorder, as has been implied when the term frontal lobe syndrome is employed. This highlights the need for detailed and thorough assessment to determine what sub-components of the dysexecutive syndrome are evident in order that effective treatment can be planned. For a wider discussion of the dysexecutive syndrome and rehabilitation see Alderman and Burgess (2003).

Treatment Options

Because behaviour disorders are likely to result from complex interactions between a wide range of factors, by necessity treatment should be designed to meet the unique needs of each separate person. There are a number of diverse methods available for the treatment of behavioural problems amongst neurological patients, including pharmacological and rehabilitative interventions (Rao & Lyketsos, 2000). However, not all of these will necessarily be appropriate to all people. For example, with regard to the UK McMillan and Oddy (2001) make the point that very few services exist that are specifically designed to meet the needs of people for whom personality changes and cognitive impairment are the primary disabilities. These authors also argue that people who present with severe behaviour disorders should always be admitted to a specialised neurobehavioural service for treatment. Whilst few units offering such a service are required, it remains the case that places may be restricted to people who happen to live within particular catchment areas (Greenwood & McMillan, 1993). Furthermore, those services that do exist in the UK fall predominantly in the independent sector where the costs necessary to deliver effective neurobehavioural programmes may serve to further exclude people who should be in receipt of them. In other countries with different funding systems, access to more specialised services may be easier in principle, but often they do not exist, or sufficient funding is not available for the time needed.

It is clearly beyond the scope of this chapter to attempt a comprehensive review of all available treatment methods available: a substantial account of the state of current practice can be found in Wood and McMillan (2001). However, principle mainstream approaches include the following:

Pharmacological

Scope for pharmacological intervention is considerable and drug therapies have an important role to play in the treatment of behaviour disorders (see Eames, 2001; Rao & Lyketsos, 2000). However, a number of factors need to be considered regarding these. First, less if known about the effectiveness of drug therapies because relatively few controlled studies have been conducted, whilst single case studies presented in the literature generally lack sufficient methodological rigour to enable objective evaluation of efficacy (Rao & Lyketsos, 2000; Alderman, Knight, & Morgan, 1997). Second, a major problem highlighted by Eames (1990, 2001) is that symptoms of organic brain injury can sometimes be mistaken as evidence of mental illness and lead to administration of an inappropriate drug regime. It is therefore essential that assessment is made by an experienced neuropsychiatrist; unfortunately, few are available at this time in the UK (Alderman, 2001).

Despite these notes of caution, it is clear that pharmacological intervention has a significant contribution to make towards the management of behaviour disturbance amongst people with brain injury. It is beyond the scope of this scope of this chapter to examine the role of medication in-depth: however, there are many examples in the literature to illustrate what benefits there might be. For example, amantadine has been shown to be beneficial in the treatment of a range of neurobehavioral sequelae, including aggression (Nickels, Schneider, Dombovy, & Wong, 1994; Gualtieri, 1991). Anticonvulsants are especially relevant in the management of irritability, aggression, and paroxysmal mood disorders (Hirsch, 1993; Mooney, & Hass, 1993; Giakas, Seibyl, & Mazure, 1990). Carbamazepine appears to have special relevance (Foster, Hillbrand, & Chi, 1989; Mattes, 1990; Azouvi, Jokic, Attral, Denys, Markabi, & Bussel, 1999). Valproic acid is also commonly used and reported to be equally as beneficial as carbamazepine (Rao & Lyketsos, 2000).

Psychotherapy

This is a broad and multiply defined concept (Jackson & Gouvier, 1992) which encompasses various therapies that have arisen from different models of psychopathology (Patterson, 1996). Certainly, successful outcomes have been reported which have lead to positive psychosocial outcomes: well known and successful programmes have been reported by Ben-Yishay, Rattock, Lakin, Piasetsky, Ross, Silver, Zide and Ezrachi (1985), and Prigatano (Prigatano, 1986; Prigatano, Fordyce, Zeiner, Roueche, Pepping, & Wood, 1984). However, Wood and Worthington (2001a) argued that these programmes can only be employed with articulate patients with less debilitating handicaps. Neurological patients with serious behaviour problems are usually excluded from them because of intransigent problems with insight and motivation (Burgess & Wood, 1990; Sazbon & Groswasser, 1991), and because the severity of the challenging behaviour they exhibit is too great (Wood, 1987).

Cognitive therapy

Despite the widespread use and well-known efficacy of the cognitive therapies based on the earlier work of influential clinicians such as Beck (1976), little is known about their effectiveness regarding behaviourally disturbed neurological patients. One reason for this, as with pharmacological interventions, is that this area remains poorly researched to date (Manchester & Wood, 2001). Other factors may also exclude people from participating. Cognitive therapy approaches are essentially concerned with information processing. Belief systems may bias interpretation of experience which in turn alters and shapes behaviour. This can sometimes account for behaviour disorders, such as aggression. Cognitive therapy is concerned with helping patients understand that thoughts and beliefs can be maladaptive, to identify their own thinking distortions, and to help them generate more rational interpretations of events. Patients are helped to become their own 'therapist' and encouraged to test the validity of their automatic thoughts; attempts are made to modify these through a process of hypothesis testing in the real world, and dysfunctional emotions and behaviours subject to change as a consequence. It is certainly the case that reduced awareness and impairment of those cognitive skills necessary to engage in the hypothesis-testing process central to cognitive therapy, create special challenges for cognitive therapy to overcome. These may impede access to this form of therapy for some neurological patients with severe behaviour disorders. However, Kinney (2001) reports methods that enable cognitive therapy to be adapted for use with people with brain injury, and parallels with its successful employment in helping people with severe learning disability (Williams & Jones, 1997; Jones, Williams, & Lowe, 1993) suggest it may prove helpful. For a more comprehensive discussion of the application of cognitive therapy to people with brain injury see Manchester and Wood (2001) and Alderman (2003).

A Neurobehavioural Approach to the Rehabilitation of Behaviour Disorders

Treatment of behaviour disorders amongst neurological patients using behaviour therapy has received considerable attention in the rehabilitation literature during the last two decades. This approach has many advantages (see Powell, 1981; Wilson, 1989): for example, there are techniques available to both increase and decrease behaviours of interest; and the methodologies routinely employed enable objective evaluation of treatment outcome to be made.

However, there are particular reasons why behaviour therapy has special relevance to this clinical population. One of the most obvious is because people have been excluded from psychotherapy and cognitive therapy through lack of awareness, poor motivation, cognitive impairment, or the severity of behaviour disorder. These problems do not necessarily constitute a barrier to the effective use of behaviour therapy.

Neurobehavioural rehabilitation

A problem emphasised earlier in this chapter was lack of homogeneity within the neurological population. This was illustrated with reference to behaviour disorders where the complexity of reasons driving behaviour disorders was emphasised. Poor homogeneity necessitates individual assessment so that treatment is designed to meet the unique needs of every person. However, lack of homogeneity, the sheer number of possible variables concerned, and their complex interactions renders assessment itself highly problematic. Wood and Eames (Wood, 1987, 1990; Wood & Eames, 1981) argued that this problem can be countered in part by casting the brain itself in the role of dependent variable, subjecting it to environmental manipulation, and then studying the effects. In this way the nature of causative factors which underlie behaviour disorders are more likely to be determined, and inferences drawn about the nature of brain-behaviour relationships. This data-driven, objective, analytic approach to the study of brain-behaviour relationships is of course borrowed directly from behaviour therapy. An extension of this model, which incorporates principles from behaviour therapy, neuropsychology and behavioural neurology, are combined to form what Wood has described as a *neurobehavioural paradigm* to rehabilitation (Wood, 1987, 1990; Wood & Worthington, 2001a, 2001b). Neurobehavioural rehabilitation encompasses systems that address cognitive and physical sequelae of brain injury, in addition to targeting behaviour disorders.

It is beyond the scope of this chapter to provide a very detailed description of the neurobehavioural model, or how different therapy disciplines function within this. The most recent comprehensive accounts of the paradigm and the ways in which it is operationalised can be found in Wood and Worthington (2001a; 2001b), and Alderman (2001); Giles and Clark Wilson (1999) provided specific explanations of the ways in which wider therapy requirements (physical and functional) are met within services that are organised to meet social and behavioural needs using neurobehavioural principles. Concepts that differentiate neurobehavioural practice from both the medical model and traditional clinical rehabilitation (Wood & Worthington, 2001a) are that it happens post-acutely (i.e. when medical management is no longer the priority), it is community based, it employs an inter- or transdisciplinary team, and it demands a structured environment. Behaviour modification techniques are used, including stimulus control methods, chaining and shaping, and response-consequence learning technologies (Wood, 1990).

The importance of structure
The concept of structure is of paramount importance within neurobehavioural practice; consequently, this will be elaborated here. Alderman (2001) conceptualised structure within specialised neurobehavioural units as falling at four levels:

1) Structure Provided by the Physical Environment
The goal of neurobehavioural practice is the resolution of handicaps that result from disorders of social behaviour; learning plays a central role, whether it be in reacquiring old skills, or gaining new ones (Wood & Worthington, 2001a). As persistent cognitive problems, including difficulties with attention and memory, are endemic to many chronic neurological conditions, the process of learning is both slow and fragile (Wood, 1987). Given these constraints it is therefore essential that the physical environment is organised in such a way to maximise learning. For example, it should be as quiet as possible and free from extraneous 'clutter' to minimise problems with distractibility. The layout of the unit should be unambiguous and locations of bedrooms, therapy rooms, and so on, should be clear-cut. It is particularly important that the physical environment should emphasise cue-saliency, a subject matter we shall return to again later.

The three remaining levels of structure refer to what happens within the physical environment.

2) Structure Provided by a Transdisciplinary Team
Within neurorehabilitation units the clinical team should be transdisciplinary in organisation so that a unified, seamless service is provided to each patient, focussing on their individual needs (Doyle, 1997; Wood & Worthington, 2001a). Within these teams there is substantial blurring and sharing of roles. Therapists and nurses work within the same physical environment together to achieve the same set of shared goals for each patient. Achieving behavioural goals early in admission is the priority; without this, the ability of the team to engage the patient in wider rehabilitation will remain compromised. Consequently, all staff act as behaviour therapists and have an equal and joint responsibility for ensuring behaviour modification interventions are implemented as and when necessary. An transdisciplinary team facilitates good communication, a co-ordinated approach to rehabilitation, and maximises consistency.

3) Structure Provided by the Routine Imposed on the Day
A timetable of events throughout the day is employed to provide structure through routine. This typical consists of meal times, formal sessions and

'free' time. Routine facilitates a means through which individual rehabilitation needs are met and provides opportunities to practice skills throughout the day. It promotes consistency and facilitates creation of an environment in which there is an expectation for people to attend sessions and participate at an appropriate level.

4) Structure Imposed Through Behaviour Modification Interventions
This serves to provide a framework through which appropriate behaviour and effort are actively encouraged. Probably most importantly, these interventions are vehicles which facilitate appropriate interactions between staff with patients in a way that is helpful and therapeutic, as the experience of the latter is likely to have been negative (see Alderman, 2001; Alderman, Davies, Jones, & McDonnell, 1999). In addition, behaviour modification interventions raise the saliency of cues that normally regulate social behaviour; variable monitoring and poor processing of these cues can explain some of the behaviour disorders exhibited by this clinical group (see Alderman, 1996, 2001; Alderman & Knight, 1997). Utilisation of behaviour modification interventions also increases the likelihood that new learning will take place, even in the presence of cognitive impairment, through increased consistency in how staff interact with patients, by ensuring clarity of rehabilitation goals and the means by which these are achieved, and by knowing what the contingencies to patients' actions and behaviour are (Alderman, 2001).

When services are organised in this way, the net effect is the provision of a daily routine within which skills that aim to maximise independence and quality of life are repeatedly practised and acquired through procedural learning in the form of new habits. Effective communication within the transdisciplinary team, together with a programme that is grounded in behavioural methods, helps ensure rehabilitation is established at an appropriate level for each individual, that goals are shared, and that management, including contingencies to behaviour, is consistent. Good outcomes have been demonstrated regarding reduction of behaviour disorders amongst neurological patients admitted to specialised units which have operationalised the neurobehavioural paradigm (for example see Eames & Wood, 1985a, 1985b; Eames, Cotterill, Kneale, Storrar, & Yeomans, 1996).

Examples of Reduction of Behaviour Disorders

1) Inappropriate Means of Obtaining Attention from Other People
Some 'problematic' behaviours arise in part through how the environment responds to the actions of the person with brain injury. The point was previously made that people with TBI are not popular among rehabilitation professionals because of their often irritating, threatening and embarrassing behaviour, as well as their general lack of motivation (Miller & Cruzat, 1981). This can lead to situations where such people are routinely ignored.

However, one consequence of this may be that other people may inadvertently reinforce less desirable behaviours intermittently shown by a patient. For example, a natural response elicited by shouting, screaming, masturbation and aggression may be a social reprimand , such as being told '...don't do that'. Whilst feedback which takes this form would normally be expected to lead to a change in behaviour, under circumstances devoid of regular positive social contact the attention received by the person, even when it is delivered in the form of criticism, may be welcome. When this is the case, behaviour disorders can become reinforced and thus inadvertently maintained.

Figure 1 illustrates this point. It concerns HC, a young man who had sustained TBI and had acquired a range of characteristic cognitive and behavioural problems. Sequelae of his injury included coarsening of his social behaviour and a general reduction in inhibitory control. HC was noted to be unresponsive to normal social cues; a particular handicap was his lack of ability to join social interaction appropriately. In particular, he failed to wait

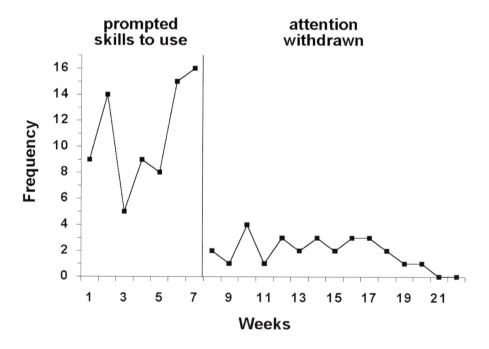

Fig. 1. Reduction in the frequency with which HC interrupted conversation. (NB. Data reflects frequency 15 minute periods in which this behaviour was observed at least once.) Contingent response to interruption in the second half of the figure was withdrawal of attention by means of TOOTS; however, appropriate skills were taught in specific sessions for this purpose, and subsequent use of these skills was reinforced through enriched social praise and attention.

for an appropriate pause in conversation and interrupted others constantly. Staff felt HC needed to relearn the rules which govern social behaviour which it was believed had been lost as a result of his brain injury. It was therefore decided that every time HC interrupted conversation, he would be consistently reminded by staff what these rules were, and what he should do to obtain attention appropriately. On the face of it this plan seems perfectly reasonable, and most people would probably take such feedback on board and use it to modify their behaviour. However, Figure 1 shows this response did not lead to a reduction in the frequency with which HC inappropriately interrupted others conversations (note that data points reflect the number of fifteen minute periods in the day in which HC engaged in this behaviour: the actual frequency was much higher). If anything, Figure 1 suggests the frequency of the behaviour increased.

Of course, what was probably happening was that HC's poor social skills were being reinforced because staff consistently gave him attention every time he interrupted. In contrast, his coarse social behaviour and general lack of inhibition rendered him unpopular with other people to the extent that his social needs were poorly met. Under these conditions, it is easy to understand how reprimand, criticism, or, as in this case, instruction intended to correct undesirable behaviour, might actually work to reinforce it. Accordingly, an intervention was designed whose aim was to change the contingencies to HC's behaviour. The principle of "Time-Out-On-The-Spot' from positive reinforcement' (abridged to 'TOOTS': see Wood, 1987; Burgess & Wood, 1990) was used: as staff attention was maintaining HC's inappropriate behaviour, they were required to consistently withdraw giving him attention whilst he attempted to interrupt conversation. In this way, reinforcement was no longer available. In addition, HC was taught the correct skills to use in formal social skills training sessions. Most importantly, staff were required to consistently reinforce use of appropriate means of getting other peoples attention whenever HC chose to use them. Figure 1 confirms that the frequency of interrupting decreased in response to this intervention.

2) Reduction in Physically Aggressive Behaviour
HC illustrates how the environment may reinforce inappropriate social behaviour and how a simple intervention can be used to reverse contingencies maintaining it. Aggressive behaviour disorders represent the greatest challenge to rehabilitation services, especially when this involves physical assaults on other people (Burke, Wesolowski, & Lane, 1988) and it is this, probably more than any other behaviour disorder, that is likely to result in exclusion from rehabilitation. However, within specialised services, the neurobehavioural paradigm may be sufficiently embraced to enable management of severe aggressive behaviour disorders (see Alderman, 2001, for a description of the requirements of such a service).

There are many reasons why neurological patients exhibit aggression. Miller (1994) summarised three of the most cited. First, it may be attributable to an episodic dyscontrol syndrome, in which disturbance of mood and behaviour is a consequence of electrophysiological brain disturbance. Second, damage to anterior brain structures decreases ability to inhibit or regulate emotional responses, leading to a lower threshold for aggressive behaviour. Third, brain injury exacerbates negative premorbid personality traits: people who were aggressive are likely to be more so as a consequence of neurological damage. An additional reason is that aggression may be negatively reinforced as it leads to avoidance of, or escape from, situations which are perceived as threatening or undesirable. For example, poor awareness and lack of insight regarding extent of disability amongst neurological patients may result in poor motivation to engage in the rehabilitation process (Prigatano, 1991; Wood, 1988; Sazbon, & Groswasser, 1991). Spontaneous bouts of aggression directed at a source of frustration, usually a nurse or therapist, may initially occur because of reduced tolerance levels. The understandable response of staff will be to withdraw. When this takes place in therapy situations the patient with little insight regarding the need for this may learn that purposefully aggressing against staff will lead to withdrawal of treatment: this behaviour may consequently become negatively reinforced (see Alderman, 1991; Alderman, Shepherd, & Youngson, 1994).

In these cases, treatment of patients within a specialised neurobehavioural service in which expectations are gradually increased, has been demonstrated to be effective in reducing aggressive behaviour disorders (Alderman, Davies, Jones, & McDonnell, 1999). The net effect of the levels of structure described by Alderman (2001) and summarised earlier will be to provide a therapeutic framework within which aggression may be safely managed. Methods are employed whose purpose is to reverse contingencies which have led to avoidance and escape from rehabilitation activities in order to deliberately elicit aggressive behaviour (with the minimum of risk). Use of behaviour modification methods is fundamental. They are used to create conditions which encourage motivation and success, by reinforcing appropriate behaviour and skills. Whenever possible, the desirable consequence to aggression is the withdrawal of attention through TOOTS whilst maintaining the required level of expectation. In this way, only behaviours that are consistent with the aims of rehabilitation are reinforced. One way of achieving this is by using a token economy (Wood, 1987), or programmes based on the principles of differential reinforcement (Alderman & Knight, 1997; Knight, Rutterford, Alderman, & Swan, 2002).

An example of the effectiveness of such an approach is illustrated in Figure 2. This concerns MW, a 43-year-old male who had sustained TBI two years previously. Severity of neurobehavioural disability proved sufficient to exclude him from the usual range of rehabilitation services, and a placement in the community proved untenable. Neuropsychological problems were evident, especially with regard to memory and executive function. He was consequently admitted to a specialised neurobehavioural unit and his aggressive behaviour monitored using the Overt Aggression Scale – Modified

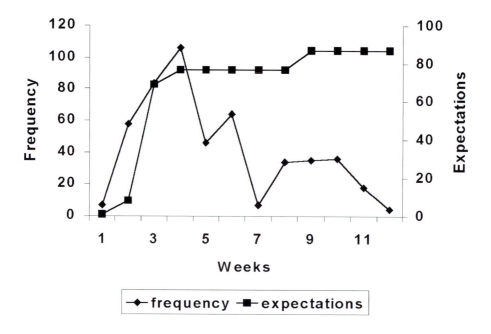

Fig. 2. Reduction in the frequency of physical aggression directed at other people by
MW. Concurrent measurement of rehabilitation demands shows that aggressive behaviour decreased despite gradual increase in expectations.

for Neurorehabilitation (OAS-MNR: Alderman, Knight, & Morgan, 1997).
The OAS-MNR enables recording of type of aggression, its frequency, severity, and methods used to manage/treat it. It also enables recording of ante-
cedents, and quantifies the intrusiveness of interventions employed. It has
proved useful in clinical work with aggressive patients (Alderman, Davies,
Jones, & McDonnell, 1999), and in audit and research (Alderman, Knight,
& Henman, 2002). In addition, the levels of expectation placed on MW in
rehabilitation are also represented in Figure 2, through ratings made using the
Neurorehabilitation Expectations Scale (NES: Swan & Alderman, in press).
In brief, the NES consists of ten activities and demands that most patients
admitted to neurobehavioural units would be exposed to. They are ranked
from least demanding (1 – 'invited to attend meals') to most demanding
(10 – 'each separate behaviour modification programme used'). Other examples of items include having a toileting programme (ranked 5) and having a
formal supervised hygiene programme (ranked 8). A gross indication of the
level of expectation for any patient can thus be obtained by summing the
ranks of those items that apply for each week of admission.

During the twelve-week assessment period represented by Figure 2,
recordings made on the OAS-MNR showed MW was frequently aggressive.

Physical aggression towards other people was the main category of aggressive behaviour recorded: of the 1138 recordings made, 53% (603) were assaults on others. Figure 2 confirms that expectations regarding MW were initially low during the first week of admission, but gradually increased thereafter (see Alderman, Davies, Jones, & McDonnell, 1999, for details of the admission process concerned). Figure 2 also shows a concurrent increase in the frequency of physically aggressive behaviour, peaking in week 4. OAS-MNR recordings suggested that increased aggression was primarily a function of rising expectations as 66% of this behaviour followed prompts and requests made by staff. However, Figure 2 confirms that whilst levels of expectation remained consistently high, the number of times MW was physically aggressive substantially decreased after the fourth week.

This brief account confirms findings reported elsewhere that aggressive behaviour disorders can be successfully reduced through exposure to a holistic neurobehavioural programme (Wood, 1987; Alderman, Davies, Jones, & McDonnell, 1999; Alderman, Bentley, & Dawson, 1999; Swan & Alderman, submitted). When aggression has previously been reinforced because it has led to avoidance of or escape from rehabilitation activities, a gradual increase in expectations, reinforcement of behaviours incompatible with aggression, and consistency of staff response, all combine to promote conditions which promote co-operation.

One major advantage of a behaviour modification approach is the substantial effect it has on achieving consistent response-sets from staff interacting with people who present with challenging behaviour (Alderman & Knight, 1997; Alderman, 2001). An important outcome in substituting what Alderman (2001) called a spontaneous, or natural, system of feedback, with a structured system, is to change staff behaviour. In the absence of structured feedback systems (of which behaviour modification interventions are part) differing staff expectations and responses will contribute to the evolution and maintenance of aggression. Variability attributable to individual staff differences will be significantly reduced through adherence to a prescribed intervention. The programme becomes a vehicle to achieve consistency amongst staff which ultimately has an impact on patient behaviour. The philosophy of the neurobehavioural approach is the reinforcement of positive behaviour, whereby behavioural programmes are vehicles that facilitate positive staff-patient interaction where previously the tendency would have been to avoid interaction or for it to be negative. When this is the case, as MW has shown, the likelihood of successful outcome in the treatment of aggression is optimised.

3) Remediation of Behaviour Disorders Resulting from Monitoring Difficulties
Enhanced cue-saliency is an integral feature of neurobehavioural rehabilitation. A consequence of enhanced structure and the availability of regular feedback is the ability to maintain a prosthetic environment. Inappropriate

behaviour can arise when social cues are missed. In addition, neurological patients may have poor awareness and lack insight regarding behaviour problems, and thus lack motivation to change. Both inefficient processing of cues and reduced awareness regarding consequences of behaviour may be the result of monitoring impairment. Both these difficulties are likely to diminish when people are immersed within the specialised environment of a neurobehavioural service because cues are exaggerated. This may be one reason why token economies and differential reinforcement programmes are successful, as they enable feedback about behaviour to be presented clearly, frequently and regularly (see Wood, 1987; Alderman & Knight, 1997). In this way, behavioural strategies enable individuals to obtain feedback from the environment which they may otherwise miss; the net effect of the prosthetic environment in which rehabilitation takes place will be to circumvent difficulties with monitoring, enabling greater recognition of cues and awareness of the impact of behaviour to take place. It could be said that the regular feedback provided to patients by staff through the structure of the behavioural programmes circumvents cognitive problems, especially those concerned with attention and memory, which would normally give rise to symptoms characteristic of the dysexecutive syndrome.

For many patients, the structure of the neurobehavioural service described earlier is sufficient to enable management of behaviour disorder and full exploitation of individual rehabilitation potential. However, it was recognised some time ago that some patients remain unresponsive to neurobehavioural paradigms in which feedback is managed using various forms of positive reinforcement programme (Alderman & Burgess, 1990).

Impairments in attention and working memory have been especially highlighted in relation to the evolution and maintenance of some behavioural problems. Explanations for these have recently been proposed using the concept of working memory proposed by Baddeley and Hitch (1974). This is conceptualised as consisting of several temporary storage systems whose activities are co-ordinated by a central executive (CE), aided by a number of subsystems which include the articulatory loop (which deals with verbal information) and the visuospatial sketchpad (which processes non-verbal material). The CE allocates attentional resources to these subsystems. CE impairment results in inefficiencies in the allocation of attentional resources which are evidenced in a range of behavioural and other symptoms seen in patients that are characteristic of the 'dysexecutive syndrome' (Baddeley, 1986; Baddeley, & Wilson, 1988). Impairment of CE functioning may result in difficulties in scheduling two or more concurrent tasks, distractibility, poor monitoring of performance, problems utilising feedback, and attention and memory problems.

Alderman and colleagues (Alderman, 1996; Alderman, Fry, & Youngson, 1995) attributed some behaviour disorders amongst neurological patients to deficits in CE function, whereby difficulties with attending to multiple events are evident functionally through people having problems in monitoring changes in the environment, their own behaviour, and internal (physiological) changes. Opportunities to receive and process feedback are reduced which results in failure to modify behaviour in response to changing circumstances: individuals with the dysexecutive syndrome therefore present as impulsive, distractible, unresponsive to cues from others, and behave inappropriately in social situations. For many patients, the provision of feedback provided through the combination of the structure and positive reinforcement programmes within a neurobehavioural unit, is sufficient to circumvent the cognitive impairment which underlies some behaviour disorders. However, Alderman (1996) argued that when CE deficit is severe only one stimulus set at a time may be routinely attended to. This may be explain why a characteristic feature of the dysexecutive syndrome is a reduced ability to change behaviour in an adaptive, flexible way, in response to changes in the environment. It has also been used to account for why some patients do not respond to use of positive reinforcement methods, a hypothesis which has received some experimental validation (Alderman, 1996).

Consequently, specific approaches have been used in the treatment of behaviour disorders thought to arise from profound difficulty in the allocation of attentional resources to the extent that only one stimulus set at a time may be routinely attended to. Use of a behaviour modification technique known as response cost is believed to have particular relevance and a number of single case studies with intransigent behaviour disorders have been described in the literature which have been successfully treated using this method (for example see Alderman & Ward, 1991; Alderman & Burgess,1990; 1994). Typically, the person who is the recipient of treatment is given a number of 'tokens' (plastic discs, or whatever else is appropriate). One of these can be subsequently removed on each occasion a target behaviour (for example aggression) is observed (see Alderman, 2001, Table 9.3, p. 195 for an illustration of the operational procedure concerning removal of tokens). After a predefined time has elapsed the number of tokens left in the persons possession are checked; providing these exceed or equal a specified target (for example 10/20) they are exchanged for an agreed reinforcer.

It has been argued response cost benefits patients with severe CE deficit because feedback is immediately contingent on behaviour (thereby reducing memory load), requires little understanding of reward contingencies, and has both verbal mediation and procedural learning components.

Alderman, Fry and Youngson (1995) used the CE model to successfully develop what is arguably a five stage cognitive rehabilitation technique used for the treatment of behaviour disorders that are secondary to severe impairment of monitoring function. Their programme of Self Monitoring Training (SMT) has some advantages over response cost, both ethically and practically; as it is directly concerned with developing cognitive skills in order to produce behaviour change, rather than simply trying to change behaviour alone, SMT is also believed to be more advantageous than response cost in that its benefits are more likely to maintain and generalise (see Knight, Rutterford, Alderman,

Table 1.   Summary of the five stages of self-monitoring training.
(*Differential Reinforcement of Low rates of behaviour: see Alderman &
Knight, 1997)

Each session within which SMT is conducted lasts the same time (for example, 20
minutes) and takes place within the context of some secondary task (for example, an
orientation session). The frequency with which target behaviours occur are usually
recorded by both patient and therapist using hand-held mechanical tally counters.

Stage 1   *Baseline*
           Therapist maintains covert frequency count of target behaviour.

Stage 2   *Spontaneous Self-monitoring*
           Patient asked at beginning of session to maintain frequency count of target
           behaviour; therapist also maintains covert count. At end of session thera-
           pist shares and compares their recording with that of the patient.

Stage 3   *Prompted Self-monitoring*
           As stage 2: however, when the therapist observes that the patient does not
           make a record of a target behaviour immediately after they have engaged
           in it, they are given one clear verbal prompt that they should do so.

Stage 4   *Independent Self-monitoring and Accuracy Reward*
           As stage 2 (therapist prompts are now withdrawn). Reinforcer available to
           patient dependent on the accuracy with which they have self-recorded the
           target behaviour (for example, if within 50% of that made by the thera-
           pist).

Stage 5   *Independent Self-monitoring and DRL**
           As stage 2 with the addition of a DRL intervention. Reinforcement is now
           available only if frequency of the target behaviour (as determined by thera-
           pist recording) has not exceeded a specified target.

& Swan, 2002, regarding a further example of use of SMT). Table 1 outlines
in brief what is entailed in each of the five stages of SMT.

The potential success of using treatment programmes which provide consistent feedback to patients immediately contingent upon behaviour disorders
secondary to poor monitoring is well illustrated by the case of FO. FO was a
27 year old male who sustained very severe brain damage through viral infection. He presented with a wide range of behaviour disorders which prevented
him exploiting his rehabilitation potential in all but a specialised neurobehavioural service. Neuropsychological examination reflected memory and executive difficulties: problems with the ability to monitor both his own behaviour
and cues within the environment were especially highlighted. Behavioural
assessment suggested the latter played a key role in the maintenance of the
problems with behaviour he showed (see Alderman, 2002, for details of this).
Accordingly, two interventions were successfully employed which aimed to
reduce the frequency of behaviour disorder through enhancing FO's monitor-

ing skills. First, response cost was employed for the purpose of decreasing the rate of occurrence of a number of bizarre behaviours. Frequency counts made during the course of a week prior to intervention clearly convey the detrimental impact these behaviours were having on his rehabilitation: hip thrusting (2050); intermittent use of a bizarre gait pattern (769); and body patting/rubbing (77). Use of response cost proved highly successful (see Alderman, in 2002).

Second, SMT was used in an attempt to reduce the frequency of self-initiated verbal output evident in structured rehabilitation activities. This was pretty much constant and served to distract both FO and others, thereby interfering with skill acquisition. It proved unresponsive to a range of reinforcement and other behaviour modification interventions. As both behavioural and neuropsychological assessment had highlighted the role of poor monitoring, it was hypothesised that impairment of this important cognitive skill accounted for both the maintenance of this problem and FO's poor response to differential reinforcement. Consequently, an attempt was made to enhance monitoring skills using SMT. FO was exposed to stages 1–4 of this as described by Alderman, Fry and Youngson (1995). Training further highlighted the magnitude of FO's monitoring difficulties: initially, he underestimated the frequency with which he initiated verbal output by as much as 161 times within a 15 minute period (average discrepancy = 84.4). By stage 4 of training, his ability to self-monitor this aspect of his behaviour had significantly improved (median discrepancy between FO's recording of initiated verbal output and that of staff = 0). Stages 1–4 of SMT are directly concerned with improving self-monitoring skills; stage 5 then attempts to successfully use these skills to reduce the target behaviour using a differential reinforcement of low rates of behaviour (DRL) programme. Equipped with new skills, this stage of training was carried out within other rehabilitation sessions from which he had previously been excluded because of the disruption he caused. Figure 3 demonstrates the success achieved.

It can clearly be seen that during the pre-treatment baseline period (in which the target behaviour was given as little social attention as possible) the frequency of FO's self-initiated verbal output was increasing. Following training of monitoring skills in separate sessions, stage 5 of SMT was carried out in-situ in a range of other rehabilitation sessions. Figure 3 demonstrates that the upward trend in this behaviour was reversed and its frequency significantly reduced. Stage 5 was stopped after FO had participated in 186 such sessions (each an hour in duration). Follow-up three months after SMT had been withdrawn confirmed that the frequency of self-initiated verbal output remained low and the improvement seen during training had maintained.

The net effects of using both response cost and SMT were that FO was able to successfully participate in the wider rehabilitation programme. Through this he acquired sufficient behavioural controls and new skills to enable him to be discharged to a smaller, less structured unit for long-term placement which otherwise his behaviour would have denied him.

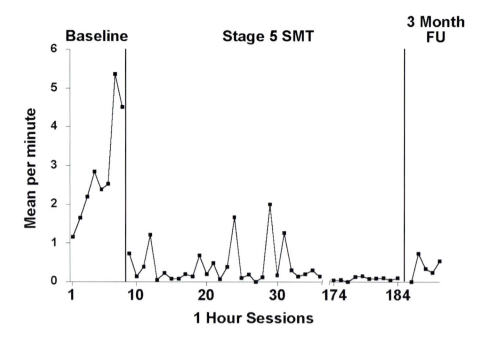

Fig. 3. Reduction in the frequency of self-initiated verbal output made by FO during rehabilitation sessions using SMT. Note that stages 1-4 of SMT were conducted in specific daily sessions for this purpose after data shown in the baseline stage were collected. Increased inhibition of verbal output had maintained relative to baseline three months after SMT had been withdrawn.

Concluding Remarks

In this chapter a very brief review of a range of treatment options available for the management of behaviour disorders characteristic of people with acquired brain injury has been attempted. Given the complexity of the population and the reasons underlying why behaviour disorders arise and are maintained, little will have been achieved other than to equip the reader with all but the minimum of knowledge regarding the issues touched upon here.

Whilst a rich variety of different types of treatment, arising from a number of diverse theoretical and applied frameworks have been put forward as options, interventions arising from the neurobehavioural paradigm have been especially highlighted. In part, this reflects the authors own clinical training and experience. However, this is also because many people referred for treatment because of behavioural problems will be excluded from participation in other types of programme. This may be because they lack the necessary cognitive skills to take part in cognitive and other verbal psychotherapies, or because they do not have the necessary insight, awareness of deficit, or motivation to undertake the active role required. However, probably the most common reason is that people are excluded from such programmes because they are behaviourally disturbed. Whilst medicine has much to offer, shortage of sufficiently trained and experienced specialised practitioners, and the relative lack of good empirical evidence regarding different pharmacological interventions, limits this at present. However, as Wood and Worthington (2001a) have argued, lack of homogeneity within the acquired neurological population and the multivariate nature as to reasons underlying behaviour disorders, renders a purely medical approach to the problem inappropriate.

The neurobehavioural paradigm can be successfully applied partly because it integrates medical, psychological and cognitive approaches under one theoretical umbrella. In addition, cognitive impairment, lack of insight and awareness, poor motivation, and severity of behavioural disturbance do not necessarily lead to exclusion. On the contrary, neurorehabilitation programmes lend themselves well to the challenges imposed by the very factors that prevent access to more traditional therapeutic orientations. In part, this is because the structures within neurobehavioural programmes act in such a way that cognitive problems that can drive and maintain behaviour disorders are circumvented. However, equally important is the influence they exert on the rehabilitation environment itself in that provision of programmed feedback systems through behaviour modification interventions changes the behaviour of those people working with a patient. The tremendous impact this can have on behaviour and functioning cannot be overstated.

Whilst neurobehavioural rehabilitation has much to offer in the treatment of this very challenging clinical population, it is not without its critics, both on ethical and practical grounds. For example, the demands of the neurobehavioural approach are such that although there are exceptions (for example, see Wood, 1988; Goll & Hawley, 1989; Watson, Rutterford, Shortland, Williamson, & Alderman, 2001) it requires establishment of specialised units because of the amount of resources and specialised knowledge required (Alderman, 2001). Behaviour modification interventions, a key component in neurobehavioural rehabilitation, have also been criticised in that they fail to generalise to other environments (McGlynn, 1990). However, it may be the case that when cognitive impairment is the major contributing factor to maintenance of behaviour disorder, the highly structured environment acts as a prosthetic in that it facilitates the effective delivery of feedback through operation of behaviour modification interventions. When people are discharged and this prosthetic is no longer available, problems with monitoring return and behaviour deteriorates. It may be that when people are no longer within the specialised environment of the neurobehavioural unit, contingencies change in such a way that behaviour disorders are re-reinforced (Alderman, 2001). It may also be that when cognitive systems are severely damaged, people will be dependent for life on systems that are placed around them which circumvent the difficulties arising from their breakdown. If so, generalisation is an unrealistic expectation; instead, finding the least intrusive level of support that enables the best quality of life becomes the goal rather than preoccupation with the idealistic aim of completely removing all structure, including behavioural programmes. When this proves to be the case, those environmental modifications necessary to achieve this aim must be implemented and maintained in order to support appropriate behaviour.

It is a reassuring reality that medical and rehabilitation expertise will continue to evolve. In the future it may be that progress in areas such as intracerebral and fetal brain cell implantation will have radical consequences for outcome after neurological insult (for example, see Elsayed, Hogan, Shaw, & Castro, 1996; Barami, Hao, Lotoczky, Diaz, & Lyman, 2001), and the blight of behaviour disorder becomes a thing of the past. In the meantime, the neurobehavioural paradigm gives clinicians a practical framework within which to work, and patients those opportunities required to maximise independence and ensure optimum quality of life.

References

Alderman, N. (1991). The treatment of avoidance behaviour following severe brain injury by satiation through negative practice. *Brain Injury, 5,* 77-86.

Alderman, N. (1996). Central executive deficit and response to operant conditioning methods. *Neuropsychological Rehabilitation, 6,* 161-186.

Alderman, N. (2001). Management of challenging behaviour. In R.L.I.Wood & T. McMillan (Eds.), *Neurobehavioural Disability and Social Handicap Following Traumatic Brain Injury.* Hove, Psychology Press.

Alderman, N. (2002). Individual case studies. In S. Priebe and M. Slade (Eds.), *Evidence in Mental Health Care.* Routledge.

Alderman, N. (2003). Contemporary approaches to the management of irritability and aggression following traumatic brain injury. *Neuropsychological Rehabilitation, 13,* 211-240.

Alderman, N. (submitted). Disorders of Behaviour. In J. Ponsford (Ed.), *Rehabilitation of Neurobehavioural Disorders.* Guilford Press.

Alderman, N. & Burgess, P.W. (1990). Integrating cognition and behaviour: a pragmatic approach to brain-injury rehabilitation. In R.L I.Wood & I. Fussey (Eds.), *Cognitive Rehabilitation in Perspective.* Basingstoke: Taylor & Francis Ltd.

Alderman, N. & Burgess, P. (1994). A comparison of treatment methods for behaviour disorders following herpes simplex encephalitis. *Neuropsychological Rehabilitation, 4,* 31-48.

Alderman, N. & Ward, A. (1991). Behavioural treatment of the dysexecutive syndrome: reduction of repetitive speech using response cost and cognitive overlearning. *Neuropsychological Rehabilitation, 1,* 65-80.

Alderman, N. & Burgess, P.W. (2003). Assessment and rehabilitation of the dysexecutive syndrome. In R. Greenwood, M.P. Barns, T. McMillan and T. Ward (Eds.), *Neurological Rehabilitation.* Hove: Psychology Press.

Alderman, N., Shepherd, J., & Youngson, H.A. (1992). Increasing standing tolerance and posture quality following severe brain injury using a behaviour modification approach. *Physiotherapy, 78,* 335-343.

Alderman, N., Fry, R.K. & Youngson, H.A. (1995). Improvement of self-monitoring skills, reduction of behaviour disturbance and the dysexecutive syndrome: comparison of response cost and a new programme of self-monitoring training. *Neuropsychological Rehabilitation, 5,* 193-221.

Alderman, N. & Knight, C. (1997). The effectiveness of DRL in the management and treatment of severe behaviour disorders following brain injury. *Brain Injury, 11,* 79-101.

Alderman, N., Knight, C., & Morgan, C. (1997). Use of a modified version of the Overt Aggression Scale in the measurement and assessment of aggressive behaviours following brain injury. *Brain Injury, 11,* 503-523.

Alderman, N., Bentley, J., & Dawson, K. (1999). Issues and practice regarding behavioural outcome measurement undertaken by a specialised service provider. *Neuropsychological Rehabilitation, 9,* 385-400.

Alderman, N., Davies, J.A., Jones, C., & McDonnell, P. (1999). Reduction of severe aggressive behaviour in acquired brain injury: case studies illustrating clinical use of the OAS-MNR in the management of challenging behaviours. *Brain Injury, 13,* 669-704.

Alderman, N., Knight, C., & Henman, C. (2002). Aggressive behaviours observed within a neurobehavioural rehabilitation service: utility of the OAS-MNR in clinical audit and applied research. *Brain Injury, 16,* 469-489.

Azouvi, P., Jokic, C., Attral, N., Denys, P., Markabi, S., & Bussel, B. (1999). Carbamazepine in agitation and aggressive behaviour following severe closed-head injury: results of an open trial. *Brain Injury, 13,* 797-804.

Baddeley, A.D. (1986). *Working Memory.* Oxford: Clarendon Press.

Baddeley, A.D. & Hitch, G.J. (1974). Working memory. In G. Bower (Ed.), *Recent advances in learning and motivation, Vol. VIII.* New York: Academic Press.

Baddeley, A.D. & Wilson, B. (1988). Frontal amnesia and the dysexecutive syndrome. *Brain and Cognition, 7,* 212-230.

Baddeley, A.D. & Wilson, B. (1988). Frontal amnesia and the dysexecutive syndrome. *Brain and Cognition, 7,* 212-230.

Barami, K., Hao, H.N., Lotoczky, G.A., Diaz, F.G., & Lyman, W.D. (2001). Transplantation of human fetal brain cells into ischemic lesion of adult gerbil hippocampus. *Journal of Neurosurgery, 95,* 308-315.

Beck, A.T. (1976). *Cognitive therapy and the emotional disorders.* Madison, C.T.: International Universities Press.

Ben-Yishay, Y., Rattock, J., Lakin, P., Piasetsky, E.B., Ross, B., Silver, S., Zide, E., & Ezrachi, O. (1985). Neuropsychologic rehabilitation: quest for a holistic approach. *Seminars in Neurology, 5,* 252-258.

Bigler, E.D. (1990). Neuropathology of traumatic brain injury. In E.D. Bigler (Ed.), *Traumatic brain injury: mechanisms of damage, assessment, intervention, and outcome.* Austin, Texas: Pro-ed.

Brooks, D.N., McKinlay, W., Symington, C., Beattie, A., & Campsie, L. (1987). The effects of severe head injury upon patient and relative within seven years of injury. *Journal of Head Trauma Rehabilitation, 2,* 1-13.

Burgess, P.W. & Alderman, N. (1990). Rehabilitation of dyscontrol syndromes following frontal lobe damage: a cognitive neuropsychological approach. In R.L.I. Wood and I. Fussey (Ed.), *Cognitive Rehabilitation in Perspective.* Basingstoke: Taylor & Francis Ltd.

Burgess, P.W. & Wood, R.L.I. (1990). Neuropsychology of behaviour disorders following brain injury. In R.L.I.Wood (Ed.), *Neurobehavioural sequelae of traumatic brain injury.* London: Taylor and Francis Ltd.

Burgess, P.W., Alderman, N., Evans, J.J., Emslie, H., & Wilson, B.A. (1998). The ecological validity of tests of executive function. *Journal of the International Neuropsychological Society, 4,* 547-558.

Burke, H.H., Wesolowski, M.D., & Lane, I. (1988). A positive approach to the treatment of aggressive brain injured clients. *International Journal of Rehabilitation Research, 11,* 235-241.

Colthart, M. (1991). Cognitive psychology applied to the treatment of acquired language disorders. In P.R. Martin (Ed.), *Handbook of behavior therapy and psychological science: an integrative approach*. New York: Pergamon Press.

Doyle, B. (1997). Transdisciplinary approaches to working with families. In B. Carpenter (Ed.), *Families in context: emerging trends in family support and early intervention*. London: David Fulton.

Eames, P.G. (1990). Organic bases of behaviour disorders after traumatic brain injury. In R.L.I. Wood (Ed.), *Neurobehavioural sequelae of traumatic brain injury*. London: Taylor and Francis Ltd.

Eames, P.G. (2001). Distinguishing the neuropsychiatric, psychiatric, and psychological consequences of acquired brain injury. In R.L.I. Wood and T. McMillan (Eds.), *Neurobehavioural Disability and Social Handicap Following Traumatic Brain Injury*. Hove, Psychology Press.

Eames, P., Cotterill, G., Kneale, T.A., Storrar, A.L., & Yeomans, P. (1996). Outcome of intensive rehabilitation after severe brain injury: a long-term follow-up study. *Brain Injury, 10*, 631-650.

Eames, P. & Wood, R.L.I. (1985a). Rehabilitation after severe brain injury: a follow-up study of a behaviour modification approach. *Journal of Neurology, Neurosurgery, and Psychiatry, 48*, 613-619.

Eames, P. & Wood, R.L.I (1985b). Rehabilitation after severe brain injury: a special-unit approach to behaviour disorders. *International Rehabilitation Medicine, 7*, 130-133.

Elsayed, M.H., Hogan, T.P., Shaw, P.L., & Castro, A.J. (1996). Use of fetal cortical grafts in hypoxic-ischemic brain injury in neonatal rats. *Experimental Neurology, 137*, 127-141.

Emerson, E., Barrett, S., Bell, C., Cummings, R., McCool, C., Toogood, A., & Mansell, J. (1987). *Developing services for people with severe learning difficulties and challenging behaviours*. University of Kent at Canterbury, Institute of Social and Applied Psychology.

Foster, H.G., Hillbrand, M., & Chi, C.C. (1989). Efficacy of carbamazepine in assaultive patients with frontal lobe dysfunction. *Progress in Neuro-Psychopharmaco,logy and Biological Psychiatry, 13*, 865-874.

Giakas, W.J., Seibyl, J.P., & Mazure, C.M. (1990). Valporate in the treatment of temper outburst. *Journal of Clinical Psychiatry, 51*, 525.

Giles, G.M. & Clark-Wilson, J. (1999). *Rehabilitation of the severely brain-injured adult: a practical approach* (2nd edn.). Cheltenham: Stanley Thornes.

Goll, S. & Hawley, K. (1988). Social rehabilitation: the role of the transitional living centre. In R.L.I. Wood & P.G. Eames (Eds.), *Models of brain injury rehabilitation*. London: Chapman Hall.

Greenwood, R.J. & McMillan, T.M. (1993). Models of rehabilitation programmes for the brain-injured adult: I. Current provision, efficacy, and good practice. *Clinical Rehabilitation, 7*, 248-255.

Gualtieri, C.T. (1991). *Neuropsychiatry and behavioral pharmacology*. New York: Springer-Verlag.

Hirsch, J. (1993). Promising drugs for neurobehavioural treatment. *Headlines*, March/April, 10-11.

Jackson, W.T. & Gouvier, W.D. (1992). Group psychotherapy with brain-damaged adults and their families. In C.J. Lang & L.K. Ross (Eds.), *Handbook of head trauma, acute care to recovery*. New York: Plenum Press.

Johnson, R. & Balleny, H. (1996). Behaviour problems after brain injury: incidence and need for treatment. *Clinical Rehabilitation, 10*, 173-181.

Jones, R.S.P., Williams, H., & Lowe, F. (1993). Verbal self-regulation. In I. Fleming & B. Stenfert-Kroese (Eds.), *People with severe learning disability and challenging behaviour: new developments in services and therapy*. Manchester: Manchester University Press.

Kimble, D.P. (1963). *Physiological psychology*. Reading, MA: Addison-Wesley.

Kinney, A. (2001). Cognitive therapy and brain injury: theoretical and conceptual issues. *Journal of Contemporary Psychotherapy, 31*, 89-102.

Knight, C., Rutterford, N., Alderman, N., & Swan, L. (2002). Is accurate self-monitoring necessary for people with acquired neurological problems to benefit from the use of differential reinforcement methods? *Brain Injury, 16*, 75-87.

Levin, H.S., Eisenberg, H.M., & Benton, A.L. (Eds.) (1991*). Frontal lobe function and dysfunction*. New York: Oxford University Press.

Manchester, D. & Wood, R.L.I. (2001). Applying cognitive therapy in neuropsychological rehabilitation. In R.L.I. Wood & T.M. McMillan (Eds.), *Neurobehavioural Disability and Social Handicap Following Traumatic Brain Injury*. Hove, Psychology Press.

Mateer, C.A. & Ruff, R.M. (1990). Effectiveness of behavioral management procedures in the rehabilitation of head-injured patients. In R.L.I. Wood (Ed.) *Neurobehavioural sequelae of traumatic brain injury*. New York: Taylor Francis.

Mattes, J.A. (1990). Comparative effectiveness of carbamazepine and propranolol for rage outburst. *Journal of Neuropsychiatry and Clinical Neuroscience, 2*, 159-164.

McGlynn, S.M. (1990). Behavioural approaches to neuropsychological rehabilitation. *Psychological Bulletin, 108*, 420-441.

McKinlay, W.W, Brooks, D.N., Bond, M.R., Martinage, D.P., & Marshall, M.M. (1981). The short term outcome of severe blunt head injury as reported by the relatives of the injured person. *Journal of Neurology, Neurosurgery and Psychiatry, 44*, 527-533.

McMillan, T.M. & Oddy, M. (2001). Service provision for social disability and handicap after acquired brain injury. In R.L.I. Wood & T.M. McMillan (Eds.), *Neurobehavioural Disability and Social Handicap Following Traumatic Brain Injury*. Hove, Psychology Press.

Miller, L. (1994). Traumatic brain injury and aggression. *Journal of Offender Rehabilitation, 2*, 91-103.

Miller, E. & Cruzat, A. (1981). A note on the effects of irrelevant information on task performance after mild and severe head injury. *British Journal of Social and Clinical Psychology, 20*, 69-70.

Mooney, G.F. & Hass, L.J. (1993). Effect of methylphenidate on brain injury-related anger. *Archives of Physical Medicine and Rehabilitation, 74*, 153-160.

Nickels, J.L., Schneider, W.N., Dombovy, M.L., & Wong, T.M. (1994). Clinical use of amantadine in brain injury rehabilitation. *Brain Injury, 8*, 709-718.

Oddy, M., Coughlan, T., Tyerman, A., & Jenkins, D. (1985). Social adjustment after closed head injury: a further follow-up seven years after injury. *Journal of Neurology, Neurosurgery and Psychiatry, 48*, 564-568.

Patterson, C.H. (1986). *Theories of counselling and psychotherapy* (4th Ed.). New York: Harper and Row.

Powell, G.E. (1981). *Brain function therapy*. Aldershot, England: Gower Press.

Prigatano, G.P. (1986). Psychotherapy after brain injury. In G.P. Prigatano, D.J. Fordyce, H.K. Zeiner, J.R. Roeche, M. Pepping & B.C. Wood (Eds.), *Neuropsychological rehabilitation after brain injury*. Baltimore: John Hopkins University Press.

Prigatano, G.P. (1991). Disturbances of self awareness of deficit after traumatic brain injury. In G.P. Prigatano & D.L. Schacter (Eds.), *Awareness of deficit after brain injury: clinical and theoretical issues*. New York: Oxford University Press.

Prigatano, G.P., Fordyce, D.J., Zeiner, H.K., Roueche, J.R., Pepping, M., & Wood, B.C. (1984). Neuropsychological rehabilitation after closed head injury in young adults. *Journal of Neurology, Neurosurgery and Psychiatry, 47*, 505-513.

Rao, V.R. & Lyketsos, M.D. (2000). Neuropsychiatric sequelae of traumatic brain injury. *Psychosomatics, 41*, 95-103.

Sazbon, L. & Groswasser, Z. (1991). Time-related sequelae of TBI in patients with prolonged post-comatose unawareness (PC-U) state. *Brain Injury, 5,* 3-8.

Shallice, T. (1982). Specific impairments of planning. *Philosophical transactions of the Royal Society of London, B, 298,* 199-209.

Shallice, T. (1988). *From neuropsychology to mental structure.* New York: Cambridge University Press.

Stuss, D.T. & Benson, D.F. (1984). Neuropsychological studies of the frontal lobes. *Psychological Bulletin, 95,* 3-28.

Stuss, D.T. & Benson, D.F. (1986). *The frontal lobes.* New York: Raven Press.

Swan, L. & Alderman, N. (in press). Measuring the relationship between overt aggression and expectations: a methodology for determining clinical outcomes.

Watson, C., Rutterford, N., Shortland, D., Williamson, N., & Alderman, N. (2001). Reduction of chronic aggressive behaviour ten years after brain injury. *Brain Injury, 15,* 1003-1015.

Williams, W.H. & Jones, R.S.P. (1997). Teaching cognitive self-regulation of independence and emotion control skills. In B. Stenfert-Kroese, D. Dagnan & K. Loumidis (Eds.), *Cognitive behaviour therapy for people with learning disabilities.* London: Routledge.

Wilson, B. (1989). Injury to the central nervous system. In S. Pearce and J. Wardle (Eds.), *The practice of behavioural medicine.* Oxford: University Press.

Wilson, B.A. (1991). Behavior therapy in the treatment of neurologically impaired adults. In P.R. Martin (Ed.), *Handbook of behavior therapy and psychological science: an integrative approach.* New York: Pergamon Press.

Wood, R.L.I. (1987). *Brain injury rehabilitation: a neurobehavioural approach.* London: Croom Helm.

Wood, R.L.I. (1988). Management of behaviour disorders in a day treatment setting. *Journal of Head Trauma Rehabilitation, 3,* 53-62.

Wood, R.L.I. (1990). Conditioning procedures in brain injury rehabilitation. In R.L.I. Wood (Ed.), *Neurobehavioural sequelae of traumatic brain injury.* London: Taylor and Francis Ltd.

Wood, R.L.I. (2001). Understanding neurobehavioural disability. In R.L.I. Wood and T. McMillan (Eds.), *Neurobehavioural Disability and Social Handicap Following Traumatic Brain Injury.* Hove, Psychology Press.

Wood, R.L.I. & Eames, P. (1981). Application of behaviour modification in the rehabilitation of traumatically brain injured patients. In G. Davey (Ed.), *Applications of conditioning theory.* London: Methuen.

Wood, R.L.I. & McMillan, T.M. (Eds.) (2001), *Neurobehavioural Disability and Social Handicap Following Traumatic Brain Injury.* Hove, Psychology Press.

Wood, R.L.I. & Worthington, A.D. (2001a). Neurobehavioural rehabilitation: a conceptual paradigm. In R.L.I. Wood and T. McMillan (Eds.), *Neurobehavioural Disability and Social Handicap Following Traumatic Brain Injury.* Hove, Psychology Press.

Wood, R.L.I. & Worthington, A.D. (2001b). Neurobehavioural rehabilitation in practice. In R.L.I. Wood and T. McMillan (Eds.), *Neurobehavioural Disability and Social Handicap Following Traumatic Brain Injury.* Hove, Psychology Press.

Chapter 10

REHABILITATION FOR PEOPLE WITH DEMENTIA

Linda Clare

University College London, UK

Neuropsychological rehabilitation is just as relevant for people with progressive disorders affecting cognitive functioning as it is for people with non-progressive brain injury. If we define the goal of rehabilitation as enabling people to 'achieve an optimal level of physical, psychological and social functioning', given any limitations imposed by injury or illness (McLellan, 1991 p. 785), then it is clear that this is an appropriate goal at any stage of a progressive disorder. Improving well-being implies an enhancement in quality of life, not only for the person with dementia but also for his or her family or caregivers. Indeed, it has been suggested that the broad concept of rehabilitation provides a suitable unifying framework for conceptualising intervention in dementia (Cohen & Eisdorfer, 1986), and within this broad framework an understanding of neuropsychological functioning is an essential element in addressing the needs of the person and his or her caregivers.

In this chapter, following a brief overview of dementia, I will focus on four key questions:

- Why is neuropsychological rehabilitation relevant for people with dementia?
- Can people with dementia benefit from neuropsychological rehabilitation?
- What is the role of neuropsychological rehabilitation in clinical practice?
- The way forward: where do we go from here?

Dementia: a Brief Overview

Dementia has been defined as 'a clinical syndrome characterised by loss of function in multiple cognitive abilities in an individual with previously normal (or at least higher) intellectual abilities and occurring in clear consciousness' (Whitehouse, Lerner, & Hedera, 1993). By implication, this decline in cognitive function will also impact on functioning in various domains of daily living and social interaction. There are numerous possible causes of dementia, but the most frequent dementia diagnosis is that of Alzheimer's disease (Morris, 1996a; 1996b; McKhann et al., 1984), followed by vascular dementia or a mixture of the two types. Less frequently diagnosed sub-types of dementia include dementia with Lewy bodies and the frontal and temporal (semantic) variants of frontotemporal dementia; these have different neuropsychological profiles, particularly in the earlier stages, and consequently somewhat different implications for rehabilitation interventions (Brandt & Rich, 1995; Hodges et al., 1999; Graham, Patterson, Pratt, & Hodges, 2001). The main focus here will be on interventions for people with Alzheimer's disease, vascular dementia or mixed dementia, reflecting the current evidence-base. Much of the work described will also be relevant for people with mild cognitive impairment or age-associated memory difficulties.

Even within a single sub-type of dementia such as Alzheimer's disease, there is considerable heterogeneity in both initial presentation (Neary et al., 1986) and course (Wild & Kaye, 1998; Storandt, Morris, Rubin, Coben, & Berg, 1992). The rate of progression of dementia is very variable, with some individuals staying in the mild stages for a number of years and others progressing more rapidly to severe impairment (e.g. Bowen et al., 1997). Some individuals develop mild cognitive impairment, with significant difficulties in the domain of episodic memory, but do not show any progression to dementia. Therefore, needs will differ according to both the neuropsychological profile and the extent to which the cognitive impairments have progressed in severity. Individual assessment, formulation and goal planning is always necessary, and a diagnostic or staging label does not suffice as a basis for developing rehabilitation plans.

Why is Neuropsychological Rehabilitation Relevant for People with Dementia?

In recent years a quiet revolution has been taking place in dementia care, and this has brought to the fore the concepts of personhood and person-centred care (Kitwood, 1997). The perspective of the person with dementia, hitherto largely neglected (Cotrell & Schulz, 1993), is now being explored and valued (Sabat, 2001; Allan, 2001; Harris, 2002) alongside that of the family member or caregiver. Psychosocial and social constructionist models of dementia (Sabat, Wiggs, & Pinizzotto, 1984; Kitwood, 1997) highlight the importance of the unique set of life experiences and coping strategies that each individual brings to the challenge of living with dementia, and the impact of the social environment on the expression and course of neurological impairment. Social and psychological factors are understood to interact with the effects of neurological impairment in a dialectical process, so that a person surrounded by a 'malignant social psychology' is likely to show 'excess disability' (Reifler & Larson, 1990) and appear more disabled than the extent of any brain pathology would indicate ought to be the case. Reducing excess disability is therefore an important target for intervention. Rehabilitation has an important role to play in tackling excess disability and enhancing well-being and quality of life for the person with dementia and his or her family. Further, it has been argued that selfhood should not be thought of as lost in dementia (Sabat, 1995), and rehabilitation may help to maintain both sense of self for the person with dementia and the perception of selfhood by others (Romero & Eder, 1992).

The context in which rehabilitation occurs is therefore crucial. In developing a model for neuropsychological rehabilitation in dementia a range of factors need to be taken into account above and beyond the person's neuropsychological profile. I have argued elsewhere (Clare, 2000) that neuropsychological rehabilitation in dementia requires a psychotherapeutic framework, equivalent to the 'holistic' approach taken in brain injury rehabilitation by Prigatano (1999). It is essential to acknowledge the person's emotional responses and coping strategies, and to work with these (Clare, 2002). Equally, rehabilitation in dementia requires a systemic perspective, in which the person and the impact of dementia can be viewed in the context of the person's network of support and care. In many cases, caregivers will be essential allies if the rehabilitation process is to be effective. It is also vital to consider that dementia is typically – although not always – a problem of later life. Rehabilitation for older people with dementia should not be undertaken without an understanding of ageing and its psychological and social implications. Finally, it is necessary to be sensitive to differences in the way dementia is perceived across diverse cultural and religious groups, and to respect values and expectations that may diverge from the way in which dementia is typically viewed by western health professionals.

The essentially collaborative and individually-targeted nature of rehabilitation means that it sits easily within this contextual framework. In addition, there is a strong rationale for the specific relevance of neuropsychological rehabilitation for people with at least some forms of dementia. This derives from evidence regarding the neuropsychology and neuroanatomy of cognitive impairments, and the capacity of the person with dementia for new learning.

Learning and Relearning: Possibilities for Intervention

Experimental studies of learning confirm that learning is possible in people with dementia. Both classical and operant conditioning of responses has been demonstrated (Camp et al., 1993; Burgess, Wearden, Cox, & Rae, 1992), as has retention of verbal information (Little, Volans, Hemsley, & Levy, 1986). However, explicit learning will be seen only where the conditions are favourable; Bäckman (1992) argues that appropriate support for memory must be provided both at encoding and at retrieval (termed 'dual cognitive support'), and notes that the level of support required will increase as the severity of dementia increases. A number of experimental studies demonstrate beneficial effects of different types of cognitive support. For example, memory performance is facilitated when multiple sensory modalities are involved at encoding (Karlsson et al., 1989) or where participants physically enact the target task at encoding (Bird & Kinsella, 1996). Similarly, in accordance with the encoding-specificity principle, provision of retrieval cues that are compatible with conditions at encoding assists recall (Herlitz & Viitanen, 1991); an example would be where a semantic orienting task is used at encoding (e.g. categorising 'apple' as 'fruit') followed by provision of category cues at retrieval (e.g. 'it's a kind of fruit') (Lipinska & Bäckman, 1997; Bird & Luszcz, 1991; Bird & Luszcz, 1993). Results presented by Lipinska and colleagues (Lipinska, Bäckman, Mantyla, & Viitanen, 1994) indicate that participants perform better with self-generated than with experimenter-provided cues. Perlmuter and Monty (1989) emphasise that personalising a task by allowing the participant to make choices about it increases perceived control and motivation, and consequently is likely to benefit performance.

A number of studies, then, demonstrate that elaboration and effortful processing can improve memory performance. At the same time, this needs to be balanced with the goal of reducing or eliminating errors during the learning process (Komatsu, Mimura, Kato, Wakamatsu, & Kashima, 2000), as the principle of errorless learning has also been shown to be useful in improving memory performance in early-stage Alzheimer's (Clare, Wilson, Breen, & Hodges, 1999; Clare et al., 2000; Clare, Wilson, Carter, Hodges, & Adams, 2001).

This growing body of evidence about the parameters that can help to facilitate successful learning or relearning for people with dementia provides important empirical support for the development of clinical rehabilitation practice. Before considering how neuropsychological rehabilitation can best be put into practice in dementia care, however, it is important to understand something of the history of psychological interventions in dementia, and to consider how neuropsychological rehabilitation relates to other approaches.

Relationship of Neuropsychological Rehabilitation to Other Psychological Interventions

One of the earliest approaches to psychological intervention was the adaptation of reality orientation (RO) for use with people who have dementia (Woods, 1992). This represented a major breakthrough as it demonstrated the possibility that psychological approaches had something to offer. The concept of reality orientation attained widespread acceptance in long-term care settings, but its implementation was not always of a high standard, with interventions sometimes applied in a rather insensitive manner. Subsequently the approach was heavily criticised for overlooking the emotional needs of the person with dementia, and alternative methods emerged in the form of practices such as validation therapy (Feil, 1992). More recent work has demonstrated that interventions based on the principles of reality orientation can have positive effects on cognition and behaviour in people with dementia (Spector, Orrell, Davies, & Woods, 1998), and has attempted to 'rehabilitate' reality orientation through the development of group interventions for people with severe dementia in residential settings (Spector, Orrell, Davies, & Woods, 2001). Similarly, evaluation of 'cognitive stimulation' group interventions for people with dementia shows positive results (Breuil et al., 1994; Vidal, Lavieille-Letan, Fleury, & de Rotrou, 1998; de Rotrou et al., 1999). Because interventions based on RO or cognitive stimulation typically incorporate a number of elements, however, it remains difficult to determine the relative contribution of different components to the positive outcomes observed, or to derive a theoretical understanding of the mechanisms by which the interventions exert their positive effects.

In the meantime, the reality orientation tradition was succeeded by a related body of work focused on 'memory training' or 'memory retraining' for people with dementia. Memory training is similar to cognitive stimulation approaches, in that the goals set and tasks used are general rather than individually-designed, but differs in that there is a more specific focus on one or more aspects of memory functioning. Memory training has been criticised in turn, firstly on the basis that gains are limited and maintenance is poor, and secondly because it is said to have negative effects on mood and well-being for people with dementia or their caregivers (Rabins, 1996; Small et al., 1997). It should be noted that these criticisms were made in the context of a strong emphasis on the value of pharmacological treatments, although the effectiveness of the pharmacological treatments currently available for people with dementia is modest (Royal College of Psychiatrists, 1997). Other reviews, in contrast, have argued that this kind of approach may be beneficial; for example, Gatz and colleagues (Gatz et al., 1998) classify 'memory retraining' as a 'probably efficacious' form of intervention which warrants more research. One reason for this divergence of views may be that increased understanding of the conditions required in order for people with dementia to learn effectively has resulted in more appropriate intervention protocols, as indicated by Bäckman (1992). There is a continuing interest in 'memory training' for people with dementia, with a variety of methods in evidence. For example, a recent randomised controlled trial (Davis, Massman, & Doody, 2001) reported gains in performance on targeted areas, but no generalised improvements. There is also a growing interest in computerised cognitive training for people with dementia (e.g. Hofmann, Hock, Kuhler, & Muller-Spahn, 1996).

In the last few years, the focus has shifted once again and researchers have begun to apply the concepts of cognitive or neuropsychological rehabilitation to dementia care (Clare & Woods, 2001). This strand of research draws extensively on the concept and practice of neuropsychological rehabilitation with brain-injured people. Interventions are devised on the basis of theoretical principles derived from neuropsychology, cognitive psychology and learning theory, and are targeted specifically to the individual on the basis of the person's neuropsychological profile. In addition, following Prigatano's holistic model of neuropsychological rehabilitation (Prigatano, 1999), they should endeavour to take into account the person's emotional and practical needs and social context, drawing on perspectives from psychotherapy and systems theory.

It is necessary to distinguish the work carried out in the tradition of reality orientation, encompassing memory training and cognitive stimulation, from attempts at implementing neuropsychological or cognitive rehabilitation. At the same time, it is important to acknowledge that there are some shared elements and that knowledge or evidence derived from one can sometimes be applicable to the other. The review that follows will focus primarily on neuropsychological rehabilitation rather than on memory training and cognitive stimulation.

What is the role of neuropsychological rehabilitation in clinical practice?

Neuropsychological rehabilitation can provide both a general framework for intervention and a means of tackling specific issues. As a general framework, it allows for a biopsychosocial formulation within which an understanding and acknowledgement of the person's cognitive impairments is central. This means, for example, that explanations and advice can be provided to the person and his or her carers, helping them to make sense of some of their difficult and distressing experiences. Specific difficulties can be addressed using methods devised for people with dementia or adapted from those reported to be useful for people with brain injury. The way in which these two aspects of neuropsychological rehabilitation are implemented in practice varies according to the needs of the individual, so that the emphasis is likely to be quite different in early- and later-stage dementia.

Interventions for people with early stage dementia

In the early stages of dementia, the main focus for intervention is likely to be everyday problems arising from difficulties with long-term episodic memory or executive function. The discussion here will concentrate on memory functioning.

The most appropriate approach will be determined through a careful assessment of the neuropsychological profile and the person's everyday functioning. This assessment should be made in the context of a broader evaluation encompassing the person's past experience and preferred ways of coping, psychological well-being, awareness of difficulties and readiness to address them, and any other possible blocks to successful outcome that may need to be overcome before the intervention begins. The way in which the person perceives his or her difficulties is likely to be particularly important here, as it has been demonstrated that expressed awareness of memory difficulties and their impact is associated with better outcome in cognitive rehabilitation interventions in the early stages of dementia (Clare, 2000; 2001; Koltai, Welsh-Bohmer, & Schmechel, 2001). The person's support systems also need to be considered, along with the willingness of family members or friends to be involved. The assessment should lead to a collaborative exercise in setting goals for intervention, in which the person with dementia plays a full part. Interventions are most likely to be effective when they address issues that are important to the person and family, and relevant to everyday life. Where the goals of the person with dementia and the family are markedly discrepant, careful and sensitive negotiation is required in order to try to reach a consensus that is acceptable to both parties, acknowledging the different emotional and practical needs of all involved.

Some people with early-stage dementia may already be engaging in self-help activities, for example those provided in books about improving memory. This can be facilitated through provision of appropriate material or suggestions. Information about memory problems and how these may be tackled (e.g. Clare & Wilson, 1997) can be helpful for the individual and for family members, empowering them to identify their own solutions to specific issues or problems.

Consistent with memory rehabilitation in brain injury, specific interventions for memory difficulties in early-stage dementia take two main forms (Franzen & Haut, 1991). Firstly, assistance can be given with learning or relearning information and skills, in order to enhance residual episodic or procedural memory performance. Secondly, strategies can be developed that enable the person to compensate for aspects of memory that are impaired and functioning poorly.

Facilitating Residual Memory Functioning

Interventions aimed at facilitating residual memory performance need to incorporate the twin guiding principles of effortfulness and errorlessness in the learning process. This can be achieved in practice by using one or more of a number of methods.

Expanding rehearsal, or spaced retrieval, has been used extensively with people who have dementia. The act of retrieving an item of information is a powerful aid to subsequent retention under any conditions. In addition, the temporal sequencing of retrieval attempts affects the extent to which benefits are observed as a result of retrieval practice, with maximum benefit occurring when test trials are spaced at gradually expanding intervals (Landauer & Bjork, 1978). Experimental studies have demonstrated that expanding rehearsal can aid new learning in people with memory disorders following brain injury (Schacter, Rich, & Stampp, 1985). The method has been adapted for use in Alzheimer's disease (Camp, 1989; Camp, Bird, & Cherry, 2000), with very short retrieval intervals – typically the first interval is 15 or 30 seconds long, and the length is repeatedly doubled. A series of studies has demonstrated clear benefits in teaching face-name associations, object naming (Abrahams & Camp, 1993; Moffat, 1989), memory for object location, and prospective memory assignments (Camp, 1989). A further advantage of the expanding rehearsal method is that it can easily be used by caregivers, with back-up support from professionals as required (Camp et al., 2000; McKitrick & Camp, 1993). Expanding rehearsal does not rule out the possibility of errors occurring, but in practice, because the initial recall intervals are so short, errors are rare. It therefore approximates well to an errorless learning procedure, while also requiring the effort of retrieving the information.

Another method that can be applied is the use of cueing (Glisky, Schacter, & Tulving, 1986; Thoene & Glisky, 1995). This can take various forms. In one version, termed 'vanishing cues' or 'decreasing assistance' (Riley & Heaton, 2000), the number of cues is gradually reduced. When learning a name, for example, this would mean that at each presentation an additional letter was removed from the end of the name. Another version, termed 'forward cueing' or 'increasing assistance' begins by offering just the initial letter and adds a letter on each subsequent presentation until the word or name is correctly given, after which the cues may be faded again as in the vanishing cues method. Cueing methods were used by Clare and colleagues (Clare et al., 2000), and were directly compared in one single case study, where forward cueing was found to be more effective than vanishing cues.

Strategies such as visual imagery mnemonics, chunking of information, the method of loci, the story method and initial letter cueing have been described in relation to the cognitive rehabilitation of memory disorders following brain injury, although some of these strategies may prove too difficult or demanding for many brain injured patients (Wilson, 1995; Moffat, 1992). There is limited evidence for the success of strategies of this kind when used with people who have Alzheimer's disease, who are likely to have difficulty both in learning an explicit mnemonic strategy and in remembering to use it appropriately (Woods, 1996; Bäckman, 1992). In some cases, however, simple strategies may be remembered and implemented. It is important to distinguish between the use of mnemonic strategies as a way of facilitating learning in specific tasks and the aim of developing spontaneous and independent use of the strategy in a wider sphere. The former is often a more appropriate goal in memory rehabilitation, and clinicians can draw on a number of strategies to facilitate learning for the person with dementia.

One report of successful use of a mnemonic strategy is provided by Hill and colleagues (Hill, Evankovich, Sheikh, & Yesavage, 1987). They describe a single case experiment in which a 66 year old man with Alzheimer's was taught to use visual imagery to extend his retention interval for names associated with photographs of faces. In an attempt to replicate the findings in a case series of eight participants, which included seven people with Alzheimer's (Bäckman, Josephsson, Herlitz, Stigsdotter, & Viitanen, 1991), only one of the participants with Alzheimer's showed training gains similar to those demonstrated by Hill et al. (1987). The remaining patients failed to benefit from training. The authors conclude that the generalisability of the approach appears limited, but comment that there might be a subgroup of people with Alzheimer's disease who respond well to this form of memory training.

This finding was supported by the results of a single case study (Clare et al., 1999) which demonstrated effective relearning of names that the participant wished to know. These were names of members of his club, and relearning them helped him to continue his engagement in this social activity. The names were relearnt from photographs, using a combination of mnemonic, vanishing cues and expanding rehearsal techniques which was intended to provide an optimal combination of errorless and effortful processes. One name was taught per session. The procedure began with a discussion leading to choice of a suitable mnemonic, linking some feature of the person's appearance with the sound of their name ('Caroline with the curly fringe'). Next, a vanishing cues process was used to encourage the participant to retrieve the name with less and less assistance; initially the name was presented minus the final letter for him to complete, and a further letter was removed on each presentation until he retrieved the name with no cues at all. After this, expanding rehearsal was used to increase the time intervals between successful attempts at retrieval, with the interval starting at 30 seconds and expanding each time the name was recalled, up to a maximum of 10 minutes. Between sessions, the participant practised the names following a carefully-devised practice procedure that he was able to undertake alone. Once all the names had been trained, generalisation to the club setting was undertaken. The participant was asked, at the club, to match each photograph to the relevant person and say the person's name. Using these methods, the participant was able to improve his recall of the names from 20% at initial baseline to 98% following the intervention. In follow up sessions conducted one, three, six and nine months after the intervention, the participant scored 100% on each occasion. He continued to practise the names during this follow up period. A further study evaluated forgetting in the absence of home practice over the subsequent two years and found that performance remained well above initial baseline levels three years after the end of the intervention (Clare et al., 2001a). He continued to enjoy attending his club and participating in activities there.

A similar approach taken with other participants again targeted goals identified by the participants, but explored the feasibility of different techniques in isolation (Clare et al., 2000; Clare et al., 2001a). Good results were obtained for mnemonic, expanding rehearsal and forward cueing strategies, with vanishing cues proving less effective, as noted above. This is in accordance with the findings of Thoene & Glisky (1995), which showed that visual imagery was a more effective strategy than vanishing cues for the acquisition of face-name associations in memory-impaired participants (the sample included one man with dementia). Thoene & Glisky argued that this was because the mnemonic strategy was able to optimise the use of residual explicit memory, in addition to encouraging deep levels of processing and the development of associations with existing knowledge.

The ability to perform everyday skills is particularly important in maintaining independence. Zanetti and colleagues (Zanetti et al., 2001; Zanetti et al., 1997; Zanetti, Magni, Binetti, Bianchetti, & Trabucchi, 1994) used a training method based on preserved procedural memory for rehabilitation of ADL skills in people with mild-to-moderate Alzheimer's. Training involved comprehensive prompting, with subsequent fading out of prompts. Preliminary results suggested this approach could be effective and produced some generalisation of improvements to untrained tasks. Another study (Josephsson et al., 1993) used individualised training programmes for activities of daily living and showed improvements in three out of four participants, although only one maintained the gains two months later. An important feature of this study was the selection of tasks which were part of the patient's usual routine and which the patient was motivated to carry out; the value of considering motivational factors in designing interventions was emphasised.

Providing External Support for Remembering

Providing external support for remembering in the form of compensatory memory aids can help to reduce the demands on memory. The selection and introduction of external memory aids requires careful consideration, and aids should be targeted as specifically as possible, rather than simply providing a generalised reminder, the reason for which may be unclear to the person with dementia (Woods, 1996). Many people who develop dementia will already be used to relying on external memory aids such as diaries and lists, and it is helpful to build on this and try to ensure that these aids are used to maximum effectiveness; for example, a diary with unstructured pages may be replaced by one that has times of day listed. People with memory impairments are unlikely to start to use new memory aids spontaneously and usually need training in their use, for example by means of prompting and fading of cues, or expanding rehearsal. Effective use of an errorless prompting and fading method to help a woman with dementia use a calendar to find out what day it was instead of repeatedly questioning her husband was reported by Clare and colleagues (Clare et al., 2000). This was a relatively simple intervention which consisted of ensuring that a suitable day-per-view calendar was placed in a prominent position and then supporting the participant's husband in carrying out a schedule of prompting in which he reminded her three times a day to look at the calendar and find out what day it was. This was intended to enable her to establish a habit of looking at the calendar. Once this habit was established, the prompts were gradually faded out. Using this method, the frequency with which the participant repetitively questioned her husband decreased significantly, and this decrease was maintained at follow up three and six months later. Both the participant and her husband were very pleased with this result and, interestingly, the gains from this simple intervention did appear to generalise to other situations as similar problem-solving strategies were spontaneously applied.

Developing technology offers increasing opportunities for identification of ingenious aids to remembering. In an early example (Kurlychek, 1983), a digital watch was set to beep every hour as a cue to prompt engagement in a predetermined activity. Use of technology is now being extended beyond the realm of specific memory aids by developing computer and video equipment to monitor and control the environment of the person with dementia in order to support independent functioning (Marshall, 1999).

Practical Implementation in Early-Stage Dementia

In clinical practice with people who have early-stage dementia, the methods and techniques of neuropsychological rehabilitation have been implemented in a variety of ways. As well as individual interventions such as those described above, a number of centres have developed group programmes aimed at helping people with early-stage dementia to cope with memory difficulties (e.g. Koltai et al., 2001). Some programmes offer parallel sessions for participants with dementia and caregivers, while in others couples attend sessions together (e.g. Sandman, 1993). Group programmes typically incorporate information and education about memory and cognitive problems as well as identification of individual goals, introduction of suitable strategies or aids, and practice in their use. When they work well, groups provide an opportunity for members to support and encourage one another, and perhaps develop friendships and social contacts. However, some people with early-stage dementia may be reluctant to attend a group, preferring one-to-one sessions, and individual preferences should be respected. Elements of cognitive rehabilitation have been incorporated in broad-based community rehabilitation programmes which also incorporate aspects such as partnered volunteering (Arkin, 1996), and in psychosocial early intervention programmes (e.g. Moniz-Cook, Agar, Gibson, Win, & Wang, 1998).

Interventions for people with later stage dementia

As dementia progresses, the focus of neuropsychological rehabilitation is likely to change to some extent. There is likely to be more emphasis on addressing behavioural issues and on enhancing well-being through maintaining interaction and engagement.

An understanding of the neuropsychological profile and the possibilities for new learning can be coupled with a behavioural approach that views behaviour as having a meaning or function rather than as a 'symptom'. This provides a framework for generating creative but highly practical solutions where cognitive impairments appear to play a part in producing 'problem' behaviour. This framework has been used, for example, to teach patients to associate a cue with an adaptive behaviour as a means of reducing behaviours that are regarded as problematic (Bird, 2001; Bird, 2000).

In some situations, rehabilitation of basic skills is an important focus. Camp and colleagues (Camp et al., 1997) describe the application of Montessori activities, designed to build skills in a developmental sequence in young children, to dementia care. An example here might be reinstating the ability to feed oneself with a spoon through a sequence of tasks starting with scooping beads with a large scoop, and progressing through scooping rice, sand and eventually liquids with gradually smaller scoops, and so on until a spoon can be used to spoon up soup.

A number of studies have demonstrated improvements resulting from the use of various external memory aids or equivalent environmental support for people with later stage dementia. In some cases these improvements have been maintained after the support has been withdrawn, while in other cases ongoing support has been required. Hanley (1986) trained in-patients with moderately advanced Alzheimer's to use a diary, reality orientation board or personal notebook to find out important information, although it is unclear to what extent the improvement was maintained. Bourgeois (1990) evaluated the effectiveness of memory wallets in enhancing conversational ability in a small sample of people with moderately advanced Alzheimer's, and reported significant improvements, with evidence of generalisation to novel utterances. Benefits were maintained at six-week follow up, and for three individuals benefits were retained after 30 months (Bourgeois, 1992). This finding has recently been replicated with people who have severe dementia (McPherson et al., 2001). As well as helping the memory-impaired person, memory wallets or memory books offer care staff a means of learning about, and engaging with, the person (Woods, Portnoy, Head, & Jones, 1992), and can be especially helpful at times of transition, such as the move into residential care. Romero and Wenz (2001) emphasise the importance of helping the person with dementia to maintain a sense of self, using materials such as memory books in a structured way to facilitate engagement with, and processing of, those aspects of self that are currently most salient for the individual. In this approach, too, memory books can become the focus for constructive interaction between the person with dementia and family members or carers.

Implementing cognitive rehabilitation in later-stage dementia requires particular attention to, and skill in, working with systems. Camp has taken an important lead in addressing practical issues regarding the implementation of rehabilitation interventions in long-term care settings (Camp, 2001), including issues of cultural and linguistic difference.

The way forward: where do we go from here?
This chapter has shown that neuropsychological rehabilitation can be applied in the context of progressive disorders such as dementia with beneficial results. The approach is relevant for both earlier and later stages of dementia, but the focus differs according to the needs of the individual and his or her carers at any given point. Comprehensive recent reviews of the literature support the relevance of this kind of approach in dementia care (De Vreese, Neri, Fioravanti, Belloi, & Zanetti, 2001), suggesting that further research is warranted, and a systematic review is in preparation (Clare, Woods, Moniz-Cook, Spector, & Orrell, 2001b).

The application of neuropsychological rehabilitation for people with progressive disorders such as dementia is a relatively recent development, and there are a number of issues that future research will need to address. At a conceptual level it will be important to ensure that cognitive rehabilitation is clearly distinguished from related, but different, approaches such as reality orientation or memory training. At a practical level, it will be necessary to continue refining our knowledge of methods and techniques that may assist in achieving specific goals. Equally, it will be important to further develop the 'holistic' framework for cognitive rehabilitation with people who have progressive disorders, ensuring that emotional needs and responses are attended to, and that the person is considered in the context of his or her social system. It will be vital to identify more clearly the factors that indicate whether or not this kind of approach is likely to be suitable for a given individual at a given time, or whether some other form of support or intervention would be more appropriate. Finally, it will be necessary to situate neuropsychological rehabilitation within a coherent approach to supporting people with progressive disorders that reflects a genuinely biopsychosocial model and espouses the aims and values of person-centred care.

References

Abrahams, J.P., & Camp, C.J. (1993). Maintenance and generalisation of object naming training in anomia associated with degenerative dementia. *Clinical Gerontologist, 12(3)*, 57-72.

Allan, K. (2001). *Communication and consultation: exploring ways for staff to involve people with dementia in developing services*. Bristol: The Policy Press.

Arkin, S.M. (1996). Volunteers in partnership: an Alzheimer's rehabilitation program delivered by students. *The American Journal of Alzheimer's Disease, 11*(Jan/Feb), 12-22.

Bäckman, L. (1992). Memory training and memory improvement in Alzheimer's disease: rules and exceptions. *Acta Neurologica Scandinavica,* Supplement *139,* 84-89.

Bäckman, L., Josephsson, S., Herlitz, A., Stigsdotter, A., & Viitanen, M. (1991). The generalisability of training gains in dementia: effects of an imagery-based mnemonic on face-name retention duration. *Psychology and Aging, 6,* 489-492.

Bird, M. (2001). Behavioural difficulties and cued recall of adaptive behaviour in dementia: experimental and clinical evidence. *Neuropsychological Rehabilitation, 11,* 357-375.

Bird, M., & Kinsella, G. (1996). Long-term cued recall of tasks in senile dementia. *Psychology and Aging, 11,* 45-56.

Bird, M., & Luszcz, M. (1991). Encoding specificity, depth of processing, and cued recall in Alzheimer's disease. *Journal of Clinical and Experimental Neuropsychology, 13,* 508-520.

Bird, M., & Luszcz, M. (1993). Enhancing memory performance in Alzheimer's disease: acquisition assistance and cue effectiveness. *Journal of Clinical and Experimental Neuropsychology, 15,* 921-932.

Bird, M.J. (2000). Psychosocial rehabilitation for problems arising from cognitive deficits in dementia. In R.D. Hill, L. Bäckman, & A.S. Neely (Eds.), *Cognitive Rehabilitation in Old Age.* Oxford: Oxford University Press.

Bourgeois, M.S. (1990). Enhancing conversation skills in patients with Alzheimer's disease using a prosthetic memory aid. *Journal of Applied Behavior Analysis, 23,* 29-42.

Bourgeois, M.S. (1992). Evaluating memory wallets in conversations with persons with dementia. *Journal of Speech and Hearing Research, 35,* 1344-1357.

Bowen, J., Teri, L., Kukull, W., McCormick, W., McCurry, S.M., & Larson, E.B. (1997). Progression to dementia in patients with isolated memory loss. *The Lancet, 349,* 763-765.

Brandt, J., & Rich, J.B. (1995). Memory disorders in the dementias. In A.D. Baddeley, B.A. Wilson, & F.N. Watts (Eds.), *Handbook of Memory Disorders.* Chichester: John Wiley & Sons Ltd.

Breuil, V., de Rotrou, J., Forette, F., Tortrat, D., Ganasia-Ganem, A., Frambourt, A., Moulin, F., & Boller, F. (1994). Cognitive stimulation of patients with dementia: preliminary results. *International Journal of Geriatric Psychiatry, 9,* 211-217.

Burgess, I.S., Wearden, J.H., Cox, T., & Rae, M. (1992). Operant conditioning with subjects suffering from dementia. *Behavioural Psychotherapy, 20,* 219-237.

Camp, C.J. (1989). Facilitation of new learning in Alzheimer's disease. In G. Gilmore, P. Whitehouse, & M. Wykle (Eds.), *Memory and Aging: Theory, Research and Practice* (pp. 212-225). New York: Springer.

Camp, C.J. (2001). From efficacy to effectiveness to diffusion: making the transitions in dementia intervention research. *Neuropsychological Rehabilitation. Special Issue: Cognitive Rehabilitation in Dementia, 11,* 495-517.

Camp, C.J., Bird, M.J., & Cherry, K.E. (2000). Retrieval strategies as a rehabilitation aid for cognitive loss in pathological aging. In R.D. Hill, L. Bäckman, & A.S. Neely (Eds.), *Cognitive Rehabilitation in Old Age.* Oxford: Oxford University Press.

Camp, C.J., Foss, J.W., Stevens, A.B., Reichard, C.C., McKitrick, L.A., & O'Hanlon, A.M. (1993). Memory training in normal and demented elderly populations: the E-I-E-I-O model. *Experimental Aging Research, 19,* 277-290.

Camp, C.J., Judge, K.S., Bye, C., Fox, K., Bowden, J., Bell, M., Valencic, K., & Mattern, J. (1997). An intergenerational program for persons with dementia using Montessori methods. *The Gerontologist, 37,* 688-692.

Clare, L. (2000). *Cognitive rehabilitation in early-stage Alzheimer's disease: learning and the impact of awareness.* Unpublished PhD thesis, The Open University, Milton Keynes.

Clare, L. (2001). Awareness of memory functioning in early-stage Alzheimer's disease: concept, assessment and relationship to the outcome of cognitive rehabilitation interventions. *Proceedings of the Alzheimer Europe 10th Anniversary Meeting, Munich, 12-15 October 2000,* 195-207, Berlin: Deutsche Alzheimer Gesellschaft e. V.

Clare, L. (2002). We'll fight it as long as we can: coping with the onset of Alzheimer's disease. *Aging and Mental Health, 6,* 139-148.

Clare, L., & Wilson, B.A. (1997). *Coping with Memory Problems: a Practical Guide for People with Memory Impairments and their Relatives and Friends.* Bury St Edmunds: Thames Valley Test Company.

Clare, L., Wilson, B.A., Breen, K., & Hodges, J.R. (1999). Errorless learning of face-name associations in early Alzheimer's disease. *Neurocase, 5,* 37-46.

Clare, L., Wilson, B.A., Carter, G., Gosses, A., Breen, K., & Hodges, J.R. (2000). Intervening with everyday memory problems in early Alzheimer's disease: an errorless learning approach. *Journal of Clinical and Experimental Neuropsychology, 22,* 132-146.

Clare, L., Wilson, B.A., Carter, G., Hodges, J.R., & Adams, M. (2001a). Long-term maintenance of treatment gains following a cognitive rehabilitation intervention in early dementia of Alzheimer type: a single case study. *Cognitive Rehabilitation in Dementia, 11,* 477-494.

Clare, L., Woods, B., Moniz-Cook, E.D., Spector, A., & Orrell, M. (2001b). Cognitive rehabilitation interventions targeting memory functioning in early-stage Alzheimer's disease and vascular dementia. *A systematic review.* Protocol., Cochrane Library. Oxford: Update Software.

Clare, L., & Woods, R.T. (Eds.). (2001). *Cognitive Rehabilitation in Dementia: a Special Issue of Neuropsychological Rehabilitation.* Hove: Psychology Press.

Cohen, D., & Eisdorfer, C. (1986). *The Loss of Self: a Family Resource for the Care of Alzheimer's Disease and Related Disorders.* New York: W W Norton & Company.

Cotrell, V., & Schulz, R. (1993). The perspective of the patient with Alzheimer's disease: a neglected dimension of dementia research. *The Gerontologist, 33,* 205-211.

de Rotrou, J., Frambourt, A., de Susbielle, D., Gelee, S., Vidal, J.C., Diehl, P.P., & Forette, F. (1999). La stimulation cognitive. In *Fondation Nationale de Gerontologie (Ed.), La maladie d'Alzheimer: prediction, prevention, prise en charge.* dixième congres de la Fondation Nationale de Gerontologie. Paris: Fondation Nationale de Gerontologie.

de Vreese, L.P., Neri, M., Fioravanti, M., Belloi, L., & Zanetti, O. (2001). Memory rehabilitation in Alzheimer's disease: a review of progress. *International Journal of Geriatric Psychiatry, 16,* 794-809.

Davis, R.N., Massman, P.J., & Doody, R.S. (2001). Cognitive intervention in Alzheimer disease: a randomised placebo-controlled study. *Alzheimer Disease and Associated Disorders, 15,* 1-9.

Feil, N. (1992). Validation therapy with late-onset dementia populations. In G.M.M. Jones & B.M.L. Miesen (Eds.), *Care-giving in Dementia: Research and Applications (Vol. 1).* London: Tavistock/Routledge.

Franzen, M.D., & Haut, M.W. (1991). The psychological treatment of memory impairment: a review of empirical studies. *Neuropsychology Review, 2,* 29-63.

Gatz, M., Fiske, A., Fox, L., Kaskie, B., Kasl-Godley, J.E., McCallum, T.J., & Wetherell, J.L. (1998). Empirically validated psychological treatments for older adults. *Journal of Mental Health and Aging, 4,* 9-45.

Glisky, E.L., Schacter, D.L., & Tulving, E. (1986). Learning and retention of computer-related vocabulary in memory impaired patients: method of vanishing cues. *Journal of Clinical and Experimental Neuropsychology, 8,* 292-312.

Graham, K.S., Patterson, K., Pratt, K.H., & Hodges, J.R. (2001). Can repeated exposure to 'forgotten' vocabulary help alleviate word-finding difficulties in semantic
dementia? An illustrative case study. *Neuropsychological Rehabilitation, 11,*
429-454.

Hanley, I. (1986). Reality orientation in the care of the elderly patient with dementia
– three case studies. In I. Hanley & M. Gilhooly (Eds.), *Psychological Therapies
for the Elderly* (pp. 65-79). Beckenham: Croom Helm Ltd.

Harris, P.B. (Ed.). (2002). *The person with Alzheimer's Disease: Pathways to Understanding the Experience.* Baltimore: Johns Hopkins University Press.

Herlitz, A., & Viitanen, M. (1991). Semantic organisation and verbal episodic memory in patients with mild and moderate Alzheimer's disease. *Journal of Clinical
and Experimental Neuropsychology, 13,* 559-574.

Hill, R.D., Evankovich, K.D., Sheikh, J.I., & Yesavage, J.A. (1987). Imagery mnemonic training in a patient with primary degenerative dementia. *Psychology and
Aging, 2,* 204-205.

Hodges, J.R., Patterson, K., Ward, R., Garrard, P., Bak, T., Perry, R., & Gregory, C.
(1999). The differentiation of semantic dementia and frontal lobe dementia (temporal and frontal variants of frontotemporal dementia) from early Alzheimer's
disease: a comparative neuropsychological study. *Neuropsychology, 13,* 31-40.

Hofmann, M., Hock, C., Kuhler, A., & Muller-Spahn, F. (1996). Interactive com-
puter-based cognitive training in patients with Alzheimer's disease. *Journal of
Psychiatric Research, 30,* 493-501.

Josephsson, S., Bäckman, L., Borell, L., Bernspang, B., Nygard, L., & Ronnberg, L.
(1993). Supporting everyday activities in dementia: an intervention study. *International Journal of Geriatric Psychiatry, 8,* 395-400.

Karlsson, T., Bäckman, L., Herlitz, A., Nilsson, L.-G., Winblad, B., & Osterlind,
P.-O. (1989). Memory improvement at different stages of Alzheimer's disease.
Neuropsychologia, 27, 737-742.

Kitwood, T. (1997). *Dementia Reconsidered: the Person Comes First.* Buckingham:
Open University Press.

Koltai, D.C., Welsh-Bohmer, K.A., & Schmechel, D.E. (2001). Influence of anosognosia on treatment outcome among dementia patients. *Neuropsychological
Rehabilitation, 11,* 455-475.

Komatsu, S.-I., Mimura, M., Kato, M., Wakamatsu, N., & Kashima, H. (2000). Errorless and effortful processes involved in the learning of face-name associations by
patients with alcoholic Korsakoff's syndrome. *Neuropsychological Rehabilitation, 10,* 113-208.

Kurlychek, R.T. (1983). Use of a digital alarm chronograph as a memory aid in early
dementia. *Clinical Gerontologist, 1,* 93-94.

Landauer, T.K., & Bjork, R.A. (1978). Optimum rehearsal patterns and name learning. In K.M. Gruneberg, P.E. Morris, & R.N. Sykes (Eds.), *Practical Aspects of
Memory* (pp. 625-632). New York: Academic Press.

Lipinska, B., & Bäckman, L. (1997). Encoding-retrieval interactions in mild Alzheimer's disease: the role of access to categorical information. *Brain and Cognition,
34,* 274-286.

Lipinska, B., Bäckman, L., Mantyla, T., & Viitanen, M. (1994). Effectiveness of self-
generated cues in early Alzheimer's disease. *Journal of Clinical and Experimental
Neuropsychology, 16,* 809-819.

Little, A.G., Volans, P.J., Hemsley, D.R., & Levy, R. (1986). The retention of new
information in senile dementia. *British Journal of Clinical Psychology, 25,* 71-
72.

Marshall, M. (1999). Person centred technology? *Signpost, 3(4),* 4-5.

McKhann, G., Drachman, D., Folstein, M., Katzman, R., Price, D., & Stadlan, E.M.
(1984). Clinical diagnosis of Alzheimer's disease: report of the NINCDS-ADRDA

Work Group under the auspices of Department of Health and Human Services task force on Alzheimer's disease. *Neurology, 34,* 939-944.

McKitrick, L.A., & Camp, C.J. (1993). Relearning the names of things: the spaced-retrieval intervention implemented by a caregiver. *Clinical Gerontologist, 14,* 60-62.

McLellan, D.L. (1991). Functional recovery and the principles of disability medicine. In M. Swash & J. Oxbury (Eds.), *Clinical Neurology, Vol. 1* (pp. 768-790). London: Churchill Livingstone.

McPherson, A., Furniss, F.G., Sdogati, C., Cesaroni, F., Tartaglini, B., & Lindesay, J. (2001). Effects of individualised memory aids on the conversation of patients with severe dementia: a pilot study. *Aging and Mental Health, 5,* 289-294.

Moffat, N. (1992). Strategies of memory therapy. In B.A. Wilson & N. Moffat (Eds.), *Clinical Management of Memory Problems, 2nd ed.* (pp. 86-119). London: Chapman & Hall.

Moffat, N.J. (1989). Home-based cognitive rehabilitation with the elderly. In L. W. Poon, D.C. Rubin, & B.A. Wilson (Eds.), *Everyday Cognition in Adulthood and Late Life* (pp. 659-680). Cambridge: Cambridge University Press.

Moniz-Cook, E., Agar, S., Gibson, G., Win, T., & Wang, M. (1998). A preliminary study of the effects of early intervention with people with dementia and their families in a memory clinic. *Aging and Mental Health, 2,* 199-211.

Morris, J.C. (1996a). Classification of dementia and Alzheimer's disease. *Acta Neurologica Scandinavica,* Supplement *165,* 41-50.

Morris, R.G. (1996b). The neuropsychology of Alzheimer's disease and related dementias. In R.T. Woods (Ed.), *Handbook of the Clinical Psychology of Ageing.* Chichester: John Wiley & Sons Ltd.

Neary, D., Snowden, J.S., Bowen, D.M., Sims, N.R., Mann, D.M.A., Benton, J.S., Northen, B., Yates, P.O., & Davison, A.N. (1986). Neuropsychological syndromes in presenile dementia due to cerebral atrophy. *Journal of Neurology, Neurosurgery, and Psychiatry, 49,* 163-174.

Perlmuter, L.C., & Monty, R.A. (1989). Motivation and aging. In L.W. Poon, D.C. Rubin, & B.A. Wilson (Eds.), *Everyday Cognition in Adulthood and Late Life* . Cambridge: Cambridge University Press.

Prigatano, G.P. (1999). *Principles of Neuropsychological Rehabilitation.* New York: Oxford University Press.

Rabins, P.V. (1996). Developing treatment guidelines for Alzheimer's disease and other dementias. *Journal of Clinical Psychiatry, 57* (suppl 14), 37-38.

Reifler, B.V., & Larson, E. (1990). Excess disability in dementia of the Alzheimer's type. In E. Light & B.D. Lebowitz (Eds.), *Alzheimer's Disease Treatment and Family Stress.* New York: Hemisphere.

Riley, G.A., & Heaton, S. (2000). Guidelines for the selection of a method of fading cues. *Neuropsychological Rehabilitation, 10,* 133-149.

Romero, B., & Eder, G. (1992). Selbst-Erhaltungs-Therapie (SET): Konzept einer neuropsychologischen Therapie bei Alzheimer-Kranken. *Zeitschrift fur Gerontopsychologie und -psychiatrie, 5,* 267-282.

Romero, B., & Wenz, M. (2001). Self-maintenance therapy in Alzheimer's disease. *Neuropsychological Rehabilitation, 11,* 333-355.

Royal College of Psychiatrists. (1997). Interim statement on anti-dementia drugs: implications, concerns and policy proposals. *Psychiatric Bulletin, 21,* 586-587.

Sabat, S. (1995). The Alzheimer's disease sufferer as a semiotic subject. *Philosophy, Psychiatry, and Psychology, 1,* 145-160.

Sabat, S. (2001). *The Experience of Alzheimer's Disease: Life Through a Tangled Veil.* Oxford: Blackwell.

Sabat, S.B., Wiggs, C., & Pinizzotto, A. (1984). Alzheimer's disease: clinical vs observational studies of cognitive ability. *Journal of Clinical and Experimental Gerontology, 6,* 337-359.

Sandman, C.A. (1993). Memory rehabilitation in Alzheimer's disease: preliminary findings. *Clinical Gerontologist, 13,* 19-33.

Schacter, D.L., Rich, S.A., & Stampp, M.S. (1985). Remediation of memory disorders: experimental evaluation of the spaced-retrieval technique. *Journal of Clinical and Experimental Neuropsychology, 7,* 79-96.

Small, G.W., Rabins, P.V., Barry, P.P., Buckholtz, N.S., DeKosky, S.T., Ferris, S.H., Finkel, S.I., Gwyther, L.P., Khachaturian, Z.S., Lebowitz, B.D., McRae, T.D., Morris, J.C., Oakley, F., Schneider, L.S., Streim, J.E., Sunderland, T., Teri, L.A., & Tune, L.E. (1997). Diagnosis and treatment of Alzheimer disease and related disorders: consensus statement of the American Association for Geriatric Psychiatry, the Alzheimer's Association and the American Geriatric Society. *Journal of the American Medical Association, 278,* 1363-1371.

Spector, A., Orrell, M., Davies, S., & Woods, B. (2001). Can reality orientation be rehabilitated? Development and piloting of an evidence-based programme of cognition-based therapies for people with dementia. *Neuropsychological Rehabilitation, 11,* 377-397.

Spector, A., Orrell, M., Davies, S., & Woods, R.T. (1998). Reality orientation for dementia: a review of the evidence for its effectiveness. *Cochrane Library* (Issue 4). Oxford: Update Software.

Storandt, M., Morris, J.C., Rubin, E.H., Coben, L.A., & Berg, L. (1992). Progression of senile dementia of the Alzheimer type on a battery of psychometric tests. In L. Bäckman (Ed.), *Memory Functioning in Dementia.* Amsterdam: Elsevier Science Publications.

Thoene, A.I.T., & Glisky, E.L. (1995). Learning of face-name associations in memory impaired patients: a comparison of different training procedures. *Journal of the International Neuropsychological Society, 1,* 29-38.

Vidal, J.C., Lavieille-Letan, S., Fleury, A.O., & Rotrou, J.D. (1998). Stimulation cognitive et psychosociale des patients dements en institution. *La Revue de Geriatrie, 23,* 199-206.

Whitehouse, P.J., Lerner, A., & Hedera, P. (1993). Dementia. In K.M. Heilman & E. Valenstein (Eds.), *Clinical Neuropsychology.* Oxford: Oxford University Press.

Wild, K.V., & Kaye, J.A. (1998). The rate of progression of Alzheimer's disease in the later stages: evidence from the Severe Impairment Battery. *Journal of the International Neuropsychological Society, 4,* 512-516.

Wilson, B.A. (1995). Management and remediation of memory problems in brain-injured adults. In A.D. Baddeley, B.A. Wilson, & F.N. Watts (Eds.), *Handbook of Memory Disorders* (pp. 451-479). Chichester: John Wiley & Sons.

Woods, B. (1992). What can be learned from studies on reality orientation? In G.M.M. Jones & B.M.L. Miesen (Eds.), *Care-giving in Dementia: Research and Applications, Vol. 1.* London: Tavistock/Routledge.

Woods, B., Portnoy, S., Head, D., & Jones, G. (1992). Reminiscence and life review with persons with dementia: which way forward? In G.M.M. Jones & B.M.L. Miesen (Eds.), *Care-Giving in Dementia: Research and Applications, Vol. 1.* London: Tavistock/Routledge.

Woods, R.T. (1996). Cognitive approaches to the management of dementia. In R.G. Morris (Ed.), *The Cognitive Neuropsychology of Alzheimer-type Dementia.* Oxford: Oxford University Press.

Zanetti, O., Binetti, G., Magni, E., Rozzini, L., Bianchetti, A., & Trabucchi, M. (1997). Procedural memory stimulation in Alzheimer's disease: impact of a training programme. *Acta Neurologica Scandinavica, 95,* 152-157.

Zanetti, O., Magni, E., Binetti, G., Bianchetti, A., & Trabucchi, M. (1994). Is procedural memory stimulation effective in Alzheimer's disease? *International Journal of Geriatric Psychiatry, 9,* 1006-1007.

Zanetti, O., Zanieri, G., Giovanni, G. d., Vreese, L.P.D., Pezzini, A., Metitieri, T., & Trabucchi, M. (2001). Effectiveness of procedural memory stimulation in mild Alzheimer's disease patients: a controlled study. *Neuropsychological Rehabilitation, 11*, 263-272.

Chapter 11

OUTCOME AND MANAGEMENT OF TRAUMATIC BRAIN INJURY IN CHILDHOOD: THE NEUROPSYCHOLOGIST'S CONTRIBUTION

Vicki A. Anderson

University of Melbourne, Australia,
Murdoch Children's Research Institute, Melbourne

Introduction

Childhood traumatic brain injury (TBI) is a frequent cause of acquired disability in childhood. While most such injuries are mild, with few sequelae, children sustaining more severe TBI may suffer permanent cognitive and behavioural impairment. Neuropsychological studies now consistently report residual problems in a range of domains, including information processing, attention, memory and learning, and executive abilities. These deficits may limit the child's ability to function effectively in day-to-day life, resulting in lags in the acquisition of skills and knowledge, with common difficulties noted in areas such as educational proficiency and social interactions. Secondary deficits may also emerge, relating to family stress and adjustment difficulties. Treatment and management of the head-injured child and family requires long-term involvement. As for adults, the aim is to understand the cognitive and behavioural consequences of the child's injuries, how they impact on the child's day-to-day life, to liaise with teachers and rehabilitation workers, to design academic interventions and behaviour management programs, and to provide counseling with respect to adjustment issues for the child and family.

This chapter aims to review current knowledge with respect to recovery trajectories and residual sequelae following childhood TBI, and to discuss the nature and process of providing rehabilitation and management within the context of the child and family. While there is a large body of knowledge addressing these issues within the adult literature, as is evident from the various chapters in the current text, paediatric rehabilitation theory and practice has received much less attention. Many rehabilitation practices employed in adult TBI can be translated into work with children, however, there are important developmental issues, which need to be considered when designing intervention models in a paediatric context.

Epidemiology

While epidemiological data on childhood TBI is scarce, findings from research in the U.S.A. has found that approximately 250 : 100,000 children suffer TBI each year. Of these, half will not seek medical attention, between 5 and 10 percent will suffer temporary and/or permanent neuropsychological impairment, and 5 to 10 percent will sustain fatal injuries (Goldstein & Levin, 1987). Examination of data specific to severe TBI shows that the mortality rate is approximately one third, with another third of children making a good recovery. The last third will exhibit residual disability (Michaud, Rivara, Grady, & Reay, 1992), and will benefit from ongoing management and rehabilitation.

The nature of childhood TBI varies with age. Infants are more likely to present due to falls or child abuse (Holloway, Bye, & Moran, 1994). The preschool stage is a high risk period, with the majority of injuries caused by falls and pedestrian accidents, consistent with increased mobility and lack of awareness of danger in this age group (Anderson, Morse et al., 1997; Lehr, 1990). Older children and adolescents tend to be victims of sporting, cycling or pedestrian accidents. Boys and girls are not equally at risk of injury. In preschool children, the male to female ratio is approximately 1.5 : 1 (Hayes & Jackson, 1989; Horowitz et. al., 1983), and by school-age males are more than twice as likely to suffer TBI (Kraus, 1995). The incidence of TBI increases in males through childhood and adolescence, with a contrasting decline for females over this period (Kraus, Fife, Ramstein, & Conroy, 1986).

TBI in childhood is more likely to occur on weekends, afternoons, and holidays, when children are involved in leisure pursuits or travelling to and from school, suggesting that many injuries may result from reckless behaviours, in poorly supervised environments (Chadwick, Rutter, Brown, Shaffer, & Traub, 1981b; Dalby & Obrzut, 1991). Some research has suggested that TBI is more common in socially disadvantaged families (Anderson, Morse, et al., 1997; Brown, Chadwick, Shaffer, Rutter, & Traub, 1981; Klonoff, 1971; Rivara et al., 1993; Taylor et al., 1995) and in children with pre-existing learning and behavioural deficits (Asarnow, Satz, Light, Lewis, & Neumann, 1991; Brown et al., 1981; Craft, Shaw, & Cartlidge, 1972), however, recent research has failed to support such findings, arguing that children who sustain injury cannot be differentiated from the general population (Perrot, Taylor, & Montes, 1991; Prior, Kinsella, Sawyer, Bryan, & Anderson, 1994).

Pathophysiology

Traumatic brain injury refers to a traumatic insult to the brain, usually due to a blow or wound to the head, and causing altered consciousness (Begali, 1992). TBI may be classified as penetrating (or open) head injury or closed head injury. Penetrating injuries account for approximately 10 percent of all childhood TBI. Primary cerebral pathology tends to be localized, while secondary damage may occur due to cerebral infection, swelling, bleeding, and raised intra-cranial pressure. Loss of consciousness is relatively uncommon, however neurologic deficits and post-traumatic epilepsy are frequently observed. Neurobehavioral sequelae tend to reflect the focal nature of the insult, and children often exhibit specific deficits consistent with the localization of the lesion, with other skills intact. Closed head injury refers to an insult where the skull is not penetrated, but rather the brain is shaken within the skull cavity, resulting in multiple injury sites, as well as diffuse axonal damage. The primary pathology includes contusion, or bruising, at point of impact of the blow and at other cerebral sites. Specific areas of the brain are particularly vulnerable to such damage, including the temporal lobes and basal frontal regions (Amacher, 1988; Courville, 1945). Secondary mechanisms, including neurochemical imbalance, haematoma, cerebral oedema, and raised intra-cranial pressure, may also occur, and are predictive of poor outcome in children (Baker, Moulton, MacMillan, & Sheddon, 1993; Quattrocchi, Prasad, Willits, & Wagner, 1991). Delayed complications may develop in the sub-acute stages post-injury, including communicating hydrocephalus, infections and there is an increased risk of epilepsy (Jennett, 1979; Pang, 1985; Ponsford, Sloan, & Snow, 1995; Raimondi & Hirschauer, 1984). Secondary injuries are more amenable to appropriate and timely medical interventions.

Mechanics, pathophysiology and age at insult

A variety of mechanisms may be acting, depending upon the maturity of the CNS at the time of injury. The skull and brain develop through childhood, resulting in different injury consequences at different developmental stages. For example, during infancy neck muscles are relatively weak, and do not adequately support a proportionately large head, leading to less resistance to force of impact. Further, the infant and toddler possess a relatively thin skull, easily deformed by a direct blow, and resulting in more frequent skull fractures. Over one third of young children who sustain TBI will have skull fractures. In contrast, contusions, lacerations and haematomas are rare (Berney, Favier, & Froidevaux, 1994; Choux, 1986; Sharma & Sharma, 1994). For older children and adolescents, intra-cranial mass lesions (haematomas, contusions) are more common, although not as common as in adult samples (Berger, Pitts, Lovely, Edwards, & Bartkowsky, 1985; Bruce, Schut, Bruno, Wood, & Sutton, 1978). Contrecoup lesions are relatively rare in all age groups (Berney et al., 1994).

The relative lack of myelination present in the immature CNS causes the cerebral hemispheres to be soft and pliable, allowing absorption of the force of impact best during infancy and early childhood. However, unmyelinated fibres are vulnerable to shearing effects, rendering the younger child at greater risk for diffuse axonal injury (Zimmerman & Bilaniuk, 1994). Reports suggest that TBI in children is more likely to result in diffuse cerebral swelling associated with vascular disruptions, with such pathology identified in one-third of the children examined by Bruce and colleagues (Bruce et al., 1978; Jennett et al., 1977). Outcomes are also different. Babies and toddlers lose consciousness less frequently than other age groups, however post-traumatic epilepsy is more common following early TBI (Berney et al., 1994; Raimondi & Hirschauer, 1984). The implications of these age-related differences are important, and suggest that pathophysiology, sequelae, recovery and outcome from childhood TBI cannot be readily extrapolated from adult findings.

Recovery from childhood TBI

The consequences of brain insult sustained early in life have long been regarded as both qualitatively and quantitatively distinct from those documented in adulthood. Pathological conditions that would almost certainly lead to severe cognitive dysfunction in an adult, such as severe unilateral brain disease or localised cerebrovascular accidents, can have quite different consequences for children. Children with focal brain injuries, for example, may go on to acquire many age appropriate abilities, free from deficits observed following similar insults in adulthood (Taylor & Alden, 1997). In contrast, children sustaining generalized cerebral insult, such as TBI, have been shown to have slower recovery and poorer outcomes than adults with similar insults (Anderson & Moore, 1995; Anderson & Taylor, 1999; Gronwall, Wrightson, & McGinn, 1997; Taylor & Alden, 1997). The timing of CNS insult is particularly important within the immature brain. The consequences of trauma are dependent upon the developmental processes underway in the CNS at time of insult. It is generally accepted that early trauma has greater potential influence, impacting on the basic structure of the brain. Further, if insult occurs at a sensitive or critical developmental period specific structures or functions may be disrupted. As the child moves through later childhood and adolescence, the nature of impairment comes to resemble the adult picture more closely, reflecting the more mature CNS, and the associated reduction in plasticity/flexibility for recovery and reorganization.

There has been much research directed to establishing a fuller understanding of the recovery process, both in children and adults. Today, we are aware of many of the physiological consequences of brain insult and the underlying aspects of recovery. There is some dispute regarding the relative efficiency of these processes in the immature child's brain versus the fully developed adult brain, with some evidence for greater recovery following early brain insult. Brain damage results in a number of changes to brain tissue, depending on the type of damage incurred. Once a lesion occurs, be it vascular, traumatic, or aplastic, a number of degenerative events follow. These events involve the death and shrinkage of axons and associated neural structures, and the consequent actions of glial cells in repairing the damage as much as possible. While these degenerative processes may occur primarily in the acute phases post-injury, there is some evidence for ongoing degeneration and cumulative pathology in children following cerebral insult (Anderson et al., 2001; Anderson & Pentland, 1998; Paakko et al., 1992; Stein & Spettell, 1995). These mechanisms are well demonstrated in the case of 'Thomas', a toddler who sustained a severe traumatic brain injury, with focal frontal damage at age three years, as a result of motor vehicle accident. The brain scans illustrated in Figure 1 were obtained immediately post-injury, and ten years later. The initial CT scan (A) shows the extent of the initial injury, particularly within the right frontal lobe. MR scans conducted ten years later clearly demonstrate the original frontal lobe injury, and subcortical pathology (B). In addition, the right hemisphere now shows evidence of generalized atrophy (C), suggestive of abnormal development post-injury.

ACUTE   10 YEARS POSTINJURY

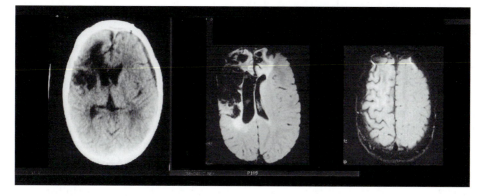

Fig. 1. Brain scans depicting pathology following severe TBI in a 3 year old child. (A) Acute CT scan, demonstrating extent of initial injury, which includes extensive right frontal damage. (B) and (C) MRI scans seven years post-injury, illustrating the initial pathology, as well as generalized right hemisphere atrophy.

Despite these various pathologic processes, some recovery of function is evident, both biologically and functionally. The proposed mechanisms of recovery can be grouped into two general classes – restitution theories and substitution theories (Kolb & Gibb, 1999; Laurence & Stein, 1978; Rothi & Horner, 1983). Restitution of function suggests that spontaneous physiological recovery occurs after brain damage. As damaged brain tissue heals, neural pathways are reactivated and so functions are restored. In contrast, substitution theories refer to restoration via transfer of functions from damaged brain tissue to healthy sites.

Restitution of function

Following injury, an initial period of diaschisis occurs, a kind of general inertia which temporarily suppresses cerebral activity in regions far from injury site, because of widespread effects on processes such as blood flow, intracranial pressure, and neurotransmitter release. A number of additional recovery processes have been described. Regeneration, the process by which damaged neurons, axons, and terminals regrow and re-establish previous of neuronal connections, is the best documented, and has been demonstrated to be functionally advantageous in the peripheral nervous system, as well as in the CNS in animal studies (Kolb & Gibbs, 1999). The possibilities for such regrowth in the CNS in humans are less clear (Bjorkland & Stenevi, 1971; Finger & Stein, 1982; Rothi & Horner, 1983), although it has been demonstrated that the hippocampus and the olfactory bulb may generate neurons during adulthood (Altman & Bayer, 1993; Lois & Alvarez-Buylla, 1994). A second recovery process is that of sprouting, where intact neurons develop branches that occupy regions left empty by damaged neurons, thus re-innervating unoccupied areas. Sprouting occurs quite early in the recovery process, being complete in a matter of weeks, with some evidence that it leads to associated behavioural improvement (Kolb & Wishaw, 1996). Denervation supersensitivity (Cannon & Rosenbleuth, 1949) provides another possible mechanism for restoration of function, suggesting that, in areas of damage, post-synaptic processes may become supersensitive to neurotransmitter substance leaking from pre-lesion neurons, thus allowing activation of post-lesion pathways and restitution of normal functioning. Currently much research effort is focussed on application of pharmacological treatments which may enhance these physiological recovery processes.

The underlying mechanisms described in restitution theories may be argued to be equally efficacious in the mature and the developing brain, with no clear neurophysiological evidence to support better physiological recovery in the developing brain. Finger and Stein (1982), in their work on age and recovery, argue that anomalous neural growth following CNS insult, via restitution mechanisms, is more likely in the immature brain, due to the less rigid organisation present. One of the possible mechanisms acting in the recovery process, that of neural competition, provides a basis for this vulnerability position. This competition hypothesis predicts that, following cerebral insult to the developing brain, there is a relocation of function, resulting in a decrease in synaptic sites available for mediating behaviours. The number of available synaptic sites is reduced, due to neuronal damage, and functional systems must work with a smaller number of synaptic connections, leading to reduced levels of functioning and the 'crowding' phenomenon. In the longer term, there remains less synaptic sites available to be taken up by new, emerging skills, leading to a picture of cumulative deficits and increasing problems with each developmental transition. (Aram & Eisele, 1994; Vargha-Khadem, Isaacs, Papaleloudi, Polkey, & Wilson, 1992).

Substitution of function
Substitution theories, arguing for either anatomical reorganisation or functional adaptation, provide some evidence for plasticity, based on the assumption that the relatively unspecialised state of the immature CNS allows for transfer or re-routing of behavioural functions, with little evidence of impairment. The first group of substitution theories, those supporting anatomical reorganisation, have a long history. Theorists such as Munk (1881), Lashley (1929) and Luria (1963) put forward arguments that there are large areas of the brain that are 'unoccupied' or equipotential, with the capacity to subsume functions previously the responsibility of damaged tissue. The advantages of reorganization theories are generally thought to reduce with age, with young children having more 'uncommitted' brain tissue, leading to a greater potential for reorganization of function. Recent research showing that the most dramatic effect of cerebral insult may be as a result of pre-natal pathology is not consistent with these theories, suggesting that the relationship between age at injury and outcome may not be a linear one (Anderson, Northam, Hendy, & Wrennall, 2001; Duchowny et al., 1996; Jacobs, Anderson, & Harvey, 2001).

Behavioural compensation (Kolb & Wishaw, 1996; Rothi & Horner, 1983) is a second possible mechanism for substitution of function. This model suggests that the patient develops new strategies or routes for cognitive functions which were previously dependent on damaged tissue. For example, a child with right parietal damage, resulting in visual analytic impairment, may develop a range of verbal mediation strategies to implement when faced with visually-based tasks. Alternatively, external strategies may be employed to minimise residual deficits. A child with memory deficits may employ a diary or note system to compensate for poor learning. This perspective underpins the philosophy for rehabilitation intervention following CNS insult, aiming to maximise behavioural compensation and recovery by suggesting strategies and modifying the individual's environment to their needs. As with restitution theories, while this model suggests that it may be beneficial for children following brain insult, there is no indication that children will benefit more than do adults (Anderson, 1988; Anderson et al., 2001; Taylor & Alden, 1997).

Neuropsychological consequences of paediatric TBI

Initially, research into paediatric TBI was directed towards identification of long-term sequelae from injuries. Today, this research is substantial and has established a knowledge base regarding the expectations for impairment following childhood TBI. In many respects, the characteristic impairments of childhood TBI mimic those seen in adults. However, where skills are undeveloped or immature at time of injury, research shows that these deficits may be more global and devastating for children.

Domain specific outcome studies

IQ

Patterns of intellectual function following childhood TBI are now well documented (Anderson & Moore, 1995; Brown et al., 1981; Chadwick et al., 1981a; Chadwick et al., 1981b; Ewing-Cobbs et al., 1997; Ponsford et al., 1997; Prior et al., 1994; Rutter, Chadwick, & Shaffer, 1983). In the absence of any pre-injury problems, mild TBI has little impact on intellectual skills, even in the acute recovery phase. In contrast, lowered intellectual quotients are frequently reported following moderate and severe TBI, with lowest scores immediately post-injury, and continued improvement in the first 6 to 12 months post-injury, followed by a plateauing effect thereafter. Long-term follow-up does indicate that intellectual growth may be differentially impacted in children with severe injuries, and for those injured in the preschool years, with intellectual quotients reducing with time since injury in these groups

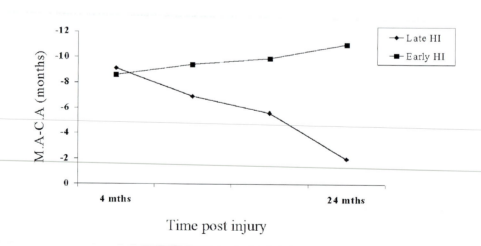

Fig. 2. Comparison of recovery trajectories for children injured before and after 7 years, represented by mental age (M.A) – chronological age (C.A) at 4 months and 24 months post head injury (HI). These findings suggest that earlier age at injury is related to poorer recovery post-injury.

(Anderson, Catroppa, Morse, Haritou, & Rosenfeld, 2000a; Jaffe, Polissar, Faye, & Liao, 1995). Figure 2 illustrates this finding, with expected results over time for older children, and those with mild to moderate injuries, but lack of recovery and/or development in the younger, severely injured children (Anderson & Moore, 1995). These results emphasize the importance of continued review and intervention in these children.

Language skills
Aphasias are rare following childhood TBI. However, clinical reports and research findings describe functional communication impairments, including slowed speech, dysfluency, poor logical sequencing of ideas and word finding difficulties (Dennis, 1989; Morse et al., 2000). Residual deficits in expressive language skills and writing abilities have also been documented (Campbell & Dolloghan, 1990; Chapman, 1995; Chapman, Levin, Wanek, Weyrauch, & Kufera, 1998; Dennis & Barnes, 1990; Didus, Anderson, & Catroppa., 2000; Ewing-Cobbs, Brookshire, Fletcher, & Scott, 1998; Ewing-Cobbs, Levin, Eisenberg, & Fletcher, 1987; Ewing-Cobbs et al., 1997; Haritou et al., 1997), with recent studies reporting high level problems with functional communication skills (Turkstra, McDonald, & DePompei, 2001). Not surprisingly, greater deficits are associated with more severe injuries. Further, younger children appear to exhibit more global language difficulties, with additional deficiencies in language comprehension observed when injuries occur in the pre-school period (Anderson et al., 1997).

Visual and motor skills
Debilitating motor and visual deficits (e.g. hemiparesis, impaired balance and steadiness, visual field defects) are common in the acute recovery stages, with rapid improvement occurring in the first few months post-injury, and systematic, but non-linear recovery up to 5 years post-injury (Thompson et al., 1994). It is only where children sustain very severe injuries, or injuries early in life, that significant motor deficits persist (Thompson et al., 1994). However, more subtle deficits, such as visuo-motor incoordination and reduced eye-hand co-ordination may be ongoing, and may occur even following relatively mild injury (Winogron, Knights, & Bawden, 1984). Such problems may limit the child's capacity for day-to-day activities such as sport and other physical pursuits and school-based skills including writing, drawing, and copying, with possible secondary implications for self-esteem, socialization, and academic development. Further, as speed requirements increase in daily life, children with significant TBI have been found to demonstrate increasing difficulties (Ewing-Cobbs, Miner, Fletcher, & Levin, 1989; Ewing-Cobbs et al., 1997).

Memory and learning
Early studies identified memory function as the most likely cognitive domain to show impairment following childhood TBI (Levin & Eisenberg, 1979;

Levin Eisenberg, Wigg, & Kobayashi, 1982; Levin et al., 1988), with greatest deficits and poorest recovery occurring following severe TBI. More recent literature has extended these findings, documenting a consistent trend for children with severe TBI to exhibit generalized deficits in learning, storage and retrieval. For children with mild/moderate injuries, consequences are less clear, but indicate that these children perform closer to normal, with perhaps some mild retrieval problems evident (Anderson, Catroppa, Morse, Haritou, & Rosenfeld, 2000b; 2001; Catroppa & Anderson, in press; Jaffe et al., 1992, 1993, 1995; Levin et al., 1993; 1994; Ong, Chandran, Zasmani, & Lye, 1999; Yeates, Blumstein, Patterson, & Delis, 1995). The implications of memory impairment in the child are likely to be substantial, given that the day-to-day tasks of childhood largely revolve around acquiring knowledge and learning and perfecting new skills. Memory problems may interfere with this process, resulting in a failure to develop at an age appropriate rate in domains such as education and social skills (Kinsella et al., 1997).

Attention skills
In contrast to the specific psychomotor slowing seen following moderate to severe adult TBI, children present with global attention deficits, with many of these problems persisting beyond the acute recovery stage (Bakker et al., 2000; Catroppa, Anderson, & Stargatt, 1999; Catroppa & Anderson, 1998; Anderson, Fenwick, Manly, & Robertson, 1998; Anderson & Pentland, 1998; Dennis et al., 1995; Ewing-Cobbs et al., 1998; Fenwick & Anderson, 1999; Kaufmann, Fletcher, Levin, Miner, & Ewing-Cobbs, 1993). These more generalized problems may reflect the relatively immature state of the attention system at the time of injury. The injury, and its associated pathology, may interrupt ongoing development, so that components of attention which usually emerge and differentiate post-injury, will fail to do so, leading to delayed or deficient performance, as for memory impairments. These problems may lead to increasing lags in the efficient acquisition of knowledge and skills, and a failure in the development and differentiation of cognitive and attentional abilities (Anderson & Moore, 1995; Dennis, Wilkinson, Koski, & Humphreys, 1995; Fletcher, Miner, & Ewing-Cobbs, 1987).

Executive functions
Deficits in executive functions, such as planning, reasoning, and self-regulation, are commonly reported in children who have suffered TBI, in keeping with the vulnerability of the pre-frontal regions in head trauma (Courville, 1945; Walsh, 1978). Despite these observations, there have been few formal studies of executive abilities, though some case descriptions do exist (Dennis, Barnes, Donnelly, Wilkinson, & Humphreys, 1996; Mateer & Williams, 1991, Passler, Isaac, & Hynd, 1985; Williams & Mateer, 1992). Neuropsychological studies have examined outcomes on traditional executive function tests, showing that performance is consistently related to injury severity, and with a trend for younger age at injury to be implicated in poorer perform-

ances (Anderson, Levin, & Jacobs, 2002; Garth, Anderson, & Wrennall, 1997; Levin et al., 1997; Levin et al., 1994; Pentland, Todd & Anderson, 1998). Children with TBI exhibit poorer reasoning skills, make more errors and use less efficient strategies, and provide ineffective or unworkable planning strategies as a result.

Functional Outcome Following TBI in Childhood

Survivors of childhood TBI frequently make a good physical recovery, and appear outwardly normal. The expectations of their abilities and behaviours are often determined by this relatively healthy presentation, despite ongoing significant cognitive and behavioural disabilities (Johnson, 1992).

Educational abilities
Academic failure has been argued to be one of the most serious consequences of paediatric TBI (Catroppa & Anderson, 2000b; Goldstein & Levin, 1985; Greenspan & MacKenzie, 1994; Levin et al., 1987). Early studies identified a relationship between injury severity and educational achievement, with Klonoff and associates (Klonoff et al., 1977) reporting that one quarter of their sample required remedial classes by five years post-injury. More recently, Kinsella et al. (1995; 1997) have found that, by two years post injury, 70 percent of children with severe injuries, and 40 percent of those with moderate injuries, were receiving special educational assistance. Socioeconomic status, male gender, maladaptive behaviours, reduced verbal learning skills and slowed psychomotor processing have been identified as predictors of poorer academic achievement post-injury (Donders, 1994; Kinsella et al., 1997; Stalings, Ewing-Cobbs, Francis, & Fletcher, 1996; Taylor et al., 2002).

Qualitative analysis of data from these studies suggests that reading accuracy skills appear to be relatively resilient in school-aged children, with arithmetic and comprehension more vulnerable (Catroppa & Anderson, 2000; Barnes, Dennis, & Wilkinson, 1999; Berger-Gross & Shackelford, 1985; Kinsella et al., 1997). Injuries sustained in the preschool period, even those of mild severity, have been associated with school failure. Despite appearing to be fully recovered immediately post-injury, these children are more likely to have reading difficulties, and require special education input as they move through the school system (Gronwall, et al., 1997; Wrightson, McGinn, & Gronwall, 1995). One possible explanation for these somewhat unexpected consequences following mild TBI, may relate to the observation that these skills must develop from scratch following a preschool injury. Thus even a mild impairment of attention and/or memory may cause disruption to this acquisition process.

Behaviour and social skills
Debate continues with respect to the aetiology of behavioural and social difficulties post-TBI. Some authors claim that these problems reflect pre-

morbid behavioural and family problems, while others support an important impact of brain injury (Donders, 1992; Farmer et al., 1996; Fletcher, Ewing-Cobbs, Miner, Levin, & Eisenberg, 1990; Max, Castillo et al., 1997a; Max, Smith et al., 1997b; Perrott, Taylor, & Montes,1991; Prior et al., 1994; Wade, Taylor, Drotar, Stancin, & Yeates, 1996). Clinical reports frequently describe behavioural change post-TBI, even in the absence of physical disability or cognitive impairment. Problems range from initial symptoms of fatigue and irritability, to more persisting deficits such as aggression, poor impulse control, hyperactivity, distractibility, depression, and anxiety (Asarnow et al., 1991; Black, Jeffries, Blumer, Wellner, & Walker, 1969; Bohnert, Parker, & Warschausky, 1997; Brink, Imbus, & Woo-Sam, 1980; Brown et al., 1981; Butler, Rourke, Fuerst, & Fisk, 1997; Cattelani, Lombardi, Brianti, & Mazzuchi, 1998; Klonoff, Clark, & Klonoff, 1995; Max, Smith et al., 1997). Reduced self-esteem and social difficulties may accompany these problems (Bohnert et al., 1997; Turkstra et al., 2001). Andrews and colleagues (Andrews, Rose, & Johnson, 1998) have identified low levels of self-esteem and adaptive behaviour and high levels of loneliness and aggression in children with TBI.

These post-injury behavioural difficulties are closely linked to injury severity. Children with severe injuries have been found to show a marked increase in psychiatric disturbance, both acutely and in the long-term post-injury. Brink and coworkers (Brink et al., 1980) report that while only 10% of their sample of severely head-injured children had any persisting neurologic impairment, 46% had severe emotional/behavioural disturbances requiring professional counselling. Brown and colleagues (Brown et al., 1981) noted that the rate of new psychiatric disorder was more than doubled in the severely injured group in comparison to controls. Within this severely injured group, history of pre-injury behavioural deficits was predictive of later psychiatric disturbance, with over half of these children developing a disturbance in the 12 months post-injury, in contrast to a figure of 29% for children with no premorbid problems.

A number of studies report increasing problems in behaviour, and increased incidence of psychiatric disturbance post-TBI (Brink et al., 1980; Brown et al., 1981; Cattelani et al., 1998; Perrot et al., 1991). This pattern may be due to the direct effects of TBI (e.g. increased impulsivity, hyperactivity associated with right frontal damage), or related to secondary factors such as family dysfunction or depression and adjustment difficulties occurring in the process of coming to terms with long-term implications of injury.

In summary, children who sustain significant TBI are at risk for cognitive, educational and behavioural problems. These problems may not be evident initially post-injury. Rather, they may develop secondary to problems of adjustment or, alternatively, they may emerge as the child fails to meet expected developmental milestones. As a consequence, rehabilitation resources need to be available to children and families throughout childhood, to ensure early identification and treatment.

Injury Related Predictors of Outcome

Variability in outcome following childhood TBI has been well documented (Fletcher, Ewing-Cobbs, Francis, & Levin, 1995). Even with our increasing understanding of the consequences of TBI in children, it remains difficult to predict which children will show good recovery, and who will require ongoing support and rehabilitation. Researchers are now beginning to address this issue, by identifying and studying potential predictors of outcome.

Injury-related factors have received most attention to date, with a clear dose-response relationship identified for injury severity and outcome at all stages of recovery. The nature of injury is also relevant, with more focal injuries generally thought to lead to better outcome than generalized insults (Anderson et al., 2001). A number of specific injury characteristics have been found to be associated with poorer prognosis in children, including depth of lesion (Ommaya & Gennarelli, 1974), presence of secondary damage due to intracranial haematomas (Berger et al., 1985; Walker, Mayer, Storrs, & Hylton, 1985), diffuse axonal injury (Filley, Cranberg, Alexander, & Hart, 1987), oedema, hypoxia, haemorrhage and herniation (Gentry, Godersky, & Thompson, 1988). Severity of total injuries and post-traumatic seizures have also been identified as predictive factors (Michaud et al., 1992).

Developmental and psychosocial factors may also contribute to long-term function. Younger age at injury has been noted to be associated with poorer recovery initially, and a failure to maintain developmental progress in the years post-injury (Anderson, 1988; Anderson et al., 2000a, 2000b; Anderson & Moore, 1995; Ewing-Cobbs et al., 1997; Gronwall et al., 1997). Psychosocial parameters, including reduced access to rehabilitation services and special education, degree of family burden and significant family dysfunction and psychiatric problems have all been found to impact on long-term recovery (Rivara et al., 1993, 1994; Taylor et al., 2002; Wade et al., 1996). Recently, gender has also been identified as a factor contributing to recovery, with females demonstrating better recovery from early childhood insult (Kolb, 1995; Raz et al., 1994, 1995).

It is probable that specific factors are predictive of recovery at different stages post-TBI. For example, injury severity is a crucial predictor of function in the acute stages of recovery, but may become less important in the long term. Longitudinal studies are underway (Anderson et al., 1997; Ewing-Cobbs et al., 1997; Jaffe et al., 1995; Kinsella et al, 1997; Taylor et al., 1995) which build on the knowledge of functional impairment gained from past research, but currently there is minimal information regarding outcome after two years post-injury.

In a recently completed study within our laboratory (Newitt, 2002), the long-term contribution of injury severity was investigated in a sample of 59 young adults who had sustained TBI in childhood. Results from the study showed that, while participants who had sustained mild or moderate TBI during childhood appeared to be functioning as independent members of the community, those with severe injuries had made a less successful transition to adulthood. Poor educational attainment, high rates of unemployment, difficulties with relationships, limited leisure activities and social isolation were commonly documented. Within this group, most participants lived with their families, and changes in family structure and function (e.g. family breakdown, marital difficulties) were common. Substance abuse and criminal behaviours, as well as psychiatric disorders, were also over-represented in this group. Greatest impairments were found for survivors who had sustained other serious injuries in addition to TBI. Similar patterns of disability have been reported in other studies (Klonoff, Clark, & Klonoff, 1995; Koshiniemi, Timo, Taina, & Leo, 1995).

Knowledge of the importance and relative contribution of injury-related, developmental and psychosocial variables is important to ensure early identification and appropriate follow-up of 'at-risk' children and families. Research suggests that additional resources may need to be directed to children with severe TBI, to younger children, who may appear to have made a good recovery acutely, but may develop problems over time since injury, and to those with multiple injuries, where physical, cognitive and emotional stressors may be present. Families experiencing high levels of stress, perhaps due to death of another family member in the accident, or to pre-existing family difficulties, may also need careful follow-up, as they may have less personal resources available to identify and act upon problems arising post-injury. Careful documentation of these potential risk factors at time of hospitalization may minimize unnecessary secondary complications of TBI.

Paediatric Rehabilitation: Theoretical Considerations

As with adult models, paediatric rehabilitation is a multidisciplinary endeavor, incorporating rehabilitation physicians, physical therapists, occupational therapists, speech therapists, play therapists, special educators, and social workers, as well as neuropsychologists, and families, in the acute stages, and providing a range of specialist interventions. Later, educational specialists and counselors may also become involved. The goals of the rehabilitation process are to promote recovery and work with the injured child and his/her family to compensate for residual deficits, to understand and treat cognitive and behavioural impairments, to recognize the role of these impairments in functional disabilities, and to monitor family and other social factors (Rourke et al., 1983; Wilson, 1997; Ylvisaker, 1998). The broad aim is to enable the child to do what he/she would like to do, or needs to do, in order to cope with life demands, but finds difficult because of the various consequences of brain injury (Ylvisaker, 1998). Thus, the emphasis of rehabilitation may vary, depending on the nature of the difficulties experienced by the individual.

Models of intervention

As for adults, approaches to paediatric rehabilitation may be divided according to the aim of the intervention. Internally focussed methods stress improving the individual's capacities, by either restoration of function via re-establishment of impaired functions, or functional adaptation, where intact abilities are utilized to 're-route' skills which have been disrupted via behavioural training. Externally focussed approaches are directed towards altering the environment to meet the child's new needs, with no intention for changing the child's actual abilities (Mateer, 1999). This environmental modification is particularly relevant once the child has returned home, and must recommence activities of daily living (Anderson et al., 2001; Park & Ingles, 2001; Ponsford et al., 1995).

For injured children additional rehabilitation options are often present. One approach focuses on acceleration of the acquisition of new skills, as well as restoration of established abilities (Ylvisaker, 1998). Such ongoing acquisition of knowledge and skills is a critical task of childhood. Unfortunately, it is the dynamic skills required for these important learning processes (e.g. attention, memory, processing speed, executive function) that are often impacted by TBI, placing children at risk for cumulative problems (Anderson et al., 2000). Thus, the treatment and optimization of these 'processing' skills is a central focus of rehabilitation. In addition, developing functional abilities, such as academic and social skills, requires particular support in the paediatric context. In many child rehabilitation centres, a combination of these intervention approaches is employed simultaneously. Currently, there is little research available on the relative efficacy of each of these models within the paediatric context. However, a recent study conducted by Selznick and Savage (2000) provides some support for such an approach. These researchers report the outcome of three single case studies where they employed behavioural methods to treat self-monitoring difficulties, which are commonly identified in children with TBI. They found that their intervention led to greater on-task behaviour and higher accuracy levels on their training tasks. Unfortunately, as with many intervention evaluations, there was no indication whether these improvements translated into day-to-day activities.

In children with TBI, a further critical intervention avenue is provided by the family unit. Parents may play a key role in the rehabilitation process, especially as early discharge to the familiarity of the home environment from acute settings is generally considered optimal in paediatric settings. Often children will return home while still suffering from the acute effects of injury (e.g. irritability, fatigue, poor attention), which are difficult to understand and manage. Detailed and realistic education for parents is an essential element of the rehabilitation program. Further, parents and families need to be informed regarding the likely physical, cognitive and emotional consequences of TBI, their impact on the child's day-to-day life, and the likely time lines for recovery. They will benefit from counseling regarding best methods for managing their child's impairments and for negotiating access of resources for their child with schools and other agencies (Holster, 1999.

Restoration of function

Restorative interventions are designed to treat the cognitive impairments, which have resulted from injury (Cicerone & Tupper, 1990: Sohlberg & Mateer, 1989). Usually, this method of intervention requires an initial neuropsychological evaluation to identify impaired cognitive abilities. The child is then trained, using specific exercises focussing on those cognitive abilities or processes, in an attempt to improve these skills, as well as to impact more generally on all cognitive functions. This method of intervention, while controversial, is probably the best evaluated rehabilitation modality. Adult results suggest that such approaches may be more effective in certain cognitive domains (e.g. attention), with small, non-significant improvements reported in other domains (Diller & Gordon, 1981; Gray, Robertson, Pentlan, & Anderson, 1992; Mateer, Kerns, & Eso, 1996; Robertson, 1990). As might be expected, there is little evidence that these approaches generalize to other cognitive domains (Miller, 1992; Park & Ingles, 2001; Ponsford et al., 1995; Wilson, 1997; Wood, 1988) or to daily functions. Further, the critical emotional, behavioural and social sequelae that often follow from brain injury are not incorporated in such approaches, despite their potential influence on the patient's capacity to benefit from treatment.

Functional adaptation

Perhaps the most popular approach to rehabilitation is to attempt to train individuals with head injury to perform various activities and tasks using alternative strategies, enabling the person to compensate for their cognitive deficits. Such intervention procedures are designed to improve or restore cognitive capacity or lessen the functional impact of the impairment (Mateer, 1996). This approach is in keeping with an emphasis on maximizing identified cognitive strengths to ensure optimal performance in everyday life. As with restorative interventions, rehabilitation needs to be preceded by a thorough evaluation of cognitive strengths and weaknesses to provide a baseline for developing appropriate compensatory strategies. Compensatory approaches are well known within the child context, and are regularly utilized in educational programs for children with developmental disorders including language delay and specific learning difficulties. For example, for children with language difficulties, teaching strategies which employ visual imagery or visual memory will provide an optional 'route' for learning skills traditionally acquired via language-based teaching strategies. Or for older children, where complex cognition may be required, training in breaking down tasks (e.g. essays, projects) into a series of steps may provide a strategy for adequate performance, which can gradually be generalized into the child/adolescent's approach to complex or novel tasks. Importantly, and as emphasized by Rourke (1989) in his treatment-orientated approach, such methods are most effective when less severe impairment is present. The more global the deficits due to TBI, the more difficult it is to identify an intact modality to employ in the design and implementation of compensatory strategies.

In addition to behavioural approaches, which emphasize changing cognitive strategies, there is also the alternative of provision of external aids or cues, such as lists, diaries or alarms. There are a number of studies within the adult literature which have suggested that application of these techniques is related to significant improvement in skills (Berg, Koning-Haanstra, & Deelman, 1991; Schmitter-Edgecombe, Fahy, Whelan, & Long, 1995; Wilson & Moffat, 1992). Until recently, external cueing has not been found to be a particularly successful approach for younger children, but becomes of increasing benefit as children reach adolescence and develop the skills necessary to use these methods to enhance memory and retention. A recent study by Wilson and colleagues (Wilson, Emslie, Quirk, & Evans, 2001) has challenged this view, showing that children as young as 8 years of age were able to benefit from a computerized reminder intervention program ('Neuropage'), showing increased ability to recall important events and information when accessing this system.

Environmental modification
Where restoration or compensation approaches are unhelpful, therapists frequently employ more external measures to minimize the functional impact of cognitive impairments. To a great extent, the emphasis of paediatric rehabilitation is on modifying the child's environment to ensure that the context is conducive to best level of function (e.g., changing school curriculum, limiting class size, ensuring law noise levels). One of the major criticisms of this method in isolation is that it makes an assumption that the child will show little 'internal improvement' post-injury (Mateer, 1996). As a result, such interventions become more important once recovery processes have stabilized and the residual deficits are apparent. To implement such environmental modifications, a thorough understanding of the individual child's cognitive strengths and weaknesses is essential. On the basis of such information, physical, contextual and educational issues can then be implemented. Such interventions rely heavily on the availability of resources, and the full support of the child's family, school and community.

Accelerating developing skills
As previously noted, the acquisition of new skills may be delayed following TBI, due to a combination of factors, including the presence of attention and memory difficulties, missed educational and social experiences, and poor self-esteem. One emphasis of rehabilitation or educational intervention, is aimed at speeding up these processes. Educational skills provide an excellent example of this. In general, with children with TBI, traditional intervention approaches are employed to help the child acquire basic academic skills of reading, spelling and mathematics, with these areas noted to be areas of

deficiency post-injury. In particular, methods which utilize individual or small group tuition, where children's processing capacities can be closely monitored, have been shown to be particularly effective (Anderson, Smibert, Godber, Ekert, & Weiskop, 2000).

Education
There is some debate regarding the efficacy of educating children with respect to the consequences of head injury, and its possible impact on their lives, with current research findings in this area being inconclusive. In a recent study by Beardmore, Tate and Liddle (1998), findings demonstrated that, while children did not show any benefit of an educational program, parents did appear to show improved understanding of their child's difficulty. These results emphasize the importance of provision of detailed and appropriate information to families. Our own experience would suggest that this information needs to be in written form, as families, affected by the stress of their child's injury and hospitalization, often have difficulty absorbing and retaining the verbal material provided by rehabilitation teams during individual consultations and family meetings. At the level of the school and community, much of the intervention effort is also focussed on providing an understanding of the child's likely deficits, those which may be explained by TBI or secondary influences, and how these may limit the child's ability to cope with routine expectations. As is the case with many aspects of intervention within the paediatric context, the educational process needs to continue over time, as children recover, and pass through various developmental stages.

Education regarding the pattern of recovery and the residual nature of deficits is of critical importance for children and families. For example, contrary to expectations for recovery post-injury, behavioural difficulties have been reported to increase with time since injury (Brink et al., 1980; Cattelani et al., 1998), associated with adjustment difficulties, or perhaps family dysfunction. Further, as children with TBI move through normal developmental transitions new cognitive problems may emerge, particularly in areas such as organization, reasoning, and problem solving. It is critical that families and survivors are aware that such problems may be head injury-based, and so seek appropriate intervention. While these difficulties may be successfully treated, specific treatment approaches need to be implemented, which account for TBI-specific effects.

Psychological treatments
Effective rehabilitation models take an holistic view of the injured child, and his/her unique profile of disabilities, taking into account behavioural and emotional functioning. Despite this, management approaches addressing the emotional, social and behavioural consequences of childhood TBI are poorly documented and evaluated. Children with TBI may exhibit such problems as a result of primary brain injury (e.g. impulsivity, inattention, hyperactivity), or secondary to hospitalization, family separation and adjustment to residual

disabilities (e.g. anxiety, depression, social isolation). An understanding of the likelihood of these problems, and their bases, need to be incorporated into rehabilitation plans, with potential for assessment and management integrated into treatment models (Anderson et al., 2001; Ponsford et al., 1995; Wilson, 1997)

Developmental issues

Approaches to paediatric rehabilitation are directed, to some extent, by the unique needs of the young child and family. Most importantly, the young child is in a state of rapid development. As a consequence, intervention strategies need to account for possible disruptions to ongoing brain development, as well as potentially cumulative cognitive and psychosocial deficits. Following TBI, children may never reach their pre-injury potential. Children with significant impairments will require long-term management and rehabilitation, with particular emphasis on developmental transitions (e.g. pre-school to school-aged, middle childhood to adolescence), where strategic shifts in approach to treatment may be required, due to changes in both contextual and cognitive demands. Further, as new skills are programmed to come 'on-line' through childhood (e.g. reasoning, planning), children with TBI may experience delayed acquisition, in association with impairments in attention, learning and processing skills. The potential for such 'emerging' deficits suggests the need for active and long-term monitoring for this group.

Assessing recovery in children is a particularly complex task. In contrast to expectations following adult TBI, simple improvement in performance is not sufficient to imply 'recovery', as developmental expectations assume ongoing improvement in abilities through childhood. Thus, when determining if a child has demonstrated recovery, or benefited from rehabilitation, developmental factors need to be carefully considered.

At a more practical level, the common practice following injury in childhood is for early discharge from hospital, usually once symptoms of post-traumatic amnesia (PTA) have subsided. The accepted view is that return to the familiar home environment will be beneficial for recovery. As a result, intensive, structured rehabilitation programs are often impractical within the paediatric context, after the acute recovery stage. Rather, the emphasis is on outpatient care, and supporting the family to cope with the child's needs. Thus, a heavy burden of care falls upon the family unit, and there is much evidence that the healthy functioning of the family is critical to good outcome for survivors of childhood TBI (Perrott et al., 1991; Wade et al., 1996).

The educational context is also important to consider. Children are encouraged to return to school, at least on a fractional basis, as early as possible, thus re-establishing a social network, and a normal daily routine, as quickly as possible. This transition is often difficult and fraught with stress for the child, family and school. For many schools, the return of the child with TBI will be their first experience of working with a brain-injured child. There is a need for close liaison between rehabilitation team, school staff and family during this gradual process, to ensure that appropriate knowledge is available regarding expectations and treatment. Often, the head-injured child appears quite normal superficially, despite significant cognitive deficits, and it important that those within the school context comprehend and act upon the child's need for special assistance. Classroom discussions may also be beneficial, providing the child's classmates with an understanding of the child's needs and problems in a manner that is readily understood, and minimizes fears associated with the child's possible disabilities.

Management and Intervention: the Process

Recovery

Assessment and management of the child who has sustained a TBI commences at the scene of the injury, where conscious state and neurological status are evaluated. By the time the child reaches hospital he/she will have sustained permanent primary impact-related brain injury, which is thought to be relatively insensitive to medical treatment. Secondary effects will also be developing, and these have been shown to be more amenable to medical intervention. Early treatment is directed towards the accurate identification of these secondary complications and their rapid treatment (Miller, 1992). A number of parameters are particularly informative for determining injury severity at this early stage: level of consciousness, duration of altered consciousness, duration of post-traumatic amnesia, clinical evidence of skull fracture or cerebral pathology, and neurological and mental status.

In paediatric patients a combination of measures is usually employed to determine the severity of the injury, as no single indicator has proven to have sufficient predictive power in isolation (Fletcher et al., 1995). The poor reliability of traditional indices may reflect the relatively recent development of tools, such as the paediatric versions of the Glasgow Coma Score, PTA scales, the range of mechanisms of injury, the developmental level of the child at time of injury, as well as pre-injury factors including environment and premorbid ability.

The recovery process

The stages of recovery following childhood TBI follow a relatively predictable path, depending on the nature and severity of injury. As for adults, there are substantial differences between the rapid and uncomplicated recovery following mild TBI, and the more protracted process associated with moderate and severe TBI.

Mild injuries

After mild TBI, there may be a brief period of altered consciousness, and perhaps a period of post-traumatic amnesia, characterized by confusion and disorientation. Children are routinely observed for a short time and discharged home without hospital admission. Clinically, children may exhibit symptoms of fatigue and irritability. Transient cognitive problems may also occur, including reduced attention, psychomotor slowing, poor memory and behavioral symptoms (Beers, 1992; Boll, 1983). More significant motor and language deficits are uncommon. Over time, these deficits reduce and, while there is ongoing debate with respect to outcome, a good recovery is common, particularly in school-aged children, and where no premorbid problems were present (Asarnow et al., 1995; Polissar et al., 1994; Ponsford et al., 1997).

Moderate and severe injuries

Recovery from moderate and severe TBI is more protracted and may be seen as a multi-phase process, where there is an interaction between the child's physical recovery and developmental level, the family response and the reintegration of the child back into the wider community. Waaland and Kreutzer (1988) describe a series of stages which families commonly experience post-TBI, beginning with shock, optimism, and denial during the early stages of recovery, followed by more realistic anger, guilt and blame, and later grief and adjustment. These phases are summarized in Table 1.

Acute phase

During this phase progress is monitored for evidence of deterioration, due to raised intra-cranial pressure or haematoma, which may require surgery. Physical rehabilitation commences at this early stage, focussing on maintaining the child's physical strength. This is a time of intense anxiety for families, where the major focus is their child's survival. Further stressors may include injuries/fatalities of other family members, financial or employment pressures, family separation, and the need to care for other siblings. Feelings may fluctuate from hope and optimism to devastation and despair. Grief, guilt and blame can also be central issues for parents and siblings during this period (Waaland & Kreutzer, 1988).

Early rehabilitation

As the child emerges from coma more active rehabilitation begins. Some children are difficult to manage at this time, when features may include restlessness, agitation, confusion and disorientation. Nursing care and therapies during this period are often limited to containing such behavioural challenges. On emergence from PTA, functional impairments may be evident, and more intensive rehabilitation, including occupational and speech therapy may be instituted. The goal is to work towards an early return home to a familiar environment. Return to school is generally a gradual process, with the child initially attending for short periods, primarily for social contact, with involvement increasing as he/she gains physical strength.

This phase of recovery tends to involve a degree of balancing between rehabilitation goals, social adjustment needs of the child, and school and family resources. It is a stressful time for the family, who must negotiate

Table 1. Issues facing children and families following TBI.

Recovery stage	Child issues & responses	Family issues & responses
Acute: survival hospitalisation	survival early rehabilitation separation from parents coping with medical procedures	hope/fear re child's survival helplessness guilt/blame over injury family separation practical pressures: child care for other siblings, financial and employment concerns
Sub-acute: recovery/adjustment discharge and rehabilitation	intensive rehabilitation adjustment of acute disability fatigue and irritability social isolation	adjusting to changes in child denial of child's disability balancing needs of injured child and other family members practical issues: ongoing financial and employment concerns stress of attending and following through on rehabilitation procedures
Chronic: acceptance reintegration into community	adjustment to residual physical & cognitive disability social rejection and isolation feelings of loss and frustration depression	practical issues: organising educational resources managing family changes accepting residual disabolities of the child & adjusting expectations managing behavioural and physical problems

and organize the various resources required for the child, as well as adjust to the child's physical and behavioral limitations. Families react in different ways to these stresses, depending upon their own strategies and coping styles (Waaland & Kreutzer, 1988). While family intervention may appear warranted, often parents are unable to take advantage of psychological resources at this early stage. Practical difficulties (e.g. limited time, lack of child care, employment responsibilities), intense focus on the rehabilitation demands of the child, and denial of the difficulties and stressors may each limit the success of such interventions.

Assessment
Evaluation of cognitive function is critical to efficacious treatment. Standardized intellectual assessment may be useful in determining global levels of function in the child, however, IQ tests alone are insufficient to demonstrate the range of impairments experienced post-injury. Research suggests that there may be specific neurobehavioural domains, which are particularly vulnerable to the impact of TBI, for example, attention, executive function, speed of processing, memory and learning (Anderson et al., 2001). The effect of deficiencies in these abilities may not be apparent on IQ testing until some time post-injury. Evaluation of functional abilities, such as academic achievement, behavioural and social skills, via direct testing, parent and teacher questionnaires or observations, may supplement test-based information regarding impairments of day to day function. Such data are critical to the accurate diagnosis of cognitive strengths and weaknesses, their impact on day-to-day functions and the subsequent design of individual treatment plans.

Return to school
Initial return to school is often on a part-time basis, and focussed on re-establishing social contacts for the child. Fatigue and poor attention frequently preclude children from full involvement in the curriculum. Glang, Singer and Todis (1997) note that during this process accommodations for the child need to be considered at a number of levels: (1) physical: incorporation of adaptive equipment, including wheelchairs, special desks, computers, communication devices; (2) environmental: provision of extra time, quiet, well structured classroom, opportunity for repetition, revision; and (3) instructional: specific educational programming, individual tuition, social skills retraining. These modifications need to be negotiated prior to school return preferably, to make the transition as smooth as possible for child, family, teachers and peers. Careful consultation and liaison is critical to the success of this process. Further, the development of a special program is frequently required, even in the case of less severe injuries. As Rourke (1989) states, the goals of such programs need to be realistic, and the process for achieving them operationalized carefully, rather than left at an abstract level.

As for the neuropsychological assessment process, educational planning and environmental modifications within the school context need to focus on the areas of neurobehavioural function which are commonly impaired as a result of TBI. Motor skills, fine motor skills and processing speed, attention and memory are important targets, with executive skills becoming more important as the young child moves through childhood into adolescence. Common examples of environmental modification include use of a personal computer for writing tasks, provision of extra time for task completion to compensate for slowed processing speed. Attentional difficulties may be supported by provision of an 'aide' who is able to work one-on–one with a child and help direct and maintain attention to task. Short days, or school weeks may be beneficial for a child suffering from fatigue, while modification to the school curriculum may also be required. For example, for a child suffering from visual and motor deficits, subjects such as graphics or art may be particularly frustrating. For the more mildly injured child, who suffers from fatigue and mild processing difficulties, reducing the curriculum, thus allowing for more time to be committed to each subject, may be all that is required to enable adequate performance. Where memory and learning problems are present, access to individual tuition which can provide repetition and revision of classwork may be helpful. A number of recent texts provide a range of practical suggestions for school re-integration of children with TBI (e.g. Begali, 1992; Glang, Singer, & Todis, 1997; Johnson, Uttley, & Wyke, 1989; Ylvisaker, 1998).

Chronic phase

Some children sustaining more severe TBI may enjoy a relatively full recovery, with little requirement for professional intervention or support. More commonly such injuries are associated with ongoing impairments necessitating life-long medical involvement and rehabilitation. Problems are often most apparent at each developmental transition. At such times the child and family may need support and professional input to negotiate new challenges, and enhance the understanding of those working with the child. School entry may emphasize the child's limitations, for example, motor incoordination may be apparent in poor sporting ability or writing and drawing difficulties. Communication and attentional difficulties may limit the child's capacity to participate fully in many academic and social activities. Children experiencing these problems may require support additional to that provided within regular school resources. Perhaps the most stressful transition of all is into adolescence, where peer pressure and issues of identity are paramount. Adolescents may refuse to accept extra therapy or intervention, which identifies them as different. They may become depressed as they begin to fully appreciate the impact that their deficits will have on their future. This pattern of recovery, with its developmental implications, argues that children sustaining moderate and severe TBI require ongoing professional support into adulthood, particularly as they and their families gradually adjust to residual physical, cognitive and behavioral sequelae, and then at critical developmental transitions.

TheNeuropsychologist and Paediatric Rehabilitation

In the context of a multidisciplinary rehabilitation team, the neuropsychologist may be minimally involved with the injured child during the acute stage of recovery. Input may be sought regarding issues such as emergence from post-traumatic amnesia or the appropriate environment for optimal recovery, but by-and-large these tasks are incorporated into other therapy programs. The neuropsychologist becomes more central once the child is able to cope with assessment procedures, and an initial evaluation may be conducted to determine early impairment. Neuropsychological findings may then be integrated into the rehabilitation and school re-integration processes. Once full re-integration has occurred, the need for extra educational support may become evident. Teaching aides, to provide individual instruction or tailoring of educational programs, are frequently employed to encourage ongoing development and recovery. The child may continue to receive therapies during this period, either at a rehabilitation facility, or via the school. Regular liaison may be established with school staff, parents and involved professionals, to ensure that programs are being implemented appropriately, and with expected impact. Ongoing neuropsychological assessment of recovery and current levels of functioning is important in order to inform those working with the child. Results will inform parents and teachers about any recovery that may have occurred, or of plateaus in recovery. Such data may provide much needed motivation, or help determine why the child is not progressing, despite enthusiastic input. In addition such reviews may alert the rehabilitation team to the need for extra therapeutic intervention.

Completion of education can also be a time of significant trauma for adolescents and families. Our own research has demonstrated that children who sustain severe TBI are more likely to leave school early, and to have difficulty finding paid employment (Newitt, 2002). This process may be supported via a range of vocational services, ranging from those which provide training for the individual to prepare curriculum vitae or to perform adequately in interviews, to liaison services where counselors discuss the individual's needs with potential employers or conduct site visits to determine any environmental modifications which may be required to enhance the individual's performance.

Depending on the resources of the rehabilitation team, the neuropsychologist may also be required to monitor family function and coping. The added demands of the child's injury, in terms of emotional, financial and physical resources may be great. Issues of blame, loss and grief may need to be addressed. Feelings of hopelessness, being trapped, and ambivalence to the child may also emerge. Even in families that cope well, behavioural difficulties exhibited by the child with TBI are often difficult to understand and manage. Treatment and education regarding these problems may be provided by the neuropsychologist, perhaps in consultation with a family therapist or individual counselor.

Conclusions

Consequences of childhood TBI are varied and difficult to predict. Research suggests that mild TBI may result in few, if any, residual impairments. In contrast, for moderate-to-severe injuries residual neurobehavioural deficits are common. Crystallized skills (e.g. well learned skills and knowledge) appear less vulnerable than fluid skills (e.g. planning, reasoning, problem solving), with greatest deficits in attention, memory speed of processing and high level language and non-verbal abilities. The common sequelae of childhood TBI appear to be qualitatively different from those described following adult TBI. While adult injury may result in immediate and devastating consequences in terms of brain injury, cognitive disability and behavioural impairment, for the child there is an ongoing interaction among these domains, potentially resulting in cumulative, and global disability. Thus, recovery is less complete, with additional deficits often 'emerging' as the child passes through each developmental stage.

Recent longitudinal research has shown that recovery and ultimate outcome are dependent on a number of biological, developmental and psychosocial factors, including nature and severity of injury, premorbid abilities, developmental level at time of injury, time since injury, stability of family unit, and access to resources. The relative importance of each of these parameters in determining outcome, the possibility that their impact may be greatest at different stages in the recovery process, and their mechanisms of interaction, are still to be determined.

Rehabilitation in the paediatric context, aimed at treating these ongoing and substantial neurobehavioural problems, is a long-term commitment. Children and families will often require ongoing support and intervention, as the child and family pass through developmental transitions and family change. Regular monitoring is required to prevent the emergence of unnecessary secondary problems, particularly in the social and emotional domains. At present, within the paediatric context specifically, there is limited direction for clinicians, with few models for child rehabilitation described in the literature, and even less data describing evaluation and efficacy of child-based interventions. Reports from outcome studies of injured children who have reached adulthood, argue strongly for more intensive and long-term intervention and education following child TBI.

References

Altman, J. & Bayer, S. (1993). Are new neurons formed in the brain of adult mammals? In C. Cuello (Ed.), *Restorative neurology: Volume 6. Neuronal cell death and repair* (pp. 203-225). Amsterdam: Elsevier.

Amacher, A.L. (1988). *Pediatric head injuries*. St Louis, Missouri: Warren H. Green Inc.

Anderson, V. (1998). Assessing executive functions in children: Biological, physiological, and developmental considerations. *Neuropsychological Rehabilitation, 8*, 319-350.

Anderson, V. (1988). Recovery of function in children: The myth of cerebral plasticity. In M. Matheson & H. Newman (Eds.), *Proceedings from the Thirteenth Annual Brain Impairment Conference* (pp. 223-247). Sydney: Academic Press.

Anderson, V., Bond, L., Catroppa, C., Grimwood, K., Keir, E., & Nolan, T. (1997). Childhood bacterial meningitis: Impact of age at illness and medical complications on long term outcome. *Journal of the International Neuropsychological Society, 3,* 147-158.

Anderson, V., Catroppa, C., Morse, S., Haritou, F., Rosenfeld, J. (2001). Outcome from mild head injury in young children: A prospective study. *Journal of Clinical and Experimental Neurospychology, 23,* 705-717.

Anderson, V., Catroppa, C., Morse, S., Haritou, F., & Rosenfeld, J. (2000a). Recovery of intellectual ability following TBI in childhood: Impact of injury severity and age at injury, *Pediatric Neurosurgery, 32,* 282-290.

Anderson, V., Catroppa, C., Morse, S., Haritou, F. & Rosenfeld, J. (2000b). Recovery of memory function following traumatic brain injury in preschool children. *Brain Injury, 8,* 679-692.

Anderson, V., Fenwick, T., Manly, T., & Robertson, I. (1998). Attentional skills following traumatic brain injury in childhood: A componential analysis. *Brain Injury, 12,* 937-949.

Anderson, V., Levin, H.S., Jacobs, R. (2002). Executive functions after frontal lobe injury. In D. Stuss and R. Knight (Eds), *Principles of Frontal Lobe Function.* NY: Oxford.

Anderson, V. & Moore, C. (1995). Age at injury as a predictor of outcome following pediatric head injury. *Child Neuropsychology, 1,* 187-202.

Anderson, V., Morse, S.A., Klug, G., Catroppa, C., Haritou, F., Rosenfeld., J., & Pentland, L. (1997). Predicting recovery from head injury in school-aged children: A prospective analysis. *Journal of the International Neuropsychological Society, 3,* 568-580.

Anderson, V., Northam, E., Hendy, J., & Wrennall, J. (2001). *Developmental neuropsychology: A clinical approach.* Hove: Psychology Press.

Anderson, V. & Pentland, L. (1998). Residual attention deficits following childhood head injury. *Neuropsychological Rehabilitation, 8,* 283-300.

Anderson, V., Smibert, E., Godber, T., Ekert, H . & Weiskop, S. (2000). Cognitive and academic outcomes following cranial irradiation and chemotherapy in children: A longitudinal study. *British Journal of Cancer, 82,* 255-262.

Anderson, V., Smibert, E., Ekert, H., & Godber, T. (1994). Intellectual, educational and behavioral sequelae following cranial irradiation and chemotherapy. *Archives of Disease in Childhood, 70,* 476-483.

Anderson, V. & Taylor, H.G. (1999). Meningitis. In Yeates, K.O., Ris, M.D., & H.G. Taylor (Eds.), *Pediatric neuropsychology: Research, theory and practice* (pp. 117-148). New York: Guilford.

Andrews, T., Rose, F., & Johnson, D. (1998). Social and behavioural effects of traumatic brain injury in children. *Brain Injury, 12,* 133-138.

Aram, D. & Eisele, J. (1994). Intellectual stability in children with unilateral brain lesions. *Neuropsychologia, 32,* 85-95.

Asarnow, R.F., Satz, P., Light, R., Lewis, R., & Neumann, E. (1991). Behavior problems and adaptive functioning in children with mild and severe closed head injury. *Journal of Pediatric Psychology, 16,* 543-555.

Asarnow, R.F., Satz, P., Light, R., Zaucha, K., Lewis, R., & McCleary, C. (1995). The UCLA study of mild head injury in children and adolescents. In S.H. Broman & M.E. Michel (Eds.), *Traumatic head injury in children* (pp. 117-146). New York: Oxford University Press.

Baker, A., Moulton, R., MacMillan, V., & Sheddon, P. (1993). Excitatory amino acid in cerebrospinal fluid following traumatic brain injury in humans. *Journal of Neurosurgery, 79,* 369-372.

Bakker, K. & Anderson, V. (2000). Assessment of attention following preschool traumatic brain injury: A behavioural attention measure. *Pediatric Rehabilitation, 3,* 149-158.

Barnes, M., Dennis, M., & Wilkinson, M. (1999). Reading after closed head injury in childhood: Effects on accuracy, fluency, and comprehension. *Developmental Neuropsychology, 15,* 1-24.

Beardmore, S., Tate, R., & Liddle, B. (1999). Does information and feedback improve children's knowledge and awareness of deficits after traumatic brain injury? *Neuropsychological Rehabilitation, 9,* 45-62.

Begali, V. (1992). *Head injury in children and adolescents* (second ed.). Brandon, VT: Clinical Psychology Publishing Company Inc.

Berg, I., Koning-Haanstra, M., & Deelman, B. (1991). Long-term effects of memory rehabilitation: A controlled study. *Neuropsychological Rehabilitation, 1,* 97-111.

Berger, M.S., Pitts, L.H., Lovely, M., Edwards, M.S., & Bartkowsky, H.M. (1985). Outcome from severe head injury in children and adolescents. *Journal of Neurosurgery, 62,* 194-198.

Berger-Gross, P., & Shackelford, M. (1985). Closed-head injury in children: neuropsychological and scholastic outcomes. *Perceptual and Motor Skills, 61,* 254.

Berney, J., Froidevaux, A., & Favier, J. (1994). Pediatric head trauma: Influence of age and sex. II. Biochemical and anatomo-clinical observations. *Child's Nervous System, 10,* 517-523.

Bjorkland, A. & Stenevi, U. (1971). Growth of central catacholamine neurons into mesencephalon. *Brain Research, 31,* 1-20.

Black, P., Jeffries, J., Blumer, D., Wellnner, A., & Walker, A. (1969). The post-traumatic syndrome in children. In A. Walker, W. Caveness, M. Critchley, & C. Charles (Eds.), *The late effects of head injury* (pp. 142-149). Springfield, Il.: Thomas.

Bohnert, A., Parker, J., & Warschausky, S. (1997). Friendship and social adjustment following traumatic brain injury: An exploratory investigation. *Developmental Neuropsychology, 13,* 477-486.

Brink, J., Imbus, C., & Woo-Sam, J. (1980). Physical recovery after closed head trauma in children and adolescents. *The Journal of Pediatrics, 97,* 721-727.

Brown, G., Chadwick, O., Shaffer, D., Rutter, M. & Traub, M. (1981). A prospective study of children with head injuries: II. Psychiatric sequelae. *Psychological Medicine, 11(1),* 49-62.

Bruce, D.A., Raphaely, R.C., Goldberg, A.I., Zimmerman, R.A., Bilaniuk., L.T., Schut, L., & Kuhl, D.E. (1979). Pathophysiology, treatment and outcome following severe head injury in children. *Child's Brain, 2,* 174-191.

Butler, K., Rourke, B., Feurst, D., & Fisk, J. (1997). A typology of psychosocial functioning in pediatric closed head injury. *Child Neuropsychology, 3,* 98-133.

Campbell, T.F. & Dollaghan, C.A. (1990). Expressive language recovery in severely brain-injured children and adolescents. *Journal of Speech and Hearing Disorders, 55,* 567-581.

Cannon, W. & Rosenbleuth, A. (1949). *The supersensitivity of denervated structures.* New York: Macmillan.

Catroppa, C. & Anderson, V. (in press). Recovery in memory function in the first year following TBI in children, *Brain Injury.*

Catroppa, V. & Anderson, V. (2000). Recovery of educational skills following pediatric head-injury. *Pediatric Rehabilitation, 3,* 167-176.

Catroppa, C. & Anderson, V. (1998). Attentional skills in the acute phase following pediatric traumatic brain injury. *Child Neuropsychology, 5,* 251-265.

Catroppa, C., Anderson, V., & Stargatt, R. (1999). A prospective analysis of the recovery of attention following pediatric head injury. *Journal of the International Neuropsychological Society, 5,* 48-57.

Cattelani, R., Lombardi, F., Brianti, R., & Mazzuchi, A. (1998). Traumatic brain injury in childhood: Intellectual, behavioral and social outcome into adulthood. *Brain Injury, 12,* 283-296.

Chadwick, O., Rutter, M., Brown, G., Shaffer, D., & Traub, M. (1981a). A prospective study of children with head injuries: II. Cognitive sequelae. *Psychological Medicine, 11,* 49-61.

Chadwick, O., Rutter, M., Shaffer, D., & Shrout, P. (1981b). A prospective study of children with head injuries: IV. Specific cognitive deficits. *Journal of Clinical Neuropsychology, 2,* 101-120.

Chapman, S. (1995). Discourse as an outcome measure in pediatric head-injured populations. In S.H. Broman & M.E. Michel (Eds.), *Traumatic head injury in children* (pp. 95-116). New York: Oxford University Press.

Chapman, S., Levin, H., Wanek, A., Weyrauch, J., & Kufera, J. (1998). Discourse after closed head injury in young children: Relationship of age to outcome. *Brain and Language, 61,* 420-449.

Choux, M. (1986). Incidence, diagnosis and management of skull fractures. In A.J. Raimondi, M. Choux, & C. DiRocco (Eds.), *Head injuries in the new born and infant* (pp. 163-182). New York: Springer-Verlag.

Cicerone, K. & Tupper, D. (1990). Neuropsychological rehabilitation: Treatment on errors in everyday function. In D. Tupper & K. Cicerone (Eds.), *The neuropsychology of everyday life: Issues in development and rehabilitation* (pp. 271-291). Boston, MA: Kluwer Academic Publishers.

Courville, C.B. (1945*). Pathology and the nervous system.* Mountain View CA: Pacific Press.

Craft, A.W., Shaw D.A., & Cartlidge, N.E. (1972). Head injuries in children. *British Medical Journal, 4,* 200-203.

Dalby, P.R. & Obrzut, J.E. (1991). Epidemiologic characteristics and sequelae of closed head-injured children and adolescents: A review. *Developmental Neuropsychology, 7,* 35-68.

Dennis, M. (1989). Language and the young damaged brain. In T. Boll & B.K. Bryant (Eds.), *Clinical neuropsychology and brain function: Research, measurement and practice* (pp. 85-124). Washington: American Psychological Association.

Dennis, M. & Barnes, M. (1990). Knowing the meaning, getting the point, bridging the gap, and carrying the message: Aspects of discourse following closed head injury in childhood and adolescence. *Brain and Language, 39,* 428-446.

Dennis, M., Barnes, M.A., Donnelly, R.E., Wilkinson, M., & Humphreys, R.P. (1996). Appraising and managing knowledge: Metacognitive skills after childhood head injury. *Developmental Neuropsychology, 12,* 77-103.

Dennis, M., Wilkinson, M., Koski, L., & Humphreys, R.P. (1995). Attention deficits in the long term after childhood head injury. In S. Broman & M.E. Michel (Eds.), *Traumatic head injury in children* (pp. 165-187). New York: Oxford University Press.

Didus, E. Anderson, V., & Catroppa, C. (2000). The development of pragmatic communication skills in head-injured children. *Pediatric Rehabilitation, 3,* 177-186.

Diller, L., & Gordon, W. (1981). Rehabilitation and clinical neuropsychology. In S. Filskov & T. Boll (Eds.), *Handbook of clinical neuropsychology* (pp. 702-733). New York: Wiley.

Donders, J. (1992). Premorbid behavioral and psychosocial adjustment of children with traumatic brain injury. *Journal of Abnormal Child Psychology, 20,* 233-246.

Donders, J. (1994). Academic placement after traumatic brain injury, *Journal of School Psychology, 32,* 53-65.

Duchowny, M., Jayakar, P., Harvey, A.S., Altman, N., Resnick, T., Levin, B. (1996). Language cortex representation: effects of developmental versus acquired pathology. *Annals of Neurology, 40,* 91-98.

Ewing-Cobbs, L., Brookshire, B., Scott, M., & Fletcher, J. (1998). Children's narratives following traumatic brain injury: Linguistic structure, cohesion, and thematic recall. *Brain and Language, 61,* 395-419.

Ewing-Cobbs, L., Fletcher, J., Levin, H., Francis, D., Davidson, K., & Miner, M. (1997). Longitudinal neuropsychological outcome in infants and preschoolers with traumatic brain injury. *Journal of the International Neuropsychological Society, 3,* 581-591.

Ewing-Cobbs, L., Levin, H., Eisenberg, H., & Fletcher, J.M. (1987). Language functions following closed head injury in children and adolescents. *Journal of Clinical and Experiemental Neuropsychology, 9,* 575-592.

Ewing-Cobbs, L., Levin, H., Fletcher, J.M., Miner, M.E., & Eisenberg, H. (1990). The Children's Orientation and Amnesia Test: Relationship to severity of acute head injury and to recovery of memory. *Neurosurgery, 27,* 683-691.

Ewing-Cobbs, L, Miner, M.E., Fletcher, J.M. & Levin, H. (1989). Intellectual, language and motor sequelae following closed head injury in infants and preschoolers. *Journal of Pediatric Psychology, 14,* 531-547.

Ewing-Cobbs, L., Prasad, M., Fletcher, J.M., Levin, H.S., Miner, E, & Eisenberg, H. (1998). Attention after pediatric traumatic brain injury: A multidimensional assessment. *Child Neuropsychology, 4,* 35-48.

Farmer, J., Haut, J., Williams, J., Kapila, C., Johnstone, B., & Kirk, K. (1996). Memory functioning in children with traumatic brain injury and premorbid learning problems. *Journal of the International Neuropsychological Society, 2,* 38-39.

Fenwick, T. & Anderson, V. (1999). Impairments of attention following childhood traumatic brain injury. *Child Neuropsychology, 5,* 213-223.

Filley, C.M., Cranberg, M.D., Alexander, M.P., & Hart, E. (1987). Neurobehavioral outcome after closed head injury in childhood and adolescence. *Archives of Neurology, 44,* 194-198.

Finger, S. & Stein, D.G. (1982). *Brain damage and recovery.* New York: Academic Press.

Fletcher, J., Ewing-Cobbs, L., Francis, D., & Levin, H. (1995). Variability in outcomes after traumatic brain injury in children: A developmental perspective. In S.H. Broman & M.E. Michel (Eds.), *Traumatic head injury in children* (pp. 3-21). New York: Oxford University Press.

Fletcher, J., Ewing-Cobbs, L., Miner, M.E., Levin, H.S., & Eisenberg, H.M. (1990). Behavioral changes after closed head injury in children. *Journal of Consulting and Clinical Psychology, 58,* 93-98.

Fletcher, J., Miner, M., & Ewing-Cobbs, L. (1987). Age and recovery from head injury in children: Developmental issues. In H. Levin., H. Eisenberg, & J. Grafman. (Eds.), *Neurobehavioral recovery from head injury* (pp. 279-291). New York: Oxford.

Garth, J., Anderson, V.A., & Wrennall, J. (1997). Executive functions following moderate to severe frontal lobe injury: Impact of injury and age at injury. *Pediatric Rehabilitation, 1,* 99-108.

Gentry, L., Godersky, J, & Thompson, B. (1988). MR imaging of head trauma: Review of the distribution and radiographic features of traumatic lesions. *Archives of Neurology, 44,* 194-198.

Glang, A., Singer, G., & Todis, B. (Eds.). (1997). *Students with acquired brain injury: The school's response.* Baltimore: Paul H. Brookes.

Goldstein, F.C. & Levin, H.S. (1987). Epidemiology of pediatric closed head injury: Incidence, clinical characteristics and risk factors. *Journal of Learning Disabilities, 20,* 518-525.

Goldstein, F.C. & Levin, H.S. (1985). Intellectual and academic outcome in children and adolescents: research and empirical findings. *Development Neuropsychology, 1,* 195-214.

Greenspan, A. & MacKenzie, E. (1994). Functional outcome after pediatric head injury. *Pediatrics, 94,* 425-432.

Gronwall, D., Wrightson, P., & McGinn, V. (1997). Effects of mild head injury during the preschool years. *Journal of the International Neuropsychological Society, 6, 592-597.*

Gray, J., Robertson, I., Pentland, B., & Anderson, S. (1992). Micro-computer based attentional training after brain damage: A randomised group controlled trial. *Neuropsychological Rehabilitation, 2, 97-115.*

Haritou, F., Ong, K., Morse, S., Anderson, V., Catroppa, C., Rosenfeld, J., Klug, G., & Bucolo, C. (1997). A syntactic and pragmatic analysis of the conversational speech of young head injured children. In J. Ponsford, P. Snow, & V. Anderson. (Eds.), *International perspective in traumatic brain injury* (pp. 187-190). Melbourne: Academic Press.

Hayes, H.R. & Jackson, R.H. (1989). The incidence and prevention of head injuries. In D.A. Johnson, D. Uttley, & M.A. Wyke (Eds.), *Children's head injury: Who cares?* (pp. 183-193). London: Taylor & Francis.

Holloway, M., Bye, A., & Moran, K. (1994). Non-accidental head injury in children. *The Medical Journal of Australia, 160,* 786-789.

Holster, S. (1999). Pediatric family-centred rehabilitation. *Journal of Head Trauma Rehabilitation, 14,* 384-393.

Horowitz, I., Costeff, H., Sadan, N., Abraham, E., Geyer, S., & Najenson, T. (1983). Childhood head injuries in Israel: Epidemiology and outcome. *International Rehabilitation Medicine, 5,* 32-36.

Jacobs, R., Anderson, V., & Harvey, A.S. (2001). Neuropsychological profile of a 9-year old child with subcortical band heteropia or 'double cortex'. *Developmental Medicine and Child Neurology, 43,* 628-633.

Jaffe, K.M., Polissar, N.L., Fay, G.C., & Liao, S. (1995). Recovery trends over three years following pediatric traumatic brain injury. *Archives of Physical Medicine and Rehabilitation, 76,* 17-26.

Jaffe, K.M., Fay, G.C., Polissar, N.L., Martin, K.M., Shurtlef, H.A., Rivara, J.B., & Winn, R. (1993). Severity of pediatric traumatic brain injury and neurobehavioral recovery at one year – A cohort study. *Archives of Physical Medicine and Rehabilitation, 74,* 587-595.

Jaffe, K.M., Fay, G.C., Polissar, N.L., Martin, K.M., Shurtlef, H.A., Rivara, J.B., & Winn, R. (1992). Severity of pediatric traumatic brain injury and neurobehavioral outcome: A cohort study. *Archives of Physical Medicine and Rehabilitation, 73,* 540-547.

Jennett, B. (1979). Post-traumatic epilepsy. *Advances in Neurology, 22,* 137-147.

Jennett, B., Teasdale, G., Galbraith, S., Pickard, J., Grant, H., Braakman, R., Avezaat, C., Maas, A., Minderhoud, J., Vecht, C., Heiden, J., Small, R., Caton, W., & Kurtz, T. (1977). Severe head injuries in three countries. *Journal of Neurology, Neurosurgery, and Psychiatry, 40,* 291-298.

Johnson, D., Uttley, D., & Wyke, M. (Eds.). (1989). *Children's head injury: Who cares?.* London: Taylor & Francis.

Kaufmann, P., Fletcher, J., Levin, H., Miner, M., & Ewing-Cobbs, L. (1993). Attention disturbance after pediatric closed head injury. *Journal of Child Neurology, 8,* 348-353.

Kinsella, G., Prior, M., Sawyer, M., Murtagh, D., Eisenmajer, R., Anderson, V., Bryan, D., & Klug, G. (1995). Neuropsychological deficit and academic performance in children and adolescents following traumatic brain injury. *Journal of Pediatric Psychology, 20,* 753-767.

Kinsella, G., Prior, M., Sawyer, M., Ong, B., Murtagh, D., Eisenmajer, R., Bryan, D., Anderson, V., & Klug, G. (1997). Predictors and indicators of academic outcome in children 2 years following traumatic head injury. *Journal of the International Neuropsychological Society, 3,* 608-616.

Klonoff, H. (1971). Head injuries in children: Predisposing factors, accident conditions, accident proneness and sequelae. *American Journal of Public Health, 61,* 2405-2417.

Klonoff, H., Clark, C., & Klonoff, P. (1995). Outcome of head injuries from childhood to adulthood: A twenty-three year follow-up study. In S.H. Broman & M.E. Michel (Eds.), *Traumatic head injury in children* (pp. 219-234). New York: Oxford University Press.

Klonoff, H., Low, M.D., & Clark, C. (1977). Head injuries in children: A prospective five year follow-up. *Journal of Neurology, Neurosurgery, and Psychiatry, 40,* 1211-1219.

Kolb, B. (1995). *Brain plasticity and behavior.* New Jersey: Erlbaum.

Kolb, B. & Gibb, R. (1999). Neuroplasticity and recovery of function after brain injury. In D. Stuss, G. Winocur, & I., Robertson (Eds.), *Cognitive neurorehabilitation.* (pp. 9-25). New York: Cambridge University Press.

Kolb, B. & Wishaw, Q. (1996). *Fundamentals of human neuropsychology (4th ed.).* New York: W.H. Freeman.

Koshiniemi, M., Timo, K., Taina, N., & Leo, J. (1995). Long-term outcome after severe brain injury in preschoolers is worse than expected. *Archives of Pediatric and Adolescent Medicine, 149,* 249-254.

Kraus, J.F. (1995). Epidemiological features of brain injury in children. In S.H. Broman & M.E. Michel (Eds.), *Traumatic head injury in children* (pp. 117-146). New York: Oxford University Press.

Kraus, J.F., Fife, D., Cox, P., Ramstein, K., & Conroy, C. (1986). Incidence, severity, and external causes of pediatric brain injury. *American Journal of Epidemiology, 119,* 186-201.

Kriel, R.L., Krach, L.E., & Panser, L.A. (1989). Closed head injury: Comparisons of children younger and older than six years of age. *Pediatric Neurology, 5,* 296-300.

Lange-Cosack, H., Wider, B., Schlesner, H.J., Grumme, T. & Kubicki, S. (1979). Prognosis of brain injuries in young children (one until five years of age). *Neuropaediatrie, 10,* 105-127.

Lashley, K. (1929). *Brain mechanisms and intelligence.* Chicago: University of Chicago Press.

Laurence, S. & Stein, D. (1978). Recovery after brain damage and the concept of localisation of function. In S. Finger (Ed.), *Recovery from brain damage* (pp. 369-407). New York: Plenum Press.

Lehr, E. (1990). *Psychological management of traumatic brain injuries in children and adolescents.* Rockville, Maryland: Aspen.

Levin, H., Culhane, K., Mendelsohn, D., Lilly, M., Bruce, D., Fletcher, J., Chapman, S., Harward, H., & Eisenberg, H. (1993). Cognition in relation to magnetic resonance imaging in head-injured children and adolescents. *Archives of Neurology, 50,* 897-905.

Levin, H. & Eisenberg, H. (1979). Neuropsychological impairment after closed head injury in children and adolescents. *Journal of Pediatric Psychology, 4,* 389-402.

Levin, H., Eisenberg, H., Wigg, N., & Kobayashi, K. (1982). Memory and intellectual ability after head injury in children and adolescents. *Neurosurgery, 11,* 668-673.

Levin, H., Grafman, J. , & Eisenberg, H. (1987). *Neurobehavioral recovery from head injury.* New York: Oxford University Press.

Levin, H.S., High, W., Ewing-Cobbs, L., Fletcher, J.M., Eisenberg, H.M., Miner, M., & Goldstein, F. (1988). Memory functioning during the first year after closed head injury in children and adolescents. *Neurosurgery, 22,* 17-34.

Levin, H., Mendelsohn, D., Lilly, M., Fletcher, J., Culhane, K., Chapman, S., Harward, H., Kusnerik, L., Bruce, D., & Eisenberg, H. (1994). Tower of London performance in relation to magnetic resonance imaging following closed head injury in children. *Neuropsychology, 8,* 171-179.

Levin, H., Song, J., Scheibel, R., Fletcher, J., Harward, H., Lilly, M., & Goldstein, F. (1997). Concept formation and problem solving following closed head injury in children. *Journal of the International Neuropsychological Society, 3,* 598-607.

Lois, C. & Alvarez-Buylla, A. (1994). Long distance neuronal migration in the adult mammalian brain. *Science, 264,* 1145-1148.

Luria, A.R. (1963). *Restoration of function after brain injury.* New York: Macmillan.

Mateer, C. (1999). Executive function disorders: Rehabilitation challenges and strategies. *Seminars in Clinical Neuropsychiatry, 4,* 50-59.

Mateer, C., Kerns, K., & Eso, K. (1996). Management of attention and memory disorders following traumatic brain injury. *Journal of Learning Disabilities, 29,* 6118-632.

Mateer, C.A. & Williams, D. (1991) Effects of frontal lobe injury in childhood. *Developmental Neuropsychology, 7,* 69-86.

Mateer, C.A. (1990). Cognitive and behavioral sequalae of face and forehead injury in childhood. *Journal of Clinical and Experimental Neuropsychology, 12,* 95.

Max, J., Smith, W., Sato, Y., Mattheis, P., Castillo, C., Lindgren, S., Robin, D., & Stierwalt, J. (1997a). Predictors of family functioning following traumatic brain injury in children and adolescents. *Journal of the Academy of Child and Adolescent Psychiatry, 37,* 83-90.

Max, J., Smith, W., Sato, Y., Mattheis, P., Castillo, C., Lindgren, S., Robin, D., & Stierwalt, J. (1997b). Traumatic brain injury in children and adolescents: Psychiatric disorders in the first three months. *Journal of the Academy of Child and Adolescent Psychiatry, 36,* 94-102.

Michaud, L.J., Rivara, F.P., Grady, M.S., & Reay, D.T. (1992). Predictors of survival and severe disability after severe brain injury in children. *Neurosurgery, 31,* 254-264.

Miller, J.D. (1992). Pathophysiology and management of head injury. *Neuropsychology, 5,* 235-261.

Munk, H. (1881). Über die Funktion der Grosshirnrinde. *Gesammelte aus den Jahren 1877-80.* Berlin: Hirschwald.

Newitt, H. (2002). *Adult outcome from childhood brain injury.* Unpublished doctoral dissertation, University of Melbourne.

Ommaya, A. & Gennarelli, T. (1974). Cerebral concussion and traumatic unconsciousness: Correlation of experimental and clinical observations on blunt head injuries. *Brain, 97,* 633-654.

Ong, L., Chandran, V., Zasmani, S., & Lye, M. (1999). Outcome of closed head injury in Malasian children: neurocognitive and behavioural sequelae. *Journal of Paediatric Child Health, 34,* 363-368.

Paakko, E., Vainionpaa, L., Lanning, M., Laitinen, J., & Pyhtinen, J. (1992). White matter changes in children treated for acute lymphoblastic leukemia. *Cancer, 70,* 2728-2733.

Pang, D. (1985). Pathophysiologic correlates of neurobehavioral syndromes following closed head injury. In M. Ylvisaker (Ed.), *Head injury rehabilitation: Children and adolescents* (pp. 3-70). London: Taylor & Francis.

Park, N. & Ingles, J. (2001). Effectiveness of attention rehabilitation after acquired brain injury: A meta-analysis. *Neuropsychology, 15,* 199-210.

Passler, M.A., Isaac, W., & Hynd, G.W. (1985). Neuropsychological development of behavior attributed to frontal lobe functioning in children, *Developmental Neuropsychology, 1,* 349-370.

Pentland, L., Todd, J.A., & Anderson, V. (1998). The impact of head injury severity on planning ability in adolescence: A functional analysis. *Neuropsychological Rehabilitation, 8,* 301-317.

Perrott, S.B., Taylor, H.G., & Montes, J.L. (1991). Neuropsychological sequelae, familial stress, and environmental adaptation following pediatric head injury. *Developmental Neuropsychology, 7*, 69-86.

Polissar, N., Fay, G., Jaffe, K., Liao, S., Martin, K., Shurtleff, H., Rivara, J., & Winn, H. (1994). mild pediatric traumatic brain injury: adjusting significance levels for multiple comparisons. *Brain Injury, 8*, 249-264.

Ponsford, J., Sloan, S., & Snow, P. (1995). *Traumatic brain injury: Rehabilitation for everyday adaptive living.* Hove, UK: Lawrence Erlbaum Associates.

Ponsford, J., Willmott, C., Rothwell, A., Cameron, P., Kelly, A., Ayton, G., Curran, C. & Nelms, R. (1997). Cognitive and behavioural outcome following mild traumatic brain injury in children. *Journal of the International Neuropsychological Society, 3*, 225.

Prior, M., Kinsella, G., Sawyer, M., Bryan, D., & Anderson, V. (1994). Cognitive and psychosocial outcomes after head injury in childhood. *Australian Psychologist, 29*, 116-123.

Quattrocchi, K., Prasad, P., Willits, N., & Wagner, F. (1991). Quantification of midline shift as a predictor of poor outcome following head injury. *Surgical Neurology, 35*, 183-188.

Raz, S., Goldstein, R., Hopkins, T., Lankerbach, M., Shah, P., Porter, C., Rigg, W., Magill., L. & Sander, C. (1994). Sex differences in early vulnerability to cerebral injury and their neurodevelopmental implications. *Psychobiology, 22*, 244-253.

Raz, S., Lankerbach, M., Hopkins, T., Glogowski, B., Porter, C., Rigg, W., & Sander, C. (1995). A female advantage in cognitive recovery from early cerebral insult. *Developmental Psychology, 31*, 958-966.

Raimondi, A. & Hirschauer, J. (1984). Head injury in the infant and toddler. *Child's Brain, 11*, 12-35.

Rivara, J.B, Jaffe, K.M., Fay, G.C., Polissar, N.L., Martin, K.M., Shurtleff, H.A., & Liao, S. (1993). Family functioning and injury severity as predictors of child functioning one year following traumatic brain injury. *Archives of Physical Medicine and Rehabilitation, 74*, 1047-1055.

Rivara, J.B., Jaffe, K.M., Polissar, N.L, Fay, G.C., Martin, K.M., Shurtleff, H.A., & Liao, S. (1994). Family functioning and children's academic performance and behavior problems in the year following traumatic brain injury. *Archives of Physical Medicine and Rehabilitation, 75*, 368-379.

Robertson, I. (1990). Does computerised cognitive rehabilitation work? A review. *Aphasiology, 4*, 381-405.

Rothi, L. & Horner, J. (1983). Restitution and substitution: Two theories of recovery with application to neurobehavioral treatment. *Journal of Clinical Neuropsychology, 3*, 73-81.

Rourke, B.P. (1989). *Nonverbal learning disabilities.* New York: Guilford.

Rourke, B.P., Bakker, D.J., Fisk, J.L., & Strang, J.D. (1983). *Child neuropsychology: An introduction to theory, research, and clinical practice.* New York: Guilford.

Rutter, M., Chadwick, O., & Shaffer, D. (1983). Head injury. In M. Rutter (Ed.), *Developmental neuropsychiatry* (pp. 83-111). New York: Guilford.

Schmitter-Edgecombe, M., Fahy, J., Whelan, J., & Long, C. (1995). Memory remediation after severe head injury: Notebook training versus supportive therapy. *Journal of Consulting and Clinical Psychology, 63*, 484-489.

Selznick, L. & Savage, R. (2000). Using self-monitoring procedures to increase on task behaviour with three adolescent boys with brain injury. *Behavioral Intervention, 15*, 243-260.

Sharma, M. & Sharma, A. (1994). Mode, presentation, CT findings and outcome of pediatric head injury. *Indian Pediatrics, 31*, 733-739.

Sohlberg, M. & Mateer, C. (1989). Training use of compensatory memory books: A three-stage *behavioral approach. Journal of Clinical and Experimental Neuropsychology, 11*, 871-891.

Stalings, G., Ewing-Cobbs, L., Francis, D., & Fletcher, J. (1996). Prediction of academic placement after pediatric head injury using neurological, demographic and neuropsychological variables. *Journal of the International Neuropsychological Society, 2,* 39.

Stein, S., Spettell, C., Young, G, & Ross, S. (1993). Delayed and progressive brain injury in closed-head trauma: Radiological demonstration. *Neurosurgery, 32,* 25-31.

Taylor, H.G. & Alden, J. (1997). Age-related differences in outcomes following childhood brain insults: An introduction and overview. *Journal of the International Neuropsychological Society, 3,* 555-567.

Taylor, H.G., Drotar, D., Wade, S., Yeates, K., Stancin, T., & Klein, S. (1995). Recovery from traumatic brain injury in children: The importance of the family. In S.H. Broman & M.E. Michel (Eds.). *Traumatic head injury in children* (pp. 188-218). New York: Oxford University Press.

Taylor, H.G., Yeates, K., Wade, S., Drotar, D., Stancin, T., & Minich, N. (2002). A prospective study of short- and long-term outcomes after traumatic brain injury in children: behavior and academic achievement. *Neuropsychology, 16,* 15-27.

Thompson, N.M., Francis, D.J., Stuebing, K.K., Fletcher, J.M, Ewing-Cobbs, L., Miner, M.E., Levin, H.S., & Eisenberg, H.M. (1994). Motor, visuo-spatial, and somatosensory skills after closed head injury in children and adolescents: A study of change. *Neuropsycholgy, 8,* 333-342.

Turkstra, L., McDonald, S., & dePompei, R. (2001). Social information processing in adolescents: Data for normally developing adolescents and preliminary data from their peers with traumatic brain injury. *Journal of Head Trauma Rehabilitation, 16,* 469-478.

Vargha-Khadem, F., Isaacs, E., Papaleloudi, H., Polkey, C., & Wilson, J. (1992). Development of intelligence and memory in children with hemiplegic cerebral palsy. *Brain, 115,* 315-329.

Waaland, P. & Kreutzer, J. (1988). Family response to childhood traumatic brain injury. *Journal of Head Trauma Rehabilitation, 3,* 51-63.

Wade, S., Taylor, H.G., Drotar, D., Stancin, T., & Yeates, K.O. (1996). Childhood traumatic brain injury: Initial impact on the family. *Journal of Learning Disabilities, 29,* 652-661.

Walker, M., Mayer, T., Storrs, B., & Hylton, P. (1985). Pediatric head injury – factors which influence outcome. In P. Chapman (Ed.*), Concepts in pediatric neurosurgery, Vol. 6,* (pp. 84-97). Basel: Karger.

Walsh, K.W. (1978). *Neuropsychology: A clinical approach.* New York: Churchill Livinstone.

Williams, D. & Mateer, C. (1992). Developmental impact of frontal lobe injury in middle childhood. *Brain and Cognition, 20,* 96-204.

Willmott, C., Anderson, V, & Anderson, P. (2000). Attention following pediatric head injury: A developmental perspective. revision submitted to *Developmental Neuropsychology, 17,* 361-379.

Wilson, B.A. (1997). Cognitive rehabilitation: How it is and how it might be. *Journal of the International Neuropsychological Society, 3,* 487-496.

Wilson, B.A., Emslie, H., Quirk., K., & Evans, J. (2001). Reducing everyday memory and planning problems by means of a pager system: A randomised control crossover study. *Journal of Neurology, Neurosurgery and Psychiatry, 70,* 477-482.

Wilson, B.A. & Moffat, M. (1992). *Clinical management of memory problems.* London: Chapman & Hall.

Wilson, J., Wiedmann, K., Hadley, D., Condon, B., Teasdale, G., & Brooks, D. (1988). Early and late magnetic resonance imaging and neuropsychological outcome after head injury. *Journal of Neurology, Neurosurgery, and Psychiatry, 51,* 391-396.

Winogron, H.W., Knights, R.M., & Bawden, H.N. (1984). Neuropsychological deficits following head injury in children. *Journal of Clinical Neuropsychology, 6,* 269-286.

Wood, R. (1988). Attention disorders in brain rehabilitation. *Journal of Learning Disabilities, 21,* 327-332.

Wrightson, P. McGinn, V., & Gronwall, D. (1995). Mild head injury in preschool children: Evidence that it can be associated with persisting cognitive defect. *Journal of Neurology, Neurosurgery, & Psychiatry, 59,* 375-380.

Yeates, K. (1999). Closed-head injury. In Yeates, K.O., Ris, M.D., & H.G. Taylor. (Eds.), *Pediatric neuropsychology: Research, theory and practice* (pp. 192-218). New York: Guilford.

Yeates, K., Blumstein, E., Patterson, C.M., & Delis, D.C. (1995). Verbal memory and learning following pediatric closed head injury. *Journal of the International Neuropsychological Society, 1,* 78-87.

Ylivasaker, M. (Ed.). (1998). *Head injury rehabilitation: Children and adolescents.* Boston: Butterworth-Heinemann.

Zimmerman, R. & Bilaniuk, L. (1994). Pediatric head trauma. *Pediatric Neuroradiology, 4,* 349-366.

Chapter 12

REHABILITATION OF PEOPLE IN STATES OF REDUCED AWARENESS

Agnes Shiel

MRC Cognition and Brain Sciences Unit, Cambridge, UK

Background

> 'No head injury is too severe to despair of, nor too trivial to ignore'
>
> Hippocrates 4th Century B.C.

Survival after very severe head injury is a relatively new phenomenon. Numbers of survivors appear to be increasing although this has not been formally evaluated. Recent advances such as the introduction of paramedics and better roadside care, improved neurosurgical techniques, development of Intensive Therapy Unit (ITU) care and greater understanding and prevention of secondary complications have contributed to this increase. These measures, while preventing or minimising some head injuries, may also have the unanticipated consequence of increasing survival among very severely injured people. Therefore a relatively new area of rehabilitation has been developing in the past ten years – the rehabilitation of people who are considered to be in a reduced state of consciousness.

Four distinct groups can be described as being in reduced states of consciousness after head injury – those in coma, those in the Vegetative State (VS), those in the Minimally Conscious State (MCS) and those who are in Post Traumatic Amnesia (PTA). Although these are four distinct groups, many of the approaches to assessment with the first three groups are similar although the treatment and the goals set may be completely different. Because of this it is essential that the diagnosis is accurate.

Coma

The word coma comes from the Greek 'Koma' meaning state of sleep. The best known definition is that of Jennett and Teasdale (1977) who describe coma as 'giving no verbal response, not obeying commands and not opening the eyes spontaneously or to stimulation' (p. 878). Other features of coma include: no arousal and no awareness; no eye opening; reflex movements only; no language comprehension and no purposeful response. Traumatic coma per se is short lived and within 2–4 weeks the patient will have progressed either to the vegetative state, the minimally conscious state or to PTA.

The Vegetative State

The vegetative state is the description most commonly used to describe the state of complete unresponsiveness observed where the patient is not in coma – i.e. eye opening is present. Jennett and Plum (1972) coined the term 'persistent vegetative state' but the term of choice in the UK and the USA at present is either 'vegetative state' or 'chronic vegetative state'. This is because the term 'persistent' implies that there will be no change. While this is undoubtedly true for the majority of patients who are vegetative after a significant period of time, a small minority may recover to some extent.

Two reports on the vegetative state are those produced by the Royal College of Physicians (RCP) (1996) and by Andrews et al. (1996). The report by the RCP state three criteria which must be met if a patient is to be diagnosed as being in VS: first, that patients show no evidence of awareness, no volitional response and no evidence of language comprehension; second that a cycle of eye opening and closure is present and third that hypothalamic and brain stem function is intact. Further behavioural features, include incontinence, spontaneous blinking, occasional movements of eyes or head, aimless movement of limbs or trunk and facial grimacing.

In contrast to this clinical description of the syndrome, Andrews et al (1996) suggest behavioural description of patients rather than distinguishing between coma, vegetative presentation and an 'undecided' category. They recommended that the most appropriate method of assessment was to describe the level of responsiveness in behavioural terms and to describe but not to interpret any movements or behaviours observed.

The Minimally Conscious state

The minimally conscious state is defined by Giacino et al. (2002) as "evidence of limited but clearly discernible self or environmental awareness on a reproducible or sustained basis by one or more of the following – simple command following; yes/no responses; intelligible verbalisation; purposeful behaviour and inconsistent but meaningful interaction" (Giacino et al. 2002). The presentation includes arousal and sustained tracking but the patient's behavioural repertoire is severely compromised. It is reported that there is limited self awareness but that patients do feel pain. As with the vegetative state, sleep wake cycles are established and many patients have severely limited movements.

Post Traumatic Amnesia (PTA)

PTA is defined as 'a period of variable length following closed head trauma when the patient is confused, disorientated, suffers from retrograde amnesia and seems to lack the capacity to store and retrieve new memories' (Schacter & Crovitz, 1977, p. 150). Although termed 'amnesia' PTA involves impairment of a number of cognitive processes. Amongst the features of PTA are disorientation, impaired day to day memory, slowed retrieval from semantic memory, slowed reaction time, slowed speed of information processing and difficulty with abstract thought (Wilson et al., 1999).

Recovery and Rehabilitation

The underlying mechanisms of recovery and response to rehabilitation after traumatic brain injury are not entirely clear but rehabilitation should not be confused with recovery. It is probable that recovery of the 'vegetative' functions such as eye opening occur purely as a result of biological recovery. On the other hand, improvements in day to day ability to function in the community are more likely to occur as a result of as a result of new learning, relearning and compensation. It is less clear how recovery and rehabilitation interact in the interim stages and it is for this reason that a number of 'theories' or models have been proposed. It is probable that a combination of factors is involved, more heavily loaded towards biological recovery in the initial stages and towards learning and compensation at the end.

Ponsford et al, (1995) identifies the following as a basis for rehabilitation after brain injury:

- restorative – theories relating to restoration of function.
- compensatory – theories of behavioural compensation and functional adaptation.
- environmental – manipulation of the environment to facilitate independence.

Restoration

The basis of restoration is that the intervention can restore or repair the lost function. This aim of restoration is to maximise the biological recovery by focusing therapy at the specific function which is impaired. The goal of treatment is for the patient to perform the activity in the same way and using the same functions (motor, cognitive, perceptual) as before. The intention is to isolate the impairment and treat using highly structured and repeated practice focusing on the impairment rather than on the disability caused by it. Examples of restorative approaches are the 'Bobath' approach to restoration of physical function (where the goal is for patients to move 'normally' rather than functionally) or computer training to restore impaired attentional skills. The theoretical basis of restorative treatment is that recovery of damaged functions may be facilitated if treatment begins early enough, but there is little evidence as to efficacy. Such approaches may bear little relationship to daily life as intervention is focused solely on impairment with little or no input at the level of disability or handicap. At present, the main restorative intervention for patients who are in coma in the vegetative state or who are minimally responsive is coma stimulation programmes.

Studies of Coma Stimulation

The concept of stimulating patients who are unresponsive after a brain injury is not a new one. Hipprocates recommended that 'the patient in a state of coma should be spoken to in a loud voice, splashed with cold water and exposed to bright light'.

Giacino (1996) reviewed studies of coma stimulation in treating patients in coma and evaluated them using a classification system developed by Woolf (1993). Experimental evidence was categorised as class I, II or III. Class I evidence was described as the 'gold standard' and comprises evidence based on randomised, prospective controlled clinical trials. Class II evidence includes descriptive studies, retrospective studies and prevalence studies as well as retrospective and cohort studies. Class III evidence includes uncontrolled studies and case reports. One study met the criteria for class I evidence (Johnson et al., 1993), three studies met the criteria for class II evidence. (Mitchell et al., 1990, Pierce et al., 1990 and Wood et al., 1993) and three others met the criteria for Class III evidence. Of the latter, two were case study series [Hall et al., (1992) and Talbot & Whitaker, (1994)] and one was a descriptive study of a clinical series (Rader et al., 1989). The only study to meet the criteria for Class I evidence evaluated the effect of a programme of multisensory stimulation to a group of patients admitted to a neurosurgical unit. Patients were randomly allocated to a treatment or non treatment group. However, no significant differences between the groups were found although this may have been because of the small sample size (n = 14).

In fact, the numbers of patients included in all studies were small. The study meeting class I criteria included only 14 patients (Johnson et al., 1993) and the studies meeting class II criteria studies included 24 (Mitchell et al, 1990), 30 (Pierce et al., 1990) and 8 (Wood et al., 1993) patients respectively. Emergence from coma was used as a measure of outcome in all studies and the studies by Pierce et al. (1990) and Wood et al. (1993) also examined length of hospital stay. Although the results of all studies except that of Johnson et al. appeared to suggest that the patients undergoing intervention – sensory stimulation or in the case of Wood et al. – (1993), sensory regulation – spent less time in hospital, the small numbers make such a conclusion debatable. The results also appear contradictory; in the study by Wood et al. (1993) patients were not stimulated; in contrast, the amount of stimulation was regulated. Hence, when the combined results of these studies are considered, in each case the group that improved most rapidly was the intervention group. This raises the question of whether the interventions (ie stimulation or regulation) were in fact effective or whether the increased time and attention given to the intervention groups was in fact more important than either of the interventions tested.

Compensation

Recovery is defined in terms of reduction of disability and handicap. In using compensation the emphasis of treatment is changed from focusing on impairment (as in restorative approaches) to focusing on intact skills and using these to compensate for limitations caused by the impairments. Patients are taught to use compensatory devices and learn to develop new strategies and skills. For example, if a patient has memory problem internal strategies such as mnemonics or imagery and external aids such as notebooks, diaries and checklists may be used. Previous research (Wilson & Hughes, 1997) demonstrated that some brain-injured patients could learn compensatory strategies. Such techniques are also acceptable to patients. Use of external aids such as notebooks and diaries is in many cases an extension of previously learned behaviour rather than introduction of new behaviour. Where it is a new behaviour it is socially acceptable in that it is an extension of everyday behaviour. However, to succeed in using compensation, patients must have some ability to learn as it involves learning new skills or applying previously learned skills to new areas. Therefore, the approach is not appropriate for patients with severe cognitive impairment or severely impaired learning skills.

Environmental Modification

An alternative compensatory approach is to modify the environment rather than the patient. Using this approach, tasks are altered and components of the environment changed to facilitate independence. This approach is particularly

appropriate for patients with severe cognitive impairment or severe dysexecutive syndrome with poor motivation and who are incapable of adapting to
changed circumstances. The benefit of such an approach is that it maximises
residual abilities but the major disadvantage is that the success or failure of
the environmental manipulation is dependent on others.

A second aspect of the environment to be considered is the effect of a
stimulating environment. Results from animal studies suggest that the environment of the patient can moderate survival and growth of nerve cells. When
rats placed in enriched or impoverished environments after brain injury were
examined it was shown that not only did the rats in the enriched environment
show evidence of improved cognitive and behavioural recovery but also that
the effect was permanent (Stein et al., 1995).

A further environmental variable often not considered is the effect of the
behaviour of other people in the patient's environment. Studies with other
patient groups e.g. people with schizophrenia have shown that changing the
behaviour of others in the patient's environment can affect the person's own
behaviour (Falloon et al. 1984), although this is an area which has not yet
been formally investigated in patients with traumatic brain injury.

Although these models of rehabilitation differ, none is used to the exclusion of the others. In fact, different approaches to rehabilitation at different
stages is probably most appropriate. Animal studies suggest that the most
rapid recovery of damaged structures occurs in the days and weeks immediately after the insult. Thus, rehabilitation programmes using a restorative
approach would be most likely to affect outcome in the early recovery period.
Compensatory approaches may be more appropriate as time passes. However, as achievement of the target goals(s) is the aim of rehabilitation, it is
rarely possible to differentiate the exact processes whereby this is achieved.

Pharmacology

The literature on pharmacological intervention for people in states of reduced
consciousness is surprisingly sparse and, as yet, there is little evidence of
efficacy. Theoretically, drugs acting on neurotransmittors could increase
arousal thereby facilitating responsivity. However, increased arousal (e.g.
increased frequency and duration of eye opening) does not necessarily result
in increased awareness. In a recent review, Giacino (2001) commented that
the dearth of literature on this topic suggests that recovery from states of
reduced consciousness mediated by drug therapy is rare.

Assessment

Once a head injured patient is medically stable, more attention turns to assessment of the consequences of the injury. A head injury may cause a variety

of physical, cognitive, social and behavioural impairments. Emergence from coma in severely injured patients may be gradual but the difficulties involved in assessing these patients (whether they are in coma, in a vegetative state or in a minimally conscious state) are similar. Unless accurate assessment takes place, small gains may be missed or misinterpreted. With such patients, it is not unusual to believe mistakenly that nothing is happening even though slow but subtle progress is being made over weeks or months. Therefore both monitoring progress and setting appropriate and achievable goals can present a challenge for the rehabilitation team working with these patients. Patients may have a very limited behavioural repertoire and these behaviours may occur at infrequent and unpredictable intervals. Furthermore, as level of consciousness fluctuates, different degrees of stimulation may be required to elicit responses at different times. For the therapist dealing with these severely compromised patients, goal setting particularly in the area of cognition may be difficult when the baseline level of functioning is not clear.

Among the scales available to assess this population are the Rancho Los Amigos Scale (Hagen et al., 1987) and the Glasgow Coma Scale (Jennett & Teasdale 1977), (GCS) (See Appendix). There are limitations to the use of these scales however, when the period of unresponsiveness continues for an extended period. Subtle changes in behaviour may not be enough to record a change – as for example with patients where there is general agreement among those caring for him/her that the patient is 'lighter' (i.e. more responsive but in an undefined manner) but the change is not enough to move categories on the GCS or the Rancho scales.

In response to the need for an assessment to fill this gap, the Wessex Head Injury Matrix (WHIM) (Shiel et al., 2000a, 2000b) was developed. The scale was developed by observing recovery after brain injury in 88 patients and dividing this into small steps or behaviours. In all, there are 62 behaviours or steps on the scale and these items can be used to monitor change from the point of admission to emergence from PTA. The scale has behaviours relating to social behaviour, cognition, attention and communication. The items on the scale are in hierarchical order – i.e. the order in which they are most likely to recover. Thus, the items on this scale can also be used to formulate short term goals for rehabilitation. The scale is designed to be used by the multidisciplinary team and is administered by observation and by presenting patients with meaningful stimuli e.g. photographs and relevant questions (identified by the patients' families) and by observing and recording their responses to these.

The scale divides clinical recovery into small steps which can be used to evaluate progress from the point of admission to emergence from PTA. It includes items of communication, social behaviour, cognition, attention and communication. All items require ability to make some kind of response but do not require any assumption to be made about the purpose of the response or the patient's level of awareness. The items on the scale are assessed by observation and items are fine grained enough to show small increments. The items on the scale also have the potential to be used to formulate short term goals for rehabilitation.

In the next section, rehabilitation programmes incorporating the approaches to assessment and rehabilitation described above will be considered in the context of specific case studies.

Coma

Many of the techniques used in rehabilitation with patients who are in coma, minimally conscious or in the vegetative state overlap. However, the goals of treatment will be very different in each of these cases. These differences will be illustrated by using a number of case descriptions. Initially, it may not be possible to elicit any meaningful response from the patient – however, changes of position or environment may alter this giving the team a focus for intervention. An example of this is given in the first case.

Case Study 1

JX, a 20 year old man was involved in a RTA and sustained a severe head injury. CT/MR showed diffuse brain injury with focal frontal and temporal lesions. GCS at the scene of the accident was 3 and increased to 4 after resuscitation. JX also had a fractured pelvis, fractured right femur and tibia, fractured ribs and a fractured clavicle. He was electively sedated, paralysed and ventilated. A bilateral frontal craniotomy was carried out to reduce intercranial pressure, and his orthopaedic injuries were fixed. 14 days after the accident, sedation was withdrawn but JX made poor respiratory efforts and GCS remained at 3. Over the next week he was gradually weaned off the ventilator but his GCS still remained at 3.

Rehabilitation commenced with JX as soon as sedation was withdrawn. In addition to the GCS he was assessed daily using the WHIM. Physiotherapy treatment commenced aiming at preventing deformity such as contractures and maintaining respiratory independence. By the 23rd day after injury JX had begun to open his eyes and was extending his limbs to painful stimuli (GCS motor score 2).

He was otherwise unresponsive while lying in bed. However, when he was seated over the side of the bed his eye gaze became more purposeful and he also tried to push the physiotherapist away from him. At this point his respiratory system was compromised so he was only able to tolerate sitting for about 4 minutes before his oxygen saturation level decreased. As his responsiveness while sitting suggested that this was crucial for his early rehabilitation, a multidisciplinary programme of rehabilitation involving nursing, OT and physiotherapy staff was commenced. The aims of the programme were as follows

- to increase sitting (and ultimately standing) tolerance.
- to monitor change in levels of arousal and determine whether this was related to posture.
- to use this information to monitor level of cognitive function during times of high and low arousal.

It transpired that JX's levels of arousal and responsiveness were consistently better while sitting upright. Furthermore, the increase in arousal was maintained for up to an hour after treatment. Although, levels of arousal at rest gradually began to 'catch up' JX continued to be more responsive when sitting and standing than when lying.

Goals for his early rehabilitation were now extended and the WHIM was used to identify the following common goals (i.e. to be addressed by all disciplines):

1) to track for 3 seconds
2) to maintain eye contact for 5 seconds
3) to make eye contact for 3 seconds
4) to look at the person giving attention

Each of the goals was time dated based on the rate of recovery which had already been observed. As the rate of recovery over the previous fortnight had been slow but steady a timespan of two weeks to achieve the goals was aimed for. In the event, JX's recovery began to speed up and all goals had been achieved a week later. At this stage also JX's condition was considered to be stable so he was moved from the ITU onto the ward. The rehabilitation procedure continued in the same manner i.e. interdisciplinary. Rehabilitation should begin in coma. As can be seen from the example above the principles are the same as in any other stage after brain injury – goal driven and multidisciplinary. However, rehabilitation during coma differs from that at a later stage in one main way – it is not possible to carry out a rehabilitation programme successfully as in a single discipline. In the example above, arousal levels only improved when the patient was seated out of bed initially. Had this observation not been made, staff motivation to continue with such an intensive programme may have been less. Later, behaviour occurred at infrequent and unpredictable intervals. The team involved worked together with the patient, thus allowing him have more intensive treatment (because a minimum of 3 disciplines were present each session). As the nursing staff monitored his progress on the WHIM on a 24 hour basis this facilitated an accurate picture of JX's cognitive level to be established making goal setting more realistic and achievable. The salient point is that none of the rehabilitation disciplines could have achieved what they did alone but as they did work in a multidisciplinary manner JX's rehabilitation programme was well underway by the time he moved to an acute neurosurgical ward. The programme provided for JX utilised the skills of all members of the team and, because the team used joint sessions, several issues were addressed in fewer interventions – for example, changes in position from lying to sitting and standing affected not only arousal levels but also benefited respiratory and urinary systems, and helped prevent development of secondary complications such as contractures. Prevention of such secondary complications is an essential part of early intervention with these patients. If such problems are allowed to develop, valuable rehabilitation resources may need to be directed towards reversing these rather than towards promoting improvement in other areas.

The Vegetative State

On the surface, it may seem as though a patient in the vegetative state is unlikely to benefit from neuropsychological rehabilitation. However, there are two main areas where input is extremely valuable – in assessment and in using observation to answer questions. These two points are illustrated in the following case description.

Case Study 2

YZ, a 41 year old man was admitted to hospital with a severe respiratory tract infection. He was homeless and had a long history of alcoholism. Following admission to hospital his condition deteriorated and he had a cardiac arrest. He was resuscitated but did not regain consciousness. A CT scan taken at the time did not identify significant abnormality but mild atrophy was noted.

YZ was nursed on an acute medical ward. Seven days after the arrest he was recorded as having his 'eyes open and looking around'. He was not referred to the rehabilitation team for another 4 months, for physical and cognitive assessment and rehabilitation. He was assessed using the WHIM and his level of function is shown below.
- eyes open
- eyes open and move
- attention held by dominant stimulus

These behaviours are consistent with a diagnosis of vegetative state. In addition, YZ had severe contractures of all 4 limbs and both hands were contracted so that spontaneous or purposeful motor activity was to all intents and purposes impossible. The rehabilitation programme designed for YZ was based on principles of environmental manipulation. As his injury was anoxic and no change had been observed for 4 months it was considered that his potential for change was low. However, this did not mean that rehabilitation was inappropriate – just that appropriate techniques and models were selected and used. The main goals of rehabilitation were to:

- identify any evidence of independent cognitive function
- identify any potential behaviours which could be exploited to set up a communication system

Again as in the previous case described, a multidisciplinary approach was required. As the patient was so severely physically compromised, the first area to be addressed was that of seating and positioning. As YZ groaned and grimaced occasionally it was difficult to determine whether he was comfortable or uncomfortable in different positions and types of seating. Therefore a series of behavioural observations using time sampling was used at rest, before changing position, after being seated and again when at rest in an attempt to find a seating system which would place him in a good posture to facilitate any purposeful movement possible and maximise arousal while causing no distress or discomfort. The results of this exercise were ambiguous – in the case of one seating position groaning and grimacing increased on two occasions out of three. In the cases of the other two systems tried no change was observed. It was concluded that the position where it was possible that he could be uncomfortable would be avoided and the other system was chosen.

Once seating had been satisfactorily addressed the next goal was to assess the level of cognitive function. Staff on the ward had reported that YZ enjoyed sitting at the ward window watching the traffic on the road below. As he had worked as a mechanic at one stage, this was of interest in that it could potentially have been an appropriate response to a meaningful stimulus. Consequently a series of behavioural observations using event sampling was undertaken. The behaviour of interest was eye movement and this was counted looking out the window, sitting in the ward, sitting in the hospital restaurant and lying in bed. The results were unequivocal – eye movement in all four conditions was the same.

During this time, observations of behaviour using the WHIM were taken weekly. No new behaviours had been recorded during his admission to rehabilitation although his posture and contractures had responded to treatment. While the assessment and treatment had been taking place a search had also been underway to find a suitable placement for the patient. He was discharged to a nursing home but the aims of rehabilitation (to set up a seating system such that any voluntary motor skills were facilitated and to identify if there were any signs of independent cognition) were achieved. Although no major gains in function were achieved by rehabilitation in this case, the benefits of intervention are clear. The patient's diagnosis was confirmed, a seating system was organised and based on the diagnosis, an appropriate placement was found.

The Minimally Conscious State

Patients who are initially in the vegetative state may improve some considerable time after the injury. This fact draws attention to the importance of reassessment of such patients as a change in awareness may allow significant progress to be made at a later stage. The third case description highlights this.

Case Study 3

GA is a 23 year old man who incurred a very severe head injury in a RTA where he was the driver. Two passengers in the car were killed in the accident and GA was admitted to hospital with GCS of 3. It was also noted that he was hypoxic in A&E. He remained in coma for 26 days when his GCS reached 9 (E4,VR M3). After 3 months his total number of behaviours on the WHIM was 3 (eyes open briefly, eyes open for an extended period and eyes open and moving). He was transferred to a rehabilitation unit and after 10 months was discharged to a nursing home. He was diagnosed as being in a vegetative state. Four years later, his family were contacted as a follow-up study of all patients admitted to a previous study was being undertaken. A health professional who was in contact with the patient wrote to the researcher with the following information 'he is in a vegetative state and will probably refuse to co-operate with your assessment'. Before seeing the patient for follow up, several members of staff were interviewed about his communicative behaviour using an adapted version of the Pragmatics Scale of Early Communication Skills. Amongst the behaviours reported were 'stiffening his limbs when being dressed by a member of staff he disliked'; 'moving his head to facilitate being shaved' and 'getting agitated when he heard his family's voices when they came to visit'.

Assessment on the WHIM demonstrated that while this man was very severely brain injured he was no longer in a vegetative state and could be more accurately described as being in the minimally conscious state (Giacino et al 2002). The behaviours observed are shown in Table 1.

Table 1. Whim Behaviours.

WHIM Behaviours
• obeying simple commands
• moving body and limbs to facilitate washing, shaving etc
• tracking source of sound
• nod/shake head
• volitional vocalization to express feelings
• silent mouthing
• selective response to preferred people
• turn head/eyes to look at when someone is talking
• watches person moving in line of vision

In this case, the change in 'label' had major consequences for the patient. He was seen by a speech and language therapist and after a number of sessions learned to indicate 'yes' and 'no' reliably. Although very dysarthric he became able to indicate preferences. He was also reassessed by OTs and physiotherapists and began attending a Day Centre for people with Head Injuries where daily therapy was provided. Reassessment some time later showed that his attention and socialisation had improved significantly.

Post Traumatic Amnesia

Another stage of recovery where the patient can be said to be in a reduced state of consciousness is the period of PTA. Patients in PTA have poor memory and are disoriented but studies by Wilson et al. (1992 and 1999) have shown that a number of other cognitive deficits are also present during this period. Behaviours observed during PTA may include any or all of the following: aggression (both verbally and physically), disinhibition, swearing, limited awareness of personal safety, no initiation of movement, passivity, lack of motivation or general lack of co-operation. Although patients in PTA manifest a large number of impairments it is not usually appropriate to assess using standard neuropsychological instruments. They have such poor attention that it is frequently difficult to test for longer than 10-15 minutes and in addition they may change so rapidly that the results of the tests are worthless by the time that testing is complete. There are a number of assessments of PTA. The best known are the Galveston Orientation and amnesia test (GOAT) (Levin et al., 1975) and the Westmead Test (Shores et al., 1986). However, both of these assessments concentrate on aspects of memory and orientation and do not address the other deficits found in patients in PTA. Thus in common with assessment of patients in the other states of reduced consciousness observation of behaviour is a valuable tool.

Although the goals and interventions used with patients in PTA will be very different, again the underlying principles will be the same. Not infrequently, referrals for patients in PTA will be prompted by difficulties in managing their behaviour in the ward environment. Many of these difficulties are caused by impaired memory, disorientation to time and place, impaired language skills, reduced reasoning, insight and judgement which leads to misperceptions causing problem behaviour. Although rehabilitation should be well underway by this stage, a large part of the intervention available here involves managing the problem, frequently by altering the environment and the behaviour of the people within it.

Many management approaches are potentially useful. Amongst the alterations, which can be made, are the following:

- Limit number of visitors – overarousal may exacerbate behaviour problems
- Treatment and assessment sessions should be for short periods

- Consistency of staff as far as possible to give a feeling of familiarity
- Therapy sessions to be carried out on the ward if possible on ward
- Simple instructions

It may also be helpful if the patient is nursed in a single room as this can decrease stimulation. However, if this is the case, care must be taken not to isolate them as this can create a whole new set of difficulties if the patient is deprived of all social contact. In those cases where physical aggression is present, simple precautions such as not treating the patient in a room alone and being aware of issues such as personal space are important.

Case Study 4

A 33-year old male jockey was racing when he was involved in an accident. The horse fell and he was kicked on the head. He sustained a severe head injury, a fractured left clavicle and scapula, a fractured pelvis, bilateral fractured femurs and a fractured right tibia and fibula. His GCS after rescusitation was 6 (E2, V1, M3). He was sedated and ventilated and the fractures were treated using external fixation among other procedures. 28 days after injury he was out of coma and in post traumatic amnesia. He believed he was on holiday in a hotel and persisted in trying to get out of bed. He was verbally and physically disinhibited and aggressive on occasion. He had removed part of the external fixation on his pelvis and had to return to theatre to have it refixed. He had an attention span of less than 30 seconds and became upset and aggressive when more than one person was present.

The main aim for this patient was to manage the behaviour in the short term by modifying the environment and modifying the behaviour of the people around the patient. He was moved to a single room but was checked every 15 minutes. His family and friends were requested to visit one at a time and for no longer than 15 minutes at a time. His family provided a television so he could watch sports programmes. Therapy sessions had already been held on the ward as he was supposed to be on complete bedrest and this was continued. Another important aspect of the intervention was to explain what was happening to the patient's family and friends who were very concerned that he had had a 'personality change'. Post traumatic amnesia was explained to them and the management regime was also described.

In terms of rehabilitation, the following cognitive goals were set and as in all other cases were addressed by the interdisciplinary team

- to be oriented in time, place and person
- to comprehend short sentences
- to attend for short periods

Progress was recorded daily and in the next few week he gradually emerged from PTA.

Conclusion

Rehabilitation of patients in reduced states of consciousness, particularly in coma, the vegetative state and the minimally conscious state is an emerging issue. Knowledge and skills in treating an assessing these groups could be considered to be in their infancy in comparison to rehabilitation of patients after head injury generally. Yet, there is enormous potential for development of the whole concept and the potential benefits are considerable if the time in hospital is reduced and the overall outcome improved. Working with relatively unresponsive patients demands particular skills but can be more rewarding than many other areas of rehabilitation. To quote a physiotherapy colleague

> *'you can be verbally and physically abused at work; you never receive positive feedback from the patient; they may never remember you; it's frustrating – the patients can be slow to recover, if they ever do, ... and I love it!'*

References

Andrews, K. and the International Working Party. (1996). *International Working Party Report On The Vegetative State.* Published by the Royal Hospital for Neurodisability.

Falloon, I.R.H., Boyd, J.L., Mcgill, C.W., Razani, J., Moss, H.B., & Gilderman, A.M. (1984). Family Management in the prevention of Exacerbations of Schizophrenia: A Controlled Study. *New England Journal Of Medicine, 306,* 1437-1440.

Giacino, J.T. (1996). Sensory Stimulation: Theoretical Perspectives and the Evidence for Effectiveness. *Neurorehabilitation, 6,* 69-78.

Giacino, J.T. (1997). Disorders of consciousness: differential diagnosis and neuropathologic features. *Semin-Neurol., 17 (2),* 105-11.

Giacino, J.T. (2001). Revisiting the vegetative state: major developments over that last decade. *Physical Medicine and Rehabilitation: State of the Art Reviews, 15,* 399-415.

Giacino, J.T., Ashwal, S., Childs, N., Cranford, R., Jennett, B., Katz, D.I., Kelly, J.P., Rosenberg, J.H., Whyte, J., Zafonte, R.D., & Zasler, N.D. (2002). The minimally conscious state: definition and diagnostic criteria. Neurology, *58 (3),* 349-53.

Giacino, J.T., & Zasler, N.D. (1995). Outcome after severe traumatic brain injury: Coma, the vegetative state, and the minimally responsive state. *Journal of Head Trauma Rehabilitation, 10 (1),* 40-56.

Hagen, C., Malkmus, D., & Durham, P. (1987). Levels Of Cognitive Functioning. Professional Staff Association of Rancho Los Amigos Hospital (Eds.) *Rehabilitation of the Head Injured Adult: Comprehensive Physical Management.* Downey, CA: Rancho Los Amigos Hospital Inc.

Hall M.E., Macdonald S., Young G.C. (1992). The Effectiveness of Directed Multisensory Stimulation versus Non-Directed Stimulation in Comatose CHI Patients: Pilot study of a single subject design. *Brain Injury, 6,* 435-445.

I Fortuny, L.A., Briggs, M., Newcombe, F., Ratcliffe, G., & Thomas, C. (1980). Measuring the duration of PostTraumatic Amnesia. *Journal of Neurology, Neurosurgery and Psychiatry, 43,* 377-79.

Jennett, B., & Plum, F. (1972). Persistent Vegetative State after Head Injury: A Syndrome In Search Of A Name. *Lancet, i,* 734-737

Jennett, B., & Teasdale, G. (1977). Aspects of Coma after Severe Head Injury. *The Lancet, i,* 878-81.

Johnson, D.A., Roethig-Johnson, K., & Richards, D. (1993). Biochemical and Physiological Patterns of Recovery in Acute Severe Head Injury: Responses to Multisensory Stimulation. *Brain Injury, 7,* 491-499

Levin, H.S., O'Donnell, V.M., & Grossman, R.G. (1975). The Galveston Orientation and Amnesia Test: A practical scale to assess cognition after head injury. *Journal of Nervous and Mental Diseases, 167,* 675-684.

Mitchell, S., Bradley, V.A., Welch, J.L., & Britton, P.G. (1990). Coma Arousal Procedure: A therapeutic intervention in the treatment of Head Injury. *Brain Injury, 4,* 273-279.

Pierce, J.P., Lyle, D.M., Quine, S., Evans, N.J., Morris, J., & Fearnside, M.R. (1990). The effectiveness of coma arousal intervention. *Brain Injury, 4,* 191-197.

Plum, F., & Posner, J.B. (1980). *The diagnosis of stupor and coma. (3rd ed).* Davies: Philadelphia.

Ponsford, J., Sloan, S., & Snow, P. (Eds) (1995). *Traumatic Brain Injury: Rehabilitation for everyday adaptive living.* Hove: Lawrence Erlbaum Associates

Rader M.A., Ellis D.W. (1994). The Sensory Stimulation Assessment Measure (SSAM): A tool for early evaluation of severely brain-injured patients. *Brain Injury, 8,* 309-321.

Royal College Of Physicians (1996). *The Permanent Vegetative State: Review Of A Working Party.* Convened By The Royal College Of Physicians and endorsed by the conference of Medical Royal Colleges and their faculties of the United Kingdom. *J.R. Coll Physicians London, 30,* 119-21.

Schacter, D.L., & Crovitz, H.F. (1977). Memory function after closed head injury; a review of quantitative research. *Cortex, 30,* 150-176.

Shiel, A., Horn, S.A., Wilson, B.A., Watson, M.J., Campbell, M., & McLellan, D.L. (2000a). The Wessex Head Injury Matrix (WHIM) main scale: a preliminary report on a scale to assess and monitor patient recovery after severe head injury. *Clin Rehabil., 14 (4),* 408-16.

Shiel, A., Wilson, B.A., Horn, S.A., Watson, M.J., & McLellan, D.L.(2000b). *The Wessex Head Injury Matrix (WHIM).* Thames Valley Test Company.

Shores, E.A., Marosszeky, J.E., Sandanam, J., & Batchelor, J. (1986). Preliminary validation of a clinical scale for measuring the duration of post-traumatic amnesia. *Med-J-Aust. 144* (11): 569-72.

Stein, D.G., & Brailowsky, S. (1995). *Brain Repair.* OUP NY.

Talbot L.R., Whitaker H.A. (1994). Brain-Injured Persons in an altered state of consciousness: Measures and intervention strategies. *Brain Injury, 8,* 689-699.

Wilson, B.A., Baddeley, A., Shiel, A., & Patton, G. (1992). How Does Post Traumatic Amnesia Differ from the Amnesic Syndrome and from Chronic Memory Impairment? *Neuropsychological Rehabilitation, 2,* 231-243.

Wilson, J.C., & Hughes, E. (1997). Coping With Amnesia: The Natural History of a Compensatory Memory System. *Neuropsychological Rehabilitation, 7,* 43-56.

Wilson, B.A., Evans, J.J., Emslie, H., Balleny, H., Watson, P.C., & Baddeley, A.D. (1999). Measuring recovery from post traumatic amnesia. *Brain Inj., 13(7),* 505-20.

Wood, R.L., Winkowski, T., Miller, J. (1993). Sensory Regulation as a method to promote recovery in patients with altered states of consciousness. *Neuropsychological Rehabilitation, 3,* 177-190.

Woolf, S.H. (1993). Practice Guidelines – A New Reality in Medicine .3. Impact on Patient Care. *Archives Of Internal Medicine, 153,* 2646- 2655.

Appendix – The Glasgow Coma Scale

EYES	4 =	Open spontaneously
	3 =	To verbal command
	2 =	To pain
	1 =	No response
MOTOR	6 =	Obeys commands
	5 =	Localises to pain
	4 =	Flexion – withdrawal
	3 =	Flexion – abnormal
	2 =	Extension
	1 =	No response
Verbal	5 =	Oriented and converses
	4 =	Disoriented and converses
	3 =	Inappropriate words
	2 =	Incomprehensible sounds
	1 =	No response

Chapter 13

NEUROREHABILITATION SERVICES AND THEIR DELIVERY

TM McMillan

Department of Psychological Medicine,
University of Glasgow, UK

Introduction

If you spend an hour leafing through this book, during that time there will have been almost 25 admissions to hospital as a result of traumatic brain injury (TBI) for every 60 million people living in a Western culture (200,000 people with TBI per year). Most of these will be people with 'minor' TBI; ie brief loss of consciousness and post-traumatic amnesia lasting less than a day. Some people with minor TBI are admitted to hospital for overnight observation and then discharged, often with little understanding of the possible impact of head injury on daily life. Many of these make a good recovery within 3 months and if then asked, many would report no persisting symptoms, but not all. For example in some urban areas, persisting disability has been reported in more than 40% of people with minor TBI, one year post-injury (Thornhill et al., 2000). Nevertheless they are not routinely offered follow-up, support, education or rehabilitation if needed. During this hour, another 4 people will have been admitted with cerebral damage (excluding stroke but including subarachnoid haemorrhage) from other causes (Langton-Hewer, 1993) and a further 2 or 3 people will have sustained a severe TBI. If they have severe physical injuries they are likely to receive rehabilitation. If not, they are likely to follow a similar path to people with minor TBI unless becoming an obvious problem because of very severe and persisting cognitive impairment, aggression or are disruptive. Even if discharged from general hospital to a nursing home, it is likely that half will receive no specialist rehabilitation before admission and few after admission (Barodawala et al., 2001, McMillan & Laurie, submitted). In the UK, hospital records will not record 20-50% of cases as having had a TBI at all, and overall, less than 30% will receive follow-up, rehabilitation or social services support (Murphy et al., 1990; Moss & Wade, 1997; Thornhill et al., 2000).

These recent studies make clear that these problems continue. What is worse, is that in the UK we know about the absence of comprehensive and well organised neurorehabilitation services, and have been reminded of this repeatedly for more than half a century (Tomlinson, 1943; Piercy, 1956; McCorquodale, 1965; Tunbridge, 1972; Royal College of Physicians, 1986, 2000; Medical Disability Society, 1988; British Psychological Society, 1989; Royal College of Psychiatrists, 1991; British Society for Rehabilitation Medicine, 1998; Royal College of Surgeons, 2000). Perhaps during this time we have learned more about what a comprehensive service needs to include (McMillan & Oddy, 2001), more about the nature and consequences of traumatic brain injury on the person and their family (Oddy, 1993; Ponsford, 1995; Willer, 2001) and more about rehabilitation and its effectiveness (Chesnut et al., 1999, Cicerone et al., 2000, Wilson, 2002).

The NIH Consensus Development Panel (National Institutes of Health, 1999) noted a number of shortcomings of current rehabilitation in the USA which are also relevant elsewhere; these include (a) the narrow focus of medical restoration approaches and the need to emphasise environmental modification to create enabling conditions, (b) the needs of high risk groups are under-represented (eg infants, adolescents and the elderly), (c) the need for rehabilitation over a lifetime, (d) difficulties in accessing rehabilitation and (e) involvement of the person with TBI and their families in decision making. It seems worthwhile therefore, to establish principles that guide services and their development.

General Principles in Developing a Comprehensive Service

1. A Comprehensive service

This should be available to all people with acquired brain injury irrespective of age. It should include a range of professional staff together with cognitive and behavioural assessments and interventions. It should include or have access to assessment and interventions for related problems such as alcohol and drug abuse.

2. Identification of Cases

It is known that many people with TBI are not identified as such and hence cannot considered for rehabilitation (Moss & Wade, 1997; Thornhill et al.,

2000). Clearly it is important to have a system which not only allows proper diagnostic labelling, but that this information is easily transferred to services that provide post acute management, treatment and support. Early after injury, some people with TBI do not think that they have problems and will not take up offers of help. However in the early stages, they can be given information about how to access appropriate services should they later wish to seek help.

3. Quality of Life and Users Views
The purpose of rehabilitation is to maximise quality of life and independence. Service development and rehabilitation programmes should take account of the views of clients and their carers.

For example, people with acquired brain injury can find it difficult to mix with other client groups such as people with learning difficulties, physical disability or those who they understand to be mentally ill. This is because they feel different from these groups–people with TBI have usually led an independent premorbid lifestyle, their problems usually stem from cognitive and emotional rather than physical problems and they themselves have organic brain injury and not mental illness.

4. Client Centred Approach
It is widely accepted that rehabilitation of people with acquired brain damage should be client centred, and adopt whenever possible a 'partnership' model between client and clinician. The importance of taking account of the view of close relatives has also been long recognised (Brooks et al., 1987b). Systems exist which incorporate this approach into the backbone of rehabilitation processes, such as client centred goal planning (McMillan & Sparkes, 2001).

5. Appropriate discharge
In most cases discharge planning should begin soon after admission. The principle is that people should be moved on to the next stage in rehabilitation when they are capable of benefiting from it, this includes discharge to home, or to specialist rehabilitation.

6. Flexibility of Approach
A service for people with acquired brain injury must provide for an immense range of disability and handicap. This extends from people with minor TBI who might require information and advice for a short time, to people with severely brain injury who are dependent for all care. A heterogeneous population of this kind needs a seamless service that is responsive to changing needs over time and can detect these needs by offering follow-up. A poor service may provide intervention that is non-specialist and dependent on availability rather than the patient's needs.

7. Community Integration

Most people with acquired brain injury return to the community within days or weeks of injury. A small but significant number require longer periods of inpatient treatment. Some require treatment after return to the community. It is important that wherever possible treatment and support services are developed in areas of reasonable geographical proximity to the person's eventual destination. This allows flexibility in terms of gradual return to the community and allows relatives easier access during inpatient stay. Historically there has tended to be a focus in the UK on hospital based rehabilitation services. These are needed but it has to be remembered that most people with brain injury spend most of their lives in the community and there is a need to have a range of services for community residents. Local proximity of services, should not however be at the expense of the effectiveness of treatment.

8. Access

Given that people with severe acquired brain injury are likely to have impairment and disability over the long term, it is important that services are accessible to them at those times in life when they are in need. It is not unusual for individuals to live in the community for some time even though their coping skills are reduced, but then cannot manage following a life event (e.g. death of a carer) when they require further help.

9. Liaison between Services

In the UK it is acknowledged that services which exist for acquired brain injury do not always communicate well with each other, or with other relevant services such as Child and Adolescent, Mental Health, Forensic, Drug and Alcohol Abuse and Older Adult. The principle should be for provision of the appropriate service(s) at a time that the client needs it; systems need to be developed to allow closer interagency and within agency working.

10. Evaluation

A key focus in Health Services now is the effectiveness of intervention. New services that are being created should have an evaluation system inbuilt at the outset and existing services need to develop such a system. Although this system should include activity (e.g. numbers and types of cases seen), it should also go beyond this to other key result areas. There should be objective indicators of change in disability or handicap for treatment services and outcome in terms of maintaining or enhancing quality of life for other services that are not treatment focussed.

Issues in Service Planning

These are considered under five main headings, which are service need, component services, liaison and communication, staffing and funding.

1) Service need

A recent study reported findings on a cohort of people with TBI admitted to Glasgow hospitals over a period of one year (Thornhill et al., 2000). The study was unusual because it included all people 14 years and over and did not exclude cases on the basis of previous history or other concurrent problems. It therefore represents the clinical load and case-mix that a service would have to deal with in practice. They found that 3,000 people with TBI were admitted in the year (approximately 330/100,000 population). About 500 remained in hospital for 48 hours or more. Of these more than half were discharged in a week or less, about 80 were admitted for more than 4 weeks and 45 were aged over 70. The admission rate found by Thornhill et al. (2000) is a little higher but not dissimilar to earlier studies (270-310) in Scotland (Jennett & MacMillan, 1981) and in England and Wales (Field, 1976), with 5-7% of people with TBI sustaining a severe injury or worse (Glasgow Coma Scale score < 8), (Lewin, 1968, Miller & Jones, 1985). Thornhill et al found more than 40 percent of their representative sample were disabled at one year follow-up of a representative sample, including more than 40% of those classified as minor brain injuries. At one year only 47% of the disabled survivors had received hospital follow-up, only 28% rehabilitation and only 15% contact from social services (see also Kay et al., 2001).

It seems that there has been a threefold decline in death/serious injury resulting from road traffic accidents between 1973 and 1993 (Broughton 1997). This is probably as a result of improved safety (such as seat belts and cycle helmets), developments in medical care and treatment-for example published guidelines for trauma care, the availability of CT scanners in local hospitals, early transfer to neurosurgery and the continuing development of pharmacological treatments (Teasdale, 1995). Nevertheless the persisting high incidence and one year prevalence of TBI reported in Thornhill et al's cohort study, means it remains the most common cause of acquired brain damage in young adults and is one of the top five most common neurological conditions overall. However caution should be applied when considering the size of service components locally, given the wide range of incidence reported in one study in the North West Region of England. Although the overall incidence of admissions of people with TBI was similar to reports from other studies (295/100,000) there was a huge range within its 19 component districts (88-885/100,000), and less than a quarter had an incidence within the range normally quoted for the UK (Tennant et al., 1995). A wide range of incidence has also been reported in the US (Kraus & McArthur, 1996).

2) Component services

In principle these are the easiest to determine, and are discussed later in this chapter. A key issue is to what extent should a planner make use of existing services-or develop these, and to what extent should new services be planned. The overall model will obviously be influenced by services already present. TBI results in disabilities which can be of relatively short duration, or which can be lifelong, which may require inpatient or residential stay or return home, which can result in difficulty with basic daily living skills ranging from minimal to complete dependence, which can end with return to previous employment or make return to work impossible. Given that outcome is so wide ranging, no single unit is likely to cater for all needs and instead a multi component system is more appropriate if a goal of providing the right input at the right time for the client is to be achieved.

3) Communication and Liaison

A system is needed for identification that distinguishes between those who have facial/head lacerations and cerebral injury, which records the fact of TBI even when there are more acute somatic issues to deal with at the time, and which routinely refers for specialist assessment or to the next stage in rehabilitation. People with brain injury may have co-existing problems that bring them into contact with other services such as drug and alcohol abuse, mental health, learning disabilities and forensic. Inter-agency liaison is needed to properly deal with these issues, and clearly worked referral pathways are required to achieve this. People may fall through a 'therapeutic net' not only between hospital and community, but also when they cross age barriers between adolescent-adult and adult-older adult. Most neurorehabilitation services are for the younger adult. Traditionally younger adult refers to people aged 16–64, the former to allow for developmental and educational considerations and the latter retirement and frailty. However given the trend for earlier retirement, and physical good health into the 70s and beyond it may be worth giving careful consideration to upper age restrictions for neurorehabilitation services. Continuity requires good liaison with child and adolescent and older adult services.

Long term needs need to be considered and account taken of vulnerability to life events that the TBI causes. Someone may do well in rehabilitation and return to the community to a good quality of life but may not be able to cope with life stresses following a bereavement, relationship difficulties, moving house or a change of job. At these times they may need further help which should not only be available but should be readily accessible and within a reasonable period of time. Hence people with acquired brain injury and their relatives have to have been told how to get help and this should be available without barriers (e.g. by self referral).

4) Staffing

Reviews of workforce planning for brain injury rehabilitation services in Scotland make clear that there is in fact little co-ordination between planning workforce numbers and service developments. Commonly services are planned locally with little consideration of where the staff might come from and this can result in problems with recruitment or retention, the latter resulting from a finite pool of trained staff circulating around services. Workforce planning is obviously a long-term issue, where the numbers of professionals needed has to be projected several years ahead of the implementation of service plans. For example, in the UK there is a shortage of clinical psychologists generally. Training psychology graduates in clinical psychology takes three years, with a further six years before they would be considered to be sufficiently experienced to take charge of a rehabilitation facility. What is needed is central co-ordination of workforce planning, informed by the professions, by training courses and by local planning initiatives and government policy for health. Difficulties caused by poor co-ordination of workforce and service planning are often greatly underestimated.

Services can founder if dependent on a charismatic and experienced individual leader who leaves. A critical staff mass reduces this possibility. It means that sufficient experienced and senior staff are available to allow for random variations in recruitment and retention without the service deteriorating catastrophically. Having a critical staff mass at key points in the Service means that less skilled staff can be given professional support and training to enable them to work effectively in parts of the Service where they may be the only professional in that discipline.

5) Funding

Obviously many initiatives have foundered here. Insurance claims can fund rehabilitation packages. Health insurance may provide funding but this is often strictly time limited. In the UK insurance funding tends to operate in the independent sector, and surprisingly is found rarely in the National Health Service; the NHS funds both NHS operated rehabilitation facilities and those in the independent sector. In Australia, the no fault compensation scheme provides rehabilitation for people with TBI resulting from accidents. In the USA rehabilitation tends to be funded by health insurance, and is often more strictly time limited for this reason. Clearly there is a political dimension to planning if funding is to become available to the extent required to provide a comprehensive service. In an era of cost constraints for health and social services, it is worth noting estimates of the financial cost to the community of people hospitalised because of TBI over their lifetime. In the mid 1980s, Max et al. (1991) estimated this to be over 115,000 US dollars per person, providing an unambiguous argument for reducing this cost, by effective neurorehabilitation.

Purchasers must be encouraged to achieve a balance between financial cost and impact of a service on disability/handicap or quality of life. This requires meaningful audit of clinical input as well as measurement of outcome. Other non-specific activities such as information giving and staff training must also be accounted for. Clearly research should be part of health planning, (e.g. the development/effectiveness of new treatment techniques).

Purchasing priorities can be altered by public policy. Legislation can provide a mandate for the development of services. For example allowing the development of state co-ordinated services in Minnesota (Murrey et al., 1998). In 1996 the US Congress passed the TBI Act, to improve access to services and enhance prevention, surveillance and research and funded government departments in order to do this; States can apply for grants and have to match funding. In some states in the USA, a proportion of fines from road traffic offences are put towards trust funds for brain injury and spinal cord injury rehabilitation (Vaughn & King, 2000). Nevertheless in the USA there remains a view that access to rehabilitation is dependent on the ability to pay, that services are patchy, may not be available for the length of time needed by the client and that the concept of a seamless service is a distant hope (Eazell, 2001). In Australia most people with brain injury receive rehabilitation automatically under the Transport Accident Commission and Work Cover schemes together with no-fault compensation; this seems to allow a more comprehensive and less time limited service than currently found in the UK or USA (Ponsford, 2001). The ratio of cost to outcome (cost-effectiveness) has been reported, although well controlled studies on brain injury rehabilitation are rare (see Cardenas et al., 2001). They could be used to argue for changes in funding priorities; however it is more likely that pressure from large and well organised voluntary groups supported by professionals and research evidence, will lead to root changes in legislation that will have a more substantial and widespread effect.

The Components of a Service (see Fig. 1)

These numbers are based on numbers of people requiring a service per one million of the population.

Early Management and Rehabilitation
Soon after trauma, a decision has to be made about whether there is a TBI and if so whether it may be severe. Given the association between TBI and alcohol drinking it may not be clear whether an individual is intoxicated, in PTA or both. In other cases there may be concern over developing intracranial complications. Hence there is a need for a short-term observation facility, for up to 48 hours in Accident and Emergency (Royal College of Surgeons, 2000). Although formal rehabilitation is usually not practical, staff require skills in managing patients who may be difficult because of being confused and disorientated, and as a result are difficult to manage.

People with multiple injuries are likely to be admitted to surgical, ortho-paedic or general medical wards. In the UK, people without severe physical trauma who remain in coma, may be admitted to any ward where a bed is available. This includes young people with TBI admitted to wards for the elderly, oncology wards and so on. Ward staff often have little experience in dealing with these cases, who can be disruptive to other patients because of post traumatic amnesia (eg getting into the wrong bed, wandering, shouting and swearing, being over familiar). Discharge can be miss-timed because of poor understanding of the likely time course of recovery, rehabilitation

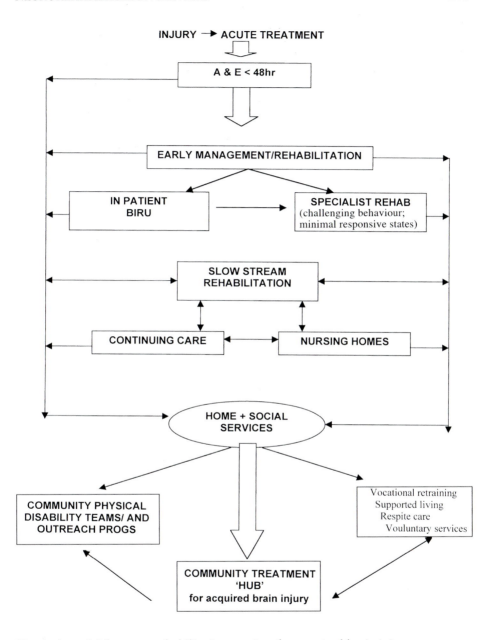

Fig. 1. A model for neurorehabilitation services for acquired brain injury.

needs and available resources. Some people are admitted to specific wards for specific interventions (eg orthopaedic) and are discharged without record or referral regarding the TBI.

For those people with TBI admitted for more than 48 hours, an early management and rehabilitation ward is needed. Staff would be experienced in dealing with these cases and the ward would have clear referral links with inpatient rehabilitation and community services. They would have an understanding of key concepts of help in managing these patients and promoting best outcome, including sensory regulation (Wood, 1991), capacity to learn even in post traumatic amnesia (Wilson et al., 1992), forestall unnecessary emergence of persisting challenging behaviour (Johnson & Balleny, 1996), appropriately use psychotropic medications and provide measured early education to relatives about brain injury. Patients would be admitted once medically stable/after surgery. The main goals would be to actively encourage referrals of all people with TBI admitted for more than 48 hours; monitor prolonged coma and gauge signs of recovery; provide an environment which is safe; prevent contractures and sores developing and maintain posture; offer active rehabilitation for those who are able, taking account of likely fatigue, poor stamina and need for rest; discharge to the next appropriate step in rehabilitation having initiated this process at an early stage in concert with social services as appropriate.

Ideally there should be one ward of this kind in each hospital where there is a major Accident and Emergency receiving unit. Hence, in a city with a population of a million there may be several such sites. One study reported over 550 people with TBI/million /annum admitted for longer than 48 hours; length of stay will vary but more than half will be discharged in 3–7 days, and 84% within a month hours (Kay et al., 2001). To prevent bed blockages, services for people who are slow to recover or in prolonged coma are needed in addition to intensive inpatient rehabilitation and community resources.

Inpatient rehabilitation

A small proportion of people with acquired brain injury require traditional residential, specialist physical therapy. Sixty-eighty beds per million are needed for rehabilitation of young adults with physical disability from all causes (Royal College of Physicians, 2000); about six would be needed for people with TBI. The treatment team consists of nurses, physiotherapists, occupational therapists, speech and language therapists, clinical psychologists, social workers and leadership by medical staff. Rehabilitation is usually intensive (eg 5 hrs/day) and may last for up to 12 months, but in the UK lasts more commonly for 2–3 months. Trends towards reducing the intensity and duration have been noted in the USA (Eazell, 2001), but there is danger that outcome will become less effective in reducing disability and handicap.

Psychosocial rehabilitation is geared towards minimising the impact of cognitive and emotional impairments prior to discharge into the community. The team would be as above, with less emphasis on physical therapy. Leadership is usually non-medical and there may be greater emphasis on generic workers. This reflects the model, which is geared towards psychological approaches to reducing dependency (Wood & Worthington, 2001). Units of this kind can usually manage challenging behaviour that is mild or moderate (ie does not involve danger to self or others). Residential units more specifically orientated towards psychosocial interventions are often based on the milieu approach, where the environment itself is devised as a therapeutic medium, in concert with specific individual and group-based programmes sometimes including psychotherapy; admission is often for 6-12 months and there is some evidence for effectiveness from controlled trials (Willer et al., 1999, Wood et al., 1999).

Severe Challenging Behaviour
About 1 person per million per annum will develop severe and persisting challenging behaviour, where the person is a danger to themself or others or their behaviour leads to significant social disadvantage. Almost ten times this number might have persisting behaviour problems that are less severe and affect daily life adversely (Johnson & Balleny, 1996), but may not need inpatient treatment. Such behaviour has traditionally been treated in specialist units, which adopt a therapeutic milieu in addition to specific behaviour modification programmes tailored to each individual. Few such units are needed, but they require high staffing ratios and high quality of intervention to be safe and effective. These units are usually staffed by clinical psychologists who commonly lead the clinical team that includes medics, occupational therapists, speech and language therapists, social workers, generic workers. They treat chronic, severe behaviour problems by designing a programme which manipulates reinforcers of behaviour and gives immediate and consistent response to inappropriate behaviour in an environment which itself operates as a therapeutic milieu. This is required especially when an individual has little or no insight into the inappropriateness of the behaviour. There is clear evidence for the effectiveness of interventions of this kind (see Alderman, 2001) although treatment can be lengthy and is often 6-12 months in duration (Eames & Wood, 1985).

Neurorehabilitation units that do not specialise in behaviour treatment might manage difficult behaviour during its natural course by providing a safe and understanding environment and a programme of care geared towards this end. Occasional cases have been reported where treatment has been successful in non-specialist inpatient units that have clinical psychology support. They often employ additional nurses to reduce disruption and who are trained to apply the behaviour programme for that client (McMillan et al., 1990, Johnston et al., 1991). Nevertheless, this can prove difficult (see Alderman, 2001), often causing tensions within these units because of the disruption to other patients and staff and the common expectations of ward staff that unless behavioural treatments show immediate effects it is inappropriate for violent patients to remain with them.

Minimally Conscious or Responsive Cases

This refers to people who are or may be in a low awareness state or where cognitive ability is unknown because of severe physical impairment. There may be a question of whether the individual is in a vegetative state. Less than one percent of hospital admissions will pass into a persisting vegetative state (Kraus & McArthur, 1996) and only a small proportion of these survive beyond 12 months, but a few survive for many years (Jennett, 2002). They tend to block acute beds in general wards for many months and are then discharged to nursing homes where they receive neither rehabilitation nor further specialist assessment. Usually there is little expert advice available with regard to whether the person is progressing and is moving out of the vegetative state, whether they would be able to communicate if the appropriate response medium was found and the person was trained to use it or whether they are not recovering. Clearly there are very different implications in terms of management for someone who is 'locked in' with relatively intact cognitive functioning and an inability to express this and someone who is in a vegetative state with absence of cognitive function. This is also a key issue for relatives who may be unable to process their grief because they maintain hope that their loved one can understand them.

A specialist unit with 3–4 beds/million is required, which will carry out repeat assessments, will give appropriate nursing care, can provide any treatments that might possibly be considered effective (such as sensory stimulation), will liase with and counsel relatives and will given an informed opinion about prognosis and needs. This could be a part of another inpatient unit such as the Early Management Unit, or an inpatient rehabilitation unit. The effectiveness of sensory stimulation treatments is not proven (McMillan & Wilson, 1993), but in the least, can allow relatives to feel they are making a contribution to care.

Community 'Hub' for Treatment of Psychosocial Problems

Traditionally, neurorehabilitation facilities have concentrated on physical rehabilitation. Over the past twenty years the need for rehabilitation of problems associated with cognitive and emotional problems has become increasingly apparent, as has awareness that most disabled people with TBI do not have debilitating physical problems and few have access to rehabilitation treatments. The problems that they have are nevertheless significant and stem from combinations of cognitive deficits, reduced motivation, impaired insight, irritability and other changes in personality. Community based treatment is needed given that these people will spend most of their lives after injury in the community. Furthermore such services may be needed intermittently over many years, because this group tends to be young, with a near normal lifespan but with reduced ability to cope with life stress. Day units specifically orientated towards psychosocial interventions are often based on a 'holistic' approach, where the individual is considered as a whole, in concert with specific individual and group-based educational and treatment programmes sometimes including psychotherapy. Admission is often for 6–12 months, and there is some evidence for overall effectiveness (Prigatano & Fordyce, 1986; Teasdale et al., 1993; Ben Yishay, 1996; Klonoff et al., 2000; Wilson et al., 2000).

A community treatment unit can act as a 'hub' for local community services. It requires a day centre base, allowing clients the option of being seen at home or at the Centre, and in this way making the most efficient use of clinical time. It also allows for group based programmes to be established and ease of access to several members of the multidisciplinary team at once. Ideally everyone admitted with TBI would be automatically referred and followed-up, (including people with minor TBI admitted to Accident and Emergency). It would act as a 'hub' for less specialised community based 'spokes'. Its six major roles are discussed below. These roles may apply to other service components, or given a different configuration of services but are given here to emphasise the way in which a unit of this kind can serve as a 'hub' for community rehabilitation.

1. Follow-up

The establishment of routine or automatic referral pathways of all people admitted to hospital after TBI is crucial. All people hospitalised after TBI would be actively followed up. This facilitates early hospital discharge as well as preventing people with TBI falling through the therapeutic net. However, to ensure this, a reliable and valid system for coding traumatic intracerebral damage is needed (Jennett, 1996).

2. Treatment

The service would offer time limited treatment interventions. These would involve support and advice to relatives. Included would be people hospitalised with minor TBI; the provision of limited/brief intervention for people admitted to hospital with less severe TBIs, can lead to fewer symptom complaints and reduced social disability at follow-up (Wade et al., 1998). Group and individual based programmes would be available to people with more severe disabilities. Physical therapy would not be offered but would be found in the community elsewhere. Deterioration of function and the development of new problems might be reduced by proactive follow-up and successful treatments are more likely to generalise to the environment in which the individual normally lives, than they would in an artificial hospital or 'hotel' based setting.

The service would offer clinical interventions designed not only to monitor and maintain function (including managing changes in circumstance), but also, where realistic, to reduce disability using rehabilitation techniques embedded in a client centred goal planning system (McMillan & Sparkes, 2001). In this way deterioration in function and the development of new problems might be minimised and successful treatments should be best placed to generalise to the actual environment in which the individual normally lives rather than an artificial hospital or 'hotel' based setting. Interventions would include functional changes in the environment to prevent problems arising, strategies to circumvent problems, treatments which might reduce cognitive impairments and psychological effects (eg depression, anxiety, PTSD) and the development of greater insight through education and role play.

3. Critical staff mass
As described above this would reduce dependency on any individual in the team and makes the effectiveness and viability of the team less vulnerable to problems resulting from acute staff retention.

4. Inter-agency liaison
People with traumatic brain injury can be involved with a number of other health provisions including mental health, drug and alcohol abuse, learning difficulties and forensic services. There is a clear need for liaison to ensure continuity of input and that the right input is provided at the right time; a key feature of the case management role of the centre. A community unit of this type is also key in liasing with adolescent services to ensure continuity of care as the individual passes in to adulthood. The same is true of older people in the adult service who become the responsibility of the older adult services.

5. Staff training
Professional training usually contains a large generic component and there is often limited training in neurorehabilitation. There is a need for training some of which has to take place locally including for staff at the 'spokes'. Training is at three levels; for local professionals who specialise in neurorehabilitation but need to keep apace of new developments; for local professionals who see people with brain injury infrequently; for care assistants/ carers who may be involved intensively with an individual with brain injury but have had no training.

6. Evaluation
Purchasers of services must be encouraged to consider costs in terms of value. This requires audit of clinical input as well as measurement of outcome. The other non-specific activities such as information giving and staff training must also be accounted for. Specific research issues should be addressed, such as the effectiveness of new treatment techniques.

Community Based Outreach and Rehabilitation
There has been a rapid expansion of community based physical therapy teams in the past decade. These are typically multidisciplinary (but are under-resourced in terms of clinical psychology), see people in their homes (but do not have opportunity to see people as groups in Centres, reducing efficiency), their main client groups are stroke and multiple sclerosis (about 5% of caseload is those with brain injury). In the UK intervention is time limited, a minority are offered routine follow-up and the intensity of input routinely

offered is limited (McMillan & Ledder, 2001; Enderby & Wade, 2001). Although this resource is used only by a small number of people with TBI it is valuable and needs to be linked not only to hospital discharge but also with the Community 'Hub' for acquired brain damage. Recent randomised control trial evidence suggests that a community based team, seeing clients usually in their own homes for 7 months can improve self-organisation and well being, with no differences found for socialising, employment or mood (Powell et al., 2002).

Vocational Re-entry
Return to competitive employment is greatly reduced following severe brain injury, with less than a third working 2–7 years after injury (Brooks et al., 1987a; McMordie et al., 1990). In addition to obvious financial implications for the person with brain injury and their family, loss of work is often associated with reduced self-esteem and feelings of lack of worth. In addition to formal rehabilitation schemes, a range of other options that include work retraining and supported work is required. Key to this is assessment of capacity and guidance about feasible options.

Supported employment schemes have been advocated in the USA, which incorporate client assessment, client advocacy, matching of client capacity to job needs, training at the job-site by a job coach, developing job retention strategies and follow-up which includes assessment of work performance (Kreutzer et al., 1988). Support may be required for 10 months, reducing in intensity during that time and with relative independence being achieved after about 5 months. Overall an average of about 300 hours of intervention is needed, but with input of this kind and for this length of time, return to work can be increased dramatically from 36% to 75%, with an average time in work of 10 months at follow-up (Wehman et al., 1993). Wall et al (1998) found greater return to work (from 32% *pre-injury* to 59%) after a 10-week community based, work retraining programme (work adjustment training and supported employment), with continued employment at 18 month follow-up. In these studies, return to work is often in a lower capacity (and with lower salaries) than pre-injury, which may lead to dissatisfaction in the longer term as suggested by one 5 year follow-up (Ashley et al., 1997).

Case Management
Where the community is geographically dispersed over a wide area, or where there are few specialists in head injury, or where an individual requires a care regime, a case management system may be effective in monitoring and maintaining the individual in the community. This is the model where the case manager acts as a co-ordinator of (community) service provision and advocate of the patient. If there is a limited rehabilitation system to refer people to Case Management may be ineffective in changing outcome (Greenwood et al., 1994) except for severely dependent cases. Nor is there compelling evidence

from studies on other patient groups, for effectiveness of case management in improving service provision or reducing costs of care and time off work (Leavitt et al., 1972; Perlmann et al., 1985; Wasylenski et al., 1985; Challis & Davies, 1986). If there is a comprehensive system as suggested here, then brain injury case management may be redundant. This may not be true where case mangers are financially empowered and can initiate an end to rehabilitation provision, such as in the USA (Dixon et al., 1988; Deutsch & Fralish, 1988).

Social Support
Social care is a key service component. The purpose is to enhance and maintain quality of life, as distinct from treatment (designed to reduce disability of handicap). Included are social services care support, day centres, sheltered work, respite care, legal advice including advice and help about benefits. In addition the voluntary sector provide services that are relevant to leisure, education and care. There are few day centres specifically for people with brain injury in the UK; Headway Houses (organised via the National Head Injuries Association) are an important exception. Day centres can at a minimum provide a routine and some sense of variety in day to day life and prevent the person with brain injury becoming effectively housebound, lonely and feeling stigmatised because they find it difficult to fit in to activities run by the able bodied and are not always well received by them. When suitable, opportunities designed to integrate people with brain injury into support systems and activities for use by the general population can be taken advantage of. However, by nature of the brain injury, these people differ from some other disabled groups. Personality and behaviour changes can cause difficulty with social integration and to avoid them withdrawing and become isolated, specific support services for people with brain injury can be a solution and are needed.

Included here must be support for relatives. Many studies attest to the strain associated with living with people whose personality has changed as a result of TBI, often accompanied by financial stringencies and social isolation (Oddy et al., 1985; Brooks et al., 1987b).

Residential Care
There is little published about people with brain injury in nursing homes. A recent study surveyed all nursing homes in Glasgow and found 100 young adults with acquired brain damage per million. Documentation provided to the nursing homes was poor. This meant that reason for placement and rationale for medication were unclear. Proactive review of needs was uncommon. Many were taking several medications prescribed preadmission and not reviewed. A minority had rehabilitation before or after admission. Many were in mixed units with older adults and people with learning disabilities. Specialist residential homes with regular Consultant review and access to rehabilitation are recommended (McMillan & Laurie, submitted).

Supported Living
A small proportion of people with TBI cannot live independently and are unable to live with relatives. In this case placement will often be in group homes or residential nursing homes. Even if suitable in principle, the latter most commonly have a mixture of residents, most of whom are elderly and some are learning disabled, and hence in practice are not ideal for young people with TBI. Group homes are more commonly found for ex-drug and alcohol abusers and people with mental health problems and less commonly for people with brain injury people specifically; this echoes disadvantages stated previously in terms of care staff not building expertise with this client group.

Respite Care
There is a need not only to provide services to allow people with brain injury and their relatives to live apart for short periods. These facilities need to be available not only for planned breaks, but for periods of family crisis. This can be difficult to achieve given the unpredictable nature of crises and the tendency for holidays to be popular at specific times of year. Included would be (traditional) residential accommodation near to the locality, sporting schemes for disabled people, which ideally specialises in brain injury and holiday centres providing breaks for people with brain injury. Short breaks can make use of day centres, sheltered or voluntary employment, sporting and leisure facilities. Social services care support or 'buddy' systems can allow people with brain injury access to leisure and shopping facilities independently from their family.

Children, adolescents and older adults
It is tragic that that most discussions about services for people with acquired brain injury focus on sub-populations, most usually young adults with TBI and older adults with stroke. This may reflect the poor service available generally. However the notion of a comprehensive service should not be that it starts at 16 and ends at the age of 65. It is not suggested that service components serve all ages, but that services are designed to be seamless across age barriers, and that artificial barriers are not maintained (e.g. excluding an active 65 year old from intensive rehabilitation with younger people). Although the incidence of TBI is greatest in young adults, there are also peaks under the age of 5 and over 75 (Kraus & McArthur, 1996).

Arguments for strictly compartmentalising these services are in part historical and based upon numbers (e.g. that there are several fold more disabled older than younger adults and limited services for the latter), outdated views of age (e.g. that people aged 65 and older are necessarily less active). It might be more equitable to work towards a system where people are included on the basis that they can benefit from the programme that has been developed for their needs. Education has to be accounted for with children, although a greater degree of flexibility, allowing access to adult services and routine referral pathways across the adolescent-adult barrier would help until a comprehensive rehabilitation service is available to children and adolescents.

References

Alderman, N. (2001). Managing challenging behaviour. In R.L.I. Wood, T.M. McMillan, *Neurobehavioural Disability and Social Handicap.* (pp. 175-208). Hove: Psychology Press.

Ashley M.J., Persel C.S., Clark M.C., & Krych D.K. (1997). Long-term follow up of post-acute traumatic brain injury rehabilitation: a statistical analysis to test for stability and predictability of outcome. *Brain Injury, 11,* 677-690.

Barodawala, S., Kesavan, S., Young, J. (2001). A survey of physiotherapy and occupational therapy provision in UK nursing homes. *Clinical Rehabilitation, 15,* 607-610.

Ben-Yishay, Y. (1996). Reflections on the evolution of the therapeutic milieu concept. *Neuropsychological Rehabilitation, 6,* 241-360.

British Association of Rehabilitation Medicine (1998) *Rehabilitation after traumatic brain injury.* BSRM c/o Royal College of Physicians, London.

British Psychological Society (1989) *Services for Young Adult Patients with Acquired Brain Damage.* Leicester: BPS.

British Society Rehabilitation Medicine (1998).

Brooks, D.N., McKinlay, W.W., Symington, C., Beattie, A., & Campsie, L. (1987a). Return to work within the first seven years of severe head injury. *Brain Injury, 1,* 5-19.

Brooks, D.N., Campsie, L., Symington, C. et al. (1987b). The effects of severe head injury on patient and relative within seven years of injury. *J Head Trauma Rehabilitation, 2,* 1-13.

Broughton J. (1997). Road accident statistics. In M. Mitchell (ed.), *The aftermath of road traffic accidents* (pp 15-32). London: Routledge.

Cardenas, D.D., Haselkorn, J.K., McElligott, J.M., & Gnatz, S.M. (2001). A bibliography of cost-effectiveness practices in physical medicine and rehabilitation: AAPM&R White Paper. *Archiv Phys Med Rehab, 82,* 711-719.

Challis, D. & Davis, B. (1986). *Case management in community care.* Aldershot, Gower.

Chesnut, R.M., Carney, N., Maynard, H., Mann, N.C., Patterson, P., & Helfland, M. (1999). Summary report: Evidence for the effectiveness of rehabilitation for persons with traumatic brain injury. *J Head Trauma Rehab., 14,* 176-188

Cicerone, K.D., Dahlberg, C., Kalmar, K., Langenbahn, P., Malec, J. et al. (2000). Evidence based cognitive rehabilitation: recommendation for clinical practice. *Arch Phys Med Rehab., 81,* 1596-1615.

Deutsch, P.M. & Fralish, K.B. (1988). Innovations in head injury rehabilitation, Mathew Bender, pp. 3-22/3-26.

Dixon, T.P., Goll, S., & Stanton, K.M. (1988). Case management issues and practices in head injury rehabilitation. *Rehabilitation Counselling Bulletin, 31,* 325-343.

Eames. P. & Wood, R. (1985). Rehabilitation after severe brain injury: A follow-up study of a behaviour modification approach. *J Neurology, Neurosurgery Psychiatry, 48,* 616-619.

Eazell, D.E. (2001). Commentary on service provision for social disability and handicap after acquired brain injury: an American perspective. In R.L.I. Wood & T.M. McMillan (eds.), *Neurobehavioural Disability and Social Handicap* (pp. 281-285). Hove: Psychology Press.

Enderby, P. & Wade, D.T. (2001). Community rehabilitation in the United Kingdom. *Clinical Rehabilitation, 15,* 577-581.

Field, H.J. (1976). *Epidemiology of Head Injuries in England and Wales with Particular Reference to Rehabilitation*. London: HMSO.

Greenwood, R.J., McMillan, T.M., Brooks, D.N., Dunn, G., Brock, D., Dinsdale, S., Murphy, L., & Price, J. (1994). Effects of case management after severe head injury. *British Medical Journal, 308,* 1199-1205.

Jennett, B. (1996). Epidemiology of head injuries. *J Neurology Neurosurgery, Psychiatry, 60,* 362-369.

Jennett, B. & MacMillan, R. (1981). Epidemiology of head injury. *BMJ 282,* 101-104.

Jennett, B. (2001). *Vegetative States*. Cambridge: Cambridge University Press.

Johnson, R., & Balleny, H. (1996). Behaviour problems after brain injury: incidence and need for treatment. *Clinical Rehabilitation, 10,* 173-181.

Johnston, S., Burgess, J., McMillan, T.M., & Greenwood, R.J. (1991). Management of adipsia by a behavioural modification technique. *J Neurology, Neurosurgery, Psychiatry, 54,* 272-274.

Kay, A.D., Thornhill, S., & Teasdale, G.M. (2001). The head injured adult-who cares? *B J Neurosurgery, 15,* 508-510.

Klonoff, P.S., Lamb, D.G., & Henderson, S.W. (2000). Milieu based rehabilitation in patients with traumatic brain injury: outcome at up to 11 years postdischarge. *Arch Phys Med Rehab., 81,* 1535-1537.

Kraus, J.F. & McArthur, D.L. (1996). Epidemiological aspects of brain injury. *Neurologic Clinics, 14,* 435-448

Kreutzer, J.S., Wehman, P., Morton, M.V., & Stonnington, H.H. (1988). Supported employment and compensatory strategies for enhancing vocational outcome following traumatic brain injury. *Brain Injury, 2,* 205-223.

Langton-Hewer, R. (1993). The epidemiology of disabling neurological disorders. In R.G. Greenwood et al. *Neurological Rehabilitation* (pp 3-12). Hove: Psychology Press.

Leavitt, S.S., Beyer, R.D., & Johnston, T.L. (1972). Monitoring the recovery process *Industrial Med., 41,* 25-30.

Lewin, W. (1968). Rehabilitation after head injury. *British Med Journal, 1,* 465-470.

Max, W., MacKenzie, E.J., & Rice, D.P. (1991). Head injuries: costs and consequences. *J Head Trauma Rehabilitation, 6,* 76-91.

McMillan, T.M., Papadopoulos, H., Cornall, C., & Greenwood, R.J. (1990). Modification of severe behaviour problems following Herpes Simplex Encephalitis. *Brain Inj., 4,* 399-406.

McMillan, T.M., Ledder, H. (2001). A survey of services provided by community neurorehabilitation teams in south east England. *Clinical Rehabilitation, 15,* 582-588.

McMillan, T.M. & Oddy, M. (2001). Service provision for social disability and handicap after acquired brain injury. In R.L.I. Wood & T.M. McMillan, *Neurobehavioural Disability and Social Handicap* (pp. 257-274). Hove: Psychology Press.

McMillan T.M. & Wilson (1993). *Neuropsychological Rehabilitation, 3,* 149-160.

McMillan, T.M. & Sparkes, C. (2001). Goal planning and neurorehabilitation: The Wolfson Neuro-Rehabilitation Centre approach. *Neuropsychological Rehabilitation, 9,* 241-252.

McMillan, T.M. & Laurie, M. (submitted). Young adults with brain injuries in nursing homes in Glasgow.

McCorquodale, Report (1965). **Cmmd**. 1867. London, HMSO.

McMordie, W., Barker, S.L., & Paolo, T.M. (1990). Return to work (RTW) after head injury. *Brain Injury, 4,* 57-69.

Medical Disability Society (1988). Report of a working party on the management of traumatic brain injury. London: *The Development Trust for the Young Disabled*.

Miller, J.D. & Jones, P.A. (1985). The work of a regional head injury service. *Lancet, 1*, 1141-1144.

Moss, N.E.G. & Wade, D.T. (1996). Admission after head injury: How many occur and how many are recorded? *Injury, 27*, 159-161.

Murrey, G.J., Helgeson, S.R., Courtney, C.T., & Starzinski, D.T. (1998). State co-ordinated services for traumatic brain injury survivors: toward a model delivery system. *J Head Trauma Rehabilitation, 13*, 72-81.

Murphy, L.D., McMillan, T.M., Greenwood, R.J., Brooks, D.N., Morris, J.R., & Dunn, G. (1989). Services for severely head injured patients in North London and environs. *Brain Injury, 4*, 95-100.

Oddy, M., Coughlan, T., Tyerman, A., & Jenkins, D. (1985). Social adjustment after closed head injury: A further follow-up seven years after injury. *J. Neurology Neurosurgery Psychiatry, 48*, 564-568.

Oddy, M. (1993). Psychosocial consequences of brain injury. In R.J. Greenwood & M. Barnes et al. (eds.), *Neurological Rehabilitation* (pp. 423-436). Edinburgh: Churchill Livingstone.

Pearcy Report (1956). *Report of the Committee of Enquiry on the rehabilitation training and resettlement of disabled persons*. Cmmd. 9883. London, HMSO.

Perlmann, B.B., Melnick, G., & Kentera, A. (1985). Assessing the effectiveness of a case management programme. *Hosp Comm Psychiatry, 36*, 405-407.

Ponsford, J. (1995). *Traumatic brain injury: rehabilitation for everyday adaptive living*. Hove: Lawrence Erlbaum Associates Ltd.

Ponsford, J.L. (2001). Commentary on service provision for social disability and handicap after acquired brain injury: An Australian perspective. In R.L.I. Wood & T.M. McMillan, *Neurobehavioural Disability and Social Handicap* (pp. 275-279). Hove: Psychology Press.

Powell, J., Heslin, J., & Greenwood, R. (2002). Community based rehabilitation after severe traumatic brain injury: a randomised control trial. *J Neurol Neurosurg Psychiatry, 72*, 193-202.

Prigatano, G.P. & Fordyce, D.J. (1986). *The Neuropsychological Rehabilitation Program at Presbyterian Hospital*. Oklahoma City: John Hopkins University Press, Baltimore.

Royal College of Physicians (1986). Physical disability in 1986 and Beyond. *J Royal College of Physicians London, 20*, 30-37.

Royal College of Physicians (2000). Medical rehabilitation for people with physical and complex disabilities. *Royal College of Physicians*, London.

Royal College of Psychiatrists (1991). services for brain injured adults. *Psychiatric Bull., 15*, 513-518.

Royal College of Surgeons (1999) Report of the working part on the management of head injuries. *Royal College of Surgeons of England*, London.

Teasdale, G.W. (1995). Head injury. *J Neurol Neurosurg Psychiatry, 58*, 526-539.

Teasdale, T.W., Christensen, A.-L., & Pinner, E.V. (1993). Psychosocial rehabilitation of cranial trauma and stroke patients. *Brain Injury, 7*, 535-542.

Tennant, A., MacDermott, N., & Neary, D. (1995). The long term outcome of head injury; implications for service planning. *Brain Injury, 9*, 595-605.

Thornhill, S., Teasdale, G., Murray, G., McEwen, J., Roy, C.W., & Kay, P. (2000). Disability in young people and adults one year after head injury: prospective cohort study. *B Med. J., 320*, 1631-1635.

Tomlinson Report (1943). *Report of the Inter-departmental Committee on the Rehabilitation and Resettlement of Disabled Persons*. Cmmd. 64115. London, HMSO.

Tunbridge Report (1972). *Rehabilitation report of a sub-committee of the standing medical advisory committee*. London, HMSO.

Vaughn, S.L. & King, A. (2000). A survey of state programmes to finance rehabilitation and community services for individuals with brain injury. *J Head Trauma Rehabilitation, 16*, 20-33.

Wade, D.T., King, N.S., Wenden, F.J., Crawford, S., & Caldwell, F.E. (1998) Routine follow-up after a head injury: a second randomised controlled trial. *J Neurology Neurosurgery, Psychiatry, 65*, 177-183.

Wall, J.R., Rosenthal, M., Niemczura, J.G. (1998). *Community based retraining after acquired brain injury. Brain Injury, 12*, 215-224.

Wasylenski, D.A., Goering, P., & Lancee, W. (1985). Community based training after acquired brain damage. *J Nervous and Mental Disease, 17*, 303-308.

Wehman, P., Kregel, J., Sherron, P., Kreutzer, J., Fry, R., & Zasler, N. (1993). Critical factors associated with the successful supported employment placement of patients with severe traumatic brain injury. *Brain Injury, 7*, 31-44.

Willer, B., Button, J., & Rempel, R. (1999). Residential and home based rehabilitation of individuals with traumatic brain injury: a case control studt. *Arch Phys Med Rehabilitation, 80*, 399-406.

Willer, B., Flaherty, P.M., & Coallier, S. (2001). Families living with the effects of acquired brain injury. In R.L.I Wood & T.M. McMillan, *Neurobehavioural Disability and Social Handicap* (pp 47-64). Hove: Psychology Press.

Wilson, B.A., Baddeley, A., Shiel, A., & Patton, G. (1992). How does post traumatic amnesia differ from amnesic syndrome and chronic memory impairment? *Neuropsychological Rehabilitation, 2*, 231-243.

Wilson, B.A., Evans, J.J., Brentnall, S., Bremner, S., Keohane, C., Williams, H. (2000). The Oliver Zangwill Centre for neuropsychological rehabilitation; a partnership between healthcare and rehabilitation research. In A.-L. Christensen & B.P. Uzzell (eds.), *International Handbook of Neuropsychological Rehabilittion* (pp. 231-246). New York: Kluwer Academic Press.

Wilson, B.A. (2002). Towards a comprehensive model of cognitive rehabilitation. *Neuropsychological Rehabilitation, 12*, 97-110.

Wood, R.L.I. (1991). Critical analysis of the concept of sensory stimulation for patients in vegetative states. *Brain Injury, 5*, 401-410.

Wood, R.L.I., McRea, J.D., Wood, L.M., & Merriman, R.N. (1999). Clinical and cost effectiveness of post-acute neurobehavioural rehabilitation. *Brain Injury, 13*, 69-88.

Wood, R.L.I. & Worthington, A. (2001). Neurobehavioural rehabilitation in practice. In: R.L.I. Wood, TM McMillan, *Neurobehavioural Disability and Social Handicap* (pp. 133-156). Hove: Psychology Press.

Chapter 14

THE FUTURE OF NEUROPSYCHOLOGICAL REHABILITATION

Barbara A. Wilson

MRC Cognition and Brain Sciences Unit, Cambridge, and The Oliver Zangwill Centre, Ely, UK

Introduction

Neuropsychological rehabilitation is coming of age. In a recent book on neuropsychological interventions, Eslinger (2002) said 'Professionals who reported psychometric testing data in relationship to a particular lesion location or disease process were somehow perceived as more experimental and scientific, while rehabilitators were perceived as seeking a therapeutic effect from a theoretical and non-experimental approach' (e.g. how can we make this person better?) (p. 4). Although this attitude still prevails in some quarters, there is increasing recognition of the value and effectiveness of rehabilitation to improve the quality of life for people with brain injury and enable them to survive in their most appropriate environments. The contributors to this book demonstrate how theory and practice inform each other and can result in the successful remediation of real life problems.

Since I started working in the field of brain injury rehabilitation twenty three years ago, I have noticed several changes and these are almost certainly changes for the better. I cannot say that all these changes are new developments as Poppelreuter, for one was describing some of them as long ago as 1917 (Poppelreuter). Indeed, the rehabilitation programmes set up for the German soldiers who survived gun shot wounds to the head in the first world war are better than many rehabilitation programmes in existence today. Nevertheless, the early twenty first century is an exciting time to be working in rehabilitation and the future looks promising. To my mind, recent changes that I feel will be most influential in neuropsychological rehabilitation for the next decade or two are:

1. Rehabilitation is now seen as a partnership between people with brain injury, their families and health service staff.
2. Goal planning is becoming increasingly established as one of the major methods for designing rehabilitation programmes.
3. Cognitive, emotional and psychosocial deficits are interlinked and all should be addressed in neuropsychological treatment programmes.
4. Technology is playing (and will continue to play) an increasing part in the understanding of brain injury and in enabling brain injured people to compensate for their difficulties.
5. Rehabilitation is beginning to take place in intensive care, it is not solely for those people who are medically stable and
6. There is a growing belief that neuropsychological rehabilitation is a field that needs a broad theoretical base incorporating frameworks, models and methodologies from a number of different fields.

Let us now consider each of these six points in turn.

Rehabilitation as a Partnership between Clients, Families and Health Care Staff

In 1991, McLellan (1991) defined rehabilitation as a two way process between people disabled by injury or disease, health care staff and members of the wider community. He believed that, unlike surgery or drugs, rehabilitation is not something we 'do' to people or 'give' to people. Instead, the disabled person is part of a two way interactive process. This represented a move forward. For many years the person with disability was told what to expect in and from rehabilitation, the rehabilitation staff determined what areas to work on, what goals to set, what was achievable and what was not. Sometime in the 1980's, the philosophy began to change – at least in some centres – so that in many rehabilitation programmes today, clients and families are asked about their expectations, rehabilitation goals are discussed and negotiated between all parties involved. The focus of treatment is on improving aspects of everyday life and, as Ylvisaker and Feeney (2000) say, rehabilitation needs to involve personally meaningful themes, activities, settings and interactions. Evans, this volume Chapter 4 illustrates this approach in his case description of David, a man with attention and planning problems following a stroke. Tate, Strettles and Oseteo, this volume Chapter 8 also imply the importance of partnership in the descriptions of their service for people with brain injury and Clare, this volume Chapter 8, describes how people with dementia select their own targets for treatments. McMillan, too, in Chapter 13 states that client centred approaches are desirable in the delivery of rehabilitation services. This is a much healthier state of affairs than providing clients with experimental or artificial material to work on. Motivation is likely to be increased because all are working on real life problems and generalisation difficulties are avoided.

Goal Planning as a Means of Designing Rehabilitation Programmes

One of the ways of ensuring a client centred approach and achieving a genuine partnership is to use goal planning to devise treatment programmes. Goal planning allows treatment to be tailored to the individual needs of people with brain injuries and their families. Although this approach is not new and has been used in rehabilitation settings for a number of years and with a number of diagnostic groups, including people with brain injury, in the last 10 years more and more centres have adopted this method to plan rehabilitation. Goal planning makes sense to staff, to clients and to families.

Houts and Scott (1975) suggest there are five principles involved in goal planning. First, involve the patient. Second, set reasonable goals. Third, describe the patient's behaviour when the goal is reached. Fourth, set a deadline. Fifth, spell out the method so that anyone reading it would know what to do. McMillan and Sparks (1999) add to this list. They say that goals should be client centred, they should be realistic and potentially attainable during admission, they should be clear and specific, have a definite time deadline and be measurable. They also say that long term and short term goals are required. Long term goals usually refer to disabilities and handicaps as the purpose of rehabilitation is to improve everyday functioning and these goals should be achieved by the time of discharge from the centre. Short term goals are the steps required to achieve the long term goals.

The process of goal planning involves allocation of a chairperson, formulation of a plan of assessment, having goal planning meetings, the drawing up of a problem list and plans of action, and the recording of whether or not the goals are achieved (or, if not achieved why not). The main advantages of this system are first, the aims of admission are made clear and explicitly documented; second, patients or clients, their families and carers are all involved; third, some outcome measures are incorporated into the treatment programmes and fourth, the artificial distinctions between outcomes and patient/ client activities are removed. Although, in principle, it is possible to make the goals too easy, there are ways round this. McMillan and Sparks (1999) believe one can avoid making goals too easy through staff training and experience while Malec (1999) describes goal attainment scaling to allow a measure of comparability between different goals. It is probably true to say that goal planning is one of the most sensible outcome measures but should be used alongside other more standardised measures such as measures of handicap, mood, psychosocial functioning and demographics. Wilson, Evans and

Keohane (2002) provide a fairly detailed description of goal planning used
in the successful treatment of a man who sustained both a head injury and
a stroke. Manly, this volume chapter 3, discusses the targeting of functional
goals in treatment; Evans, chapter 4 and Wilson, chapter 5 both refer to goal
planning in their descriptions of treatments. Williams, chapter 6 says goal
setting procedures are one of the main components of programmes dealing
with cognitive and emotional disorders and the recognition of the importance
of goal planning is directly or indirectly addressed in almost every chapter in
this volume.

Cognitive, Emotional and Psychosocial Deficits are Interlinked

Although cognitive deficits are, perhaps, the major focus of neuropsychological rehabilitation, there is a growing awareness that the emotional and
psychosocial consequences of brain injury need to be addressed in rehabilitation programmes. Furthermore, it is not always easy to separate these out
from one another. Not only does emotion affect how we think and how we
behave, cognitive deficits can be exacerbated by emotional distress and can
cause apparent behaviour problems. Psychosocial difficulties can also result
in increased emotional and behavioural problems and anxiety can reduce the
effectiveness of our intervention programmes. There is clearly an interaction
between all these aspects of human functioning as recognised by those who
argue for the holistic approach to brain injury rehabilitation. This approach,
pioneered by Diller (1976), Ben-Yishay (1978) and Prigatano (1986) is committed to the belief that the cognitive, psychiatric and functional aspects of
brain injury should not be separated from emotions, feelings and self-esteem.
Holistic programmes include group and individual therapy in which patients
are encouraged to more aware of their strengths and weaknesses, helped to
understand and accept these, given strategies to compensate for cognitive
difficulties and offered vocational guidance and support. Prigatano (1994)
suggests that such programmes appear to result in less emotional distress,
increased self-esteem and greater productivity. Prigatano (1999) and Sohlberg
and Mateer (2001) both describe the importance of dealing with the cognitive, emotional and psychosocial consequences of brain injury. Wilson et al.
(2000) present a British holistic programme based on the principles of Ben-
Yishay (1978) and Prigatano (1986). This is the Oliver Zangwill Centre for
Neuropsychological Rehabilitation in Ely, Cambridgeshire. Although, these
programmes appear to be expensive in the short term, they are probably
cost effective in the long term (see Wilson & Evans, 2003) and Prigatano
(2003).
   In this volume, several chapters are concerned with cognitive difficulties
(e.g. Chapters 3,4,5, 6 and 10). Williams, Chapter 7, is concerned with the
rehabilitation of emotional disorders following brain injury; he says that
survivors are at particular risk of developing mood disorders. He goes on

to say that this area is one of the key areas for development in neurological services. Social aspects of rehabilitation are the concern of Tate et al in Chapter 8. They describe a service in Australia that many countries must envy. Behaviour disorders are targeted by Alderman, Chapter 9. He works at The Kemsley Unit, St Andrews Hospital, Northampton – a unit that treats some of the most severely disturbed brain injured people in the United Kingdom. Anderson, Chapter 11 discusses cognitive, social and behavioural problems in children who have survived brain injury; she says that it is rare to find holistic programmes for children and McMillan Chapter 13 addresses several aspects of holistic treatment approaches.

Technology in Rehabilitation

The increasing use of sophisticated technology such as Positron Emission Tomography and Functional Magnetic Resonance Imaging is enhancing our understanding of brain damage (see for example Menon et al., 1998). To what extent these methods can improve our rehabilitation programmes remains to be seen. What is clear is the value of technology for reducing everyday problems of people with neurological damage. One of the major themes in rehabilitation is the adaptation of technology for the benefit of people with cognitive impairments. Computers, for example, may be used as cognitive prosthetics, as compensatory devices, as assessment tools or as a means for training. Given, the current expansion in information technology, this is likely to be an area of growth and increasing importance in the next decade. One of the earliest papers to use an electronic aid with a person with brain damage was Kurlychek (1983). This was important in that it tackled a real life problem as it was used to teach a man to check his timetable. In 1986 Glisky, Schacter and Tulving (1986) taught memory impaired people computer terminology and one of their participants was able to find employment as a computer operator. Kirsch and his colleagues (Kirsch, Levine, Fallon-Krueger, & Jaros, 1987) designed an interactive task guidance system to assist brain injured people perform functional tasks. Since then, there have been numerous papers reporting successful use of technology with brain injured people. A recent paper by Wilson, Emslie, Quirk and Evans (2001) used a randomised control crossover design to demonstrate that it is possible to reduce the everyday problems of neurologically impaired people with memory and/or planning difficulties with a paging system. Another area where technology is likely to play an increasing role in the future is Virtual Reality (VR). VR can be used to simulate real life situations and thus be beneficial for both assessment and treatment.

In this volume, Boake, chapter 2 includes discussion of some of the early computer based cognitive rehabilitation programmes; Manly, chapter 3, presents some discussion of technology in the remediation of attention disorders and unilateral neglect, while both Evans and Wilson also refer to technology in rehabilitation in their respective chapters.

Rehabilitation Begins in Intensive Care

Perhaps one of the greatest changes in rehabilitation over the past few years has been in the assessment and management of people in reduced states of awareness i.e those who are in coma, or who are vegetative or who are minimally conscious (Jennett, 2002). Jennett and Teasdale (1977), the authors and developers of The Glasgow Coma Scale (GCS -1977) define coma as 'giving no verbal response, not obeying commands and not opening the eyes spontaneously or to stimulation ' (p. 878). The Royal College of Physicians report (1996) describes the characteristics of people in the vegetative state and Giacino et al. (2002) discusses the Minimally Conscious State. Since the GCS appeared over a quarter of a century ago, several other assessment tools have been developed to measure the behaviour of people in reduced states of awareness. One of the most recent is The Wessex Head Injury Matrix (WHIM – Shiel et al., 2000). The WHIM can also be used to set goals for treatment. The goal planning approach is followed here in much the same way as described earlier with the exception that the client will not be able to participate in goal selection. The goals of course will be different from those set for people in the later stages of recovery. Whereas a rehabilitation goal for someone in a rehabilitation centre a year or two post injury might be to do with work or driving or using a compensatory system, the goal for someone just emerging from coma might be to increase eye contact or to establish a method of communication. The goals for this group of people might well be focussed on reducing impairments where the goals for people in the later stages are more likely to be with reducing handicap or increasing participation in society.

In this volume, Shiel, chapter 12 discusses rehabilitation of people in states of reduced awareness and presents four case studies to illustrate some of the principles involved.

Neuropsychological Rehabilitation is a Field that Needs a Broad Theoretical Base

Because people with brain injury are likely to face multiple difficulties including cognitive, social, emotional and behavioural problems, no one model or group of models is sufficient to deal with all these issues. In order to improve cognitive, social emotional and behavioural functioning in everyday life we should not be constrained by one theoretical framework. Of the many theories that impact on rehabilitation, four areas are perhaps, of particular importance namely theories of cognitive functioning, of emotion, of behaviour and of learning. Consideration should also be given to theories of assessment, recovery and compensation. All the contributors to this book have tried to make clear how their clinical practice has been shaped by different theoretical models. Wilson, Chapter 1, explicitly argues for a broad based model and refers to a recently published comprehensive model of rehabilitation (Wilson, 2002). Boake, Chapter 2, describes the different methodologies that influenced some of the historical figures in the field. In Chapter 3, Manly refers to numerous theories of attention that have guided treatment approaches to this difficult area. The same is true of Evans in Chapter 4 and Wilson Chapter 5. Raymer and Maher, Chapter 6, carefully describe language frameworks that have been used to understand language disorders and to assess these disorders and finally to treat them. Of several models of emotion, Williams, Chapter 7, is particularly influenced by Cognitive Behaviour Therapy which is certainly one of the most carefully worked out and clinically useful models of emotion at this time. Tate and her colleagues, Chapter 8, are influenced, among other things, by the World Health Organisation's International Classification of Functioning framework to address social problems faced by people with brain injury. The neurobehavioural model of Wood (1987, 1990) is one that has influenced Alderman's work, Chapter 9, in his treatment of brain injured people with severe behaviour problems. Clare, Chapter 10, in her discussion of rehabilitation for people with dementia draws upon theories of memory, psychotherapy, emotion and other work. Anderson, Chapter 11 considers the outcome and management of children with traumatic brain injury so an understanding of development along with other frameworks and models is crucial in this field. Recent frameworks of levels of awareness and recovery are incorporated into Shiel's chapter (Chapter 12) about her work with people in states of reduced awareness. Finally, McMillan in Chapter 13 is concerned with the components and frameworks of service delivery for the rehabilitation of people with brain injury. Thus, it can be seen that ethical and effective neuropsychological rehabilitation requires a synthesis and integration of several frameworks, theories and methodologies to achieve its aims and ensure the best clinical practice.

References

Ben-Yishay, Y. (Ed.). (1978). *Working approaches to remediation of cognitive deficits in brain damaged persons (Rehabilitation Monograph)*. New York: New York University Medical Center.

Diller, L.L. (1976). A model for cognitive retraining in rehabilitation. *The Clinical Psychologist, 29,* 13-15.

Eslinger, P.J. (2002). *Neuropsychological Interventions: Clinical Research and Practice*. New York: The Guilford Press.

Giacino, J.T., Ashwal, S., Childs, N., Cranford, R., Jennett, B., Katz, D.I., Kelly, J.P., Rosenberg, J.H., Whyte, J., Zafonte, R.D., & Zasler, N.D. (2002). The minimally conscious state: definintion and diagnostic criteria. *Neurology, 58,* 349-353.

Glisky, E.L., Schacter, D.L., & Tulving, E. (1986). Computer learning by memory impaired patients: Acquisition and retention of complex knowledge. *Neuropsychologia, 24,* 313-328.

Houts, P.S., & Scott, R.A. (1975). Goal planning in mental health rehabilitation. *Goal Attainment Review, 2,* 33-51.

Jennett, B. (2002). *The Vegetative State: Medical Facts, Ethical and Legal Dilemmas*. Cambridge: Cambridge University Press.

Jennett, B., & Teasdale, G. (1977). Aspects of coma after severe head injury. *Lancet*, *1*, 878-881.

Kirsch, N.L., Levine, S.P., Fallon-Krueger, M., & Jaros, L.A. (1987). The microcomputer as an 'orthotic' device for patients with cognitive deficits. *Journal of Head Trauma Rehabilitation*, *2*, 77-86.

Kurlychek, R.T. (1983). Use of a digital alarm chronograph as a memory aid in early dementia. *Clinical Gerontologist*, *1*, 93-94.

Malec, J.F. (1999). Goal attainment scaling in rehabilitation. *Neuropsychological Rehabilitation*, *9*, 253-275.

McLellan, D.L. (1991). Functional recovery and the principles of disability medicine. In M. Swash & J. Oxbury (Eds.), *Clinical neurology* (pp. 768-790). Edinburgh: Churchill Livingstone.

McMillan, T., & Sparkes, C. (1999). Goal planning and neurorehabilitation: The Wolfson Neurorehabilitation Centre approach. *Neuropsychological Rehabilitation*, *9*, 241-251.

Menon, D.K., Owen, A.M., Williams, E.J., Minhas, P.S., Allen, C.M.C., Boniface, S.J., Pickard, J.D., Kendall, I.V., Downey, S.P.M.J., Clark, J.C., Carpenter, T.A., & Antoun, N. (1998). Cortical processing in persistent vegetative state. *Lancet*, *352*, 220.

Poppelreuter, W. (1917). *Disturbances of Lower and Higher Visual Capacities Caused by Occiptal Damage* (J. Zihl & L. Weiskrantz, Trans.). Oxford: Clarendon Press.

Prigatano, G.P. (1994). Individuality, lesion location, and psychotherapy after brain injury. In A.-L. Christensen & B. P. Uzzell (Eds.), *Brain injury and neuropsychological rehabilitation* (pp. 173-186). Hillsdale, NJ: Lawrence Erlbaum Associates.

Prigatano, G.P. (1999). *Principles of neuropsychological rehabilitation*. New York: Oxford University Press.

Prigatano, G.P. & Pliskin N.H. (Eds.) (2003). *Clinical Neuropsychology and Cost-Outcome Research: An Introduction*. Hove: Psychology Press.

Prigatano, G.P., Fordyce, D.J., Zeiner, H.K., Roueche, J.R., Pepping, M., & Woods, B.C. (Eds.). (1986). *Neuropsychological rehabilitation after brain injury*. Baltimore: The Johns Hopkins University Press.

Shiel, A., Horn, S.A., Wilson, B.A., Watson, M.J., Campbell, M.J., & McLellan, D.L. (2000). The Wessex Head Injury Matrix (WHIM) main scale: A preliminary report on a scale to assess and monitor patient recovery after severe head injury. *Clinical Rehabilitation*, *14*, 408-416.

Sohlberg, M.M., & Mateer, C.A. (2001). *Cognitive rehabilitation: An Integrative Neuropsychological Approach*. New York: Guilford Press.

Wilson, B.A. (2002). Towards a comprehensive model of cognitive rehabilitation. *Neuropsychological Rehabilitation*, *12*, 97-110.

Wilson, B.A., Emslie, H.C., Quirk, K., & Evans, J.J. (2001). Reducing everyday memory and planning problems by means of a paging system: A randomised control crossover study. *Journal of Neurology, Neurosurgery and Psychiatry*, *70*, 477-482.

Wilson, B.A., & Evans, J. (2003). Does cognitive rehabilitation work? Clinical and economic considerations and outcomes. In G. Prigatano (Ed.), *Clinical neuropsychology and cost-outcome research: An introduction*. Hove: Psychology Press, 329-349.

Wilson, B.A., Evans, J., Brentnall, S., Bremner, S., Keohane, C., & Williams, H. (2000). The Oliver Zangwill Centre for Neuropsychological Rehabilitation: A partnership between health care and rehabilitation research. In A.-L. Christensen & B. P. Uzzell (Eds.), *International handbook of neuropsychological rehabilitation* (pp. 231-246). New York: Kluwer Academic/Plenum Publishers.

Wilson, B.A., Evans, J.J., & Keohane, C. (2002). Cognitive rehabilitation: A goal-planning approach with a man who sustained a head injury and cerebro-vascular complications. *Journal of Head Trauma Rehabilitation, 11*, 542-555.

Wood, R.L. (1987). *Brain injury rehabilitation: A neurobehavioural approach.* London: Croom Helm.

Wood, R.L. (1990). *Neurobehavioural sequelae of traumatic brain injury.* London: Taylor & Francis Ltd.

Ylvisaker, M., & Feeney, T. (2000). Reconstruction of identity after brain injury. *Brain Impairment, 1*, 12-28.

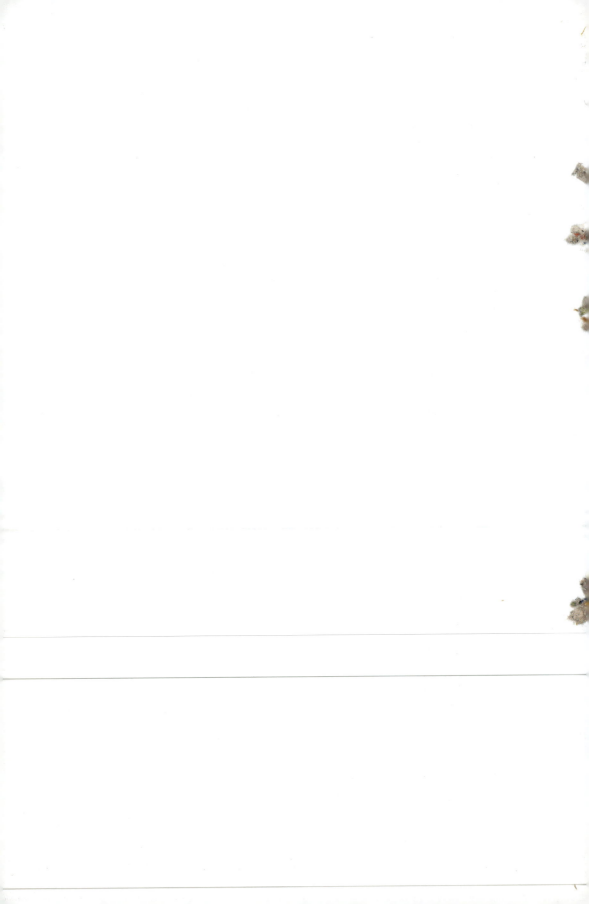

INDEX

STUDIES ON NEUROPSYCHOLOGY, DEVELOPMENT, AND COGNITION

1. *Fundamentals of Functional Brain Imaging: A Guide to the Methods and their Applications to Psychology and Behavioral Neuroscience*. Andrew C. Papanicolaou
1998. ISBN 90 265 1528 6

2. *Forensic Neuropsychology: Fundamentals and Practice*. Edited by Jerry J. Sweet
1999. ISBN 90 265 1544 8

3. *Neuropsychological Differential Diagnosis*. Konstantine K. Zakzanis, Larry Leach and Edith Kaplan
1999. ISBN 90 265 1552 9

4. *Minority and Cross-Cultural Aspects of Neuropsychological Assessment*. Edited by F. Richard Ferraro
2002. ISBN 90 265 1830 7

5. *Ethical Issues in Clinical Neuropsychology*. Edited by Shane S. Bush and Michael L. Drexler
2002. ISBN 90 265 1924 9

6. *Practice of Child-Clinical Neuropsychology: An Introduction*. Byron P. Rourke, Harry van der Vlugt and Sean B. Rourke
2002. ISBN 90 265 1929 X

7. *The Practice of Clinical Neuropsychology: A Survey of Practices and Settings*. Greg J. Lamberty, John C. Courtney and Robert L. Heilbronner
2003. ISBN 90 265 1940 0

8. *Neuropsychological Rehabilitation: Theory and Practice*. Edited by Barbara A. Wilson
2003. ISBN 90 265 1951 6

Anne Brontë

Maria H. Frawley

Elizabethtown College

Twayne Publishers
An Imprint of Simon & Schuster Macmillan
New York

Prentice Hall International
London • Mexico City • New Delhi • Singapore • Sydney • Toronto

Twayne's English Authors Series No. 524

Anne Brontë
Maria Frawley

Twayne Publishers
An Imprint of Simon & Schuster Macmillan
1633 Broadway
New York, NY 10019

Library of Congress Cataloging-in-Publication Data
Frawley, Maria H., 1961–
    Anne Brontë / Maria H. Frawley.
        p.   cm. — (Twayne's English authors series : No. 524)
    Includes bibliographical references and index.
    ISBN 0-8057-7060-7 (alk. paper)
        1. Brontë, Anne, 1820–1849—Criticism and interpretation   2. Women and
literature—England—History—19th century   3. Identity (Psychology) in literature
4. Narration (Rhetoric)   5. Self in literature.   I. Title.   II. Series: Twayne's
English authors series ; TEAS 524.
    PR4163,F73   1996
    823'.8—dc20   96–12871
                                                                                CIP

10   9   8   7   6   5   4   3   2   1

Printed in the United States of America

To my children,
Christopher Barton Frawley and Emma Sanford Frawley

Contents

Preface

Anne Brontë, the youngest child of the celebrated Brontë family, lived from 1820 until 1849 in Yorkshire, England. She wrote a significant body of poetry, some of which was copublished with her sisters Emily Brontë and Charlotte Brontë in *Poems* by Currer, Ellis and Acton Bell (1846). Brontë also published two novels, *Agnes Grey* (1847) and *The Tenant of Wildfell Hall* (1848). In the nearly 150 years since Brontë lived and wrote, literary critics and historians have come increasingly to appreciate her aesthetic and intellectual achievements. Their scholarship, however, continues to stress the autobiographical interest of her work. Brontë's life experiences, particularly her work as a governess and her relationship with her sisters, had an undeniable influence on her writing. Nevertheless, Brontë's poetry and fiction subsume a representation of personal experiences within a broader consideration of issues having to do with self-understanding, self-representation, and dilemmas of identity.

Drawing on some little-used and heretofore unknown primary sources, including Brontë's Bible, her diary papers, and her music manuscript books, *Anne Brontë* offers a detailed and comprehensive analysis of Brontë's increasingly sophisticated understanding of the psychological and social dimensions of identity. It reassesses long-standing assumptions about Brontë's use of autobiographical forms and rhetoric. Synthesizing a range of scholarship on the nature of subjectivity and on the form and function of life narratives, it elucidates Brontë's experimental approach to depicting modes of self-understanding and strategies of self-representation. The book positions Anne Brontë within the traditions of Victorian women's writing often depicted as "proto-feminist" and demonstrates in ways not yet considered the extent to which Brontë's social milieu nurtured her innovative approach to self-representation.

Acknowledgments

Many people have helped to make it possible for me to work on this book. I would like to acknowledge support from the Faculty Grants Committee at Elizabethtown College, which enabled me to begin amassing material on Anne Brontë. Members of the interlibrary loan staff of the High Library at Elizabethtown College have on many occasions expeditiously helped to locate books and articles necessary to my work. Frederick Ritsch, Provost of Elizabethtown College, has been particularly sensitive to my research needs. Thanks also to Herbert Sussman for his attentive readings of early drafts; and to my research assistant, Alison Labbate, for her indefatigable help in preparing the manuscript for production.

Librarians at the Pierpont Morgan Library in New York City provided me with crucial access to Brontë material. Ann Dinsdale and Kathryn White of the Brontë Parsonage Museum in Haworth, West Yorkshire, were accommodating, gracious, and informative in helping me to work with materials at their library. Finally, I would like to acknowledge the invaluable support of the National Endowment of the Humanities, which made it possible for me to travel to the Brontë Parsonage Museum and to spend an uninterrupted period of time on this book.

As always, I am thankful to Barbara Gates, who, in her legendary Brontë seminar at the University of Delaware, inspired my interest in the Brontë family. Most of all, I am grateful to my husband, William Frawley, for his perceptive advice and his inexhaustible encouragement and patience.

Chronology

1820 Anne Brontë born at Thornton, Bradford, Yorkshire, on 17 January.

Brontë family moves to Haworth in April.

1821 Brontë's mother, Maria Branwell Brontë, dies on 15 September.

1825 Older sister Maria Brontë dies on 6 May; older sister Elizabeth Brontë dies on 15 June.

1835 Anne Brontë takes the place of her sister Emily Brontë at Roe Head School, near Dewsbury Moor.

1837 Visits with Moravian minister James de la Trobe while at Roe Head.

Leaves Roe Head School in December.

1839 Becomes governess at the Ingham family home, Blake Hall, Mirfield, on 8 April.

William Weightman becomes curate at Haworth in April.

Leaves Blake Hall in December.

1840 Becomes governess at the Robinson family home, Thorp Green Hall, Little Ouseburn, in August.

1842 Aunt Elizabeth Branwell dies on 29 October.

1843 Branwell Brontë becomes tutor at Thorp Green in January.

1845 Anne Brontë leaves Thorp Green in June.

Branwell Brontë leaves Thorp Green in July.

1846 *Poems* by Currer, Ellis and Acton Bell published in May.

1847 *Agnes Grey* published in December.

1848 *The Tenant of Wildfell Hall* published in June. Anne Brontë and her sister Charlotte Brontë travel to London to prove separate identities to Charlotte Brontë's London publishers, Smith and Elder.

Anne Brontë writes Preface to the Second Edition of *The Tenant of Wildfell Hall* on 22 July.

1848   Anne Brontë's poem "The Three Guides" published in *Fraser's Magazine* in August.

Branwell Brontë dies on 24 September.

Emily Brontë dies on 19 December.

1849   Anne Brontë dies at Scarborough on 28 May.

Chapter One

"A Silent Invalid Stranger": Dilemmas of Identity in the Works of Anne Brontë

The 19th-century novelist and poet Anne Brontë has, in many ways, been condemned to be seen only as her family and friends saw her. Their labels are the ones that have resonated throughout nearly 150 years of scholarship on the Brontë family, especially in biographical and critical studies of Anne Brontë. "Exiled and harassed," was the way her sister Emily once described her.[1] To her sister Charlotte, on whom biographers have been most dependent for information regarding Anne, she was "a patient, persecuted stranger" (*BLFC,* I, 241), a woman who "covered her mind, and especially her feelings, with a sort of nun-like veil"[2] and who was "reserved even with her nearest of kin" (*BLFC,* II, 241). Most overtly deprecatory was her brother Branwell, who, in an often-quoted sentence, was said to have considered Anne "Nothing, absolutely nothing."[3] "Dear little Anne" to her father, Patrick Brontë (*BLFC,* I, 130), and "dear, gentle, Anne" (*BLFC,* I, 112) to the family friend Ellen Nussey, Anne Brontë—the youngest of the Brontë family—was little understood by the few people with whom she was intimate during her 29 years of life. Relatively little private writing of Brontë's remains from which to reconstruct an idea of how she might have seen herself and how she might have responded to the way others believed her to be; what does remain suggests a similar degree of inscrutability. In one of her last letters, written in May 1849 to turn down an offer to stay during her illness with the Nussey family, she describes herself simply as "a silent invalid stranger" (*BLFC,* II, 321).

The purpose of this book is not to refute the accuracy of these labels, which, for a variety of reasons, continue to influence the ways in which Anne Brontë's works are read and interpreted. Rather, its purpose is to challenge the assumption that such descriptions indicate weaknesses of Brontë or of her artistry. Indeed, by underscoring as they do the peculiar nature of Brontë's individuality—the autonomy she established and nur-

1

tured by distancing herself from those around her—such labels reveal one of the ideas most essential to her writing: *identity*. This book will explore the myriad ways that Brontë registered a concern with identity, the process and problems of self-fashioning, in her life and work. Brontë sought to preserve autonomy through a variety of distancing strategies and, in doing so, to suggest that privacy could function as a source of strength. Almost all of her work—which includes both published and unpublished poetry, two novels, private writing (i.e., diary papers, correspondence, and personal notes), and artwork (watercolor drawings and pencil sketches)—makes manifest an ongoing interest in the relationship between what today would be thought of as social, psychological, and spiritual dimensions of identity. Indeed, however frustrating it is to confront the sometimes disparaging and often inadequate labels that Brontë's family members and acquaintances used to describe her, it is clear that she cultivated an identity that both baffled and consternated others, often intentionally.

Anne Brontë's lifelong interest in dilemmas of identity led her, intellectually and emotionally, in several different directions during the course of her writing career. Much of her work—from juvenilia and early poetry to the novel she completed just two years before her death—reveals an ongoing exploration of the effort entailed in the related processes of apprehending and crafting identity. This exploration led her not to write her own autobiographical account per se, but rather to incorporate the idea of self-representation into much of her poetry, prose, and artwork, creating in the process a variety of hybrid genres. Through her innovative approach to self-representation Brontë worked toward the creation of an "axiology of the self," an understanding of identity that distinguished between private apprehension of being and public performance of self and that simultaneously accounted for such complexities as secrecy and self-deception.[4]

Several key ideas related to self-understanding and self-representation recur throughout Brontë's prose and poetry. The single most prominent of these ideas concerns the nature and function of *secrecy,* that which is either unwittingly or deliberately hidden from others. Brontë's interest in secrecy extended beyond human manifestations to the natural world: "A fine and subtle spirit dwells / in every little flower," she wrote in the poem "The Bluebell."[5] Much of Brontë's poetry suggests that secrecy can become a source of strength: "They little knew my hidden thoughts / And they will never know," the narrator of "Self-Congratulation" declares with pride (9, ll. 53–54). Yet in many other poems secrecy becomes a source of anguish; in "The Doubter's Prayer," for instance, the speaker grieves that "none can hear [her] secret call, / Or see the silent tears [she] weep[s]" (23, ll. 31–32).

The idea of secrecy is integral to Brontë's fiction as well. Her two novels—*Agnes Grey* (1847) and *The Tenant of Wildfell Hall* (1848)—both explore social, economic, and personal situations that prompt women in particular to adopt secrecy as a defense mechanism. Yet both novels also expose the extent to which secrecy becomes a form of emotional imprisonment. Agnes Grey initially keeps many of her career aspirations from her family; later, as a governess, she is routinely forced to internalize her feelings of disappointment and anger toward her employers as well as her feelings of love for the local curate. The heroine of *The Tenant of Wildfell Hall,* Helen Huntingdon, is initially unwilling to reveal to her family her doubts about her fiancé's integrity; once she has committed herself to the relationship, she internalizes her fears of a failing marriage, giving vent to her feelings only within the pages of her diary. Her subsequent—and criminal—decision to leave her husband, taking with her their young son, forces her to assume a false name, live in virtual seclusion, and keep her real identity a secret from her new community.

Related to the notion of secrecy, and equally prominent in Brontë's fiction and poetry, is the idea of *silence,* which functions most often to mark the secrecy that either protects or plagues her narrators. Like other women writers of her time, Brontë often used silence to signify a linguistic condition either willingly adopted by women or imposed on them against their will. Silence, like secrecy, simultaneously signifies within her work a form of power and a form of powerlessness. Both Agnes Grey and Helen Huntingdon make frequent use of their diaries to express concerns that they feel unable to openly relay to others. Moreover, both women, at key moments in the narratives, demonstrate their control of a situation—their power—by their refusal to speak.

Silence is central to Brontë's poetry as well. The speaker of the poem "Past Days" mourns for the time "When speech expressed the inward thought / And heart to kindred heart was bare" (26, ll. 7–8). The speaker of "Severed and Gone" prays within her "silent room" for a love relationship (55, l. 22). Most often, the women of Brontë's poems struggle to repress emotions that agitate the placid exteriors they strive to maintain. The narrator of "If This Be All" feels "powerless to quell / The silent current from within" (39, ll. 18–19). In Brontë's poetry, silence also functions as an indicator of a speaker's inability to articulate her emotions. In "Views of Life," for instance, she writes of an enthralling sunset sky that "I cannot name each lovely shade, / I cannot say how bright they shone;" (42, ll. 21–22). Brontë's poems reveal speakers who both control their world through their silence (e.g., "I would not tell") and who feel powerless in their awareness that others do not understand them (e.g., "Thou knowest not").

Another idea recurrent throughout Brontë's poetry and fiction is the experience of *isolation,* both situational and self-imposed, and its impact on the development of self. Brontë's poetic personas and fictional heroines are often women who feel physically and psychologically confined. Like the "solitary" dove of the poem "The Captive Dove," they feel condemned by circumstances to "pine neglected and alone" (24, l. 28). The women of Brontë's novels live in or are displaced to secluded regions of Britain; their jobs and marriages deprive them of close contact with their families; death separates them from loved ones; they are marginalized from society by professional occupation and social class; they lack intimate relationships outside family that would allow for emotional sharing; and they feel isolated and silenced within their families as well. In *Agnes Grey* Brontë represents in many ways the governess as working within an institution of isolation and, indeed, as embodying the concept herself. *The Tenant of Wildfell Hall,* in turn, explores the idea of isolation—both enforced and self-imposed—within marriage, within community, and, in a sense, within one's self. As Helen Huntingdon, the novel's heroine, explains to herself in her diary, "I wanted no confidant in my distress. I deserved none—and I wanted none. I had taken the burden upon myself: let me bear it alone."[6]

Predictably, situations of solitude have psychological correlates in Brontë's poetry as well, where her personas often explore the emotions that accompany their isolation. The speaker of "The Student's Serenade," for instance, revels in imagining that "O'er these wintry wilds alone / Thou wouldst joy to wander free," (29, ll. 41–42). Similarly, the speaker of a poetic fragment assumed to have been written while Brontë worked as a governess remarks, "But I would rather *weep* alone / Than *laugh* amid their revelry" (28, ll. 3–4). In many poems, Brontë explores the distinction between solitude and loneliness. The speaker of "Dreams" writes that "While on my lonely couch I lie / I seldom feel my self alone" (40, ll. 1–2). Yet, as often, Brontë's speakers feel condemned to a life of loneliness. Even "Dreams," which begins with the liberating notion that one's imagination can provide the pleasure that one's life experiences denies, ends with the speaker waking to gloom: "But then to wake and find it flown, / The dream of happiness destroyed / To find myself unloved, alone, / What tongue can speak the dreary void?" (ll. 21–24).

Binding the interrelated notions of secrecy, silence, and isolation together in Anne Brontë's work is, finally, an examination of whether individual identity is stable and consistent or whether it is malleable and inconsistent, fluctuating with different situational demands.[7] The idea that the self is in a fundamental sense malleable both intrigues and frightens Brontë, and her works consequently pose the dilemma in a variety of forms. One of her very early poems, "The Captive's Dream," begins with the narrator remarking, "Methought I saw him but I knew him not; / He was so changed from what he used to be" (4, ll. 1–2).

Brontë explores in her work a wide range of questions related to the issues of stability and malleability as they apply to selfhood. What does it mean to continually shuffle between public and private selves? What aspects of personality can or cannot change during a lifespan? How mutable is identity? What kinds of circumstances—physical, economic, social—can cause character to alter, temporarily or permanently? In *Agnes Grey,* the eponymous heroine struggles with a family that seems unwilling to recognize how she changes, and yet she herself depends upon the stability of those around her and is curiously afraid that others might change. *The Tenant of Wildfell Hall* revolves around Helen Huntingdon's gradual coming to terms with the extent to which her husband's alcohol abuse alters dimensions of his character that she once refused to acknowledge and that she has no power to change. Like Agnes Grey, she, too, is plagued by a sense that her own character is malleable in ways she little foresaw. Two years into her marriage Helen worries that is she "becoming more indifferent and insensate" and reveals her astonishment in her diary by exclaiming, "How immeasurably changed was I!" (*TWH,* 274 and 275). Brontë's concern with and beliefs about individual identity and self-representation permeate her poetry and fiction. The thematics of secrecy, silence, and isolation, and their relationship to the question of selfhood as stable or malleable, must, however, be understood as part and parcel of Brontë's overarching sense of her duty as a writer.

Brontë's primary aesthetic imperative was to be honest with her subject matter, to resist the temptation to represent human experiences, and especially women's experiences, as in any way better than they actually were. As she explained in the "Preface to the Second Edition" of *The Tenant of Wildfell Hall,* "I would rather whisper a few wholesome truths therein than much soft nonsense" (*TWH,* 29). The faithful pursuit of truth, even in fiction, was one she believed necessary because of what she understood to be the didactic purposes of fiction. In a frequently quoted portion of the "Preface," she attacked the "delicate concealment of facts" pervasive in her society by writing: "To represent a bad thing in its least offensive light is doubtless the most agreeable course for a writer of fiction to pursue; but is it the most honest, or the *safest*? Is it better to reveal the snares and pitfalls of life to the young and thoughtless traveler, or to cover them with branches and flowers?" (*TWH*, 30; emphasis mine). Here Brontë adopts a kind of maternal mantle, endowing the role of the novelist with the rhetoric of motherly duties to educate and protect, in this case by exposure to "real-life" experiences. Indeed, it was precisely her strong belief in the imperative of honest representation that enabled her to overcome the kind of silence that so constricted the women of her fictional and poetic worlds. Later in the "Preface" she proclaimed, "When I feel it my duty to speak an unpalatable truth, with the help of God, I *will* speak it" (30).

Although Brontë's quest to represent truthfully the dilemmas experienced by 19th-century women led some of her critics to accuse her of a "morbid love of the coarse, if not of the brutal," it was one that, in the end, was marked not by what one might expect—bitter resignation or angry denial—but instead by a tentative declaration of hope.[8] Brontë found hope for self-understanding and fulfillment in a variety of ways. Much of her work suggests that she believed childhood could offer a lifelong sense of confidence; that memory could provide one with unlimited access to past securities; that the imagination could offer temporary escape from a hostile environment; that nature could remind one of the possibility for transcendence; that a benevolent God offered the possibility and promise of salvation to even the most sinful of people; and finally, that the human heart, for Brontë the repository of hope, enabled one to feel love, even in the most desperate situations.

As her novels and poetry illustrate, Brontë understood the multidimensionality of human identity, its power and its powerlessness, and was keenly attentive to the many ways that experiences could impact the self in the constitution of identity. Not surprisingly, Brontë was attuned as well to the implications of this dynamic model of identity for her own sense of self. Indeed, the thematics of her fiction are the thematics of her life: there, too, she struggled with and yet embraced secrecy, silence, and solitude; there, too, she speculated about how her own "character" would change over time. Although scant, what biographical information is available about Brontë's life experiences reveals a woman well aware of the differences between her own public and private personas and attuned to the ways she had changed and would change over the years. For example, one of Brontë's diary papers, written in July 1845, surveyed a hypothetical future for herself and her family and concluded with the following question and comment: "What changes shall we have seen and known; and shall we be much changed ourselves? I hope not, for the worse at least. I for my part cannot well be flatter or older in mind than I am now" (*BLFC,* II, 53). Other portions of Brontë's writing intimate that she felt her identity within her family as daughter or sister to constitute a public "role," and that only God had access to the private being, the true self, that she sought to discern.

Existing biographical information on Brontë also reveals a person who struggled with perplexing questions about the impact of her circumstances. She pondered the impact on her identity of her position within the family as the *youngest* daughter. She explored the effects of her regional heritage—the impact of growing up in a remote, rural region of Britain. Economic circumstances—the advantages and disadvantages of having to work for a living—were also part of Brontë's ongoing inquiry into how her identity evolved over time. Adding still another level of complexity to her thinking on these matters was an abiding religious sensibility and faith that on some occasions exacerbated and at other times assuaged her concerns about the limitations of self-apprehension and self-control. Just as she provides no simplistic solutions in her poetry or fiction to the inevitable questions raised in her exploration of identity, so too does her private writing suggest an unstinting commitment to truth, even if that commitment entails accepting sometimes uncomfortable degrees of uncertainty.

One important and exciting consequence of Brontë's ongoing interest in the apprehension, development, and representation of self is the often innovative interplay in her work between fictional and autobiographical modes and materials. The interweaving between the two, while central to her methods, has nonetheless posed considerable interpretive difficulties to her biographers and critics, who all too often have felt it necessary to rely on the fiction and poetry to "reveal" and interpret Brontë's life experiences. Much Brontë scholarship is shaped by the reverse tendency as well: that is, critics have in the past relied heavily on information about her life experiences, scant as it is, to interpret her work. Brontë biographer Edward Chitham aptly summarizes these methodological difficulties when he writes, "One of our reasons for seeking a biography of any author is to help to illuminate that author's works; but if the major source for that biography *is* the corpus of those works, how can we avoid a vicious circle in which we read autobiography into the literature and then use our observations to show how the fiction grew from the life?"[9]

Such interpretive challenges are partially inevitable, given the limited nature of information on Brontë's life experiences. Nonetheless, they are intensified by an equally prevalent, if more pernicious, trend in scholarhip on Brontë: the tendency to restrict interpretation of her personality, life experiences, and artistic output to its comparative interest; that is, to study Anne Brontë and her work according to the ways she duplicates or departs from the attributes that have come to be associated with her sisters Emily Brontë and Charlotte Brontë. To a certain extent, Brontë's personality, life experiences, and artistic output were greatly affected by her relationship to her sisters: for most of her life, the sisters lived and worked together; as motherless women, they were each other's primary sources of emotional sustenance; they were each other's first readers and critics; they were arguably each other's most important literary influences. Nonetheless, the comparative analyses so endemic to scholarship on Brontë characteristically reduce the interest of their relationships to the superficial. Thus, Anne Brontë has often been described—probably from Elizabeth Gaskell's biography *The Life of Charlotte Brontë* onward—as more attractive if less engaging than her sister Charlotte and as more outgoing if less talented than her sister Emily.[10] Indeed, comparative analyses permeate all scholarship on the Brontës. As Helena Michie has wryly commented of the Brontës: "These sisters internalize the idiom of comparison; they come to life with respect to each other, sometimes without respect for each other."[11]

The related tendency to read Brontë's works against those of her sisters—for instance, to study *Agnes Grey* as Brontë's version of *Jane Eyre,* or to examine *The Tenant of Wildfell Hall* as a reworking and domestication of *Wuthering Heights*—has been equally damaging to her reputation. Even critics eager to correct the historical undervaluation of Brontë's achievements have fallen prey to the lure of comparative analysis, reproducing the approach they claim to reject.[12]

Clearly, situated as they were within Haworth Parsonage, virtually removed, except via the books and magazines they routinely read, from the kind of literary community beginning writers would have found in London, or even Manchester, the Brontë sisters created a kind of literary culture within the confines of their own home, and their close working relationship warrants a certain amount of critical comparison between their artistic output. Yet, the comparative trends pervasive in Brontë scholarship have resulted in often misguided notions of Anne Brontë's works as artistically or intellectually "lesser" than those of her sisters and have oversimplified the significance of biographical slants on and autobiographical impulses within her writing. Consequently, critics have missed the single most important dimension of her writing: that the intermingling of fact and fiction, experienced and imagined, was a necessary and deliberate feature of Brontë's work that enabled her to represent the ways in which selfhood is both experienced *and* fashioned.

An understanding of the "purely" autobiographical dimensions of Anne Brontë's work—that is, the elements of her writing that documented her own lived experiences—is, notwithstanding these drawbacks, crucial, especially given the extent to which her writing concerns itself with society's impact on identity. Autobiographical impulses—important, if sometimes difficult to discern—emerge throughout her writing, early and late; these impulses cannot be traced back to single identifiable or verifiable events, but they are critical to an understanding of her artistic efforts. To appreciate fully the myriad ways in which Brontë's work is informed by what might be thought of as autobiographical impulses requires first a clear understanding of what has been and can be meant by the term "autobiography."

Autobiographical Issues and Anne Brontë Scholarship

Interpreting Anne Brontë's work as "autobiographical" in the most traditional sense of the term—that is, as a self-composed narrative of one's life experiences, mimetically transcribed—has tended historically to eradicate important complexities of her work and to limit appreciation of her overall achievement. As one critic has summarized it, "The self who lives is not the same as the self who writes, but that is not to say that the first is simply irrelevant and 'dead.'"[13] Interpreting Brontë's work as having attributes of *life writing* allows one instead to more fully address the potential for cross-fertilization between its fictional and its nonfictional dimensions and to acknowledge the indeterminacy with which Brontë's narratives embrace subjectivity and objectivity.[14]

To appreciate the variety of ways in which life writing evidences itself in Brontë's poetry, fiction, letters, and diary passages, though, one must begin with what is most closely based on the actuality of her life. No biographer or critic of Brontë could legitimately or profitably read her work without an awareness and acknowledgement of the impact that her experiences had on her writing. These experiences range from the concrete to the less tangible. For example, Brontë's experiences as a governess first at Blake Hall in Mirfield and later at Thorp Green Hall were undeniably important determinants of plot and character in her first novel, *Agnes Grey*. Similarly, her dismay at witnessing the damaging effects of drugs and alcohol on her once talented brother Branwell undoubtedly shaped her characterization of Arthur Huntingdon in *The Tenant of Wildfell Hall*. Equally influential, though less readily identifiable, is the impact on Brontë of growing up from infancy without her mother, who died less than two years after she was born. Several of her poems, for example, "The Orphan's Lament," are surely related in some ways to her own experiences as a motherless child.

Nonetheless, many of Brontë's readers have overestimated the extent to which her works are dominated by the strictly autobiographical. Biographical scholarship about Brontë often assumes a transparent relationship between the fictional and the autobiographical.[15] The critical drive to distill out of Brontë's work that which can be clearly labeled "autobiographical" haunts interpretation of her poetry as well, which is often divided into two discrete genres, one "concerned with an imaginary environment" and the other "based on situations encountered in actual life" (Chitham, 1991, 10).

The traditional notions of what constitutes the autobiographical and what constitutes the imaginary that undergird these divisions have dictated not just biographical studies but, more important, critical interpretations of Brontë's work as well. Most often, the autobiographical impulses of Brontë's work, interpreted in the most traditional and limited sense described above, have been seen as superseding other authorial imperatives, whether they be aesthetic or didactic. Brontë's critics have resisted more broadly historical interpretations, interpreting much of her work in relation to a select number of significant life experiences, among them her experiences as a governess, her relationship to her brother Branwell, and her presumed affection for the Reverend William Weightman, who from 1839 until 1842, when he died, was her father's curate at Haworth. While these "actual life experiences" are undoubtedly important to understanding much about Brontë's life and work, they have overshadowed more subtle and more important dimensions of her writing.

Interpreting the governess's experience that Brontë explores in *Agnes Grey* simply (and simplistically) as mirroring Brontë's own often degrading experiences as a governess obscures the multiple ways that Brontë used the governess figure to introduce into her narrative a subtle examination of the fluidity of boundaries between the ostensibly rigid binary of the public and the private, to interrogate the nature of subjectivity, and to explore more broadly the notion of social invisibility, a notion that for her extended in its implications far beyond the situation of the governess. Identifying the fictional character Edward Weston in *Agnes Grey,* the man whom Agnes eventually marries, with William Weightman glosses over the many ways that Brontë uses Weston as a figure to explore the peculiar nature of Agnes's secrecy and silence and their relationship to her desire for intimacy; her drive to rescue others and to be rescued herself; and the related ideas of social position and class boundaries, particularly as they affect individual identity. Similarly, several of Brontë's poems that have to do with love relationships have been seen as mere reflections of her grief at Weightman's death and the consequent loss of any romantic prospect for herself, rather than as the sophisticated analyses of isolation and identity that they are.

While *The Tenant of Wildfell Hall* has, in general, prompted a far wider and more complex range of responses than *Agnes Grey,* it too has suffered from overly restrictive interpretations based on biographical readings of the text. Interpreting Arthur Huntingdon's demise simply as a reflection of Brontë's dismay at the physical and moral failure of Branwell ignores a number of fascinating dimensions of his character: the ways that he draws on a language that relies on Helen's silence; the ways he in turn "voices" predominantly male assumptions about the role and function of women; and the impact of his objectifying language on Helen's own subjectivity. Reading the portions of the text that concern themselves with Arthur's presumed failure to take responsibility for his self and to ask for forgiveness of his sins as mere reflections of Brontë's own reaction against the Calvinist notion of a "spiritual elect" and correlary desire to believe in universal salvation obscures the ways that Brontë uses these scenes to demarcate new stages in her heroine's understanding of her own identity and her increasing unwillingness to play the role of savior.[16]

Any discussion of Anne Brontë's critical heritage must acknowledge that Charlotte Brontë was Anne Brontë's first reader and critic and is at least partially responsible for inaugurating a reductive tradition of interpretation. In private letters to her publisher William Smith Williams as well as in the "Biographical Notice" that she appended to the 1850 edition of her sisters' work, Charlotte Brontë diminished Anne's achievement precisely by reducing it—if implicitly—to its autobiographical elements. Alluding to the spectacle of Branwell's demise and its impact on her sister's second novel, Charlotte Brontë wrote in the "Biographical Notice":

> She had, in the course of her life, been called on to contemplate, near at hand, and for a long time, the terrible effects of talents misused and faculties abused: hers was naturally a sensitive, reserved, and dejected nature; what she saw sank very deeply into her mind; it did her harm. She brooded over it till she believed it to be a duty to reproduce every detail (of course with fictitious characters, incidents, and situations) as a warning to others.[17]

Charlotte Brontë here intimates that *The Tenant of Wildfell Hall* is little more than a transcription of life into literature and that Anne Brontë's role as writer was simply to supply, as it were, fictitious names for her persons and places, easily identifiable for their "real" counterparts. Anne Brontë's critics today almost unanimously recognize the extent to which critical estimation of her artistic worth was negatively influenced by Charlotte Brontë's judgment.[18]

Brontë herself on several occasions called attention to the fact that certain portions of her fiction were based on situations she had actually experienced. For instance, when critics attacked *Agnes Grey* for exaggerating the kind of hardships to which governesses were subjected, she responded by calling attention to the painstaking efforts she had made to truthfully "mirror" her own experiences. In the "Preface to the Second Edition" of *The Tenant of Wildfell Hall,* she wrote:

> As the story of "Agnes Grey" was accused of extravagant over-colouring in those very parts that were carefully copied from the life, with a most scrupulous avoidance of all exaggeration, so, in the present work, I find myself censured for depicting *con amore,* with a "morbid love of the coarse, if not of the brutal," those scenes which, I will venture to say, have not been more painful for the most fastidious of my critics to read, than they were for me to describe. (*TWH,* 29–30)

Anne Brontë here uses language very much like that invoked by her sister Charlotte to explain the dubious motivations that led Anne to write *The Tenant of Wildfell Hall.* Brontë suggests that her aesthetic motivations were ultimately limited to the mimetic—that is, that she essentially "copied" onto paper what she had experienced in life, deliberately avoiding artistry (what she refers to as "over-colouring") precisely because she wanted only to be truthful to her subject matter, even if it were painful to do so.

One could argue that both Charlotte and Anne Brontë were driven to make their respective declarations regarding the supposed representational accuracy of *The Tenant of Wildfell Hall* by their awareness (and anticipation) of the kind of criticism to which the novel—like so much Victorian fiction of the period—was subjected, criticism underwritten by a code that Richard Altick aptly described as "circulating library morality."[18] What matters most, however, is that like many of their readers— then and now—both sisters assume in their arguments a fundamental distinction between the experienced and the imagined, the autobiographical and the fictional.

Driven in large measure by theoretical work on the complex nature of subjectivity, recent theories of autobiographical writing have challenged the assumption that there is "nothing problematical about the *autos,* no agonizing questions of identity, self-definition, self-existence, or self-deception."[20] These issues are made more perplexing when applied to women's experiences, which historically have been shaped by ideologies of selfhood and notions of what constitutes the public and the private that are different from those for men. Brontë's fiction, poetry, and personal writing is replete with subtle autobiographic maneuvers that invoke questions of self-definition and self-deception, problematizing identity in just the way that contemporary feminist theorists of autobiography have argued for. Nonetheless, any attempt to understand the complexities of self-understanding and self-representation in Brontë's work must necessarily attend to the ways that her approach to personal and social history are related. In fact, much of her fiction and poetry indicates that she wrote not to bridge the gulf between the two but rather to represent and explore their interactive relationship.

Sociohistorical Contexts of Anne Brontë's Work

Elucidating the interplay of fictional and autobiographic technique within Brontë's work would seem, at first glance, to be an end in itself, a way of capturing both the flavor and the complexity of her writing in a single sweeping critical perspective. Even the most private kinds of autobiographical writing, though, are public gestures of a sort. Despite the misleading myth of the Brontë sisters as isolated geniuses, Anne Brontë's social and historical milieu nurtured her artistry and affected in a variety of ways all of her writing, even the most ostensibly private. All forms of self-representation, Brontë's included, are in some sense products of their time, "rhetorical projects embedded in concrete material situations" (Gagnier, 1991, 31). While it is tempting—especially given her own attention to the isolating nature of her rural heritage—to view Brontë's work as the product of a self-enclosed environment, as literature only minimally impacted by the culture which surrounded it, such a perspective distorts the ways that her understanding of self was situated in relation to her social history and in relation to the ideologies of gender, class, race, and nation that underwrote that history.

Moving from autobiographical to sociohistorical contexts of Brontë's writing hence does not involve a radical change in perspective.[21] One way to view the relationship between the autobiographical and the sociohistorical contexts is by emphasizing the degree to which Brontë's understanding of her self as a woman was a product of the objectifying discourses she inhabited. Many issues that are now seen as central to Victorian social history—for example, marriage and the family, sickness and health care, religion and spiritualism, philanthropy and social reform—shared a dependency on rhetoric that exalted a domestic ideal and the nature and function of woman within the private sphere and that in the process helped to constitute the meaning of womanhood. Brontë tackled some social issues directly in her fiction; *The Tenant of Wildfell Hall,* for instance, questioned the legitimacy of laws that deprived married women of property rights. Typically, however, her writing focused not on specific social issues but more generally on the complexities of the domestic sphere and of private life. The dilemmas of identity that Brontë's heroines face—the struggles to develop adequate strategies of self-representation within a circumscribed domestic sphere—are part of a cultural critique that should be understood as rooted in the social history of her time. It is no surprise, then, that Brontë's authorial career coincides with what some literary historians have identified as the emergence of widespread cultural pressure on middle-class women to identify themselves through their "exalted mission as mother[s]."[22]

The media through which Brontë may have encountered such ideals and exhortations were legion, ranging from popular fiction and art of all kinds to an array of nonfictional sources—magazines, tracts, conduct manuals and advice books.[23] Brontë—whose family routinely supplemented a better-than-average home library with borrowings from the local library—was surely exposed to and familiar with many of these. The family library included, for example, Hannah More's *Moral Sketches of Opinions and Manners* (1819), and Anne Brontë herself owned G. Wright's *Thoughts in Younger Life on Interesting Subjects* (1778), a collection of anecdotes geared toward the proper moral development of young women. Throughout the 19th century, popular "marriage manuals" addressed to women proffered advice on family relations, roles, and lifestyles in the home; conduct books instructed women on how to keep a morally and physically healthy house; medical psychology textbooks were based on assumptions of the debilitating nature of female physiology; and a variety of legal documents—addressing, among other things, marriage and divorce, mothers and children, and ownership of property—constructed a woman essentially without rights. The same ideals promulgated in these nonfictional documents were conveyed, through other means, in the popular poetry and fiction of the period, with which the well-read Anne Brontë was familiar.

Much of the social history that is now associated with Brontë's culture was premised, then, on largely essentialistic notions of "woman" that in turn helped to naturalize a separation of public and private spheres of activity. Brontë's response to an ideology of "separate spheres" grew out of her exposure to this wide-ranging literature.[24] Sometimes she represented it as an ideology imposed on women, sometimes as a set of boundaries expected to be observed and willingly accommodated by women, and sometimes as an existence nurtured by women to preserve an autonomous existence.[25] No matter how she invoked the ideology, however, she used it to address the psychological and social realities of domestic life and to further her analysis of the implications of private life.

In relying exclusively on the notion of separate spheres to understand the gendered conditions of Victorian society, however, historians run the risk of vastly oversimplifying women's experience. This oversimplification is in turn reflected in much of the work done on 19th-century women writers, including Anne Brontë. The distinctions between the public and the private central to the ideology of separate spheres became blurred as the century progressed. It is within the historical moment at which the idea of separate spheres—with its complex network of cultural meanings—came distinctively into focus, only to then become subject to various forms of cultural debate, that one can locate Anne Brontë's work.[26]

Brontë's writing is embedded within a historical moment that marked itself both through its articulation of separate spheres and through its simultaneous engagement with the ambiguities of the ideology. She chose not to adopt the particular artistic techniques that critics have identified in the work of her sisters. She avoided the kind of approach that Charlotte Brontë used in her novel *Shirley*—an approach that explicitly situated the romance plot within the Luddite riots of the early 1800s. Nor did she consistently endow her work with the kind of regional accuracy that had a more general historical correlation—such as that Emily Brontë displayed in *Wuthering Heights*. Anne Brontë opted instead to work with the social history of her time through the use of several key figures. Stressing the ways in which Brontë constructed these figures to expose and assess ideological intersections, such as those between gender and class, can ultimately help to illuminate the historical underpinnings of her work.

Chief among the figures that Brontë worked with in her writing are the governess, the married woman, the mother, the artist, the invalid, and the "sinner." Through her often innovative representation of these figures, all to some extent recognizable "types" to a Victorian readership, Brontë layered her work with a host of cultural meanings that have specific historical relevance. Adding even greater complexity to her work, she often conflated figures precisely to expose and examine their contradictory natures: she scrutinized, for instance, the married woman and mother as artist; the mother as invalid; the artist as "sinner," and, last but not least, the surprisingly complex and problematic figure of the married woman as mother. In *Agnes Grey* and *The Tenant of Wildfell Hall,* as well as in much of her poetry, Brontë used these figures to register her concern about such issues as the social positioning of women within marriage and family; the role of women as moral, physical, and spiritual caregivers; the problem of women's rights in relation to property law; the utopian potential of feminine education; employment opportunities for middle-class women; charity as a female form of "rescue" work; the passive positioning of the female sexual subject; and the science of nature as a kind of feminine project.

Probably the figure who best illustrates Brontë's techniques and interests in this regard is that of the governess, who occupied a complex and ambiguous position in Victorian society. The contradictory position of the governess is in part exemplified in the range of responses that she elicited throughout the Victorian period, but especially in the 1830s and 1840s, when Brontë was writing. As a figure of female labor, she was an object of social condemnation as well as a social cause—a cause that organizations like the Governesses' Benevolent Institution were formed to support. The governess was not simply a figure of problematic class, however, for she also symbolized a kind of precarious relationship to the ideals of "true womanhood." She could enact her presumably inherent maternal instincts by functioning as a surrogate mother within the household, but she did so without any of the mother's authority. *Agnes Grey* in particular illustrates the ways in which issues of social status and sexual identity converge in the governess. In the novel Brontë exposes the impact of governess work on a young woman's developing psyche, and especially on her self-esteem, as well as her understanding of social roles. Brontë uses the governess figure to explore the relationship between social behavior and psychological development. *Agnes Grey* is thus much more than a *Bildungsroman*, an instructional novel, or a social problem novel—all labels that critics have reductively applied to Brontë's work. Using the governess figure, Brontë deftly moves from addressing broad social issues that impact the status of women in her society to questioning the extent to which identity is formed in response to different situational demands.

Having studied the relationship between psychological identity and social behavior in her representation of the experiences of the governess, Brontë turned to other tasks in *The Tenant of Wildfell Hall*. One of the reasons her second novel has generally been regarded as a greater artistic achievement is because of its more direct, complex, and unusually confrontational treatment of controversial Victorian social questions. *The Tenant of Wildfell Hall* explores more thoroughly the issues of gender, property, and propriety that are only hinted at in *Agnes Grey*. The differences between the titles of the two novels—one marking a secure individual and stable female identity and the other suggesting anonymity and displacement—point to Brontë's increasing awareness of the problematics of women's identities as social, political, economic, and sexual beings in Victorian England. Using a variety of narrative techniques (e.g., conflating epistolary with other classic autobiographic forms) and enclosing her heroine's voice within a small pocket of narrative reserved for the revelation of her diary, Brontë stylistically reinforces many of the political themes the novel broaches, most notably the "hidden" position of middle-class women within the confines of home, that quintessentially private sphere.[27] Brontë also found in *The Tenant of Wildfell Hall* the opportunity to examine thoroughly the ways in which traditional religious discourse encourages women both to accommodate and to subvert Victorian patriarchal ideologies. She accomplishes these ends primarily through the heroine Helen Huntingdon, who at various times within the text identifies herself—and is identified by others—as a wife, a widow, a nurse, an artist, a tenant, and an exile. While Brontë historicized her second novel through her complex treatment of the hybrid identities assumed by and imposed on Victorian middle-class women like Helen Huntingdon, she also used this character to study the relationship between privacy and personhood.

Self-Representation, History, and the Psychic Geography of Anne Brontë's Writing

Anne Brontë's writing—most pointedly her fiction—illustrates well the extent to which questions of self-understanding and strategies of self-representation are governed by historical contexts. To recognize the historical contexts of Brontë's writing is not to suggest that she simplistically responded in her work to historical events as they unfolded and "surrounded" her. Rather, it is to argue that her work is integrally related to a complex web of historical conditions and that the autobiographical dimensions of her writing were ultimately subsumed within broader historical and ontological considerations.

To fully understand and appreciate the complexities of Brontë's work necessitates attending both to its mimetic dimensions and to its semiotic appeal, the one emphasizing the ways that narrative and poetry may function as a representation of life and the other emphasizing the many ways that texts play with language.[28] Acknowledging the multiple contexts that are necessary to understanding Brontë's work and the circumstances of their production enables a more complete apprehension of the polyphony of voices within single works as well as her oeuvre. Alternatively, failing to acknowledge and analyze these contexts causes a reification of the very limitations that Brontë herself sought throughout much of her work to expose and analyze. As Joan Wallach Scott writes:

> To ignore politics in the recovery of the female subject is to accept the reality of public/private distinctions and the separate or distinctive qualities of women's character and experience. It misses the chance not only to challenge the accuracy of binary distinctions…but to expose the very political nature of a history written in those terms.[29]

As the following chapters demonstrate, Anne Brontë registered throughout her career an interest in and concern with the psychological and social underpinnings of identity, particularly as faced by individual women—whether herself, one of her poetic personas, or one of her fictional heroines. In a variety of ways, Brontë showed that these dilemmas emanate out of problematic understandings of public and private roles—

understandings that could be both accommodated and subverted. Brontë drew on and out of her own experiences precisely because doing so enabled her to purposefully intermingle fact with fiction, and to explore in the process the impact of "private" heritage on "public" persona as well as the relationship of both to social world, what the psychologist Jerome Bruner calls "psychic geography."

Brontë used self-representation as a strategy to constitute her own identity and to respond to the world in which that identity was situated. Although driven by the cultural anxieties that so often attended Victorian women who wrote, the self-proclaimed "silent invalid stranger" was also, in the end, an important public voice, one whose writing helped not just to elucidate the interactive relationship between personal and social history but to argue, if implicitly, for the complex ways in which that relationship directs the ways in which women shape—and are shaped by—their life experiences.

Chapter Two

"At the Foot of a Secret Sinai": Anne Brontë's Life

To all but a small number of people, Anne Brontë would not be known until she died, when Charlotte Brontë set to work preparing editions of her poetry and fiction and simultaneously issuing biographical statements prepared for the occasion of publication. Just a year after Anne Brontë's death in 1849, and still grieving from the almost back-to-back deaths of Branwell and Emily as well, Charlotte Brontë set to work preparing a new edition of *Wuthering Heights and Agnes Grey*.[1] The new edition included a section titled "Selections from Poems by Acton Bell," and prefixed to this section was a short introduction in which Charlotte Brontë assessed her sister Anne's personality and the meaning of her life. This introductory statement would have lasting influence not only on the way Anne Brontë's works would subsequently be read but also on the way in which Anne Brontë herself would be understood.

Charlotte Brontë began the introduction by writing:

> In looking over my sister Anne's papers, I find mournful evidence that religious feeling had been to her but too much like what it was to Cowper; I mean, of course, in a far milder form. Without rendering her a prey to those horrors that defy concealment, it subdued her mood and bearing to a perpetual pensiveness; the pillar of a cloud glided constantly before her eyes; she ever waited at the foot of a secret Sinai, listening in her heart to the voice of a trumpet sounding long and waxing louder. Some, perhaps, would rejoice over these tokens of sincere though sorrowing piety in a deceased relative: I own, to me they seem sad, as if her whole innocent life had been passed under the martyrdom of an unconfessed physical pain.[2]

What is intriguing about this assessment is the way in which a thematic of repression—of secrecy and silence—dominates Charlotte Brontë's portrait of her sister. Relying on a rhetoric of restraint, she stresses the emotional barriers that her sister constructed: the "pensiveness" that characterized her mood and bearing; the emotional "cloud" that ostensibly obstructed her view; the internal "voice" that only she could hear; the "pain" of which she never spoke. To Charlotte Brontë, her sister epitomized the silent sufferer—part victim, part saint. For generations of readers relying to a large extent on these initial biographical descriptions, Brontë would thus become a paradigmatic Victorian woman, one taught by her culture to "suffer, and be still."[3]

Perhaps most important for future biographers, Charlotte Brontë suggests that even those most intimately connected with her sister were prevented from having access to her, that no one really knew what she thought or felt. In a curious inversion, she goes on in the introduction to find a source of consolation in the death that she was unable to locate in the life, one stemming from her conviction that her sister's lurking doubts about the promise of salvation were resolved in the end and that she died "patiently—serenely—victoriously" (C. Brontë 1850, vi).

Charlotte Brontë was largely responsible for preparing the image of her sisters presented to and ultimately absorbed by the reading public. Her control extended from making many now suspect editorial decisions in the process of preparing editions of the poetry and fiction for the press to the less tangible, but no less significant, statements of character such as the one quoted above that would often be appended to these works. For example, in a letter written to her publisher William Smith Williams dated 5 September 1850, Charlotte Brontë wrote:

> "Wildfell Hall" it hardly appears to me desirable to preserve. The choice of subject in that work is a mistake: it was too little consonant with the character, tastes, and ideas of the gentle, retiring, inexperienced writer. She wrote it under a strange, conscientious, half-ascetic notion of accomplishing a painful penance and a severe duty. Blameless in deed and almost in thought, there was from her very childhood a tinge of religious melancholy in her mind. This I ever suspected, and I have found amongst her papers mournful proofs that such was the case. (*BLFC*, III, 156)

Yet while it has become a critical commonplace to approach Charlotte Brontë's editorial efforts with suspicion, her emphasis on privacy—both in the introduction to "Selections from the Poetry of Acton Bell" and in this letter to Williams—is on target, in that it points to the primacy of the private in Anne Brontë's life experiences and writing. Although Charlotte Brontë was unable to interpret this privacy except as evidence of her sister's martyrlike suffering, Anne Brontë in fact embraced and nurtured privacy for reasons whose implications range from the personal to the social, the historical, and the cultural.

Early Influences

To appreciate the multitude of ways in which Brontë came to embrace privacy and to investigate its implications in her work entails first understanding its relationship to her heritage—her position within her family, their social background, and their everyday life at Haworth Parsonage in Yorkshire. Born in Thornton, England, on 17 January 1820, Brontë moved just a few months later with her family to Haworth, where her father, the Reverend Patrick Brontë, was appointed the community's "perpetual curate," or new rector. In the years in which Brontë lived in Haworth, it was a relatively crowded industrial town populated primarily by subsistence farmers, weavers, and milliners. Less than 10 miles from Thornton, it was nonetheless "vastly different in terms of social outlook" and seemed to Brontë's mother to be "a banishment."[4] Although Haworth, high in the rugged mountains known as the Pennines, was seemingly far removed from centers of urban expansion, its population doubled in the first half of the century.

Moving into Haworth Parsonage, which had nine small but comfortable rooms, considerably improved living standards for the Brontë family, which at that time included six children in addition to the Reverend and Mrs. Brontë. Though it was an improvement, the house had only five bedrooms and had to accommodate, besides the family, two servants and a nurse for Mrs. Brontë, who was already suffering from the cancer that would kill her. Haworth itself was far from healthy; it lacked sewers, suffered from a notoriously polluted and inadequate water supply, and had an almost continuously damp climate. No visitor to the graveyard that surrounds the parsonage can help being stunned by the sheer number of people who died during the years the Brontë family resided there, as gravestone after gravestone—often carrying the dates of infant and child deaths—attests. There were 1,344 burials in the churchyard between 1840 and 1850, and the average age of death was 25 years ("Haworth," n.p.). Although all the Brontës outlived this standard, their lives were full of nearly constant reminders that life for many people was short and difficult. Nearly every window of the parsonage from which Brontë would have looked provides an overview of the graveyard.

Brontë's physical surroundings at Haworth combine in several respects to suggest a symbolic backdrop for the isolation that would come to characterize her demeanor and hence may be thought of as helping to constitute her "psychic geography." Positioned in between the front of the graveyard and the village of Haworth is the Parish Church of St. Michael and All Angels, where Brontë's father preached. Built in 1755 by William Grimshaw, a friend of John Wesley, the church was an important monument in the history of the Evangelical Revival and for Brontë would have had many associations beyond that of her father's place of employment.

If a graveyard and a church separated Brontë from neighbors and the bustle of Haworth activity, so too did the surrounding landscape seem to separate her from the rest of the world. Lying beyond the remaining sides of the graveyard as well as the back of the Parsonage itself were the moors, miles and miles of rough landscape characterized by a craggy and unkempt appearance—"an endless expanse of heather, bracken, ling, bilberry, moss and grass stretching as far as the eye could see, changing colour with the seasons."[5] Anne Brontë, like others in her family, found comfort in these harsh and austere surroundings, which would be associated for her with the freedom of childhood outings and with her relatively peaceful early years, during which family members were living together at home.

The entire family was not together for long, however, for Brontë's mother died of stomach cancer in September 1821, just a year and a half after Brontë's birth and the family's move to Haworth. During the months of illness that led to her death, she had remained isolated in her bedroom and, according to Elizabeth Gaskell, "was not very anxious to see much of her children."[6] The children kept themselves occupied with long walks over the moors. Furthermore, their father, always busy during the day with his parish duties, took his meals alone and "did not regularly converse with his children" (Gardiner, 1992, 48). Finally, Brontë's two oldest sisters, Maria and Elizabeth, both died shortly after having been sent to the Clergy Daughters' School at Cowan Bridge.[7]

The remoteness of Anne Brontë's physical surroundings may well have exacerbated a more fundamental sense of loneliness and isolation that began with her mother's death and continued in subsequent years. Although Brontë apparently did not remember her mother, she undoubtedly learned much of her from her family; the children kept the memory of their "independent-minded" mother alive with drawings and by reading letters that she had written to their father.[8] Brontë was in all likelihood more affected than her sisters by another piece of writing associated with her mother. As a young woman, Mrs. Brontë had written a short tract titled "The Advantages of Poverty in Religious Concerns," which may have later inspired Brontë to address the same topic in her own writing, particularly in *Agnes Grey.*

Although Brontë's father made several efforts to remarry after his wife died, he remained single for the rest of his life. Elizabeth Branwell, Mrs. Brontë's sister, arrived during her sister's illness to help with the children, and what initially was to have been a temporary arrangement became permanent. Elizabeth Branwell's role in the household is of special significance to understanding Brontë's development, for she seems to have thought of Anne as her special charge. The fact that for many years Brontë shared a bedroom with her aunt would seem to support the claim for their closeness. Moreover, in her biography of Charlotte Brontë, Elizabeth Gaskell writes about Aunt Branwell:

> Next to her nephew, the docile, pensive Anne was her favourite. Miss Branwell had taken charge of her from her infancy; she was always patient and tractable and would submit quietly to occasional oppression, even when she felt it keenly. (Gaskell 1985, 198)

Anne Brontë was more influenced by her aunt's religious beliefs than were any of her siblings, although she clearly developed her own independent beliefs as well.[9] Elizabeth Branwell was a devout Wesleyan; the inscription on the teapot believed to be hers illustrates the gist of her faith: "To Me / To live is Christ / To die is Gain," a favorite passage of the Methodist William Grimshaw.[10] Methodism was the center of Aunt Branwell's life, and her influence during Anne's childhood years is attested to by the samplers Anne stitched under her scrutiny. The second sampler, dated January 23, 1830, includes the following passage from Proverbs:

> Honour the LORD with thy substance and with the first fruits of all thine increase. So shall thy barns be filled with Plenty, and thy Presses shall burst out with new wine. My child despise not the chastening of the LORD, neither be weary of his correction.[11]

Aunt Branwell took over much of the children's education, not just instructing the girls in sewing and needlepoint and overseeing their samplers, but selecting much of their reading material as well. Although their father helped with arithmetic and geography, Aunt Branwell felt it her duty to keep the girls occupied with household duties and to limit the time they would have to read books borrowed from the circulating library at the local town of Keighley. Elizabeth Gaskell writes:

> Mr Brontë encouraged a taste for reading in his girls; and though Miss Branwell kept it in due bounds, by the variety of household occupations, in which she expected them not merely to take a part, but to become proficients, thereby occupying regularly a good portion of every day, they were allowed to get books from the circulating library at Keighley; and many a happy walk, up those long four miles, must they have had, burdened with some new book, into which they peeped as they hurried home. (Gaskell 1985, 146)

Despite the boundaries set by her aunt, Brontë had access throughout her years at home to a wide range of reading material. In addition to the local library—and supplementing Aunt Branwell's copies of *The Ladies Magazine* and *The Methodist Magazine*—the Brontës' home library included a good selection of biographies, poetry collections, religious and philosophical works, science and medical texts, and popular advice books. Among the specific titles owned by the Brontës, for example, were Edmund Burke's *Inquiry into the Sublime and the Beautiful;* Robert Burton's *Anatomy of Melancholy;* Sir Humphry Davy's *Elements of Chemical Philosophy;* Susanna Harrison's *Songs in the Night;* Felicia Hemans's *Songs of the Affections and Other Poems;* John Milton's *Paradise Lost;* a book entitled *The Gardens and Menagerie of the Zoological Society;* and Isaac Watts' *The Doctrine of the Passions Explained and Improved.*

Although certainly influential, Aunt Branwell was not the only adult to shape Brontë's motherless childhood. Tabitha Ackroyd, one of the women who had come to live as a servant at the parsonage in 1825, provided them with "the rich oral culture of Irish tales and north country folklore" and probably spurred the already active imaginations of the Brontë children (Gardiner 1992, 48). The Brontë children played and worked together in many ways—dividing up household chores, frolicking outdoors over the moors, sharing books and toys, and creating stories with one another in the process. These experiences became crucial springboards for their earliest literary ventures, juvenilia now known as the Angrian and Gondal chronicles.

The Gondal Sagas

Modeling stories and poetry after those that might have appeared in a popular literary journal like *Blackwood's Magazine* or a newspaper like *The Monthly Intelligencer,* all four of the remaining Brontë children—Branwell, Charlotte, Emily, and Anne—worked together on the creation of an ongoing saga. The beginnings of what would eventually be known as the Angrian and Gondal Chronicles can be traced to Mr. Brontë's pur-

chase of some toy wooden soldiers for Branwell. The soldiers were immediately allocated among the children, who then named them and began
to create stories in which their lives and experiences were traced.
Elizabeth Gaskell reports that, according to Charlotte, Anne Brontë's
choice "was a queer little thing, much like herself," a figure whom they
called "Waiting Boy" (Gaskell 1985, 117). The Angrian and Gondal
chronicles were a unique blend of fact and fiction, however, and some of
the inspiration for Anne Brontë's poetic contributions came from her
knowledge of places like the Isle of Guernsey as well as of historical figures, such as the Arctic explorers Michael Sadler, Lord Bentinck, and Sir
Henry Halford. These places and figures were transformed into an imaginary kingdom and populace. The extent of Brontë's participation in the
creation of these imaginary kingdoms is difficult to assess, but at some
point she joined with Emily to "secede" from the imaginary world the
children had begun to construct, moving in their own direction to create
the land of Gondal and leaving the Angrian world to Charlotte and
Branwell.[12]

Much of Brontë's original Gondal writing was either destroyed or
lost, and what remains is limited to a relatively small number of
poems—"far too little evidence for a confident reconstruction" of the
complete story (Chitham 1991, 201). Part of the interest of Anne
Brontë's Gondal contributions has to do with what they reveal about
relationships within the Brontë family; it appears that the joint writing
efforts of Anne and Emily consolidated a relationship already made close
by Charlotte Brontë's having left home to join the two eldest sisters at
the Cowan Bridge school. Ellen Nussey's now famous comment that
Emily and Anne Brontë were "like twins—inseparable companions, and
in the closest sympathy" may well reflect their working relationship as
well as their sisterly one.[13] Later, probably by 1845 when she had
become more involved with her life as a governess and consequently
more separated from her sisters, Anne would limit the extent of her
Gondal writing even while Emily continued to thrive with it.[14] In a diary
paper dating from this time, she wrote:

> The Gondals are at present in a sad state. The Republicans are upper-
> most, but the Royalists are not quite overcome. The young sovereigns,
> with their brothers and sisters, are still at the Palace of Instruction. The
> Unique Society, about half a year ago, were wrecked on a desert island as
> they were returning from Gaul. They are still there, but we have not
> played at them much yet. The Gondals in general are not in first-rate
> playing condition. (*BLFC*, II, 52)

Brontë then followed these comments with the simple question, "Will they improve?" (*BLFC,* II, 52)

As Brontë's diary passage illustrates, the interest of her Gondal writing extends far beyond its revelations of family dynamics. Despite the lack of interest in the saga that Brontë seems to express here, Gondal writing clearly provided her at some points of her life with the opportunity to exercise her imagination and to become adept at plotting stories. The mythical Gondal world was characterized by extremes—battles and conquests, exiles and reunions—but it also had affinities, particularly in its landscape, with the Yorkshire world Brontë knew and loved.[15] Brontë's early poetry in particular—poems such as "Verses by Lady Geralda," "Alexander and Zenobia," "A Voice from the Dungeon," and "The Captive's Dream"—shows well the ways in which her Gondal writing simultaneously absorbed and reflected her interest in situations of isolation and solitude.[16]

As important as the thematics of the Gondal writing, however, was its means of production. All the writing is in some way co-constructed. The earliest Angrian and Gondal tales were created by—or among—the four Brontë children; subsequent tales were invariably created in pairs. Although each Brontë produced his or her own pieces, whether stories or poems, the pieces were inevitably influenced by the work of the others. The stories or poems associated with the sagas thus call into question traditional notions of individual authorship. They also defy easy distinctions between public and private writing, or between the purely imaginative and the more strictly autobiographical work. The exact nature of this collaborative writing process is impossible to reconstruct, but Brontë's 1845 diary paper suggests that she had begun to shape work dating back to as early as 1831 into a coherent history.[17] What seems certain is that she worked very closely first with all of her siblings and then intensely with Emily on a project that eventually reached huge proportions, what Elizabeth Gaskell later described as "an immense amount of manuscript, in an inconceivably small space" (Gaskell 1985, 112).

The Road to Authorship

The introduction to the collaborative nature of writing that Brontë got through her Gondal writing would resonate in several ways in her later work. Her first published volume of poems, for example, was also a jointly produced work: *Poems* by Currer, Ellis and Acton Bell, first published by Aylott and Jones in 1846, presented selections from Charlotte, Emily, and Anne Brontë alternately, identifying individual authorship by

pseudonym at the end of each poem. In the introduction to the 1850
edition of *Wuthering Heights and Agnes Grey,* Charlotte Brontë explained
the evolution of the volume. After accounting for her discovery of Emily
Brontë's poetry, she wrote:

> Meantime, my younger sister quietly produced some of her own compo-
> sitions, intimating that since Emily's had given me pleasure I might like
> to look at hers. I could not but be a partial judge, yet I thought that these
> verses too had a sweet, sincere pathos of their own. We had very early
> cherished the dream of one day being authors. . . . We agreed to arrange
> a small selection of our poems, and, if possible, get them printed. (*BLFC,*
> II, 79)

Despite their patronizing tone toward Anne Brontë's poetry, Charlotte
Brontë's comments suggest that all three sisters shared in the process of
selecting and arranging material for their first volume of poetry.

Just a year after the sisters prepared their book of poetry, Charlotte
Brontë wrote, "C., E. and A. Bell are now preparing for the press a work
of fiction, consisting of three distinct and unconnected tales," a comment
that ambiguously links their efforts into one unified whole at the same
time that it asserts individuality.[18] When *Agnes Grey* was published, it
came out together with *Wuthering Heights* in a single three-volume edition, in essence ensuring that the works would be reviewed together and
that separate authorship would be questioned.

The Brontë sisters even collaborated, in a sense, in their private writing, often taking over personal correspondence duties for each other. For
example, after Branwell Brontë's death, Anne Brontë wrote a letter on
behalf of Charlotte Brontë to the publisher William Smith Williams.
Dated 2 October 1848, Brontë's letter began:

> My sister wishes me to thank you for your two letters, the receipt of
> which gave her much pleasure, though coming in a season of severe
> domestic affliction, which has so wrought upon her too delicate constitu-
> tion as to induce a rather serious indisposition, that renders her unfit for
> the slightest exertion. (*BLFC,* II, 260)

The end of Brontë's letter as well calls attention to the collaboration
among sisters. "[Charlotte] desires her kindest regards to you," Brontë
wrote, "and participates with me in sincere pleasure at the happy effects
of Mrs Williams's seaside residence" (*BLFC,* II, 261).

Yet Anne Brontë was not entirely comfortable with loss of individuality entailed in joint publishing ventures. She kept the family pseudonym

established with the poetry volume for the publication of her two novels, but when reviewers started to publicly express doubts about the existence of three separate Bells, she responded actively and vehemently to establish her own autonomous identity as an author, first traveling to London with Charlotte Brontë to prove her separate existence to a doubting publisher and later writing in the preface to the second edition of *The Tenant of Wildfell Hall* that she "would have it to be distinctly understood that Acton Bell is neither Currer nor Ellis Bell, and therefore, let not his faults be attributed to them" (*TWH,* 31).

What seems at first to be a straightforward gesture of modesty on Brontë's part calls attention nonetheless to her evolving desire to establish her own individuality and to separate herself from her family, a topic that she had taken up in the story of Agnes Grey as well. Throughout her childhood she had been closely protected, not just because of her position as the youngest of the six children but also because an asthmatic condition made her seem delicate, if not completely "helpless."[19] The extremely close living arrangements necessitated by available space in the parsonage may well have exacerbated Brontë's need both to establish an identity separate from the one given to her by her family and to nurture this autonomous identity within her own private world.

Just as Brontë's fiction and poetry provide ample evidence of her investment in this private world, so too do her other activities, especially her painting and her music. Like other middle-class Victorian young women, Brontë learned to play the piano by taking lessons from a local musician, and what began as a hobby eventually became a skill that helped her market herself as a governess. Early diary papers indicate that Brontë was practicing her music as early as 1834, but by the time she had begun her second stint as a governess for the Robinson family of Thorp Green, her interest in music had become stronger. She purchased music manuscript books and copied favorite hymns into them, sometimes setting her own poetry to these hymns. While religious music accounts for much of her work in these music manuscript books, popular songs are also among the contents. Her music manuscript book dated June 1843 includes three sections of songs: hymns, with titles such as "Communion" and "Justification"; sacred songs, among them "Thou Art O God!"; and songs such as "Come Beneath the Linden Tree" and "Auld Lang Syne." Working with her music manuscript books became one of Brontë's primary "private" occupations during the difficult years of living away from home, apparently filling much of the free time allocated to her while governessing.[20]

Brontë's interest in artwork, like her interest in music, began early. The education she received in art and music typifies thinking about feminine education in mid-Victorian England; yet it is also true that she continued to pursue this training into her adult life. Her extant artwork dates from the time she was nine, when she—like her sisters—was encouraged to learn to draw from copybooks. The Brontë children drew from live models, particularly each other, as well.[21] Here too, then, there is a dimension of artistic collaboration between family members, so much so that some critics disagree about whether certain drawings and paintings were Anne Brontë's own creations or were presents given to her by her siblings. Several of the paintings that are indisputably by Anne Brontë, though, help to suggest the nature of her artistic interests, emphasizing—as they often do—isolated, solitary individuals.

While Brontë's earliest drawings seem to have been of nonhuman forms—rural churches, solitary trees, and birds, for instance—as her skills improved, so too did her confidence in peopling her landscapes. In keeping with a tradition of landscape painting popular at this time, the human figures in her drawings are dwarfed by their environment, appearing in one work as tiny figures crossing a bridge and in another as a small figure following a wagon down a country lane.[22]

Two drawings, which are of particular interest because they depart from this tradition, are titled "Sunrise at Sea" and "What You Please." Both show in the foreground young women who occupy the center of interest but who yet exist in a distinctly unempowered relationship to the landscape they inhabit.[23] "Sunrise at Sea" depicts an elegantly if simply dressed woman standing on a rocky cliff, with one arm raised to shield her eyes from the sun as she gazes out toward the horizon. "What You Please," dated 1840, represents a similarly dressed young woman gazing through the branches of a tree in a forested area with an expression of concern. One arm holds back a branch so big it almost appears to be a separate tree, and the other arm is held up in an apparently protective gesture as the woman searches for someone or something and at the same time shields her eyes from the sun. Although in one drawing the viewer sees the woman from behind and in the other from the front, in both the subject is so preoccupied with her thoughts as to be oblivious to the gaze of the viewer. Both, moreover, suggest that the woman's position is one of suspended anticipation. In these drawings the feelings of the woman are the center of the work's interest and yet are not decipherable, suggesting only an attitude of expectation.

One additional group of Brontë's drawings of special interest depicts very young children, all apparently drawn between August and

November of 1837, just prior to an illness that resulted in what has been called a "psychosomatic crisis" (Chitham 1991, 52). (This episode in Brontë's life—in which she requested a visit with the Moravian minister James de la Trobe and discussed what he called "the main truths of the Bible respecting our salvation" [54]—is often linked to the representation of those issues in *The Tenant of Wildfell Hall*). The children of the drawings that Brontë produced during this apparently difficult time in her life are idealized and cherubic, unlike any of Brontë's other drawings or those of her siblings. Brontë made these drawings at roughly the same time that she composed the poem "A Voice from the Dungeon" (3), where the speaker dreams of holding her "darling boy" to her breast and accepting his gleeful kisses. Taken together, these works might indicate Brontë's desire for children of her own, or, more generally, a yearning to love and be loved unconditionally. Perhaps their most significant attribute is that they seem remarkably unlike Brontë's other artwork, thus indicating the breadth of her interests and suggesting her desire to keep some of those interests to herself.

Another manifestation of Brontë's desire for love outside her immediate family is her relationship with William Weightman, who had arrived in Haworth in 1839 to be Mr. Brontë's curate. Weightman came to Haworth while Brontë was working at Blake Hall, her first place of employment, and he died just a few years later, after she had again left home to work as a governess, this time at Thorp Green. During his time in Haworth, Weightman earned the respect of his community. He was gregarious and outgoing by the family's standards, and the Brontës admired his ability to reach out to his parishioners and yet not degrade his position. In the 1842 funeral sermon he composed for Weightman, Mr. Brontë wrote: "In his preaching, and practising, he was, as every clergyman ought to be, neither distant nor austere, timid nor obtrusive, nor bigoted, exclusive, nor dogmatical."[24]

There is no direct evidence from Brontë's own private writing with which to assess the extent of her feelings toward Weightman or their significance. Some of Charlotte Brontë's correspondence suggests that Weightman may have cultivated a romantic attachment with her sister. Several of Brontë's poems, in turn, might reflect her own romantic inclinations toward Weightman. An untitled poem dated December 1842 seems, for example, to have been intended as a private expression of love and grief. Inscribed at the top of the poem is a dedication intentionally left blank: "To—. The speaker of the poem proclaims her belief that the one for whom she mourns was one whose "brightest hopes were fixed above" (20, l. 19), but says "And yet I cannot check my sighs, / Thou

wert so young and fair" (20, ll. 21–22). A strict autobiographical interpretation of this and other poems, seeking only to identify Weightman
with the young man who figures in seven of Brontë's "love poems,"
would limit the poetry's interest; but it is worthwhile to note that
Brontë's feelings, whatever they were, were apparently harbored in privacy and only indirectly alluded to in some of her poetry.[25]

Weightman's more important role in terms of Brontë's artistic development may have been largely symbolic. Partly because of his relatively
early death at the age of 26 and partly because much of his time in
Haworth coincided with time Brontë spent away from home,
Weightman may well have embodied for her the idea of unfulfilled
potential. The difficulty of accepting the death of one so young and full
of promise was part of her father's message in the sermon written for
Weightman's funeral. Brontë's father wrote:

> He had not attained the meridian of man's life; amidst the joyous, and
> sanguine anticipations of friends, the good wishes of all, and, as may nat-
> urally be supposed, the glad hopes of himself, he was summoned for his
> removal from this world, to the bar of eternity. . . . When good men die
> early, in the full tide of their usefulness, there is bewildering amazement,
> till we read in the scriptures, that in mercy they are taken away from the
> evil to come. (Patrick Brontë 1898, 260–61)

Although Brontë was away from home when her father preached this
sermon, it is likely that she read it. Mr. Brontë explains in the beginning
of the printed version that he was requested to publish it and that he
complied in order to ensure that "there should be no discrepancy
between the pulpit and the press, but that what may be heard now, may
be read again, without any alteration" (258).

Anne Brontë in all likelihood agonized less over Weightman's youth
than over the loss of one committed in his profession to conveying beliefs
very much like her own. Again, her father's sermon is illustrative,
explaining that Weightman:

> . . . thought it better, and more scriptural, to make the love of God,
> rather than the fear of hell, the ruling motive for obedience. He did not
> see why true believers, having the promise of the life that now is, as well
> as that which is to come, should create unto themselves artificial sorrows,
> and disfigure the garment of gospel peace with the garb of sighing and
> sadness. (256)

Weightman's commitment to spiritual equality and universal salvation is very much like those Brontë has her two fictional heroines, Agnes Grey and Helen Huntingdon, express in the course of their respective narratives. It is also apparently very much like her own, emerging first in her encounter with the Moravian minister James de la Trobe and later becoming evident in a letter written on 30 December 1848 to the Reverend David Thom. Thom had written to Brontë to express the extent to which he agreed with some of the religious beliefs he gleaned from her writing. In a letter responding to Thom, Brontë expressed her gratification at knowing that others shared her belief in God's benevolence, whether "timidly suggested or boldly advocated" and wrote that "[she] would that all men had the same view of man's hopes and God's unbounded goodness as he has given to us."[26]

Brontë's belief in the promise of life after death did not entirely mitigate the intensity of her desire to experience fully what life on earth had to offer. Much of her writing indicates that she struggled as well with the idea of loss of the potential to engage in a love relationship. The idea that life is empty without a love relationship is central to "If This Be All" (39) and to "Dreams" (40), both written in 1845. In "Dreams," Brontë's speaker writes of her desire:

> To feel my hand so kindly pressed,
> To know myself beloved at last,
> To think my heart has found a rest,
> My life of solitude is past. (ll. 17–20)

And in "Self-Communion" Brontë writes:

> Love may be full of pain, but still,
> 'Tis sad to see it so depart,—
> To watch that fire, whose genial glow
> Was formed to comfort and to cheer,
> For want of fuel, fading so,
> Sinking to embers dull and drear,—(57, ll. 165–170)

Although we will never know for sure whether Brontë equated Weightman's death with the loss of a potential mate, it seems clear from her poetry that she was troubled by the prospect of living without a love relationship.

Brontë's Interest in Self-Development

It would do Brontë a disservice to suggest that she believed an erotic relationship would somehow make her life complete. Her interest in appreciating and fulfilling her own personal potential extended in many directions and to a large extent motivated her writing career. Brontë's diary papers especially reveal the depths of her ongoing concern with self-development and fulfillment. The papers are significant in this regard because, like so much of Brontë's early writing, they, too, are co-constructed. Of the several diary papers related to Brontë that are known to exist, one is cowritten with Emily. Others, though associated primarily with Anne Brontë, were written as part of a project between the sisters, who apparently agreed to write diary papers every four years in which they would reminisce about past experiences and speculate about their future.[27]

The first of the diary papers associated with Anne Brontë is dated 24 November 1834. Though it is in Emily Brontë's handwriting, it has Anne Brontë's signature at the top as well. The diary recounts a range of the day's activities for the two youngest Brontës—from feeding the pet animals to peeling apples in preparation for dinner. Toward its conclusion Emily writes, "Anne and I say I wonder what we shall be like and what we shall be and where we shall be, if all goes on well, in the year 1874—in which year I shall be in my 57th year. Anne will be in her 55th year Branwell will be going in his 58th year and Charlotte in her 59th year" (*BLFC*, I, 124–125). The bulk of the letter, especially that which lightly makes fun of the servant Tabby's way of pronunciation (e.g., "Taby said just now Come Anne pilloputate [i.e., peel a potato]") seems characteristic of Emily Brontë's sense of humor, but the later portion of the note—specifically its questioning of what the future would hold— seems characteristic of Anne Brontë.

Indeed, the diary papers that Brontë wrote when she was away from home, and hence by herself, reveal much of the same language. On 30 July 1841—the same day that Emily Brontë wrote a diary paper for herself while at home—Brontë wrote a diary paper while staying at the seaside town of Scarborough with the Murray family, for whom she worked as a governess. The note begins with an account of where her brother and sisters were living at the time; of her own position, she writes simply, "I dislike the situation and wish to change it for another" (*BLFC*, I, 239). As the diary continues, though, Brontë speculates on what changes are in store for her and for her family: "I wonder what will be our condition and how or where we shall all be on this day four years hence; at which time, if all be well, I shall be 25 years and 6 months old, Emily will be 27 years old, Branwell 28 years and 1 month, and Charlotte 29 years and a quarter" (239).

The precision with which Brontë attends to the exact projected age of herself and her family illustrates the intensity with which she anticipated change, an anticipation characteristically chastened by her use of the cautionary phrase "If all be well."[28] After outlining some of the "diversities" that have occupied her attention in the past four years (e.g., the acquisition of a dog and a hawk, the loss of a cat, various changes of employment for all of the family), Brontë becomes more introspective, first quoting Byron's lines as "How little know we what we are / How less what we may be!"[29] She then writes:

> What will the next four years bring forth? Providence only knows. But we ourselves have sustained very little alteration since that time. I have the same faults that I had then, only I have more wisdom and experience, and a little more self-possession than I then enjoyed. (*BLFC*, I, 239)

After speculating briefly on whether she would still be working on the Gondal saga in four years, she concludes:

> For some time I have looked upon 25 as a sort of era in my existence. It may prove a true presentiment, or it may be only a superstitious fancy; the latter seems most likely, but time will show. (*BLFC* I, 239)

In these passages Brontë invokes a rhetoric of self-development that permeates much of her writing—other diary papers and poetry as well as the fiction writing on which she would soon embark. This particular diary paper illustrates several crucial dimensions of Brontë's notion of self-development. On the one hand, she reveals a sense of resignation that she has only limited control over how experiences will shape her and a belief that "Providence" ultimately dictates her future. She also reveals a curious sense of frustration that she has changed so little. Rather than take comfort in what she refers to as a lack of "alteration," seeing it as a sign of the stability of her self, she criticizes herself for continuing to have faults despite the addition of a little "wisdom and experience" and prides herself on her ability to rein in and repress her emotions.

In some ways Brontë's self-assessment draws on a rhetoric of self-chastisement and correction that one would associate with the Wesleyan heritage of her Aunt Branwell. But much of her diary writing evokes contradictory anxieties that complicate an interpretation of her beliefs. She struggles to accept her lot in life, but repeatedly expresses a will to change and develop as well. Similarly, she expresses a desire for the momentous (e.g., an "era of my existence"), but simultaneously deplores her own indulgence in "superstitious fancy."

Similar anxieties reveal themselves in Brontë's diary paper of 31 July 1845, which was this time written from home. In this paper as well, Brontë's dominant concern is with her own self-development, although in this case her attitude regarding the extent of her experience has changed considerably. Shortly after beginning her paper, she writes:

> How many things have happened since [the last diary paper] was written—some pleasant, some far otherwise. Yet I was then at Thorp Green, and now I am only just escaped from it. I was wishing to leave it then, and if I had known that I had four years longer to stay how wretched I should have been; but during my stay I have had some very unpleasant and undreamt-of experience of human nature. Others have seen more changes. (*BLFC,* II, 52)

Much of the diary paper proceeds in a pattern in which Brontë states a simple fact about what she or one of her siblings is doing and follows it with a question about where the fact will lead; for example, "[Charlotte] wishes to go to Paris. Will she go?" (*BLFC,* II, 52). While in her questions about her siblings Brontë reveals simple curiosity, in her self-scrutiny she expresses frustration. Of her current writing project she states: "I have begun the third volume of *Passages in the Life of an Individual*. I wish I had finished it" (*BLFC,* II, 52).[30] Even the ordinary tasks that Brontë records inspired self-doubt. At another point in her paper, she writes: "I want to get a habit of early rising. Shall I succeed?" (*BLFC,* II, 52).

The 1845 diary paper ends in much the same way as Brontë's earlier papers, with speculation about how the family, and especially herself, would change over time:

> I wonder how we shall all be, and where and how situated, on the thirtieth of July 1848, when, if we are all alive, Emily will be just 30. I shall be in my 29th year, Charlotte in her 33rd, and Branwell in his 32nd; and what changes shall we have seen and known; and shall we be much

changed ourselves? I hope not, for the worse at least. I for my part cannot
well be flatter or older in mind than I am now. Hoping for the best, I
conclude. (*BLFC,* II, 53)

The paper is striking not simply for its evocation of Brontë's depressed
mood at this point in her life, but also for her anxiety about her own
development, an anxiety that again reveals itself as emerging out of contradictory desires. Although she frames her comments with an expression
of cautious anticipation, she acknowledges a fear that she and others have
the capacity to change for the worse. She distinguishes, if implicitly,
between external changes—say in place of employment or in writing project—and more fundamental change of character (i.e., "shall we be much
changed ourselves?"). Finally, her self-examination focuses in the end not
on her change of situation but on her state of mind, her interiority; here
too she reveals a level of distress. Ironically, Brontë had as a child yearned
for "age and experience." Elizabeth Gaskell tells of a time when Brontë's
father sought to lessen the timidity of his children by asking them "to
stand and speak boldly from under the cover of [a] mask" (Gaskell 1985,
94). When asked "what a child like her most wanted," Brontë—who was
then a mere four years old—responded "Age and experience" (94). By
1845, under the mask of her diary, she saw age and experience as only
having made her "older," and less hopeful, in mind.

Brontë's personal paradigm of self-examination may well have provided her with ideas for her work. Her fictional heroines scrutinize their
self-development in much the same way as she herself does in these diary
papers. She represents both Agnes Grey and Helen Huntingdon as
struggling with concern about the extent to which their surroundings
and companionship might change them for the worse. At first Agnes
Grey worries about how her home circumstances will change while she is
away. Later this anxiety extends to her self; having worked only a short
time away from home she writes, "Habitual associates are known to
exercise a great influence over each other's minds and manners. . . . I, as
I could not make my young companions better, feared exceedingly that
they would make me worse—would gradually bring my feelings, habits,
capacities, to the level of their own" (*AG,* 82).

Brontë's fictional heroines also express their hopes for self-development with cautious anticipation. Toward the end of *Agnes Grey,* the heroine thinks:

> "Yet who can tell" said I within myself, as I proceeded up the park—
> "who can tell what this one month may bring forth? I have lived nearly

three-and-twenty years, and I have suffered much, and tasted little pleasure yet: is it likely my life all through will be so clouded? Is it not possible that God may hear my prayers, disperse these gloomy shadows, and
grant me some beams of heaven's sunshine yet!" (*AG,* 137)

Significantly, Brontë demands that her character resign "fruitless dreaming" to "sober, solid, sad reality" before she experiences the pleasure she
desires (*AG,* 138).

Reading and Writing as Self-Development

Anne Brontë's interest in self-development shaped her other activities as
well. Rather than passively await her experiences to see whether and how
they would change her, she attempted in a variety of ways to exert control over how she developed. Brontë read widely and closely, often taking personal notes in the margins of her books. She read, for example,
through a series of inspirational poems, letters, and essays collected by
G. B. Wright titled *Thoughts in Younger Life,* composing an eight-line
poem of her own on the inside front cover of the book and making short
notes throughout. Wright's book may well have appealed at some point
to Brontë's desire for "age and experience"; in his preface, he writes,
"Our thoughts in younger life, are frequently very different from those
in more advanced periods, arising partly from a want of knowledge and
experience of men and things" (Wright 1778, iv). At one point, for
example, Brontë responds to an elegy included in the collection by composing four lines of poetry on the subject.[31] Thompson's "Elegy on the
Death of Miss Warren" had ended with the following moral tag:

> Learn hence ye kind and love-inspiring fair,
> Your *minds* alone, deserve your greatest care;
> Let *Virtue* prove your never-fading bloom;
> *For mental beauties will survive the tomb.* (Wright 49)

Wright's message on the dangers of vanity accords with some of Brontë's
own concerns. *Agnes Grey* treats in several ways what for Brontë was the
problem of her society's attitude toward physical beauty. All of her work
addresses in some way the life and health of the mind.

That Brontë considered reading to be an essential part of her own
self-development is evident in other ways as well. She appears to have

embarked late in 1841 on a self-constructed program of Bible reading and to have prefaced her project with a characteristic question of how it would influence her self-development. At the top of one of the flyleaves to her Bible is written: "What, Where, and How shall I be when I have got through?"[32] Brontë did not just read the Bible in its entirety; she took detailed notes from her reading, specifically cataloguing chapters and verses that she found interesting. Among the 17 books that attracted her particular attention are Job, Psalms, Proverbs, and Ecclesiastes. The specific chapters and verses that she selected from these and other biblical books indicate a concern with conduct, particularly in the face of real or perceived scorn; an awareness of the conflict between trust and doubt; and a desire for a "clean heart," all topics that she frequently addressed directly in her poetry and indirectly in her fiction.[33]

Brontë's biblical reading project would seem in some ways to reveal a deep religious commitment; it took nearly a year and a half, for she dates the end page of the Bible 30 April 1843. The project may also point to a conflict that she felt between the need to accept one's lot in life and the will to experience fully what life has to offer. Put another way, the conflict may have centered on the difficulty of accepting limitations, both of experience and of one's self. The project correlates, then, with another important dimension of her life experiences—her work as a governess. The two seemingly disparate elements of her life are related chronologically, for Brontë was working at Thorp Green during much of the time that she was reading through the Bible. More important, both seem to have been undertaken as welcome opportunities to widen her experiences and improve her self.

The Governess Experience

The naively unrealistic optimism that Brontë represents in *Agnes Grey* in all likelihood corresponded to her own attitude. Before beginning her work, Agnes thinks: "How delightful it would be to be a governess! To go out into the world; to enter upon a new life; to act for myself . . . " (*AG.* 8). Although all the Brontë sisters had been contemplating working as governesses to reduce the burden of upkeep, Anne Brontë was the first to secure a position. In April 1839, at the age of 19, she began work as a governess in the Ingham family home in Mirfield. Joshua Ingham, the head of the household, was a "local squire, magistrate and businessman" with an estate on 64 acres of property (Chitham 1991, 58). Brontë was hired to be in charge of the two oldest children, a seven-year old boy and a five-year old girl.

In a letter of 15 April 1839 to Ellen Nussey describing the news of
Anne's employment, Charlotte Brontë wrote:

> I could not well write to you in the week you requested as about that time
> we were very busy in preparing for Anne's departure—poor child! she left
> us last Monday no one went with her—it was her own wish that she
> might be allowed to go alone—as she thought she could manage better
> and summon more courage if thrown entirely upon her own resources. We
> have had one letter from her since she went—she expresses herself very
> well satisfied, and says that Mrs Ingham is extremely kind; the two eldest
> children alone are under her care, the rest are confined to the nursery—
> with which and its occupants she has nothing to do. (*BLFC*, I, 175)

Charlotte Brontë's stress on her sister's insistence on traveling alone to
Mirfield is particularly interesting, since she attributes it to a belief that
doing so would enable her to "summon more courage" (*BLFC*, I, 175).
It seems equally important to recognize that Brontë's desire to be
"thrown entirely upon her own resources" (*BLFC,* I, 175) suggests that
she thought of the position as an opportunity to establish independence
from her family—independence that she sought to demonstrate from
the very beginning. Despite the fearful and patronizing overtones of
Charlotte Brontë's letter, Anne Brontë's own attitude toward this first
venture may well have been more enthusiastic; several years earlier (in
1835) she had successfully taken Emily Brontë's place at the Roe Head
school when her sister returned to Haworth after failing to adjust to her
new situation.

Brontë's first experience as a governess was characterized mostly by
its brevity. The same letter from Charlotte Brontë to Ellen Nussey intimates that Anne Brontë from the very beginning struggled with behavioral problems on the part of her charges and that she was unable to discipline them as she saw fit. For reasons that are now impossible to
reconstruct, she was back in Haworth by the beginning of 1840.
Nonetheless, the initial experience with the Ingham family appears to
have heightened her desire to broaden her experiences and to establish a
degree of independence from her family.

Despite the fact that both of her sisters at this point had had unfa-
vorable experiences as governesses, Brontë began immediately to seek a
second position, and by May 1840 she had accepted one, this time in
Thorp Green Hall of Little Ouseburn, near York, at the home of a family headed by the parson and squire Edmund Robinson. Brontë worked
for the Robinson family for five years, first alone, and after January

1843 with her brother Branwell, who was appointed as tutor for the family's son Edmund.

At Thorp Green Hall, Brontë was in charge of two adolescent girls, Lydia and Elizabeth Robinson, and she also was initially expected to do some tutoring of the eight-year old Edmund Robinson. Brontë's experience working as a governess for the Robinson family was mixed. Evidence from the diary papers and letters of her sisters suggests that she felt isolated—both physically within the small schoolroom to which she was often confined and emotionally by not having a friendly relationship either with Mrs. Robinson or with any of the servants. Emily Brontë described Anne Brontë at this point in her life as "exiled and harassed" (*BLFC,* I, 238), and, in a letter to Ellen Nussey dated 1 July 1841, Charlotte Brontë referred to Thorp Green Hall as "the house of Bondage" (*BLFC,* I, 234). As mentioned above, Brontë's own diary paper of 1841 indicates that she "dislike[d] the situation and wish[ed] to change it for another" (*BLFC,* I, 239). Despite its hardships, life with the Robinsons offered Brontë experiences that might otherwise have eluded her. She seems to have taken her position seriously, purchasing a number of books—among them a German grammar and the Latin *Delectus Sententiarum et Historiarum ad usum Tironum Accommodatus* by R. Valpy—that would enhance her skills as an instructor. Not only did she strengthen her tutorial skills, improve her drawing and musical abilities, and increase her self-confidence, but she was able to travel with the Robinsons on their yearly trips to the seaside resort of Scarborough, a place she loved and returned to just before she died in 1849.

Brontë resigned from her position with the Robinsons in June 1845, and wrote disparagingly in her diary paper just one month later of the "unpleasant and undreamt-of experience of human nature" (*BLFC,* II, 52) that the position had afforded her. Remembering back to her 1841 paper, Brontë wrote (in a passage that has already been quoted, above): "Yet I was then at Thorp Green, and now I am only just escaped from it. I was wishing to leave it then, and if I had known that I had four years longer to stay how wretched I should have been" (*BLFC,* II, 52). Although her diary does not explain what finally prompted her to resign from her post, she was in all likelihood led to do so by the behavior of her brother, who was dismissed under disgrace from his position as tutor just one month after she herself had resigned. Branwell Brontë had become involved with Mrs. Robinson and, though he apparently harbored hopes of a permanent relationship, he departed from Thorp Green shortly after Mr. Robinson became aware of the situation.[34] Although her knowledge about what had taken place between her employer and her brother may well have been limited, Brontë was clearly embarrassed. The situation ended up being a turning point in Branwell Brontë's life; never fully recovering from his disappointment, he returned home and began what would be a downward spiral into opium and alcohol addiction that ended with his death. Whatever positive experiences Anne Brontë gained from her stint as a governess would thus be forever clouded by the association with her brother's demise.

Anne Brontë was, however, able to put the governessing experience to good use in her fiction. Her direct exposure to a wider social arena than she had hitherto experienced and her encounters with the conventions governing her working position enabled her to participate in the formation of a literary tradition by centering a narrative on the governess, what one critic has called "one of the most familiar and abiding images in nineteenth-century literature."[35] The governess had figured in English fiction since the end of the eighteenth century, and by the year 1847 she was a recognizable type frequently deployed when novelists wanted to investigate complexities of domestic ideology. Like other mid-century novelists, Brontë used her fiction in part to reveal the plight of the governess both within the home where she worked and within society at large. Many episodes in *Agnes Grey* emphasize the ambiguity of Agnes's position in the home of her employer, where she was neither a family member nor, strictly speaking, a servant. The pressures of the ambiguous social situation experienced by governesses had predictable psychological correlates: "Treated as if they were invisible, many governesses responded by removing themselves quite literally from the sight of their employers, retreating to the schoolroom during off-duty hours" (Hughes 1993, 101). Brontë also designed several scenes in *Agnes Grey* to depict the behavior of Agnes's employers toward her in public situations; these scenes enabled her to analyze more fully the attitude of a wider social arena toward the governess.

If the actual experience of governessing enabled Brontë to experience firsthand the social invisibility of governessing that she would later explore in *Agnes Grey,* it also inspired her to develop a public, authorial voice and to use it for didactic purposes. Just as Brontë sought in private to examine and better her self, so too did she envision authorship as an opportunity to examine and better society at large. Although she never again worked outside the home after the time at Thorp Green Hall, she continued to seek independence, this time through her writing. During this period the Brontë sisters apparently pondered the idea of opening a school of their own. Although they got as far as having advertisements drawn up, they were unable to secure any boarders for their school and eventually abandoned the idea.

The years immediately after Anne Brontë's experience as a governess are marked by a relatively rapid sequence of publication: *Poems* by Currer, Ellis and Acton Bell was published by Aylott and Jones in 1846; *Agnes Grey* was published by T. C. Newby of London in 1847; and *The Tenant of Wildfell Hall* followed the next year from the same publisher.

Authorship as Self-Development

Anne Brontë's fiction especially should be seen as a kind of dual enterprise, involving the improvement of both her self and her readership. She explains in the "Preface to the Second Edition" of *The Tenant of Wildfell Hall* that she undertook authorship not for personal gratification but rather for edification: "I wished to tell the truth, for truth always conveys its own moral to those who are able to receive it" (*TWH*, 29). Brontë's preface is marked initially by its overtures to modesty; she admits to seeking "the public ear," but suggests that once she has it she will only "whisper a few wholesome truths" (*TWH*, 29). Yet by its end, she both widens her net and expands on her motivations. In a passage remarkable in its assertiveness for a woman writer so widely regarded as quiet and unassuming, she writes:

> Yet, be it understood, I shall not limit my ambition to this,—or even to producing 'a perfect work of art': time and talents so spent I should consider wasted and misapplied. Such humble talents as God has given me I will endeavour to put to their greatest use; if I am able to amuse I will try to benefit too; and when I feel it my duty to speak an unpalatable truth, with the help of God, I *will* speak it, though it be to the prejudice of my name and to the detriment of my reader's immediate pleasure as well as my own. (*TWH*, 30)

Brontë makes clear here that her writing is part of an ongoing effort to develop her own individual potential as well as that of her readers, and that she feels it her primary duty to fulfill this individual potential. The potential that she envisions is one achieved not by aesthetic perfection but rather by her ability to will herself to speak the truth and benefit others.

Brontë's message in this preface may have been prompted by the criticism *Agnes Grey* had received, but it does not solely reflect her ambitions as a writer. Rather, these aspirations were shaped by and were an extension of her personal ambitions. In one of her last letters, written to Ellen Nussey on 5 April 1849, Brontë reveals the depth of her commitment to self-development and links her personal fulfillment to social good. Despite suffering from the same symptoms that just months before had resulted in the death of her brother and sister and having received word from her doctors that her only hope was a prompt change of climate, Brontë wrote:

> I wish it would please God to spare me not only for papa's and Charlotte's sakes, but because I long to do some good in the world before I leave it. I have many schemes in my head for future practice, humble and limited indeed, but still I should not like them all to come to nothing, and myself to have lived to so little purpose. But God's will be done. (*BLFC*, II, 321)

Brontë's message reveals both the resiliency of her ambitions and, at the same time, a remarkably profound despair at her own accomplishments thus far in life. After all, by the age of twenty-nine not only had she lived successfully away from home and family for extended periods on several occasions; she had also contributed to a published volume of poetry and published two novels.

Brontë's despair can most effectively be understood as emanating out of her sense that her potential could not simply be fulfilled professionally, whether through working or through writing. Nor did she derive comfort from her financial independence. (Although royalties from her publications had added little to the savings she had accumulated during her six years as a governess, she had been left legacies by her Aunt Branwell and by a godmother.) Much of her poetry and fiction suggests instead an ongoing concern with the role of private life in providing the ingredients necessary to self-fulfillment. Peaceful and honest relationships within the home, a love relationship beyond one's immediate family, and a child with whom to experience unconditional love all seem from Brontë's writing to have been part of her paradigm of a personal situation conducive to self-fulfillment.

Brontë's own private life denied her many of these ingredients, of course. For a host of reasons, Branwell Brontë failed to live up to his own potential and his eventual decline into opium and alcohol addiction inevitably colored Brontë's own years of professional achievement. Emily Brontë's now well-known refusal to seek help or accept comfort for her own illness must have exacerbated Anne Brontë's frustration. The relative isolation of Haworth restricted Anne Brontë's opportunities for establishing relationships beyond her family. Perhaps most significantly, she was struggling with a chronically debilitating health problem. She had suffered from asthma throughout her life, and she became seriously ill shortly after Emily Brontë's death in December, 1848. Although she actively sought the help of a variety of physicians, she eventually succumbed to consumption on 28 May 1849.

Brontë did not die at home, like the rest of her family, but rather in Scarborough, where she had gone just days before her death, accompanied by Charlotte Brontë and Ellen Nussey. Brontë's decision to travel to Scarborough at this point reveals several important dimensions of her character. On the one hand, she aspired to accept what she thought of as the will of God; her last letter to Ellen Nussey (quoted earlier in this chapter) ends with just such a declaration. An account that Nussey later gave of Anne Brontë's death would seem to confirm this dimension of her faith. Nussey reported to Elizabeth Gaskell that, when a doctor was consulted in Scarborough, Brontë commanded him to tell her how long she might live and told him "not to fear speaking the truth, for she was not afraid to die" (*BLFC*, II, 335). Despite the courage that Brontë showed in facing death, even at the very end, throughout her illness she refused to relinquish hope that she would be allowed to live longer. In the last months of her life, she tried a variety of medical treatments, even though she had been warned by her doctors not to hope for recovery.

Whether Brontë determined to go to Scarborough in hope of a cure or simply to find a more comfortable place to die will never be known for sure. Nussey's account of the Scarborough journey emphasizes Anne Brontë's emotional stamina: "Her life was calm, quiet, spiritual: *such* was her end," Nussey wrote. "Through the trials and fatigues of the journey she evinced the pious courage and fortitude of a martyr" (*BLFC*, II, 333). The "death scene," which was orchestrated by Anne Brontë herself, suggests that she died peacefully, without any doubt of the promise of salvation. After arriving in Scarborough, having stopped briefly to see York Minster, she took a donkey ride on the sands, went for a short walk, and then retired for the night. The next day, she reportedly felt a change and called for a doctor. According to Nussey, after being informed that she would soon die, Brontë:

. . . clasped her hands, and reverently invoked a blessing from on high;
first upon her sister, then upon her friend, to whom she said, "Be a sister
in my stead. Give Charlotte as much of your company as you can."
(*BLFC*, II, 335)

In another gesture of faith, she soon after remarked that "all will be well
through the merits of our Redeemer" (*BLFC*, II, 336). She tried briefly
to comfort Charlotte by saying, "Take courage," and then she died.
Nussey summarized her death by writing at the end of her account to
Gaskell, "She thought not of the grave, for that is but the body's gaol,
but of all that is beyond it" (*BLFC*, II, 336).

Anne Brontë's body was not transported back to Haworth; rather,
she was buried at Scarborough. Brontë's attraction to Scarborough had
always been based on the refuge that she found in the wildness of the
sea—not on the society offered by the resort community. Her burial
there marks, thus, a kind of permanent place of exile from society and
home, as well as a separation from her family. In this sense, it memorial-
izes the individuality that her family and friends seem always to have
recognized, if not to have understood.

In several ways, Brontë's death and burial at Scarborough bring us
back to the thematics of her life itself, dominated as it was by an interest
in the private life. This interest encouraged her to create her own distancing strategies, to nurture her privacy with secrecy and silence. Yet it
also ultimately inspired her to develop representational strategies that
enabled her to explore the complex interconnections between psychological and social identity.

Chapter Three

"The Language of My Inmost Heart": Anne Brontë's Poetics of Interiority

Anne Brontë composed poetry throughout her writing career. Her earliest "fair copy books," into which she carefully transcribed her poems from draft copy, date from 1836, when she was 16 years old, although she began writing poetry well before this date. Her last poem was written in January 1849, just a few months before her death. In the introduction to the 1850 edition of *Wuthering Heights and Agnes Grey,* Charlotte Brontë recalled a day in the autumn of 1845 when her youngest sister "quietly produced some of her own compositions" for presentation, with the hope that Charlotte would judge her works as favorably as she had judged those written by Emily Brontë (*BLFC,* II, 79). These "compositions"—poems that Brontë had apparently written in privacy—were among those eventually published in the 1846 volume *Poems* by Currer, Ellis and Acton Bell.

From the very beginning, Brontë's poetry was written with an awareness of her elders' presence. On the first page of her 1836 poetry book the following directive was recorded by her father, Patrick Brontë:

See all that is written in this Book, must be in a good, plain and legible hand.—P. B. (Chitham 1979, 27)

Brontë's father disapproved of his children's writing in small script and insisted on "normal handwriting" (Chitham 1979, 31). The slightly threatening tone of his warning implies not just that he would oversee and scrutinize his daughter's writing, but also that he would judge it according to somewhat puritanical standards. Since he must have known that his children wrote in small script to imitate the professional type they saw in literary publications, his directive seems designed in part to discourage early on any pretensions to a public forum for their writing. In a sense, Brontë's father served as her symbolic supervisor, a kind of exemplary figure of patriarchal attitudes toward the woman writer.

While all the Brontë daughters were apparently subject to the same directive from their father, Anne Brontë alone seems to have followed his wishes. Charlotte and Emily Brontë both either consistently or occasionally recorded their poetry in the characteristically minute script despite his admonition. Although Brontë used the script for her drafts, her fair copies were recorded in the "normal" handwriting that her father desired. That she used this approach seems to suggest that she valued obedience to her father more than experimental play with her sisters, or at least enough to resist any impulse to rebellion. A careful reading of her poetry, however, reveals instead an independence of thought that undercuts the view of her as orthodox daughter and writer.

The idea of obedience is central to much of Brontë's poetry. Rather than simply paying homage to the concept, though, she makes it problematic by repeatedly tackling difficult issues of obedience to God and to oneself. It seems likely that she would not have viewed her father's directive about proper handwriting as a challenge to her freedom of self-expression. On the contrary, she may well have taken it as a reminder that submission is a necessary, if perplexing, facet of self-understanding. Brontë's choice of writing for her copybooks affirms her sense that the subject matter of her poetry, much of which relates to dilemmas of identity, was most effectively presented not in the imitative script endorsed by her sisters but rather in her own personal handwriting.

By disengaging her poetry from its overtly public mode (as represented by the formal script) and adopting instead for her formal copybooks the more conventional mode of private expression (as represented by her handwriting), Brontë marked her work as distinctly her own, as different both from the "tradition" that her sisters were attempting to establish within the family and the tradition that they sought to imitate. In other ways as well, she found in writing poetry the opportunity to interrogate the demands of traditions—traditions literary and religious in orientation as well as those based on gender. Like other poets writing during the Victorian period, Brontë investigated "the terms of both self and other" and foregrounded the instability of their relationship, in the process "making the act of representation itself a focus of anxiety."[1]

Brontë's writing might profitably be understood as evidencing not just interests and techniques associated with Victorian poetry in general but also those affiliated more particularly with women's poetry of the period. The tradition of women's poetry that emerged during the period may well have provided Brontë with "a subtly determining myth of what being a woman poet means."[2] Avid readers of gift books and annuals such as *Friendship's Offerings* as well as popular periodicals, the Brontë sisters were exposed to a wide range of poetry written by women. As already mentioned, they owned collections of the works of the popular poet Felicia Hemans as well as several more general anthologies of contemporary poetry.

This tradition of women's poetry—which by the century's end would include not only Hemans's poetry but also the works of such poets as Laetitia Landon, Elizabeth Barrett Browning, Alice Meynell, and Charlotte Mew—is characterized in part by the deliberately provocative stance it takes toward the myth of female sensibility. This myth disassociated women from the material world and constructed them as symbolic representatives of moral purity. Although the topics that Victorian women poets took up were varied, their works tend collectively to suggest both a common commitment to the depiction of social injustices and a "duty to reveal women's deepest emotional reality."[3] Many Victorian women poets wrote "not from, but against the heart" (Leighton 1992, 3), in essence revolutionizing the "aesthetic of the feminine" from within (Isobel Armstrong 1993, 323–24).

Like other women poets of the period, Anne Brontë made the idea and ideal of femininity problematic in several ways—both through her investigation of the challenges to obedience and through her representation of the heart as an arena of emotional turmoil. Brontë's analysis of feminine sensibility, and of domestic ideology more generally, is in turn made more complex because it depends on a rhetoric also associated with Evangelicalism, "the religion of the heart."[4] While Brontë represented the heart as a locus of woman's feeling, she concerned herself as well with the ways self-understanding requires a personal relationship to God. This Evangelical dimension of her writing depended on an exploration of the heart as a barometer with which to monitor the inevitably unstable emotions encountered in the effort to understand the self in relation to God. Thus, when she refers, as she often does, to the hearts of her poetic personas, she characterizes them as "pensive," "burdened," "drooping," "polluted," "weary," "inconstant," "fainting," "throbbing," "hard," and "black," rhetoric frequently employed by Evangelicals to describe the difficulty of maintaining faith.

Far more than an easily identifiable symbol of idealized femininity, then, the heart for Brontë was simultaneously a source of power and of powerlessness. Symbolizing the center of the individual's emotional identity, it functioned as a secret "place" to retreat to in introspective silence and as a dimension of identity over which one had some control. Yet it was also the locus of powerful feelings that threatened to dismantle that control and to disrupt the placid surface that the individual often sought to present to others.

"Verses by Lady Geralda" (1) the earliest poem that has been attributed to Brontë, illustrates some of her concerns with emotional instability and self-understanding. Charting her journey from childhood innocence to adult experience by monitoring changes in her heart, the narrator begins by bemoaning the sadness that fills her mind when she hears the "wild winter wind / Rushing o'er the mountain heath" (ll. 2–3) and recognizes that the same sound once made her "heart beat exultingly" (l. 11) and her "whole soul rejoice" (l. 12). The narrator then reveals that she has returned to the places of her childhood expecting there to "soothe [her] weary heart" (l. 34), only to discover that "What gave [her] joy before / Now fills [her] heart with misery" (ll. 58–59). She locates the source of the change not within her surroundings but rather within herself:

> And why are all the beauties gone
> From this my native hill?
> Alas! my heart is changed alone:
> Nature is constant still. (ll. 61–64)

Nature represents here not just the natural world but rather all that is outside the speaker. Brontë's speaker questions the extent to which circumstances and experiences can completely account for her attitudinal changes, concluding that her own emotional anxieties are to blame:

> For when the heart is free from care,
> Whatever meets the eye
> Is bright, and every sound we hear
> Is full of melody. (ll. 65–68)

The burdens of adulthood have changed her, perhaps irrevocably, and it is with this idea that she struggles. Aligning herself with postlapsarian Eve, she says "But the world's before me now / Why should I despair?" (ll. 81–82). Although "left alone" (l. 76) and disconsolate, she strives instead to nurture the "cherished hope" (l. 85) that "is burning in [her] heart" (l. 87). The poem concludes:

> From such a hopeless home to part
> Is happiness to me,
> For nought can charm my weary heart
> Except activity. (ll. 97–100)

Although "Verses by Lady Geralda" was written when Brontë was 16 years old, its concern with the evocation of emotional reality is typical of much of the poetry she wrote over the next 13 years. Brontë writes "against the heart," so to speak, in "Verses by Lady Geralda" by using the language of the affective mode to reveal the process through which individuals become exiled from themselves and isolation becomes self-imposed. The final words of the poem's speaker convey at best a sense of resignation, a commitment only to activity that will allow her temporary respite from self-examination.

Bringing the feelings of her characters to the foreground enabled Brontë to distinguish between the emotional and intellectual dimensions of self-examination. Her treatment of her trademark thematic concerns—secrecy, silence, and solitude—furthered this distinction between the emotional and intellectual as well. Brontë wrote often of the difficulties of reading one's heart, of understanding one's feelings, in order to stress the emotional work entailed in self-scrunity. These emotional difficulties are characteristically marked by a retreat into secrecy or silence, a comfort in solitude, or an acceptance of geographic and psychological exile. In much of her best poetry she explores complex gestures such as sharing secrecy or giving expression to silence, as in the "silent eloquence" of "The Bluebell" (10). Brontë's interest in self-scrutiny can be seen in poems identified with the Gondal saga as well as in other poetry.[5] Her use of imaginative and autobiographic modes and a range of dialogic techniques enabled her to study secrecy, silence, solitude, and exile as strategies of self-understanding and self-representation. Understanding her methods thus allows one to see "Gondal" and "non-Gondal" poems as ultimately part of the same project.

Secrecy as Strategy: The Poetry of the Hidden

Anne Brontë was preoccupied in all her writing with secrecy, silence, and solitude as modes of self-understanding and as means of self-representation. Biographical evidence of Brontë's own demeanor lends added interest to these thematic preoccupations: both Brontë family correspondence and books written about the Brontë family suggest that Anne Brontë was markedly reserved and often silent in the presence of others, and the most reclusive member of a family notorious for their preservation of privacy.

More important, Brontë identified poetry—both as a form to read and one to write—with the province of secrecy. In a long passage in her first novel, Brontë has Agnes Grey write of the ways in which poetry serves as her "secret source of consolation." Explaining her strategies for survival as a governess, Agnes writes:

> When we are harrassed by sorrows or anxieties, or long oppressed by any powerful feelings which we must keep to ourselves, for which we can obtain and seek no sympathy from any living creature, and which yet we cannot, or will not wholly crush, we often naturally seek relief in poetry—and often find it, too—whether in the effusions of others, which seem to harmonize with our existing case, or in our own attempts to give utterance to those thoughts and feelings in strains less musical, perchance, but more appropriate, and therefore more penetrating and sympathetic, and, for the time, more soothing, or more powerful to rouse and to unburden the oppressed and swollen heart. Before this time, at Wellwood House and here, when suffering from home-sick melancholy, I had sought relief twice or thrice at this secret source of consolation; and now I flew to it again, with greater avidity than ever, because I seemed to need it more. I still preserve those relics of past sufferings and experiences, like pillars of witness set up in travelling through the vale of life, to mark particular occurrences. (*AG*, 121)[6]

What stands out most in the passage is Brontë's representation, via the character of Agnes, of secrecy as a mode of being that can be imposed on one by circumstances and yet be deliberately adopted as well. Even before Agnes mentions that poetry became her secret occupation, she writes of the "powerful feelings" that she chose not to share with others, both because she assumed that sympathetic ears would not be offered and because she chose not to seek them out. Poetry becomes an alternative outlet, a medium for dialogue with self, enabling the poet to relieve her "oppressed and swollen heart" without talking to others. At the end of the passage, Brontë subtly suggests that circumstances have made Agnes addicted to her poetry, that she increasingly needs the satisfaction of this secret outlet to survive. Even after she has left her situation, she continues, apparently, to harbor this need, for her passage implies that the poems themselves, as "relics of past sufferings," are preserved in secrecy for Agnes's private use. Although Agnes shares her diary with readers, the poems she refers to are never fully revealed.

"Self-Congratulation" (9), another early poem of Brontë's, illustrates her interest in secrecy also.[7] Well accustomed to marking new beginnings in her own spiritual and emotional development, Brontë composed this poem on 1 January 1840.[8] "Self-Congratulation" introduces a theme common to Brontë's poetry, that of the instability of selfhood—the ways individuals change over time and the ways these changes are consciously and unconsciously made manifest. Invoking the dialogue form characteristic of other poems, Brontë begins by having the speaker address a woman who is unable to hide her internal feelings:

> Maiden, thou wert thoughtless once
> > Of beauty or of grace,
> Simple and homely in attire
> > Careless of form and face.
> Then whence this change, and why so oft
> > Dost smooth thy hazel hair?
> And wherefore deck thy youthful form
> > With such unwearied care? (ll. 1–8)

The maiden's subsequent response to the question fails to satisfy the speaker, but she takes advantage of the opportunity to champion her own ability to keep her thoughts and feelings hidden from those around:

> I answered and it was enough;
> > They turned them to depart;
> They could not read my secret thoughts,
> > Nor see my throbbing heart. (ll. 21–24)

Brontë undercuts assumptions about the passivity of woman by turning the attention of the poem from the presumably romantic inclinations of the subject to the subject's ability to repress her emotions and in doing so control the self she presents to others. The speaker then suggests that the maiden's inability to exert this kind of control is quite common:

> I've noticed many a youthful form
> > Upon whose changeful face

> The inmost workings of the soul
>> The gazer's eye might trace.
> The speaking eye, the changing lip,
>> The ready blushing cheek,
> The smiling or beclouded brow
>> Their different feelings speak. (ll. 25–32)

Brontë's speaker again does not specify what feelings the eye, lip, cheek, and brow reveal, suggesting that it is their inability to hide their feelings, rather than the feelings themselves, that is at issue. Moreover, she prides herself on her own imperviousness to the scrutiny of others:

> But thank God! you might gaze on mine
>> For hours and never know
> The secret changes of my soul
>> From joy to bitter woe.
> Last night as we set round the fire
>> Conversing merrily,
> We heard without approaching steps
>> Of one well known to me.
> There was no trembling in my voice,
>> No blush upon my cheek,
> No lustrous sparkle in my eyes
>> Of hope or joy to speak.
> But O my spirit burned within,
>> My heart beat thick and fast.
> He came not nigh—he went away
>> And then my joy was past.
> And yet my comrades marked it not,
>> My voice was still the same;
> They saw me smile, and o'er my face—
>> No signs of sadness came; (ll. 33–52)

The speaker of the poem congratulates herself on her ability to keep the "feelings of her secret soul" hidden from those she sits with, presumably her friends and family. The feelings that she hides are evidently those of sexual desire, and the erotic interest of the poem is intensified by her emphasis on the repression and control of those desires.

The emotional irony of "Self-Congratulation" resides in the speaker's predicament: while feeling proud that she is inscrutable to others, she acknowledges that what she protects from their scrutiny, ultimately, is not the fulfillment but rather the painful thwarting of desire:

> They little knew my hidden thoughts
> And they will never know
> The anguish of my drooping heart,
> The bitter aching woe! (ll. 53–56)

In the end it is difficult to tell whether the speaker is triumphant or defeated in her assurance that "they will never know," but this ambiguity ultimately helps Brontë to expose the gap between the way one understands the self and the way that self is presented to others.

Another poem that evidences Brontë's interest in secrecy as a mode of self-understanding is "The Doubter's Prayer" (23), dated 10 September 1843, roughly midway through her poetic career. Composed on a Sunday, the 12-quatrain poem was originally titled simply "A Hymn." Like other Brontë poems written in an evangelical hymn tradition, this cloaks private material ostensibly unsuitable for congregational use in a public form.[9] The first stanza of "The Doubter's Prayer" invokes God as an "Eternal power of earth and air, / Unseen, yet seen in all around" (ll. 1–2) and asks him to hear the speaker's prayer for faith. In this poem the heart, an emblem of the speaker's troubled emotional life, functions as well as a symbol of her weak faith: she writes that "every fiend of Hell methinks / Enjoys the anguish of my heart" (ll. 23–24). Yet while the heart is associated with weak faith, it is also her potential salvation:

> Without some glimmering in my heart,
> I could not raise this fervent prayer;
> But O a stronger light impart,
> And in thy mercy fix it there! (ll. 13–16)

The thematic of secrecy plays an important part in the poem. The speaker momentarily wonders what she would do if she discovered that no God existed to hear or bless her:

> If this be vain delusion all,
> If death be an eternal sleep,
> And none can hear my secret call,
> Or see the silent tears I weep. (ll. 29–32)

While such doubts are almost immediately interrupted by pleas to God for help, it is noteworthy that God functions as an entity with powerful insight into her hidden feelings, as the one who could potentially "hear" her "secret call" and "see" her "silent tears." "The Doubter's Prayer" concludes with the speaker suggesting that "If [she] believe[s] that Jesus died / And waking rose to reign above" (ll. 41–42), then surely God will impart "A spring of comfort in [her] heart" (l. 48). The tone of the "doubter" is—like that of the speaker of "Self-Congratulation"—difficult to read; she could be still doubting (hence her use of the conditional "if"), or she could mean by her use of "if" to imply a logical conclusion—that *because* she believes, it necessarily follows that God will provide the comfort she seeks.

We can see in "The Doubter's Prayer" the same distillation of ideas that were explored, though to different ends, in "Self Congratulation." Even while kneeling in earnest prayer, Brontë's speaker acknowledges her inability to be obedient to faith, calling herself a "lost sinner" (23, l. 8) and describing herself as "distracted" (l. 34) and "weak, yet longing to believe" (l. 36). Her sense of the challenges of obedience is tied once again to her emotional life: she registers and responds to the loss of faith with "anguish of [her] heart" (l. 24), as opposed to her mind, and she hypothesizes that by revisiting the "blessed words" of Jesus she will find "a spring of comfort" (l. 48). Finally, she implies that God alone has access to her weaknesses, that her "secret call" and "silent tears" are registered by no one else. Here, too, her secrecy is presented as a measure of self-control and hence as a source of comfort, despite the undesirable feelings they shroud.

"The Doubter's Prayer" shows as well the ways in which Brontë's notion of secrecy as a self-representational strategy relates to the idea of silence, which is as salient a feature of her poetry. The speaker's appeal for faith is marked by a "secret call" and "silent tears" that work mutually to constitute and signify her desires. Like secrecy, silence is represented in Brontë's poetry as a condition that can be imposed on an individual and yet simultaneously adopted as a defensive gesture of self-preservation.

Silence as Speech: The Poetry of Expression

Silence achieves a special valence in Anne Brontë's works because of its relevance to women's writing in general. Largely because of patriarchal social structures that historically have restricted women's symbolic and literal access to public arenas for self-expression, many women writers developed "strategies of reticence" to challenge the very structures that silenced them.[10] Brontë dealt with the issue of woman's silence in two crucial ways. On the one hand, she empowered many of her poetic personas and fictional heroines by giving them opportunities to develop confidence in self-expression. Perhaps more important, she sought in a variety of ways to explore how silence itself empowered her female characters to exert control over their worlds. She used silence as a way of investigating more fully the private dynamics of individual experience. For Brontë the challenge of writing poetry was not really with restrictive societal definitions of femininity or with overcoming barriers to authorship—to public voice—set by the patriarchal culture that surrounded her. The very realm in which femininity was constructed—the private sphere—interested her as an emotional and cognitive domain.

Not surprisingly, silence performs an important function within this domain. In much of Brontë's poetry, silence becomes a means through which to understand and represent one's self. On occasion her personas confront the silence of others; in the 1845 poem "Night" (37), the speaker recounts dreams in which "a voice may meet my ear / That death has silenced long ago" (ll. 5–6).

More often, however, Brontë's speakers struggle with their own silence. In the 27-line poem "The Captive's Dream" (4), Brontë's speaker repeatedly tells her readers that she cannot voice the words she longs to speak. The poem tells the story of an encounter the speaker, a Gondal character identified as Alexandrina Zenobia, has with a man whom she barely recognizes, so changed in physical appearance seems he. "Woe-worn," "haggard," and stricken with grief, he prays for death and the speaker struggles but fails to respond: "I had no power to speak," she simply notes (l. 9). She knows she has the ability to save him but is unable to access that power and avail herself of it:

> And yet I might not speak one single word;
> I might not even tell him that I lived
> And that it might be possible if search were made,

> To find out where I was and set me free,
> O how I longed to clasp him to my heart,
> Or but to hold his trembling hand in mine,
> And speak one word of comfort to his mind. (ll. 11–17)

The interest of the poem turns on its exploration of the speaker's thwarted desires. Nowhere in the poem is her linguistic predicament explained; she simply reiterates five times that she cannot speak. Her physical powers of utterance are inexplicably gone:

> I struggled wildly but it was in vain,
> I could not rise from my dark dungeon floor,
> And the dear name I vainly strove to speak,
> Died in a voiceless whisper on my tongue. (4, ll. 18–21)

The emphasis on the speaker's voicelessness is critical.[11] The agony that the poem seeks to represent has not been brought on by her separation from her companion or from the apparently dire circumstances that he has found himself in. Rather, Brontë stresses the speaker's acute awareness of her own inability to respond and to express herself. Indeed, if Victorian poetry can be characterized by the "representational anxiety" it exhibits (Isobel Armstrong 1993, 7), Brontë's poetry might be said to depict the anxiety of self-representation.

"The Captive's Dream" illustrates as well how exile from others can lead to exile from self, a topic Brontë would take up in both of her novels. Though the experience of exile was a critical feature of the Gondal saga, it worked its way into "non-Gondal" poems as well. Dated 12 November 1843, "Past Days" (26) has traditionally been interpreted as a poem that registers Brontë's dismay at a change in the atmosphere of her own household, presumably her estrangement from Emily. The poem begins with the speaker lamenting the emotional emptiness of her home:

> 'Tis strange to think there was a time
> When mirth was not an empty name,
> When laughter really cheered the heart
> And frequent smiles unbidden came,

> And tears of grief would only flow
> In sympathy for others' woe. (ll. 1–6)

The theme of this opening stanza is played out in other ways for the remaining four stanzas; the characterization of what life has instead become remains unspoken but implied.

That Brontë's characterization of household life should be "unspoken" is in keeping with the way that silence itself works its way into the textual fabric of the poem, marking by both its presence and its absence unwelcome changes in relationships. The speaker remembers a time "When speech expressed the inward thought / And heart to kindred heart was bare" (26, ll. 7–8); a time when "silence, solitude and rest" were welcome features of day-to-day life (l. 11); and when night was dreaded because "friendly intercourse must cease / And silence must resume her power" (ll. 21–22).

"The Captive's Dream" and "Past Days" are alike in their focus on the discomfort of silence when imposed by circumstances rather than willingly adopted as a strategy for oneself. The two poems share as well an exploration of character change that enables Brontë to begin questioning the stability of selfhood. Just as the speaker of "The Captive's Dream" agonizes over her difficulty in recognizing a long-lost companion, so altered is his appearance, so too does the speaker of "Past Days" mourn the changes in her household companions. In both works, the speakers struggle with accepting changes in others; their struggle is made worse by the silence that seems to have been imposed on them. Other poems by Brontë, however, take up the topic of silence as a barrier to self-development by examining the emotional pain entailed in maintaining silence and the deeply isolating effects of verbal distance. In this way, Brontë's evocation of silence led her naturally to explore as well the situation of solitude.

Situating Solitude: The Poetry of Isolation

Anne Brontë's use of secrecy and silence in her poetry suggests that she was also interested in the situations associated with this interiority. The 12–line poem "Night" (37) reveals well the interconnectedness of secrecy, silence, and solitude in Brontë's thought. A poem about dreaming, it explores an individual's attempt to come to terms with her private desires. She begins by writing "I love the silent hour of night" (l. 1); she also acknowledges that in her dreams she hears "a voice . . . / That death has silenced long ago" (ll. 4–5). Hearing this voice through her dreams enables her to experience "hope and rapture" . . . / Instead of solitude and woe" (ll. 7–8).

Just as secrecy and silence functioned in Brontë's poems as linguistic conditions that could be either adopted by one or imposed on one, so too could solitude be simultaneously desired and abhorred, as "The Captive Dove" (24), written on 31 October 1845, illustrates. Brontë invokes a traditional symbol of woman common in the 19th century, the caged bird, to explore captivity and solitude. In this case, the speaker projects her own sense of isolation onto the dove that she addresses in the poem:

> Poor restless Dove, I pity thee,
> And when I hear thy plaintive moan
> I'll mourn for thy captivity
> And in thy woes forget mine own. (ll. 1–4)

In the last line of this opening stanza the speaker implies that her own woes are also woes of captivity, understood in a less literal sense. She intimates that the dove's unfulfilled potential and thwarted efforts speak to her own emotional stagnation:

> To see thee stand prepared to fly,
> And flap those useless wings of thine,
> And gaze into the distant sky
> Would melt a harder heart than mine. (ll. 4–8)

In a gesture Brontë used in a variety of poems, the speaker abruptly interrupts her address to the dove and contemplation of its predicament to issue the following rebuke:

> In vain! In vain! Thou canst not rise—
> Thy prison roof confines thee there;
> Its slender wires delude thine eyes,
> And quench thy longing with despair. (24, ll. 9–12)

The reprimand is asserted in such a way as to leave open to interpretation whether the speaker is chastising herself or the dove for believing in the possibility of escape and liberty. In the process Brontë destabilizes the opposition between self and other, creating within the poem a dialogue through which the speaker engages with several "selves."

Although the fourth stanza of the poem suggests that the speaker imagines the dove as "made to wander" (24, l. 13), a being with "the will to rove" (l. 16) and hence content with its liberty, the fifth stanza more overtly projects the speaker's own desires onto the dove:

> Yet hadst thou but one gentle mate
> Thy little drooping heart to cheer
> And share with thee thy captive state,
> Thou couldst be happy even there. (ll. 17–20)

It is not the condition of captivity that accounts for the unhappiness of either the dove or the speaker, but rather the solitude that is a consequence of the captivity. With companionship, she argues, would come emotional health and fulfillment, so much so that the dove "mightst forget [its] native wood" (l. 24).[12]

Nonetheless, the concluding stanza of the poem negates the possibility suggested in the preceding two stanzas:

> But thou, poor solitary dove,
> Must make unheard thy joyless moan;
> The heart that nature formed to love
> Must pine neglected and alone. (24, ll. 25–28)

The "restless dove" of the opening invocation becomes, by the poem's conclusion, "solitary," and its solitude is further characterized by a condition of voicelessness much like that endured by the speaker of "The Captive's Dream." The final two lines of the poem reflect the speaker's own sense of her self as unfulfilled. In introducing the idea of the unfulfilled individual, the self conflicted by an awareness of instincts and desires that experience does not provide outlets for, "The Captive Dove" presents a theme that Brontë would take up in more depth in several other poems, among them "If This Be All" (39) and "Dreams" (40).

In its representation of solitude as a psychological state, as opposed to simply a physical condition, "The Captive Dove" suggests that solitude can so affect an individual who experiences it that it completely colors the way that individual relates to the world. In subsequent poems, Brontë moves away from figures, such as the dove, that allow her speakers to distance themselves, even obliquely, from self-examination. These poems more directly represent their subjects as undergoing an often painful process of self-scrutiny.

The speaker of "Dreams" (40), written in the spring of 1845, begins her exploration of dreams as an escape from a "life of solitude" (l. 20) with the following stanza:

> While on my lonely couch I lie
> I seldom feel myself alone,
> For fancy fills my dreaming eye
> With scenes and pleasures of its own. (ll. 1–4)

The dream functions as an escape from self. After establishing her predilection to escape loneliness by dreaming, the speaker examines her recurrent dream of being a mother. She associates maternity with nurturing and with the opportunity to be entirely responsible for another being:

> How sweet to feel its helpless form
> Depending thus on me alone;
> And while I hold it safe and warm,
> What bliss to think it is my own! (ll. 9–12)

The dream manifests her attraction to the ownership and control associated with motherhood, hence the speaker's use of "me alone" to describe her role as caretaker and "my own" to describe the infant. The poem then suggests that the speaker desires a child not just to satisfy unfulfilled nurturing instincts, but also to alleviate her solitude:

> To feel my hand so kindly pressed,
> To know myself beloved at last,
> To think my heart has found a rest,
> My life of solitude is past. (ll. 17–20)

Far from simply endorsing the domestic ideology that championed motherhood as a natural role for women, Brontë emphasizes the emotional and psychological needs that produce the desire of her speaker. The speaker imagines that not until she has a child of her own will she know herself to be loved and will her isolation end. The last two stanzas

represents herself as controlled against her will by those around her and as unable to create for herself a sense of autonomy. Yet the second of these stanzas turns from placing blame on those around her to focusing on the internal dynamic that has left her in stasis: "the silent current from within" (39, l. 19) that is as powerful as "the outward torrent's swell" (l. 20). The last stanza then suggests that though the speaker is uncomfortable with her alienation, her desires for relationships are turned on her, "driven backward to [her] heart," and "turned to wormwood there" (l. 24).

Concluding this section with imagery of waste and decay within her heart, she turns back at the poem's conclusion to readdress God:

> If clouds must ever keep from sight
>   The glories of the sun;
> And I must suffer Winter's blight
>   Ere Summer is begun:
>
> If life must be so full of care,
>   Then call me soon to Thee;
> Or give me strength enough to bear
>   My load of misery. (39, ll. 25–32)

In no other single poem is the feeling of private anguish so intense as in "If This Be All." The first two lines of the last stanza express a sentiment that might almost be labeled suicidal; the speaker would rather die and be with God than continue a life seemingly fraught with problems. Yet rather than end the poem with an expression of those feelings, she asks only for the strength to continue living.

Like "If This Be All," "Severed and Gone" (55) expresses a speaker's yearning for a relationship that is impossible. Written in April 1847 and often interpreted as Brontë's reaction to the death of William Weightman, the poem examines a woman who privately harbors feelings for a man long dead and who feels isolated yet, because of her access to memories, not alone.[13] The poem begins with the speaker linking her own solitude on earth and her correlative intensity of emotion with the isolation of her lost loved one:

> Severed and gone, so many years!
> And art thou still so dear to me,

> That throbbing heart and burning tears
> Can witness how I clung to thee?
>
> I know that in the narrow tomb
> The form I loved was buried deep,
> And left, in silence and in gloom,
> To slumber out its dreamless sleep. (ll. 1–8)

The silence of the crypt is associated in the sixth stanza of the poem with the speaker's own bedroom, where she prays at night for a vision of her lover:

> For ever gone; for I, by night,
> Have prayed, within my silent room,
> That Heaven would grant a burst of light
> Its cheerless darkness to illume;
>
> And give thee to my longing eyes,
> A moment, as thou shinest now,
> Fresh from thy mansion in the skies,
> With all its glories on thy brow. (ll. 21–28)

Brontë makes use of additional motifs established as well in "Night" (37), written nearly two years earlier, in which the speaker rhapsodizes about the "blissful dreams" (l. 2) that appear in the "silent hour of night" (l. 1). In "Severed and Gone," the speaker abruptly interrupts her prayers in much the same way as the speaker of "Dreams." She chastises herself for indulging in such desires:

> False hope! vain prayer! it might not be
> That thou shouldst visit earth again.
> I called on Heaven—I called on thee,
> And watched, and waited—all in vain. (55, ll. 37–40)

In her drive to find some way out of her solitude, the speaker turns from God to her self, suggesting that the memory of her lover inhabits her heart:

> Thou breathest in my bosom yet,
> And dwellest in my beating heart;
> And, while I cannot quite forget,
> Thou, darling, canst not quite depart. (ll. 53–56)

Here again, then, Brontë subordinates the sentimental tradition with which women writers were presumed to be associated by exploiting its psychological and emotional interest.

While "Severed and Gone" might be said to champion "the permanence of love in the face of transience" (Langland 1989, 75), it also concerns itself with the uniquely isolated position of the one who continues to love, despite the loss of an object of love. The speaker concludes:

> Earth hath received thine earthly part;
> Thine heavenly flame has heavenward flown;
> But both still linger in my heart,
> Still live, and not in mine alone. (55, ll. 65–68)

The repetition of "still" in the last two lines is significant. It represents the constancy of feelings in the speaker, who from the very beginning of the poem emphasizes that her feelings have withstood "slow decay" (l. 18). Yet Brontë's use of "still" helps also to underscore the silent situation of the speaker, who seems to have harbored the emotional impact of her loss and grief alone. Brontë used "still" to help convey situations of problematic communication in other poems as well; in "The Three Guides" (56), written in August 1847, she writes "Dull is thine ear; unheard by thee / The still small voice of Heaven" (ll. 49–50).

Although Brontë represented solitude as painful isolation, she also explored its potential to nurture an individual's privacy and to enable self-examination. In this way, her poetry, like that of other Victorian women poets, participates in her culture's "discussion of the nature of the nineteenth-century female imagination" (Leighton 1992, 3). Even in poems that tackle the challenges of loneliness, Brontë's speakers often acknowledge the comfort of their isolation.

One poem that stresses the pleasures of privacy is "The Arbour" (38), which begins with a description of luxurious physical surroundings:

> I'll rest me in this sheltered bower,
> And look upon the clear blue sky

That smiles upon me through the trees,
Which stand so thickly clustering by;

And view their green and glossy leaves,
All glistening in the sunshine fair;
And list the rustling of their boughs,
So softly whispering through the air. (ll. 1–8)

The speaker of "The Arbour" is led, like so many of Brontë's poetic personas, to interrogate her self for indulging in comforting thoughts. In
the fifth stanza of the poem she interrupts herself to begin such a
process:

Oh, list! 'tis summer's very breath
That gently shakes the rustling trees—
But look! The snow is on the ground—
How can I think of scenes like these? (ll. 17–20)

Brontë's speaker treats imaginative escape as an occasion for guilt.
The poem concludes by invoking a characteristic pattern: after her
speaker scolds herself for turning away from reality, she turns inward to
her heart to assess her own isolation:

'Tis but the *frost* that clears the air,
And gives the sky that lovely blue;
They're smiling in a *winter's* sun,
Those evergreens of sombre hue.

And winter's chill is on my heart—
How can I dream of future bliss?
How can my spirit soar away,
Confined by such a chain as this? (38, ll. 21–28)

Although "The Arbour" ends with an allusion to the speaker's sense of
psychological imprisonment, many other nature poems written by
Brontë demonstrate an alternative impulse, one that Brontë typically
expressed through her use of the adjective "wild" and through the
related thematic of exile.

The Poetry of Exile and Its Alternatives

From the very beginning of her career, Anne Brontë was attracted to the psychological and emotional interest of exile. She frequently created characters in her poems who were captives, as in "The Captive's Dream" (37), "A Voice from the Dungeon" (3), "The North Wind" (5), and the untitled poem that begins "A Prisoner in a dungeon deep" (48). Many other poems created situations of exile less explicitly—often, for example, by using representations of the undomesticated, of wildness, to help describe an individual's distance or alienation from something, whether that something be one's past, one's home, one's loved ones, or one's self. These less tangible situations of solitude are incorporated in Gondal poems as well, often helping to underscore the less concrete emotional and psychological implications of the speaker's predicament.

In "Verses by Lady Geralda" (1), for instance, the speaker begins her study of how she has changed by examining her reactions to the places of her past. She hears "the wild winter wind" (l. 2), remembers how she used to rejoice in "its wild and lofty voice" (l. 10), and recollects childhood journeys to vales "of wild and lovely flowers" (l. 30). When she comes to understand that she, not Nature, has changed, she concludes that, because of her anxieties, "The sweetest strain, the wildest wind . . . Like doleful death knells seem" (ll. 69–73). The poem associates her loss of pleasure in wilderness with her loss of family:

> Father! thou hast long been dead,
> Mother! thou art gone,
> Brother! thou art far away,
> And I am left alone. (ll. 73–76)

In another maneuver that subtly questions the legitimacy of a domestic ideology that idealized the home, Brontë concludes the poem with her speaker's decision to embrace a life of exile, a life as a wanderer, as the only acceptable solution. As she explains it, "From such a hopeless home to part / Is happiness to me" (ll. 97–98). In "Verses by Lady Geralda," Brontë avoids creating a false binary where "the wild" functions in simplistic opposition to home. Rather, both are seen as psychological constructs, as perceptions of the speaker's consciousness that over time have changed.

Homelessness is not often accepted as easily as it seems to be in "Verses by Lady Geralda," despite the agony that the speaker expresses midway through her story. In "A Voice from the Dungeon" (3), the speaker, in typical Brontë fashion, wakes from a dream of domestic bliss (i.e., she dreams of clasping her "darling boy" to her breast and of his childish laughter), uttering "one long piercing shriek" (l. 48) to "wild despair" (l. 51):

> Alas! Alas! That cursed scream
> Aroused me from my heavenly dream;
> I looked around in wild despair,
> I called them, but they were not there;
> The father and the child are gone,
> And I must live and die alone. (ll. 49–54)

The speaker's "wild despair" conveys the agony with which she experiences waking from her dream and the concomitant loss of pleasure, illusory though it was, as well as her concurrent realization that she is condemned to loneliness.

Another poem that illustrates the ways Brontë integrated secrecy, silence, and solitude into her poetry of exile is "The North Wind" (5). Like "A Voice from the Dungeon," "The North Wind" is a relatively early poem. Dated 26 January 1838, it is "signed" by the Gondal character Alexandrina Zenobia. Throughout the poem she describes the "language" of the wind, which, as it "moans and murmurs mournfully," "speaks to [her]" (ll. 6–7). The wind is forceful and undomesticated; as the speaker explains, "No other breeze could have so wild a swell" (l. 2) Brontë creates a level of dialogue within the poem by using the speaker's narrative as a frame to surround three stanzas of monologue associated with the wind itself. The speaker languishes in a dungeon, and the wind helps her to recollect her past:

> When thou, a young enthusiast,
> As wild and free as they,
> O'er rocks and glens and snowy heights
> Didst often love to stray. (ll. 12–15)

The wind continues to remind the speaker of her affiliation with the wilderness that it represents:

> I have howled in caverns wild
> Where thou, a joyous mountain child,
> Didst dearly love to be. (ll. 18–20)

She responds with an invocation to continue its work:

> Blow on, wild wind, thy solemn voice,
> However sad and drear,
> Is nothing to the gloomy silence
> I have had to bear. (ll. 29–32)

The poem concludes with her reluctant admission that, although "Confined and hopeless" (l. 37), she yearns to be told of "liberty" and her "mountain home" (ll. 38–39).

Just as the speaker of "The Arbour" (38) found in her surroundings the emblems of her own "chill" heart, so too does the speaker of "The North Wind" hear in the wind's message a reflection of her own desires. In "The North Wind," Brontë repeats as well the dynamic found in "Verses by Lady Geralda" (1), a dynamic in which the wild symbolizes the distance of the speaker from the domestic. The poem then underscores the thematic of homelessness by revealing that the speaker's exile is constituted both by her captivity and by her banishment from a childhood pleasure in the wild.

The same cluster of ideas—the wild, home and homelessness, and exile— manifest themselves in non-Gondal poems as well. The speaker of "Home" (30), an undated poem published in the 1846 collection, begins by surveying the natural wonders and comfort that surround her; in the opening stanzas her eyes pass over the glistening sun, woodland ivy, and the silver rays of beech trees. Though seemingly a gentle scene, the second stanza notes that "wildly through unnumbered trees / The wind of winter sighs" (ll. 7–8). The recognition of this wild wind prompts Brontë's speaker to break from her ruminations and to call for an even less domesticated scene:

> But give me back my barren hills
> Where colder breezes rise:
> Where scarce the scattered, stunted trees
> Can yield an answering swell,

But where a wilderness of heath
Returns the sound as well. (ll. 11–16)

Although the speaker is surrounded by a cultivated and comfortable
kind of nature (in the form of "a garden," "groves," and "velvet lawns"),
she is more attracted to a place she associates with her past, and presumably with her childhood. She describes a "little spot" that is surrounded
by "gray walls" and "Where knotted grass neglected lies, / And weeds
usurp the ground" (ll. 23–24). She associates this wilderness with home,
and the poem ends by emphasizing her distance from it:

Though all around this mansion high
Invites the foot to roam,
And though its halls are fair within—
Oh, give me back my home! (ll. 25–28)

"Home" lends itself to an autobiographical reading that focuses on
the homesickness Brontë experienced on leaving Haworth for Thorp
Green.[14] Yet it seems equally important to stress the ways in which the
speaker of the poem uses the thematic alternatives of wilderness and cultivated nature, of home and exile, to convey her sense of identity. By
repudiating any desire to live within a "mansion high," however fair its
halls, or to roam about groves and gardens, no matter how attractive the
landscaping, she embraces a more humble rural and class heritage,
implicitly identifying that heritage as essential to her self-understanding.

Although Brontë continued to work with concepts of home and
homelessness throughout her poetic career, she came increasingly to
associate home with "a place of eternal rest" (Langland 1989, 82). The
home that had been affiliated in earlier work with family becomes in
later poems simply a house that lacks the shared thoughts and mutual
understanding that for Brontë defined the family. Challenging an idealized version of domesticity, "Monday Night May 11th 1846" (49)
implicitly makes just such a distinction between house and home:

Why should such gloomy silence reign;
And why is all the house so drear,
When neither danger, sickness, pain,
Nor death, nor want have entered here? (ll. 1–4)

Brontë's speaker looks first outside her self to her external surroundings to uncover the source of change. When her search fails to identify a cause, she is led to speculate on the isolating effects of empathy that goes unexpressed. She thinks she understands the emotions of others in her house, but feels powerless to convey her empathy:

> The moon without as pure and calm
> Is shining as that night she shone;
> But now, to us she brings no balm,
> For something from our hearts is gone.
>
> Something whose absence leaves a void,
> A cheerless want in every heart.
> Each feels the bliss of all destroyed
> And mourns the change—but each apart. (ll. 9–16)

The heart functions here not just as the barometer with which the speaker measures change. What the heart does register, in other words, is emptiness or a lack—a "want"—that is felt because of the obliteration of what was once there. Emphasizing this lack, Brontë is able to suggest an "existential emptying" of domestic sensibility, one that is characteristic not just of her poetry but of Victorian women's poetry in general (Leighton 1989, 298). In the last two stanzas of the poem, Brontë's speaker suggests that the change is irrevocable:

> 'Twas *Peace* that flowed from heart to heart
> With looks and smiles that spoke of Heaven,
> And gave us language to impart
> The blissful thoughts itself had given.
>
> Sweet child of Heaven, and joy of earth!
> O, when will Man thy value learn?
> We rudely drove thee from our hearth,
> And vainly sigh for thy return. (49, ll. 21–28)

In the concluding stanzas of "Monday Night May 11 1846," Brontë returns to themes already well established in her work: the idea that language, the ability to express oneself and communicate effectively, is dependent upon emotional stability. In this poem, it is emotional stability itself—represented here as Peace—that is exiled, driven from the home. The desire to return to the past, in whatever form, is illusory, Brontë suggests.

As "Home" and "Monday Night May 11th 1846" make clear, Brontë's use of exile, of motifs that included in various ways garden and wilderness, home and homelessness, extended into all her work, not simply the extreme situations of captivity and imprisonment typical of the Gondal poems. "Monday Night May 11th 1846" chronicles an emotional withdrawal from home, a recognition that the sanctuary it might once have represented is tenuous and, once gone, impossible to reestablish. The movement away from home as a sanctuary seems to result in an even greater retreat into interiority and helps to illustrate the ways that Brontë used exile, secrecy, silence, and solitude, as strategies of self-examination.

Reticence and Retreat: A Gendered Reading of Brontë's Poetry

Anne Brontë represented secrecy, silence, solitude, and exile as strategies for self-understanding and as tools for self-representation. The importance of these themes to Brontë is suggested by the manuscript copies of her poems, many of which show that she originally capitalized the words "silence" and "solitude," perhaps to emphasize the powerful capacity of each to shape identity. She was well aware, however, of the broader cultural forces that impacted the dynamics of private experience. To ask what Brontë's poetry can teach us about the material conditions shaping the identities of Victorian women would seem in some ways to contradict her own poetic aims. For Brontë, the end of poetry was to have located and understood the "language of [her] inmost heart," as she wrote in "To Cowper" (19, l. 5). Yet even this identification of poetry with the realm of the private is a gesture generated in part by 19th-century ideologies of femininity and by the lived experience of many Victorian middle-class women. As Brontë's poetry so clearly shows, that "inmost heart" was much more than an uncomplicated symbol of woman's destiny; for Brontë, the heart was also an emblem of the emotional dilemmas encountered in the discovery of identity and in the representation of that identity to others.

One of Brontë's last poems, "Self-Communion" (57), [15] introduces via its very title the psychological complexity typical of her work. Written between November 1847 and April 1848, "Self-Communion" grapples with the multidimensionality of identity and the corresponding possibility for multiple levels of dialogue with the self. Suggesting as it does both the act of sharing and the idea of common faith, the notion of "self-communion" implies a divided or fractured identity, whose component parts engage with one another rather than with those outside the self. Furthermore, just as "communion" refers as well to the act of receiving the Eucharist and becoming transformed in the process, so too does "self-communion" imply a process of personal transformation.

"Self-Communion" stands apart from Brontë's other poetry in several ways, most notably in its uncharacteristic length. The 334–line poem proceeds in dialogue form. Although initially the speaker seems to engage in dialogue with someone else, by the poem's end it becomes clear that the conversation is entirely self-constructed, with each "speaker" representing a dimension of the subject's identity. The poem begins with an eight-line stanza in which the subject of the poem is directed by one side of her self to seek repose:

> "The mist is resting on the hill;
> The smoke is hanging in the air;
> The very clouds are standing still;
> A breathless calm broods everywhere.
> Thou pilgrim through this vale of tears
> Thou, too, a little moment cease
> Thy anxious toil and fluttering fears,
> And rest thee, for a while, in peace." (ll. 1–8)

The repetition in the first three lines of participles in the present progressive form help to create an aura of indefinite suspension that the speaker of this stanza identifies with her natural surroundings. Furthermore, the compatibility between the denotions of the verbs "rest," "hang," and "stand" complicates the action implied by the participle form, creating in the process an almost oxymoronic sense of suspended or arrested movement. This somewhat confused state is underscored by the haziness of the setting itself—the mist, smoke, and clouds. The subject of the poem is constructed as a product of this environment; as a "pilgrim," she is associated with movement and change, yet she is also advised to stop "a little moment" and rest "for a while" from the psychological turmoil of her journey.

The response of the subject of the poem to this request introduces a number of issues, but most prominent is the idea of loss, which she associates with the nature of temporality itself: "'I would, but Time keeps working still / And moving on for good or ill: / *He* will not rest nor stay'" (57, ll. 9–11). Within the span of her first 11 lines, Brontë experiments with the multiple meanings of "still," in much the same way as in "Severed and Gone" (55). With yet another use of "still," the subject of the poem goes on to distinguish between the idea of time as an accumulation of experience and time as a measure of lost possibility: "In pain or ease, in smile or tears, / He still keeps adding to my years / And stealing life away" (57, ll. 12–14). She laments her lost childhood and early youth, and acknowledges that though she "cannot see how fast it goes" (l. 26), her "inward spirit knows / The wasting power of time" (ll. 27–28).

In response to this expression of regret and fear, the subject of "Self-Communion" is told that the "inward spirit" of which she spoke is ultimately immune to the ravages of time:

> Time steals thy moments, drinks thy breath,
> Changes and wastes thy mortal frame;
> But though he gives the clay to death,
> He cannot touch the inward flame. (57, ll. 29–32)

She is advised to allay her fears by turning to memory as a source of permanent inspiration and knowledge: "The wise will find in Memory's store / A help for that which lies before / To guide their course aright" (ll. 37–39). Here again "Self-Communion" addresses ideas that Brontë had explored in earlier poems, among them "Severed and Gone."

Following this advice, the subject of the poem begins to analyze her childhood, which, she suggests, introduces her to the difficulty of truthfully representing her self to others. From lines 43 through 128, the alternative voice in the poem functions merely as a prod, only once interrupting to encourage further introspection: "Look back again—What dost thou see?" (57, l. 92). The self that the subject of the poem constructs during this portion of her introspective process is akin to the personas Brontë developed in other poems. On four occasions in 41 lines she characterizes her self by reference to her heart: she has "A tender heart too prone to weep" (l. 54), "A heart so ready to believe / And willing to admire" (l. 66–67), a "heart so prone to overflow / E'en at the *thought* of other's woe" (ll. 82–83), and "A young heart feeling after God" (l. 95). To cope with the "sin and falsehood" (l. 65) that surround her, she turns inward, adopting secrecy and silence as protective shields: she acknowledges that "The only bliss its soul can know:—" is "Still hiding in its breast" (ll. 52, 53) and that her heart harbors "A love so earnest, strong and deep / It could not be expressed" (ll. 55–56). This idea of self-imposed isolation and silence dominates the remainder of her portions of the poem. Much later, for instance, she acknowledges the pain she experienced upon learning the "truth" that she "must check, or nurse apart / Full many an impulse of the heart" (ll. 190–191), but then she writes:

> Until, at last, I learned to bear
> A colder heart within my breast;
> To share such thoughts as I could share,
> And calmly keep the rest. (ll. 200–203)

Not surprisingly, the speaker's emotional predicament condemns her to a solitude that she sees as at once inevitable and intolerable. She asserts her belief that her "inner life of strife and tears, / Of kindling hopes and lowering fears, / To none but God is known" (57, ll. 100–102) and proclaims that "'Tis better thus: for *man* would scorn . . . But *God* will not despise!" (ll. 103, 106). Yet at the same time the speaker asks how "That soul, that clings to sympathy / As ivy clasps the forest tree, / How can it stand alone?" (ll. 79–81). Invoking a similar metaphor later in the poem, she suggests that her solitude is a natural result of outside forces:

> I saw that they were sundered now,
> The trees that at the root were one:
> They yet might mingle leaf and bough,
> But still the stems must stand alone. (ll. 204–207)[16]

Although the subject of the poem occasionally expresses unequivocal confidence in God, several important portions of the poem illustrate the ways her understanding of God challenges her understanding of self. Throughout these portions, the alternative voice in the poem functions not just to prod the subject to further introspection but also to encourage the subject's faith. In a short stanza following the subject's investigation of her childhood and youth, this voice reminds her to find assurance in God:

> 'So was it, and so will it be;
> Thy God will guide and strengthen thee;
>   His goodness cannot fail.
> The sun that on thy morning rose
> Will light thee to the evening's close,
>   Whatever storms assail. (57, ll. 129–134)

In language reminiscent of that used by the speaker of "The Doubter's Prayer" (23), the response of the subject to this reminder indicates that a part of her is unwilling to accept such easy assurances. Her reluctance stems from an uneasiness with accepting changes in her self, and in an important portion of the poem she counters with a declaration that implies that God is not all-powerful:

> '*God* alters not; but Time on me
> A wide and wondrous change has wrought;
> And in these parted years I see
> Cause for grave care and saddening thought.
> I see that time, and toil, and truth
> An inward hardness can impart,—
> Can freeze the generous blood of youth,
> And steel full fast the tender heart. (57, ll. 135–142)

By personifying Time (as she had personified Memory at an earlier point in the poem), the subject of the poem constructs counterforces to God and represents herself as unable to exert any control over processes much larger than herself. Her sense of self is dominated by her interior landscape, one that has become irrevocably "hardened" by experience.

Although she is encouraged to believe that her sense of a "hardened" heart is a God-given tool to protect her from pain and to enable her to approach difficult experiences with reason rather than with feeling, she finds herself unable to do so, again turning to her heart as a barometer of her capacities (or lack thereof): "'Nay, but 'tis hard to *feel* that chill / Come creeping o'er the shuddering heart" (57, ll. 163–64). For nearly a hundred lines after this point, the subject of the poem discusses the meaning of love in her life, arguing both for its role in saving her from anguish and for its failure to sustain her in times of need. Once again countering an idealized and sentimental version of the restorative power of love, Brontë invokes the concept instead to analyze the idea of the lost potential for self-fulfillment:

> Love may be full of pain, but still,
> 'Tis sad to see it so depart,—
> To watch that fire, whose genial glow
> Was formed to comfort and to cheer,
> For want of fuel, fading so,
> Sinking to embers dull and drear,—
> To see the soil turned to stone
>   For lack of kindly showers,—
> To see those yearnings of the breast,
> Pining to bless and to be blessed,
> Drop withered, frozen one by one,
> Till centred in itself alone,
> It wastes its blighted powers. (57, ll. 165–177)

Reason, she subsequently argues, has functioned in her life not as an instrument of learning but rather as a source of mockery and derision (57, l. 221). Returning to the technique established in earlier poems, she interrupts her thoughts of love's potential to chide her self:

> O vainly might I seek to show
> The joys from happy love that flow!
> The warmest words are all too cold
> The secret transports to unfold
> Of simplest word or softest sigh,
> Or from the glancing of an eye
>   To say what rapture beams;
> One look that bids our fears depart,
> And well assures the trusting heart
> It beats not in the world alone—
> Such speechless raptures I have known,
>   But only in my dreams. (ll. 233–244)

Allowing the subject to interrupt her self not with the alternative voice
that has already engaged her in dialogue but rather with an additional
voice, Brontë adds complexity to the poem's heteroglossic or multivoiced
representation of dilemmas of identity. The dynamics of "Self-
Communion" change dramatically soon after this expression of anguish,
with the alternative voice of the poem becoming increasingly dominant
and the subject's hesitant and sorrowful voice becoming increasingly
recessive.

In lines 261 through 296, the alternative is noticeably less patient
with the subject, bluntly telling her, "'So must it fare will all thy race /
Who seek in earthly things their joy'" (ll. 261–62), scolding her with the
label "weak of heart" (l. 271), and commanding her to prepare for a battle and to "strive" for "'Love and Wisdom's sake!'" (l. 296). The harsh-
ness of this message prompts the subject of the poem to admit in
response that her "worst enemies" are "within [her] breast" (ll.
301–302), another implicit reference to her divided identity. When told
that her rest will not be found in this world but rather "beyond the
grave" (l. 306), she asks simply for direction: "Show me that rest—I ask
no more" (l. 310) and seemingly gives up her introspective quest for self-
understanding.

Furthermore, she accepts, if only partially, the comfort in God that
her alternative voice had earlier offered. To manifest this process of
acceptance, Brontë adds yet another layer of voice to the poem, this one
the subject's hypothetical version of something God might say:

> Could I but hear my Saviour say,—
> "I know thy patience and thy love;
> How thou has held the narrow way,
> For my sake laboured night and day,
> And watched, and striven with them that strove;
> And still hast borne, and didst not faint,"—
> Oh, this would be reward indeed! (57, ll. 326–32)[17]

Just as in earlier poems Brontë used the conditional "if" to suggest the
coexistence of a kind of logical assurance and mere possibility, so too do
the modal verbs of "could" and "would" that frame the speech that she
imagines is spoken by God suggest cautious hypotheticality. The poem
does not conclude with this passage, which would in essence make what

had been the dominant voice of the subject through much of the poem the "last word." Rather the poem ends with a brief, two-line directive from the alternative voice, commanding her simply and somewhat brusquely to "'Press forward, then, without complaint; / Labour and love—and such shall be thy meed'" (ll. 333–34).

Read as autobiography, the ending of "Self-Communion" helps to reinforce the popular image of Anne Brontë as a quiet sufferer, determined to hide emotional turmoil beneath a "placid exterior" (Langland 1989, 63). Yet Brontë clearly uses the poem as an opportunity to explore the roles of secrecy, silence, solitude, and exile in the formation of identity and in the subsequent apprehension of that identity that the speaker comes to in the process of the poem. In its heteroglossic evocation of this process of self-exploration and self-representation, "Self-Communion," like many Victorian poems, "renegotiat[es] the terms of self and world" and creates what is "simultaneously a personal and cultural project" (Isobel Armstrong 1993, 7). Brontë's poem challenges the notion of a unified self by representing instead a consciousness interrogating itself; in doing so, she represents self-awareness as a recognition of a multilayered and often conflicted identity. Yet because the several layers of voice that are made manifest in "Self-Communion" emanate presumably from the same source, and the subject of the poem is one who understands her identity as evolving along a continuum of time, the poem simultaneously asserts a unified self, stable in some respects despite changes brought by experience.[18]

As "Self-Communion" illustrates so well, Anne Brontë concerned herself as a poet with a wide range of emotional and behavioral issues related to what she saw as fundamental dilemmas of identity—the difficulties of understanding the self and its development over time, of maintaining self-control in the face of social pressure, and of representing the self truthfully to others. These issues were further complicated by her awareness of the challenges to the relationship of the individual, even the believing individual, with God. As chapters 4 and 5 will show, Brontë's understanding of the complexity of the inner life—of the private life as a dynamic arena within which many dimensions of experience contribute to the formation of consciousness and self-understanding as well as to modes of self-representation—was critical to her fiction as well. Together, these next chapers indicate her enduring interest in the strategies that human beings employ in their sometimes futile efforts to know themselves and their place in history.

Chapter Four

"An Alien among Strangers": The Governess as Narrator in *Agnes Grey*

Anne Brontë's poetry hints at the social conditions that underwrote her depiction of the dilemmas encountered in a process of self-understanding and self-representation. In her fiction, these social conditions figure much more prominently, so much so that they often dominate the interpretation of her novels. For many readers, *Agnes Grey* seems on first encounter to be an exemplary type of social protest writing popular in the early and mid-Victorian period—the governess novel. Figuring in many novels of the 1830s, by 1847, when *Agnes Grey* was published, the governess stood "at the very heart of the English novel" (Hughes 1993, 1). Her ascent to this position is partly accounted for by the Governesses' Benevolent Institution, which was founded in the 1840s and issued reports on the status of the governess that in turn prompted periodical essayists to take up her cause as a subject of social concern.[1] The governess was a victim of a range of economic and social hardships, and the stories written about her became part of the "Condition of England" literature associated with these years in Great Britain.

Like many of these works, *Agnes Grey* attends to the economic conditions that precipitate the central character's decision to seek work as a governess. It documents the physical hardships that she confronts once employed and explores the social implications of her "reduced" position in society. Like most authors of governess novels, Brontë used the governess to demarcate and study the boundaries between the domestic woman and the working woman.[2] In *Agnes Grey,* however, these concerns are ultimately subsumed by Brontë's interest in dramatizing the interior world of her heroine. This interior world is made turbulent by Agnes Grey's private sense of her successes and failures in the public world. Her interior world is further characterized by an overwhelming sense of isolation that reveals itself in her secrecy and silence. Indeed, what distinguishes Brontë's novel most from other novels that describe the experiences of governesses is the attention she pays to the psychological domain inhabited by her heroine.[3] By emphasizing her heroine's lack of presence and voice, Brontë represents the condition of the governess as one of social and psychological invisibility. Yet, by representing that invisibility, by presenting it to a readership for consideration, she in essence makes it visible and makes it spoken.

The novel's status as social protest fiction is partly a consequence of the didactic overtones that dominate Brontë's narrative. Both in its evocation of Agnes Grey's work as a governess and in the style Agnes adopts as a narrator, the novel encourages readers to speculate on the educational work performed by fiction.[4] Indeed, Brontë invited such an approach in the opening paragraph of the novel, which begins with Agnes telling her readers:

> All true histories contain instruction; though, in some, the treasure may be hard to find, and, when found, so trivial in quantity, that the dry, shrivelled kernel scarcely compensates for the trouble of cracking the nut. Whether this be the case with my history or not, I am hardly competent to judge. I sometimes think it might prove useful to some, and entertaining to others; but the world may judge for itself. Shielded by my own obscurity, and by the lapse of years, and a few fictitious names, I do not fear to venture; and will candidly lay before the public what I would not disclose to the most intimate friend. (*AG*, 1)

Brontë continues through the novel to stress the instructional motivations that influence both what experiences Agnes selects for her readers and how she presents those experiences. As Agnes later explains:

> I have not enumerated half the vexatious propensities of my pupils, or half the troubles resulting from my heavy responsibilities, for fear of trespassing too much upon the reader's patience; as, perhaps, I have already done: but my design, in writing the few last pages, was not to amuse, but to benefit those whom it might concern: he that has no interest in such matters will doubtless have skipped them over with a cursory glance, and, perhaps, a malediction against the prolixity of the writer; but if a parent has, therefrom, gathered any useful hint, or an unfortunate governess received thereby the slightest benefit, I am well rewarded for my pains. (*AG*, 29)

Both of the passages quoted above are important—not simply in their invocation of the narrative's educational imperative, but also in the way they reveal an overlapping of social and psychological concerns.

Although her public duties as author are foremost in Agnes's explanation of her methods, her underlying beliefs about privacy emerge
through her references to her own "obscurity," the fears and pain that
accompany her work as an author, and the intimacy that she establishes
with her readers.

Brontë distinguishes Agnes's readership into two discernible types,
one clearly more ideal than the other: those who will approach the story
as a utilitarian tool (represented in the second passage by the parents and
governesses) and those who will seek from the narrative only amuse-
ment. Brontë uses these passages to underscore the kind of identity that
Agnes attempts to construct for herself in relationship to her readers as
well. In the first passage she projects herself as fundamentally cautious;
though ironic in her allusion to the demands of interpretation that novels exact of their readers, she clearly wants to be seen as circumspect and
self-effacing, "daring" to present her work to the public only because she
can do so anonymously. In the second passage she comes across as a martyr, willing to suffer the "pains" of writing for the benefit of others and
immune to the criticisms of those who deride her efforts.

That these two "selves" seem in some respects incongruous should not
surprise, for Brontë used the character of Agnes Grey to explore many of
the issues of individuality and of conflicted identity that permeate her
poetry as well. Just as Agnes as governess has a complicated relationship
to the families for whom she works, so too does Agnes as narrator have a
complicated relationship to her readers. Although she pledges in her
opening paragraph to "candidly lay before the public" her most private
experiences, she later reneges on her promise. Roughly midway through
her narrative, she explains:

> I began this book with the intention of concealing nothing; that those
> who liked might have the benefit of perusing a fellow creature's heart:
> but we have *some* thoughts that all the angels in heaven are welcome to
> behold, but not our brother-men—not even the best and kindest
> amongst them. (*AG,* 91)

Brontë uses Agnes's declaration to stress the power that she exerts as a
narrator, power that functions within the novel as a counterpoint to the
lack of authority she associates with her position as a governess. Equally
important is Brontë's association of Agnes's narrative with the domain of
the private: Brontë implies that her readers have been exposed not just
to Agnes's external activities, but to the emotional turmoil of her interior world as well. This interior world is multilayered; while Agnes

reveals some of its dimensions to her readers, others are ostensibly too sacrosanct for public display. In constructing a kind of "semi-private narration," then, Brontë has Agnes act as her own censor, choosing what and what not to reveal to her designated audience.[5]

Brontë adds another layer of complexity to our understanding of Agnes's identity in this passage by describing her narrative methods as well. Although Agnes suggests that some of her private thoughts will remain private, her readers clearly know by this point in the narrative that she is alluding to the romantic feelings she harbors for Edward Weston, the curate she has come to know while working for the Murray family. The passage functions more, then, to remind readers of her ostensible power to control the narrative than to actually exert that control. As a deliberate intrusion into the narration of the story itself, the passage calls attention to the command that Agnes has achieved as a writer (and in retrospect, presumably when her "true history" is culled from the pages of a diary) at precisely the point in the story when she begins to feel most her lack of control as a woman. In its manifestation of the imprecise boundaries between the public and the private, the passage points to part of the feminist interest of Brontë's work. Moreover, in its attention to the tribulations of Agnes's interior world, it exemplifies well the ways that social and psychological concerns coexist in Brontë's novel and, in doing so, may help to elucidate why Charlotte Brontë would once have described *Agnes Grey* as the "mirror of the mind of its author."[6]

Brontë's concerns with her character's psychological development emerge most clearly during episodes devoted to Agnes's experiences as a governess. Shortly after beginning her second appointment as a governess and meeting her new supervisor, the chilly Mrs. Murray, mother of the children for whom she would be responsible, Agnes describes herself as "an alien among strangers" (*AG,* 52). Capturing as it does the extreme feelings of estrangement and exile that haunt Agnes as she encounters a world emotionally and culturally remote from that which she had known, the phrase resonates throughout the entire novel. Although she at one point readies herself to "stand alone" among "strange inhabitants" (*AG,* 12), she is not prepared for the assaults to her sense of self that she experiences as a governess, as for instance when she overhears the senior Mrs. Bloomfield, mother of her first employer, questioning whether she is "a *proper person*" (*AG,* 31).

Brontë's rhetoric enables her to emphasize the issues of autonomy and self-understanding at stake in Agnes's quest to define herself through her experiences as a governess. Because Brontë worked as a governess herself, first at Blake Hall in Mirfield and then at Thorp Green, *Agnes Grey* has often been used to recreate Brontë's own experiences.[7] The novel clearly has autobiographical correlates, both in its evocation of the governess experience and in its rendering of Agnes's position within and feelings about her family. Yet the tangible details that Brontë uses to describe Agnes's position at home or at work are ultimately subsumed within a more profound investigation of how that position impacts her emotional development and sense of self. Brontë is careful to locate the roots of this emotional development within Agnes's own home.

Agnes Grey and the Family Plot

The domestic ideology to which Brontë responded in her novel represented the nuclear family as a panacea for most social ills. In many ways, the married woman and mother stood at the center of this idealized family, for she was keeper of the home and selfless beholder of the moral virtues associated with family life. In its evocation of Agnes's family life, *Agnes Grey* participates in an important cultural moment in the history of the family, one that complicates this sentimental picture of the traditional Victorian family. Through the structure of the novel itself, as well as in the selection of materials she attributed to Agnes, Brontë ensured that her heroine's experiences as a governess would be read as related to—even an outgrowth of—her experiences within her family.

First and foremost among these is her experience as a daughter. After the opening paragraph that invokes the novel's claim to "true history," Agnes situates her self in relation to her parents. Significantly, she begins with her father, subtly linking his moral character with his economic position: "My father was a clergyman of the north of England, who was deservedly respected by all who knew him; and, in his younger days, lived pretty comfortably on the joint income of a small incumbency and a snug little property of his own" (*AG,* 1). Of her mother, Agnes writes:

> My mother, who married him against the wishes of her friends, was a squire's daughter, and a woman of spirit. In vain it was represented to her that, if she became the poor parson's wife, she must relinquish her carriage and her lady's-maid and all the luxuries and elegances of affluence; which to her were little less than the necessaries of life. (*AG,* 1)

The way in which Agnes positions her parents enables Brontë to demarcate several class boundaries. Her father clearly belongs to the middle class, although at its lower end; he is a respected person by the standards of his own neighborhood, if a poor parson by the standards of those above him on the social scale. Whereas Agnes characterizes her father by the dual standards of his morality and his economic position, her mother's class is modified by a characterization of her personality. Twice in her opening narrative she refers to her mother's "high spirit," representing it as that which, in combination with her aversion to the attraction of riches, accounts for her otherwise unthinkable decision to "bury herself" in a "homely village" (*AG*, 2). Agnes's narrative of her parents' marriage tells an ambiguous story of social slippage. She proclaims that "you might search all England through and fail to find a happier couple" (*AG*, 2), evidently wanting her readers to respect the standards by which her mother chose to live. Yet, at the same time, she documents the process by which her family and especially her father were tempted to speculate away their little wealth in hopes of improving their economic standards, and describes the "bitterness" and "distress" that ensue (*AG*, 5).

Emphasizing self-sacrifice, Brontë uses Agnes's narrative to show the ways that she defines herself as submissive. She relates this submissiveness to Agnes's sense of daughterly duty. Agnes carefully documents the family's lowered living conditions and the sacrifices made as a result of her father's mistakes:

> The useful pony phaeton was sold, together with the stout well-fed pony—the old favourite that we had fully determined should end its days in peace, and never pass from our hands; . . . Our clothes were mended, turned, and darned to the utmost verge of decency; our food, always plain, was now simplified to an unprecedented degree—except my father's favourite dishes; our coals and candles were painfully economized—the pair of candles reduced to one, and that most sparingly used; the coals carefully husbanded in the half-empty grate: especially when my father·was out on his parish duties, or confined to bed through illness. . . . As for our carpets, they in time were worn threadbare, and patched and darned even to a greater extent than our garments. (*AG*, 5–6)

Agnes's catalog of sufferings stands out from other episodes recounted in her narrative both in its precision and in its breadth; on few other occasions does she pay so much attention to supplying her readers with so many specific instances of the point she wants to make. Noteworthy in her account is the attention she pays to the sacrifices her family makes in order that her father's pride not be further damaged. Significantly, their sacrifices involve more than simply relinquishing material goods; their morality itself is compromised, Agnes implies, in several ways. Giving up plans to save a horse from overwork or early death is, in Agnes's mind, comparable to a spiritual sacrifice, as later passages detailing her intense feelings about cruelty to animals reveal; wearing clothes that hover near the "verge of decency" places her family in a precarious moral status as well.

Brontë paves the way for Agnes's account of life as a governess via this story of her parents and her life at home during her formative years. Just as Agnes's mother survives her journey down the social ladder through a combination of middle-class resourcefulness and evangelical morality, so too does Agnes illustrate her own ability to withstand economic and social hardships by enacting the very same virtues her mother represented.[8] This opening portion of the novel further enables Brontë to introduce a theme of social isolation. Although Agnes carefully accounts for the temptations that led to her father's unfortunate financial mistakes, the focus of her narrative of family history is on their social isolation, first that endured by her mother after she had agreed to marry a "poor parson," and later by the entire family as they deliberately alienated maternal relations by refusing offers of financial help that were contingent on an admission that the marriage was ill-founded. In both instances, the social isolation is imposed on them by outsiders but is willingly accepted as well. Just as Brontë's poetic personas found that situations of exile facilitated an exploration of self, so too does Agnes Grey eventually discover reasons to embrace the isolation she experiences as a governess.

Brontë suggests that Agnes is able to accept the social isolation of governessing because it is part of her heritage. One of the features of her family life that Agnes selects for emphasis is her rural heritage, which Brontë presents through the familiar rhetoric of solitude and isolation. Agnes presents her rural heritage as a function of her father's position—and hence, indirectly, her family's social isolation—but also as a more essential part of her identity. As the narrative progresses, Brontë implies that Agnes's rural heritage helps to account for her naivete and lack of preparation for the world that awaits her as a governess. Indeed, at first they threaten to prevent her access to that world: awaiting a response to her inquiries regarding governess work, she writes, "But so long and so entire had been my parents' seclusion from the world, that many weeks elapsed before a suitable situation could be procured" (*AG*, 9). Her sense of an experientially impoverished background continues to haunt her once she leaves. As she explains to herself upon arrival at the Bloomfield residence, "True, I was near nineteen; but, thanks to my retired life and the protecting care of my mother and sister, I well knew that many a girl of fifteen, or under, was gifted with a more womanly address, and greater ease and self-possession" (*AG*, 12). These concerns are reiterated in her account of life with the Murray family, where she writes, "But this gives no proper idea of my feelings at all; and no one that has not lived such a retired, stationary life as mine can possibly imagine what they were: hardly even if he has known what it is to awake some morning and find himself in Port Nelson, in New Zealand, with a world of waters between himself and all that knew him" (*AG*, 49).[9]

Significantly, Brontë locates Agnes's experience with social isolation not just with her parents but with her rendering of childhood itself. Agnes's sense of her secluded childhood leads her to long for its metonymic equivalent in nature—the "woody dales or green hill-sides" or "brown moorlands" that she reminisces about (*AG*, 88). More often, though, she refers obliquely to the social isolation that characterized her own upbringing. As she explains early in the novel:

> Mary and I were brought up in the strictest seclusion. My mother . . . took the whole charge of our education on herself, with the exception of Latin—which my father undertook to teach us—so that we never even went to school; and, as there was no society in the neighbourhood, our only intercourse with the world consisted in a stately tea-party, now and then, with the principal farmers and tradespeople of the vicinity (just to avoid being stigmatized as too proud to consort with our neighbours), and an annual visit to our paternal grandfather's; where himself, our kind grandmamma, a maiden aunt, and two or three elderly ladies and gentlemen, were the only persons we ever saw. (*AG*, 2)

As Brontë has Agnes explain it, the social isolation endured by the family is partly chosen and shapes Agnes's experiences as a child in several ways. Although her account of family heritage had earlier emphasized her mother's disregard for the social hierarchy of which she was a part, this anecdote, by distinguishing between "neighbours" and "society," reveals just the opposite. Agnes implies that her family's encounters with local farmers and tradespeople were artificial, designed to hide the social pride that they really felt.

Most important, Brontë links the social isolation of Agnes's family not only to Agnes's developing class-consciousness but also to her own sense of a private life. Although Agnes hints at regret at not attending school as other children in the neighborhood do, her account reveals a more tangible level of discomfort with her background:

> Sometimes our mother would amuse us with stories and anecdotes of her younger days, which, while they entertained us amazingly, frequently awoke—in *me,* at least—a secret wish to see a little more of the world. (*AG,* 2)

Agnes admits here to a latent attribute of her identity, a desire for experience beyond that provided within the confines of her home. She ensures that this desire is unknown to those closest to her. Brontë's use of italic to emphasize Agnes's sense of separation from her sister ("in *me,* at least,") is also noteworthy, underscoring as it does divisions within the seemingly homogeneous unit of the family. Agnes's sense of her self as separate from her family parallels as well certain moments in the text when she reveals her discomfort with the kind of attention her family gives her.

Throughout the opening portion of the novel, Brontë uses rhetoric to reveal that Agnes commands little respect as an individual within her family. Agnes occupies—in her own mind, at least—an almost invisible place in the family. Early on in her narrative, Agnes explains that being the youngest child, and only one of two from an original group of six to survive "the perils of infancy and early childhood," she "was always regarded as the *child,* and the pet of the family," a designation that resulted in making her "too helpless and dependent—too unfit for buffeting with the cares and turmoils of life" (*AG,* 2). When the financial woes brought on by her father's speculations begin, opportunities for her sister Mary to help out by painting are encouraged, but Agnes is passed over without a word, told only to "Go and practise [her] music, or play with the kitten" (*AG,* 6). As Agnes explains, "though a woman in my own estimation, I was still a child in theirs" (*AG,* 6).

The Grey family's reaction to her suggestion, revealing the extent to which her lack of status has become deeply inculcated in their thinking, is a key feature of Brontë's critique of the family, which shows the extent to which Agnes's sense of self is at stake in the debate about whether she should work as a governess. When Agnes initially announces her presence by saying, "I wish *I* could do something," her family reacts negatively both to the idea of working as a governess and, significantly, to the idea of Agnes's working at all. As Agnes writes, "My mother uttered an exclamation of surprise, and laughed. My sister dropped her work in astonishment, exclaiming, '*You* a governess, Agnes! What *can* you be dreaming of!'"(*AG,* 7). Further countering her suggestion, her mother says, "'But, my love, you have not learned to take care of *yourself* yet: and young children require more judgment and experience to manage than elder ones'"(*AG,* 7). Recollecting her father's reaction, Agnes writes: "'What, my little Agnes a governess!' cried he, and, in spite of his dejection, he laughed at the idea" (*AG,* 8). In the first two of these instances, Mary's emphasis on *you* and Mrs. Grey's emphasis on *yourself* call into question Agnes's status as an autonomous individual with her own independent identity, which she had put forward with her own emphasis on *I.* Although attuned to the implications of her family's behavior (at least in retrospect), Agnes absorbs some of their patterns of thought—patterns that deny her an independence and maturity comparable to her age, and result in her seeing herself as somehow less than fully developed and able to act on her own.

The family plot that opens the novel introduces other themes as well, among them Agnes's affinities with the natural world and especially with animals. Clearly the most important theme, in terms of setting the stage for her subsequent experiences, has to do with the sense of self that Agnes develops within her family and with how it determines the effect her work experiences will have on her. In many ways, the novel's emphasis on Agnes's subsequent psychological development once she has left home becomes a commentary on the home life she left. In doing so, Brontë deepens the interpretive interest of Agnes's subsequent governess experience by linking it to a broader critique of the domestic ideal and of related ideologies of gender and class that sentimentalized the family and that restricted societal understandings of a woman's capacity for self-determination.

"A Stranger in a Strange Land": The Governess Story

The phrase "a stranger in a strange land" would seem at home in almost any episode in *Agnes Grey* devoted to the heroine's life as a governess. It comes in fact from the correspondence of Brontë's father. In response to a letter he had received from a fellow clergyman expressing sympathy on the death of his wife, Maria Branwell Brontë, Patrick Brontë wrote, "Had I been at D[ewsbury] I should not have wanted kind friends; had I been at H[artshead] I should have seen them and others occasionally; or had I been at T[hornton] a family there who were ever truly kind would have soothed my sorrows; but I was at H[aworth], a stranger in a strange land" (*BLFC,* I, 58). The phrase captures his sense of exile as an Irishman living in Yorkshire as well as the overwhelming emotional alienation of losing his wife, an alienation only partially mitigated, his later comments imply, by his religious faith.

It is this combined sense of geographic exile and emotional or psychological alienation that plague Agnes Grey as she struggles to survive in a world that she feels is radically unfamiliar to her. Perhaps no other theme so preoccupied Brontë. As the title implies, *The Tenant of Wildfell Hall* would bring exile and alienation to the foreground: Helen Huntingdon is both physically banished from her home and alienated, by virtue of her alias as the widow Mrs. Graham, from her self. Just as Brontë in her poetry created characters who were exiled from their home and family to explore the process of self-examination that inevitably ensued, so too in *Agnes Grey* she uses Agnes's sense of alienation as a springboard for self-scrutiny. Indeed, Agnes describes the "strange feeling of desolation" with which she greeted her first morning in the Murray home as follows:

> I awoke . . . feeling like one whirled away by enchantment, and suddenly dropped from the clouds into a remote and unknown land, widely and completely isolated from all he had ever seen or known before; or like a thistle-seed borne on the wind to some strange nook of uncongenial soil, where it must lie long enough before it can take root and germinate, extracting nourishment from what appears so alien to its nature: if, indeed, it ever can. (*AG,* 49)

Although Brontë has Agnes reveal a cynicism born out of her difficult experiences with the Bloomfield family, the young woman who commences a career as a governess is not yet disillusioned. The young woman who leaves her home to begin work as a governess is not simply one who has not been provided with sufficient opportunities to establish an autonomous identity. Brontë represents Agnes's condition in almost pathological terms; she is passive—at least on the outside—to an extreme degree. Although she expresses her inward determination to persevere in her plans for work despite the obstacles presented at home, she manages to act on that determination only indirectly, pressuring her mother to approve her plans and obtain her father's consent. Significantly, when the plans finally come to fruition, Brontë uses the passive voice; Agnes says, "At last, to my great joy, it was decreed that I should take charge of the young family of a certain Mrs. Bloomfield" (*AG,* 9). Most often, Brontë establishes Agnes's passivity by calling attention to her voice—or, more precisely, to her lack of voice. Upon hearing her family's arguments against her desire to work, she writes, "I was silenced for that day, and for many succeeding ones" (*AG*, 8). Perhaps more pointedly, Agnes's sister asks her "Only think . . . what would you do in a house full of strangers, without me or mamma to speak and act for you— . . . ?" (*AG*, 8).

Such comments help the reader to understand that because Agnes's background is so empty of opportunities for autonomous action, or self-government, she is especially unprepared for governess work—for work that will, literally, require her to govern others. Brontë ironically suggests that her awareness of what she lacks ultimately drives her to governessing. Imagining herself as a governess, Agnes writes:

> How delightful it would be to be a governess! To go out into the world; to enter upon a new life; to act for myself; to exercise my unused faculties; to try my unknown powers; to earn my own maintenance, and something to comfort and help my father, mother, and sister, beside exonerating them from the provision of my food and clothing; to show papa what his little Agnes could do; to convince mamma and Mary that I was not quite the helpless, thoughtless being they supposed. (*AG*, 8)

The dire economic circumstances of her family and her potential role in alleviating their stress function within this passage as little more than an afterthought. Her primary incentive, Brontë implies, is self-oriented; she wants to establish independence and to prove that her identity is not that which her family has accorded her.

Adding to the reader's sense of Agnes's unrealistic optimism are the naiveté and idealism that Brontë reveals in her anticipation of her actual duties as a governess:

> And then, how charming to be entrusted with the care and education of children! Whatever others said, I felt I was fully competent to the task: The clear remembrance of my own thoughts in early childhood would be a surer guide than the instructions of the most mature adviser. I had but to turn from my little pupils to myself at their age, and I should know, at once, how to win their confidence and affections: how to waken the contrition of the erring; how to embolden the timid, and console the afflicted; how to make Virtue practicable, Instruction desirable, and Religion lovely and comprehensible. (*AG*, 8–9)

Undercutting the domestic ideology that revealed itself in 19th-century conduct books and works of instruction for women, Brontë ensures that Agnes uses the same idealistic rhetoric to approach the task of governessing.[10] According to Agnes's internal logic, the skills she already possesses as a woman will be exactly the skills that she will need in her work. In this passage Brontë foreshadows as well the impact that Agnes's negative experience as a governess will have on her self-esteem; anticipating only success, she draws here on her "own thoughts," likens her future pupils to herself, and fantasizes about proving others wrong. The narrative that follows is at least partly predictable: Agnes discovers that her own childhood has little prepared her to understand the childhood experiences of others, still less to impart her own values to those children. But just as Agnes's anticipation of life as a governess revolves at least as much around her own potential growth as around issues of work, so too does the narrative of her experience turn inward. In the process, Brontë reveals the ways in which Agnes's expectations about self-development are both achieved and disappointed.

While Agnes delineates her goals for governessing along two distinct lines—one having to do with her success as a teacher, the other involving more personal goals—Brontë shows that the important thing was that the strands are interwoven. On one level, for instance, Agnes evidences a strong desire for children of her own, which reveals itself early in her encounter with the Bloomfield family when she meets the children: "The remaining one was Harriet, a little broad, fat, merry, playful thing of scarcely two, that I coveted more than all the rest—but with her I had nothing to do" (*AG*, 14). Her desire for a child of her own turns more bitterly ironic late in the novel when she is confronted with Lady Ashby's indifference to her own infant girl. Since Agnes is unaware during these episodes that she will in fact one day have children of her own, she is reduced first through her role as a governess and later as a teacher to accepting a very limited role in relation to children.

Another way that Brontë relates Agnes's personal and career goals for self-development is through the concept of reform. Brontë stresses the extent to which Agnes approaches governessing as an opportunity for self-reform, a chance to develop those attributes she feels confident that she has but has yet to develop and perfect. While she recognizes that the children for whom she will be responsible pose serious challenges, she is—at least for a time—confident that she will be able to alter their personalities and to reform their characters. The language and behavior of the Bloomfield children shock her, but, she writes, "I hoped in time to be able to work a reformation" (*AG*, 15). Later, of "Master" Bloomfield she writes, "in time, I might be able to show him the error of his ways" (*AG*,

17). Despite continued failure to achieve her goals, she persists in her belief that reformation of character is possible: "irksome as my situation was," she writes, "I earnestly wished to retain it. I thought, if I could struggle on with unremitting firmness and integrity, the children would in time become more humanized"(*AG,* 27).

Agnes's efforts at reform enable Brontë to analyze the expectations that domestic ideology placed on the middle-class woman by virtue of her role as moral educator. Brontë shows that Agnes is most frustrated by her sense that what reformation she does achieve is fragile at best; bad examples from a father or uncle are all it takes to negate the progress she thought she had achieved. Although Agnes gradually relinquishes her belief in her own powers to effect fundamental change, Brontë shows the impact of her subsequent sense of failure. The attraction that Agnes eventually develops for the curate Edward Weston may be related to his own desire to reform his parishioners and his relative success at it; at the conclusion of her narrative, for instance, Agnes reports with pride that "Edward, by his strenuous exertions, has worked surprising reforms in his parish" (*AG,* 164). Her sometimes excessive admiration of her mother may also relate to her sense that her mother manages others more effectively than she herself is able to do. The possibilities and problems of reform—of self, of the children one supervises and instructs, or of the parishoners one oversees—manifest another way in which Brontë used her writing to question the stability of selfhood over time. In *Agnes Grey,* Brontë shows that failure to change—literally to re-form and to better one's self—can have disastrous consequences.

Agnes's relative failure to achieve the reforms she had so desired in her students is not surprising. Brontë provides so much evidence of the horrific behavior of Agnes's charges and the physical hardships she endures that the reader cannot doubt that she was faced with an impossible task. Although Agnes hints at her own lack of confidence, Brontë ensures that Agnes's readers will not doubt her. The children she tends pull her hair, threaten to destroy her personal belongings (including her cherished writing desk), affront her conscience and sensibilities with their abhorrent conduct toward the natural world (e.g., maliciously whipping horses, beating dogs, and torturing young birds), and ignore her warnings and threats. Throughout these episodes, Brontë draws the reader's attention not to the children themselves (who seem larger than life in their faults) but to Agnes as she reacts to her experiences and develops as a result.

Brontë signals the emotional implications of Agnes's experiences through her physical changes, which her family notices when she returns home on vacation and, at the end of the novel, after permanently resigning from her position. Brontë prepares readers to anticipate that Agnes will be "a good deal paler and thinner than when [she] first left home" (*AG,* 44), through a series of references to her hunger. Agnes's stint at the Bloomfield residence is marked by many occasions during which she fails to eat: when she arrives for the first time after an arduous journey she is presented with "beefsteaks and half-cold potatoes," which she finds inedible (*AG,* 13); later in her stay she notes the "frugal supper of cold meat and bread" she is invited to partake of (*AG,* 18); on still another occasion, after struggling to get the children dressed and prepared for breakfast, she finds the breakfast food cold on the table. In these and other instances, the cold food that Agnes fails to eat parallels the frigid demeanor of her employers, and particularly of Mrs. Bloomfield, whom she describes as "cold, grave, and forbidding—the very opposite of the kind, warm-hearted matron my hopes had depicted her to be" (*AG,* 18). Her subsequent stay at Horton Lodge, the Murray family residence, is little better. Of her first meal there, Agnes writes: "Having broken my long fast on a cup of tea and a little thin bread and butter, I sat down beside the small, smouldering fire, and amused myself with a hearty fit of crying" (*AG,* 48).

In these instances, Brontë invokes a trope of nourishment common in women's writing of the 19th century. Agnes herself recognizes that the nourishment she needs is emotional, writing at one point in her stay with the Bloomfields: "Kindness, which had been the food of my life through so many years, had lately been so entirely denied me, that I welcomed with grateful joy the slightest semblance of it" (*AG,* 31). Later, she describes a short stay at home as "quiet enjoyment of liberty and rest, and genuine friendship, from all of which I had fasted so long" (*AG,* 41). The references in *Agnes Grey* to nourishment, both physical and emotional, are legion and help Brontë to show the impact of Agnes's diminished social status as a governess. Indeed, the process by which Agnes literally becomes thinner parallels the process by which the reader becomes increasingly aware of her social invisibility.

Throughout the novel, Brontë marks Agnes's social invisibility in two important and interrelated ways, both of which reveal the dissonance of class status for the governess. Agnes's sense of her status manifests itself through her preoccupation with her visible presence or lack of it. She discovers as a governess that her presence in a variety of public settings is necessary to make manifest the social status of her employers, but that her presence must also be unacknowledged. The situation that Brontë depicted in *Agnes Grey* was, in fact, fairly realistic; explaining the dilemmas of social status introduced by the figure of the governess, one historian has written, "So excruciating was the problem to all concerned that many employers and their friends adopted the cowardly, though effective, tactic of simply pretending not to 'notice' the governess on those occasions when she was obliged to be in their company" (Hughes 1993, 99–100). Brontë presents similar situations, using them to reveal the emotional anguish that they engender in her heroine. For example, describing Mr. Robson—Mrs. Bloomfield's brother—Agnes writes, "He seldom deigned to notice me; and, when he did, it was with a certain supercilious insolence of tone and manner that convinced me he was no gentleman: though it was intended to have a contrary effect" (*AG,* 36). Although Agnes seems on the surface to recognize and disparage the pretensions of Mr. Robson and others like him, the very frequency with which she notes encounters like this point to an unresolved bitterness as well.

Another strategy that Brontë uses to manifest Agnes's social invisibility is emphasizing her lack of an effective voice. Agnes's awareness of her own sense of "voicelessness," for which she accepts partial responsibility, becomes a major subject of the narrative itself and ultimately enables Brontë to explore through her representation of Agnes, situated as she was in the private sphere, the unempowered position of middle-class women. The related issues of social invisibility and voicelessness so dominate Agnes's narrative that they—rather than, for example, the physical conditions of her life as a governess—become the actual subject of the novel.

Brontë's preoccupation with Agnes's developing sense of presence and voice reveals itself early on in her account of governessing—in fact, in the same episode in which she is first presented with a meal that she is unable to eat. While she attempts out of politeness to eat her meal, she becomes self-conscious about the conversation with Mrs. Bloomfield, noting both that lady's "succession of commonplace remarks, expressed with frigid formality" as well as her own failure to respond: "I really *could* not converse," she writes (*AG,* 13)—a statement that she would echo at several other points in her narrative. Introducing a situation that would recur in other portions of the narrative, Brontë exacerbates Agnes's sense of self-consciousness by making her the object of another's gaze. Adding to her sense of discomfort at this point is an awareness that Mrs.

Bloomfield is watching her eat: "sensible that the awful lady was spectator to the whole transaction, I at last desperately grasped the knife and
fork in my fists, like a child of two years old" (*AG,* 13). In her own estimation, Agnes is reduced to a child—just the thing she had hoped to
disprove through her venture into governessing in the first place. She
accounts for her behavior in several ways: she is physically cold from her
journey and her hands are literally "benumbed" from the long drive (*AG,*
13). At the same time, she is nervous about what her new life will be like
and already disheartened by her encounters with Mrs. Bloomfield. Most
obviously, though, she begins to become conscious of her self as powerless.

Agnes's self-consciousness escalates as the weeks go on. Her difficulties with the unruly Bloomfield children are made worse by her worry
about what their parents will think, or—to be more precise—see.
Struggling to keep up with Tom and Mary Ann on a walk outside, she
thinks: "But there was no remedy; either I must follow them, or keep
entirely apart from them, and thus appear neglectful of my charge. . . . I
was in constant fear that their mother would see them from the window,
and blame me. . . . If *she* did not see them, some one else did"(*AG,* 19).
Agnes's fears seem justified: her actions and behaviors are closely monitored. Brontë repeatedly represents the Bloomfield estate or rooms
within the estate as panoptic; no matter what her position, Agnes is subject to the constant surveillance of her employers. Just as Mrs.
Bloomfield watched her in the dining room, Mr. Bloomfield watches
from the window as the children play outdoors and is "continually looking in to see if the schoolroom [is] in order" (*AG,* 34). Even visitors to
the home scrutinize Agnes's actions; she spitefully characterizes the
senior Mrs. Bloomfield as "a spy upon my words and deeds" (*AG,* 31).

Brontë counterbalances in several ways Agnes's painful sense that she
is being watched. Although Agnes doesn't directly acknowledge the
irony of it, her work policing her charges entails a good deal of espionage
as well. She at one point characterizes her job as one of "instruction and
surveillance," implying that the two were equally weighted. Some of this
is, in fact, commanded of her, as when Mrs. Murray directs her to follow
Rosalie in the park to ensure that she doesn't have an "unsightly"
encounter with the Reverend Hatfield. Yet from her ostensibly invisible
position Agnes also monitors the behavior of those around her and
records it, often in minute detail.

The emphasis that Brontë narrative places on Agnes's sense of presence, of watching and being watched, shifts slightly in the second half of

the novel, when the character Edward Weston is introduced. Some of Agnes's self-consciousness about her lack of presence persists, as for example when she records Hatfield's failure to notice her while handing the Murray girls into their carriage after the church service. In characteristic fashion, Agnes accepts some of the blame for her situation, attributing it in part to her personality and in part to her role as a governess: "I liked walking better, but a sense of reluctance to obtrude my presence on any one who did not desire it always kept me passive on these and similar occasions," she writes. "Indeed, this was the best policy—for to submit and oblige was the governess's part, to consult their own pleasure was that of the pupils" (*AG,* 87).

Nonetheless, Agnes wants her readers to blame others; describing the "great nuisance" of walking home from church with others, she notes:

> As none of the before-mentioned ladies and gentlemen ever noticed me, it was disagreeable to walk beside them, as if listening to what they said, or wishing to be thought one of them, while they talked over me, or across; and if their eyes, in speaking, chanced to fall on me, it seemed as if they looked on vacancy—as if they either did not see me, or were very desirous to make it appear so. (*AG,* 87)

The passage clearly reveals Agnes's self-consciousness about her lack of social visibility, but it also suggests that she, too, is driven by pride. Rather than simply walk at the pace that would occur naturally, she refuses to do anything that would allow others to think she cared what they said. As she continues:

> It was disagreeable, too, to walk behind, and thus appear to acknowledge my own inferiority; for, in truth, I considered myself pretty nearly as good as the best of them, and wished them to know that I did so, and not to imagine that I looked upon myself as a mere domestic, who knew her own place too well to walk beside such fine ladies and gentlemen as they were. (*AG,* 88)

At this point in her narrative, Agnes "shamefully" acknowledges that she worked hard "to appear perfectly unconscious or regardless of their presence" (*AG,* 88)—an ironic confession, given her bitterness about similar treatment on their part.

Part of the role that Weston serves is to allow Brontë to curb what Agnes at one point refers to as her "spirit of misanthropy" (*AG,* 88). Significantly, he does so by noticing Agnes, thus enabling Brontë to symbolically subvert the class-consciousness that would make her, as a governess, unworthy of public attention. Not surprisingly, Agnes registers his notice immediately. She describes their accidental encounter at the cottage of Nancy Brown, for example, as follows:

> "I've done you a piece of good service, Nancy," he began: then seeing me, he acknowledged my presence by a slight bow. I should have been invisible to Hatfield, or any other gentleman of those parts. (*AG,* 84).

Brontë stresses Agnes's level of self-esteem by having her insist on remaining hidden from view, refusing to accept a chair by the fire with Weston and Nancy Brown and continuing to sew silently by a window in the corner of the cottage. But it is significant that she gradually takes measures to make her presence known. In chapter 17, "Confessions," she writes, "I may as well acknowledge that, about this time, I paid more attention to dress than ever I had done before" (*AG,* 114). Her success in doing so is established in the narrative when the Murray sisters effectively bar her from going with them to church, ensuring that she won't be seen by Weston and that all of his attention will thus be reserved for them. When Agnes finally does meet him again after this point, she writes, "it was something to find my unimportant saying so well remembered: it was something that he had noticed so accurately the time I had ceased to be visible" (*AG,* 129).

Although throughout the narrative Brontë shows Agnes struggling with an inability to make her presence felt, this passage suggests that her sense of presence is tied to a sense of voice. Both are intimately connected to a sense of self that, at this point in the narrative, is beleaguered at best. From the very beginning of Agnes's account of life as a governess, Brontë emphasizes voicelessness as the distinguishing feature of her work. Remembering some warnings from her mother, she vows to "keep silence" on the faults of her charges (*AG,* 18), a decision reinforced early on by Mrs. Bloomfield's directive in regard to handling problems with the children. She effectively censors Agnes by saying, "If persuasion and gentle remonstrance will not do, let one of the others come and tell me; for I can speak to them more plainly than it would be proper for you to do" (*AG,* 52). Brontë reintroduces the theme of censorship with Mrs. Murray. As Agnes writes, "Having said what she wished, it was no part of her plan to wait my answer: it was my business to hear, and not to speak" (*AG,* 127). Although Agnes is "roused to speak" in her own defense on more than one occasion with both the Bloomfield and the Murray families, she consistently decides to "subdue" and "suppress" her impulses (*AG,* 27). What makes governessing difficult, she implies, is less the physical hardships or the embarrassment of lowered social status than the stress of having to continually restrain herself.

The emphasis on repression that is at the heart of Brontë's account of Agnes's experiences as a governess is central to the novel's romance plot as well. Like other Victorian writers, Brontë understood the power of sexuality and of sexual impulses to determine behavior and yet at the same time appreciated its "fugitive nature," its "resistan[ce] to definition, examination, and regulation."[11] Brontë showed further how the challenges of understanding and regulating erotic impulses were especially formidable for a woman like Agnes Grey, whose gender and status as a governess combined to render her passive. The challenge of exercising restraint in the presence of her charges and superiors becomes exacerbated for Agnes by the necessity of repressing her feelings for Weston. Listening to Rosalie chatter about her conversation with Weston during one of the Sundays in which she had been prevented from attending church, Agnes thinks:

> I was accustomed, now, to keeping silence when things distasteful to my ear were uttered; and now, too, I was used to wearing a placid smiling countenance when my heart was bitter within me. . . . Other things I heard, which I felt or feared were indeed too true: but I must still conceal my anxiety respecting him, in indignation against them, beneath a careless aspect; others, again, mere hints of something said or done, which I longed to hear more of, but could not venture to inquire. So passed the weary time. (*AG,* 120)

Although Agnes's situation is clearly painful, Brontë heightens the reader's appreciation of the intensity of Agnes's desire by focusing on the extent to which she controls that desire, choosing to keep her thoughts and feelings to herself rather than risking an open confession. Agnes's repression becomes a mechanism of self-control and a means of self-identification. In another important passage, she admits that not even her mother or her sister could be privy to her thoughts:

> I fear, by this time, the reader is well-nigh disgusted with the folly and weakness I have so freely laid before him. I never disclosed it then, and would not have done so had my own sister or my mother been with me in the house. I was a close and resolute dissembler—in this one case at least. My prayers, my tears, my wishes, fears, and lamentations, were witnessed by myself and Heaven alone. (*AG,* 121)

Curiously, Agnes does not explore why she felt so strongly about keeping her emotions to herself. Providing a small source of consolation is her religious faith, which enables her to feel that even in this silence she is not alone.

Brontë shows that, although silence is partially imposed upon Agnes, it is also a position that she adopts in self-defense. The politics of speaking out or choosing not to speak enter Brontë's narrative in other ways as well, as for example in the story of Rosalie's flirtation with Hatfield. When the flirtation comes to its end, Hatfield requests that Rosalie "keep silent" about his proposal of marriage, threatening her by remarking that "if you add to [my injury] by giving publicity to this unfortunate affair, or naming it *at all,* you will find that I too can speak" (*AG,* 101). The self-deprecating Agnes cannot, of course, wield power through speech in the same way as Rosalie. When she is dismissed from the services of the Bloomfield family, for instance, she writes:

> I wished to say something in my own justification: but in attempting to speak, I felt my voice falter; and rather than testify any emotion, or suffer the tears to overflow that were already gathering in my eyes, I chose to keep silence, and bear all like a self-convicted culprit. (*AG,* 41)

Brontë advances her study of the social and psychological implications of Agnes's silence in several ways. On many occasions throughout the narrative, Agnes admits that she cannot hold others entirely responsible for her silence. Of Mrs. Bloomfield's failure to allow her more than two weeks' vacation time during her first earned holiday, she notes:

> Yet she was not to blame in this; I had never told her my feelings, and she could not be expected to divine them; I had not been with her a full term, and she was justified in not allowing me a full vacation. (*AG,* 28)

Such self-critical gestures recur throughout Agnes's narrative and enable Brontë to bring to the foreground the issue of Agnes's reliability as a narrator and enhance the reader's understanding of the extent to which the nature of subjectivity itself is under scrutiny in the novel. Of the Murray children's desire to take lessons in the open air and on damp grass, which frequently made Agnes catch a cold, she writes, "But I must not blame them for what was, perhaps, my own fault; for I never made any particular objections to sitting where they pleased; foolishly choosing to risk the consequences, rather than trouble them for my convenience" (*AG,* 58–59). Here as elsewhere Agnes conveys an attitude of both martyrdom and self-deprecation.

Weston's role is again crucial to Brontë's exploration of Agnes's self-deprecating nature, for he openly expresses that which Agnes only partially accepts about her own role in representing herself as beleaguered. On one of the occasions when the two walk home together after church, he introduces the topic of social disposition and when she complains that her position denies her opportunities to make friends, he responds, "The fault is partly in society, and partly, I should think, in your immediate neighbours: and partly, too, in yourself; for many ladies, in your position, would make themselves be noticed and accounted of" (*AG,* 108). Although Weston is not saying here anything that Agnes has not already thought to herself, it is significant that he voices her thoughts, that he feels open enough with her to do so, and that he is unencumbered by social decorum, a trait she appreciates. As she subsequently thinks, "such single-minded straightforwardness could not possibly offend me" (*AG,* 109).

Nonetheless, it is precisely the fact that Weston is *not* what he initially seems that makes him attractive to Agnes. Although she is immediately drawn to him as a clergyman, approving his style of delivering a sermon and revering his "strong sense, firm faith, and ardent piety" (*AG,* 83), it is not until she hears of his attentions to the poor cottager Nancy Brown that he becomes "like the morning-star in [her] horizon" and a "subject for contemplation" (*AG,* 82). As Agnes explains it, "when I found that to his other good qualities was added that of true benevolence and gentle, considerate kindness, the discovery, perhaps, delighted me the more, as I had not been prepared to expect it" (*AG,* 83). Shortly after this admission, Agnes recollects her encounter with Weston at Nancy Brown's cottage and reminds her readers that he—unlike others—openly acknowledges her presence and speaks to her. Here, as elsewhere in the novel, Brontë stresses the importance of such attention in encouraging Agnes to distinguish Weston from others. As she had earlier emphasized, "Mr Hatfield never spoke to me, neither did Sir Hugh or Lady Meltham, nor Mr Harry or Miss Meltham, nor Mr Green or his sisters, nor any other lady or gentleman who frequented that church: nor, in fact, any one that visited Horton Lodge" (*AG,* 67).

The story of Agnes's visits to Nancy's cottage and to other homes of poor laborers also enables Brontë to explore how Agnes represents herself to others when divested of the governess role. Just as her family's fall into poverty had seemed to Agnes to be an opportunity to better herself, so too does her friendship with Nancy Brown allow her to improve herself. Even before the arrival of Weston, Agnes recognizes that Nancy Brown is the one person that she is open with, the one to whom she could "freely speak [her] thoughts" (*AG*, 81). Importantly, Agnes sees her relationship with Nancy as mutually beneficial; she seeks to help her, but she also realizes that Nancy's "conversation was calculated to render me better, wiser, or happier than before" (*AG*, 81). Like Helen Huntingdon in *The Tenant of Wildfell Hall,* Agnes worries that her association with people unworthy of her respect will inevitably exert an adverse influence on her, that the alliance with the Bloomfields and Murrays "[will] gradually bring [her] feelings, habits, capacities, to the level of their own" (*AG*, 82). Here again Agnes's expression of self-doubts exemplifies the ways that Brontë used her writing to question the stability of selfhood. Whereas earlier in the narrative Agnes had felt dismayed at her failure to reform her charges, here her frustration with governessing concerns the malleability of her self. Nancy Brown unwittingly enables Agnes to believe in its stability.

Brontë fulfills a variety of additional functions through the character of Nancy Brown. Nancy's story enables Brontë to invert the commonly held association of poverty with immorality by suggesting that Agnes's sense of morality is better served in the company of the impoverished. She also facilitates Agnes's growing recognition of what it means to speak "freely," as she apparently does with Nancy Brown, and as Weston eventually does with her. The story of Nancy Brown thus indirectly reintroduces the thematic of voice and voicelessness that runs throughout *Agnes Grey,* and indeed throughout all of Brontë's writing. Although Agnes does not realize it, her readers have become increasingly aware that while governessing has censored Agnes's public voice, it has also facilitated the emergence of an important internal voice. Agnes does speak "freely" with someone other than Nancy Brown, in other words; as her narrative progresses, she develops an ongoing conversation with her self.

Private Speech in *Agnes Grey*

Throughout her novel, Anne Brontë shows that Agnes Grey has thoughts that she keeps to herself when she lives at home with her family. It is not until Agnes recounts her experiences as a governess that her readers appreciate the function of her internal voice. Governessing so often forces her into situations in which she must keep silent that she comes increasingly to rely on expressing her thoughts only to herself, thus developing a kind of "private speech." This kind of speech, as Brontë shows, is self-directed, overt talk that enables an individual to achieve self-control in times of difficulty.[12] Throughout *Agnes Grey,* Brontë uses private speech to distinguish between various levels of voice that emerge in Agnes's narrative as she records the social difficulties associated with governessing. Distinguishing between the various levels of voice that become apparent in Agnes's narrative further enables Brontë to reveal that private speech ultimately facilitates her ability to speak more publicly, first through sermonizing passages directed at her readers and, in an important instance late in the narrative, to the character of Lady Ashby. That her attempts to write letters to her family are so often interrupted by her charges and consequently aborted increases Agnes's need for internal dialogue.

Brontë shows how Agnes's private speech, which is designed to be heard only, as it were, by herself, becomes a part of her strategy for regulating her behavior and keeping up her morale. For example, explaining her efforts to bolster her determination to bear the "tribulation" she had brought upon herself, she writes:

> I longed to show my friends that, even now, I was competent to undertake the charge, and able to acquit myself honourably to the end; and if ever I felt it degrading to submit so quietly, or intolerable to toil so constantly, I would turn towards my home, and say within myself—
> They may crush, but they shall not subdue me!
> 'Tis of thee that I think, not of them. (AG, 27–28)

Brontë reveals here that Agnes is prompted to develop private speech by both external and internal sources: while her degrading work and submissive posture play a role, so too does her sense that her family is judging her.

Brontë illustrates as well the range of functions that Agnes's private speech serves. Agnes occasionally makes reference to her thoughts simply to distinguish herself from others, as when she writes "I alone thought otherwise" (*AG,* 51) to distinguish herself from Mrs. Bloomfield and her children. At other times, her references to her private thoughts are used to reveal herself more truthfully to her readers, as when she writes "Amid all this, I confess, I wondered, too, in secret, whether we should meet or catch a glimpse of somebody else" (*AG,* 107). On other occasions, she represents her interior thoughts as hypothetical dialogue with others—what she might have said had she been in a position that allowed her freedom of expression. When the Murray girls ask her about how she bears the uncomfortable carriage ride to and from church, she writes, "'I am obliged to bear it, since no choice is left me,' I might have answered; but in tenderness for their feelings I only replied — 'Oh! it is but a short way, and if I am not sick in church, I don't mind it'" (*AG*, 58). In this instance, Agnes uses her internal voice to share with her readers a side of her self that she feels she cannot present to her charges.

Brontë implies that, for Agnes, private speech becomes a source of consolation and a mechanism of empowerment. Often, Agnes represents her private thoughts as actual, though unspoken, dialogue conducted within her own mind. When Rosalie attempts to force her to acknowledge that Mr. Hatfield is attracted to her, Brontë represents Agnes's response as follows:

> "Yes," answered I; internally adding, "and I thought it somewhat derogatory to his dignity as a clergyman to come flying from the pulpit in such eager haste to shake hands with the squire, and hand his wife and daughters into their carriage: and, moreover, I owe him a grudge for nearly shutting me out of it"; for, in fact, though I was standing before his face, close beside the carriage steps, waiting to get in, he would persist in putting them up and closing the door . . . (*AG*, 67)

Brontë's narrative moves from Agnes's explicit dialogue with Rosalie to her implicit internal dialogue with herself, and from that dialogue back into Agnes's more typical form of address to her readers.

As a mechanism of self-control, Agnes's use of private speech enhances Brontë's study of Agnes's emerging erotic impulses as well. Just as the social restraint necessitated by her role as a governess encourages Agnes to develop an internal voice, so too does the emotional restraint of her courtship with Weston facilitate situations of private speech. Becoming gradually aware that Weston may feel affectionate toward her, she writes, "'And why should he interest himself at all in my moral and intellectual capacities: what is it to him what I think or feel?' I asked myself. And my heart throbbed in answer to the question" (*AG*, 109). Brontë shows that Agnes's use of internal dialogue need not always be prompted by her interactions with those around her, for she invokes it in situations in which she is alone as well. Describing a time when Weston had walked some way with her but then took another direction, Agnes writes:

"But," thought I, "he is not so miserable as I should be under such a deprivation: he leads an active life; and a wide field for useful exertion lies before him. He can make friends; and he can *make* a home too, if he pleases; and, doubtless, he will please some time. God grant the partner of that home may be worthy of his choice, and make it a happy one— such a home as he deserves to have! And how delightful it would be to"—But no matter what I thought. (*AG,* 91)

Brontë uses this passage to underscore the distinction between Agnes's roles as an actor in the story she tells and as a narrator writing retrospectively for the reader. Agnes's private thoughts, which appear in dialogue form, with quotation marks, occurred while the situation she recounts was taking place. But the last sentence of the passage returns her to the role of narrator and illustrates her control in determining exactly how much access her readers are to have to her private thoughts.

Situations in which Agnes interrupts her thoughts (and, consequently, the flow of narrative) recur throughout *Agnes Grey* and are reminiscent of the poems in which Brontë depicted characters interrupting their own dreams and fantasies to regulate themselves and issue rebukes. Through these interruptions, Brontë reveals yet another level of complexity in the voice that Agnes develops as the novel proceeds. Although such narrative interruptions are sometimes used simply to switch directions, they always call attention to her role in directing the narrative, as, for instance, when she turns from an introductory description of Rosalie Murray to Matilda: "But enough of her: now let us turn to her sister" (*AG,* 54). Often, Agnes's interruptions suggest a more complicated relationship to her readers. Introducing Weston, she writes, "But I will not speak of that yet, for, at the time I mention, I had never seen him smile" (*AG,* 83), thereby creating a kind of narrative tension predicated on an anticipation of what will follow. At other times, her interruptions reveal themselves as mock expressions of humility: "I spare my readers the account of my delight on coming home, my happiness while there—" (*AG,* 28) and "I will not inflict upon my readers an account of my leaving home on that dark winter morning: the fond farewells, the long, long journey to O— with Mr Murray's servant" (*AG,* 47). Similarly, on one occasion when Agnes and Weston meet on their way to visit a consumptive laborer, she writes, "I have omitted to give a detail of his words, from a notion that they would not interest the reader as they did me, and not because I have forgotten them. No; I remember them well; for I thought them over and over again in the course of that day and many succeeding ones" (*AG,* 99). With such passages Brontë illustrates how Agnes routinely omits what she considers to be evidence of an emotional extreme. Through her meta-commentary on her own status as narrator, however, Agnes manages to partially reveal what she claims to be withholding. Thus, Brontë asks us to recognize Agnes's narrative control at the same time that she introduces questions about her reliability as narrator. In doing so, she places the nature of subjectivity itself at the heart of her novel.

Brontë intersperses throughout the novel many such passages bringing Agnes's narrative control and self-revelatory tactics to the foreground. When she returns to Horton Lodge after her father's death, for instance, she writes, "I will not dilate upon the feelings with which I left the old house, the well-known garden, the little village church" (*AG*, 135). As the narrative develops, however, Agnes becomes increasingly less likely to censor her thoughts. Rather than interrupt her thoughts or explicitly refuse to impart certain information to her readers, she indulges in lengthy pronouncements that are almost sermonlike in their rhetoric and effect. These pronouncements are never openly expressed to other characters in the novel or rendered in the form of dialogue; rather, they are intended only for Agnes's readers. Occurring in the text after Agnes has become influenced by Weston, they seem in some sense to be a consequence of her relationship with him. Through these homiletic passages, Brontë suggests that Agnes comes to recognize the power of her own voice by witnessing Weston in the pulpit. Yet, by restricting the reach of Agnes's voice to her fictional readership (as opposed to the characters with whom she interacts), Brontë reminds us that, as a woman, Agnes speaks with a voice that is nonetheless indirect, anonymous, and private.

An example of Agnes's sermonlike voice occurs in chapter 17, "Confessions." After beginning on a personal note and acknowledging her increased attention to dress, she moves into a disquisition on the nature of beauty. Her rhetorical strategy is to introduce an idea as a truth learned from childhood, and then to open the supposed truth to questioning: "So said the teachers of our childhood; and so say we to the children of the present day. All very judicious and proper, no doubt; but are such assertions supported by actual experience?" (*AG*, 114). Her question is followed by a long reflection on the nature of pleasure and love that invokes a range of rhetorical tactics. She writes, for example:

> A little girl loves her bird—why? Because it lives and feels; because it is
> helpless and harmless? A toad, likewise, lives and feels, and is equally

helpless and harmless; but though she would not hurt a toad, she cannot love it like the bird, with its graceful form, soft feathers, and bright speaking eyes. (*AG,* 115)

Brontë shows Agnes moving by analogy from birds and toads to women, and then from women in general to particular women who seem very much like herself. Espousing yet another version of Brontë's concern with the idea of unfulfilled potential, Agnes suggests that "if [a woman] is plain and good, provided she is a person of retired manners and secluded life, no one ever knows of her goodness, except her immediate connections" (*AG,* 115). Brontë extends the argument with examples that are couched in generality but that have specific applicability to Agnes's own situation. Expressing the same ideas that Brontë had explored in her poem "If This Be All" (39), Agnes writes, "Many will feel this who have felt that they could love, and whose hearts tell them that they are worthy to be loved again; while yet they are debarred by the lack of this or some such seeming trifle, from giving and receiving that happiness they seem almost made to feel and to impart" (*AG,* 115). She laments the plight of the "humble glow worm" and "roving fly" with "no power to make her presence known, no voice to call him, no wings to follow his flight" (*AG,* 115). Agnes preserves a certain amount of anonymity through this analogic technique, yet her message endows what might seem to be an individual problem with great consequence. Stated in terms of presence and voice, the individual problem of the powerless fly is clearly her own problem. Although she interrupts herself somewhat abruptly at the end of this passage (e.g., "I might go on prosing more and more, I might dive much deeper . . . but I forbear" [115]), she expresses herself with an uncharacteristic degree of freedom.

As Brontë's narrative winds to its conclusion, Agnes's sermonlike reflections increase in frequency and help her readers situate her individual experience within a broader frame of understanding, as for example when Brontë presents Agnes's reasons for writing poetry: "When we are harrassed by sorrows or anxieties, or long oppressed by any powerful feelings which we must keep to ourselves . . . we often naturally seek relief in poetry"(*AG,* 121). Similarly, Agnes asks us to refrain from pitying her mother after her father's death by couching their particular circumstances in a "sermon" on the advantages of "active employment":

We often pity the poor, because they have no leisure to mourn their departed relatives, and necessity obliges them to labour through their severest afflictions: but is not active employment the best remedy for overwhelming sorrow—the surest antidote for despair? (*AG*, 134)

The homiletic tone of this passage, which is reminiscent of Maria Branwell Brontë's message in her tract "The Advantages of Poverty in Religious Concerns," enables Brontë to suggest that Agnes enacts her role as a teacher less through her actual role as a governess than through her role as a narrator. Her "teachings," moreover, serve a dual purpose, for while they clearly enable her to convey what she considers to be important truths to her readers, they also implicitly allow her to under- stand her self and to "improve" it in the ways she had anticipated before she began her journey from home into governessing. Through her role as a narrator, if not as a governess, Agnes acts and speaks for her self.[13]

Brontë emphasizes Weston's role in facilitating this process. Brontë's critics have tended to downplay Weston's function within the plot, seeing him as "intrinsically un-exciting" and as little more than a device to allow Agnes "quiet" romance and modest happiness at the novel's conclusion (P. J. M. Scott 1983, 38). Yet Weston teaches Agnes, if indirectly, how to teach. From him, she learns to recognize the power and force of what seems on its surface to be quiet and ineffectual. As Nancy Brown has said of him, "when he comes into a poor body's house a-seein' sick folk, he like notices what they most stand i' need on; an' if he thinks they can't readily get it therseln, he never says nowt about it, but just gets it for 'em" (*AG*, 81). Most importantly, Weston forces Agnes to identify her strengths and to overcome her perceived weaknesses. In her creation of Weston, Brontë undercut traditional literary conventions that valorized the hero by repre- senting him in relation to a dependent heroine, the proverbial "damsel in distress." Discussing Agnes's perceived need for a home, Weston says, "You might be miserable without a home, but even *you* could live, and not *so* miserably as you suppose" (*AG*, 90). Encouraging Agnes to believe in her ability to survive on her own, Weston enables Brontë to create a different kind of female *Bildungsroman*, one not premised on the assump- tion that a woman's educational journey must end with home and fam- ily. Whereas Agnes Grey's family long before had singled her out as an object of ridicule (i.e., "*You* a governess, Agnes! What *can* you be dream- ing of?" [*AG*, 7]), Weston's emphasis on her individuality—i.e., "even *you* could live"—is undergirded by an assumption of her autonomy, rather than its opposite.

It is a measure of Brontë's commitment to psychological realism that she represents Agnes's self-doubts as so deeply inculcated in her thinking that Weston is unable to effect an immediate transformation. Of his offer to pick for her some flowers that are out of her reach, she writes: "It was Mr Weston, of course—who else would trouble himself to do so much for *me?*" (*AG,* 89). Even when he later presents her with a handful of bluebells, one of her favorite flowers, her immediate reaction is to think "it was something to find my unimportant saying so well remembered" (*AG,* 129). In both cases, Brontë reveals the extent to which self-deprecation and self-effacement are part of Agnes's consciousness. Weston contributes to the process by which Agnes gradually comes to identify her self as autonomous, but he cannot, Brontë implies, take responsibility for her self-understanding.

A Selfhood Sufficient: The Ending of *Agnes Grey*

The concluding portion of *Agnes Grey,* which chronicles Agnes's experiences once she has quit governessing to join her mother and begin teaching in "a school of [their] own" (*AG,* 139), is every bit as important to Brontë's novel as were the opening chapters devoted to Agnes's family life. Although Agnes takes home with her high hopes for meeting Weston again, she is powerless to facilitate such a meeting. Brontë stresses that Agnes's lack of control is not simply due to circumstance but is also a consequence of her passivity. Even were Agnes to find herself in close physical proximity to Weston, she would not feel herself able to act on her desires. Using the rhetoric of presence and voice so central to the governessing portion of the novel, Brontë indicates the depths of Agnes's passivity just prior to her departure from Horton Lodge, when Agnes thinks, "To be near him, to hear him talk as he did talk; and to feel that he thought me worthy to be so spoken to—capable of understanding and duly appreciating such discourse—was enough" (*AG,* 137).

The last several chapters of *Agnes Grey* are skillfully interwoven with themes established from the novel's beginning, among them Agnes's struggle with self-doubts that go back to her childhood and her reliance on an internal voice to regulate her feelings and behavior. Rather than simply following Agnes along a yellow brick road to recovery and happiness, one that leads directly to Weston and the promise of marital bliss, Brontë charts her continuing reliance on childhood habits. Her memories of his words become a "secret solace and support" (*AG,* 139), and when those memories gradually but inevitably fail to sustain her morale, she reverts to the self-deprecating behavior that he had earlier sought to eradicate. Again manifesting a reliance on private speech, Agnes writes:

I was inwardly taking myself to task with far sterner severity. "What a fool you must be," said my head to my heart, or my sterner to my softer self;—"how could you ever dream that he would write to *you?* What grounds have you for such a hope—or that he will see you, or give himself any trouble about you—or even think of you again?" (*AG,* 140)

Agnes's rhetoric of head and heart enable Brontë to distinguish between the intellectual and the emotional dimensions of self-understanding in much the same way as she did in her poetry. Addressing the themes of poems such as "Dreams" (40) and "If This Be All" (39), Brontë shows Agnes becoming so desperate that she desires death. Agnes writes, "if I was forbidden to minister to his happiness—forbidden, for ever, to taste the joys of love, to bless and to be blessed—then, life must be a burden, and if my Heavenly Father would call me away, I should be glad to rest" (*AG,* 141).

Agnes regains self-control by immediately censoring her thoughts, invoking her role as dutiful daughter as a means of salvaging a purposeful self. Although Agnes's sense of daughterly duty would seem to validate patriarchal ideology, Brontë stresses that Agnes's sense of obligation is toward her mother: "But it would not do to die and leave my mother. Selfish, unworthy daughter, to forget her for a moment!" (*AG,* 141). Relying on an interior voice to construct a dialogue with her self, Agnes resolves to make Christian duty her cause:

Did not He know best what I should do, and where I ought to labour? and should I long to quit His service before I had finished my task, and expect to enter into His rest without having laboured to earn it? 'No; by His help I will arise and address myself diligently to my appointed duty. If happiness in this world is not for me, I will endeavour to promote the welfare of those around me, and my reward shall be hereafter.' So said I in my heart. (*AG,* 141–42)

While Agnes admits to only limited success in following her own "injunctions" (*AG,* 141), she reports that "tranquility of mind was soon restored; and bodily health and vigour began likewise, slowly but surely, to return" (*AG,* 142). She alone is responsible for her recovery, Brontë implies; it is only at this point that she can begin to comprehend autonomy.

Not surprisingly, then, it is after this point in the narrative that Brontë begins to depict Agnes as able to effect change in others. Her visit to "Lady Ashby," the former Rosalie Murray, is marked by several occasions in which she openly voices the sermonlike messages that hitherto had been reserved for her anonymous readers. "'The best way to enjoy yourself is to do what is right and hate nobody. The end of Religion is not to teach us how to die, but how to live; and the earlier you become wise and good, the more of happiness you secure," she tells Rosalie (*AG,* 153).

The final two chapters of the novel represent Agnes's newfound autonomy and its limits. Chapter 24, "The Sands," begins with a simple description of Agnes's walk to the sea, but it is noteworthy that she prefaces the account of her "solitary ramble" by writing, "I was not long in forming the resolution, nor slow to act upon it" (*AG,* 155). The sea and its surroundings serve a critical function, helping Brontë to underscore the ways that Agnes's sense of her presence is tied to her understanding of autonomy. At the sea, Agnes first experiences the sensation of being completely comfortable with and by herself. Arriving early in the morning, she writes:

> Nothing else was stirring—no living creature was visible besides myself. My footsteps were the first to press the firm, unbroken sands; —nothing before had trampled them since last night's flowing tide had obliterated the deepest marks of yesterday, and left it fair and even, except where the subsiding water had left behind it the traces of dimpled pools and little running streams. (*AG,* 155)

Brontë underscores here the importance of Agnes's sense of her own visibility and of the impact of her presence on her surroundings. The experience is not just refreshing; it allows her to experience "a sense of exhilaration to which [she] had been an entire stranger since the days of early youth" (*AG,* 155). Suggesting that, having finally achieved a sense of her self as autonomous, Agnes can now be rewarded with the relationships she had so desired, Brontë then reunites her first with her terrier Snap, the "little creature" that she had earlier reported "carefully nursing . . . from infancy to adolescence" (*AG,* 93), and then with Weston himself, who in a symbolically resonant moment brings Snap—the object of Agnes's maternal instincts—to her.

Weston's return into Agnes's life is important from other standpoints as well. While he had always had the self-confidence and autonomy that Agnes lacked, he now has achieved a level of material independence as well, as Agnes notes by reporting that a gold watch has replaced his ear-

lier silver one. Brontë used watches throughout her narrative as indicators of wealth, having Agnes self-consciously note at one point that she
was "not rich enough" to own one (*AG,* 156). Like other Victorian novelists, Brontë believed in the potential of poverty to nurture self-development and she waited until the closure of *Agnes Grey* to reward Agnes
for her spiritual, emotional, and psychological development with material independence. Unlike other Victorian novelists, though, Brontë chose
not to give her heroine an abundance of riches at the end of her narrative, deliberately limiting instead the extent of Agnes's material com-
forts. In doing so, she stressed that wealth alone could not guarantee
female self-sufficiency and that the maintenance of autonomy entailed
much more than material independence.

Brontë extended her analysis of self-sufficiency in the concluding
chapter of *Agnes Grey.* While this chapter documents Weston's subsequent proposal of marriage and encapsulates the story of Agnes's life as
his wife and the mother of three children, it also picks up on the issues of
voice and presence that so dominated earlier portions of her narrative.
Again grappling with the question of how stable or malleable selfhood
is, Brontë shows that, while Agnes has progressed substantially from the
state of passive dependency that had earlier characterized her experiences, she is not completely transformed. In a revealing passage telling
of Weston's visits to her home, Agnes notes:

> He generally addressed most of his conversation to my mother: and no
> wonder, for she *could* converse. I almost envied the unfettered, vigorous
> fluency of her discourse, and the strong sense evinced by everything she
> said—and yet, I did not; for, though I occasionally regretted my own
> deficiencies for his sake, it gave me very great pleasure to sit and hear the
> two beings I loved and honoured above every one else in the world dis-
> coursing together so amicably, so wisely, and so well. I was not always
> silent, however: nor was I at all neglected. I was quite as much noticed as
> I would wish to be: there was no lack of kind words and kinder looks, no
> end of delicate attentions, too fine and subtle to be grasped by words, and
> therefore indescribable—but deeply felt at heart. (*AG,* 161)

Brontë illustrates a new dimension of Agnes's self-understanding here:
she still characterizes herself as "deficient" in terms of presence and voice,
but she is now comfortable with and confident that her position is where
she wants to be. The passage is marked throughout by important quali-
fiers: "I almost envied," "not always silent," and so forth. Although still

passive in her posture, Agnes feels herself ratified by "words" and "looks" nonetheless. Her self-understanding, Brontë implies, is sufficient.

The final section of the novel begins in a gesture Brontë frequently used to represent a process of self-regulation: Agnes overtly interrupts the flow of her narrative, writing simply, "Here I pause" (*AG,* 163). Rather than explain her interruption with an expression of concern for the reader's patience or an account of her desire to protect her privacy, however, she expresses self-satisfaction as her only imperative: "I will content myself with adding that I shall never forget that glorious summer evening" (*AG,* 163).

Brontë's summary of succeeding years is not one of total ease and untarnished happiness: Agnes acknowledges the trials that she and Weston face and stresses the limits of their successes. Their story reproduces certain aspects of Agnes's own childhood and yet improves upon it in important ways: like her own mother, Agnes takes over responsibility for educating her children, but unlike her parents, Agnes and Weston aspire to nothing more than what she describes as that which is "sufficient."

The last lines of *Agnes Grey* turn, in fact, to a thematic of satisfaction that readdresses the thematic of female self-sufficiency and, in doing so, links the social and psychological dimensions of Brontë's study of identity. Agnes writes:

> Our modest income is amply sufficient for our requirements: and by practising the economy we learnt in harder times, and never attempting to imitate our richer neighbours, we manage not only to enjoy comfort and contentment ourselves, but to have every year something to lay by for our children, and something to give to those who need it.
>
> And now I think I have said sufficient. (*AG,* 164)

Brontë reminds us here that self-sufficiency has been the goal of Agnes's narrative all along. As her last paean to frugal living, modest desires, and charitable impulses implies, self-sufficiency requires that an individual both have self-understanding and be comfortable with his or her position in society. The verbal economy implied in Agnes's declaration that she has "said sufficient" points not only to Agnes's editorial decision to end her narrative but also to Brontë's sense that the story of self-sufficiency, a narrative with social and psychological implications, has been told.

Gesturing as they do toward her own propensity to be quiet, Agnes's

closing words—"I think I have said sufficient"—remind us as well that
Brontë's novel has been about the multiple meanings of silence for
women. In *Agnes Grey,* Brontë exposed the social conditions that give rise
to a woman's silence as well as the psychological implications of that
silence. Her focus on Agnes's silence and on the social and psychological
conditions that account for her disposition and behavior may in some
measure account for the novel's critical reputation as a work of "quiet
realism" (Langland 1989, 114). Nearly every aspect of the novel, in fact,
has at some point been described as quiet; Agnes's narrative style has
been described as "a direct quiet manner" (P. J. M. Scott 1983, 14),[14] and
her narrative itself as "the quiet story of an unassuming young woman"
(Langland 1989, 117). Arnold Craig Bell, discussing Anne Brontë's role
as author, draws on Charlotte Brontë's reference to the novel as the
"mirror" of her sister's "mind," and writes, "That mind is a quiet, controlled, realistic, detached one, but searching nonetheless."[15]

Yet if *Agnes Grey* seems to Brontë's critics to embody quiet, so too
does it speak ultimately about voice. Through a range of narrative
devices, among them the representation of Agnes's private speech,
Brontë reveals the active, powerful consciousness of a woman silenced
from without but full of voice within. Brontë's decision to present the
story of Agnes Grey through a first-person narrative is important in this
respect; Agnes's decision to cull from her diary pages material with
which to construct a public narrative reveals an important assumption
on her part—that her experience is worthy of being brought forward
and told to the public. Brontë's narrative technique implies that, for
Agnes, the public presentation of her narrative is her most significant
statement of self-empowerment. Agnes's story, ending as it does in marriage, motherhood, and a relatively "hidden" life within the domestic
sphere, hardly overturns the conventions associated with Victorian
domestic realism. But Brontë's innovative methods in representing the
relationship between Agnes's mind and her voice evidence an astute
awareness both of the complex nature of subjectivity and of the relationship of that subjectivity to historical issues of visibility for women.[16]
History undergirds *Agnes Grey,* then, not just in terms of its overt subject
matter—the condition of the governess—but also in its study of subjectivity. In *The Tenant of Wildfell Hall,* Brontë would extend her analysis of
the narrative and identity even further.

Chapter Five

"The Fair Unknown":
Privacy and Personhood in
The Tenant of Wildfell Hall

Near the beginning of Anne Brontë's last novel, *The Tenant of Wildfell Hall,* the narrator Gilbert Markham describes to his friend and correspondent J. Halford the mystique of a young widow newly arrived in his community of Linden-Car. The woman has occupied several rooms in a previously uninhabited house known as Wildfell Hall and has made her desire for privacy known to her new neighbors, overly eager to obtain information about her past. Referring to this woman first as "the fair recluse" (*TWH,* 39), Markham describes the gossip promoted in the community by the woman's arrival and her subsequent failure to attend church on the first Sunday. He adds that on the following Sunday "everybody wondered whether or not the fair unknown would profit by the vicar's remonstrance, and come to church" (*TWH,* 40).[1] Markham's language—his description of the woman first as a "fair recluse" and then as a "fair unknown"—suggests that his narrative will center on ascertaining the identity of one who seems to be identifiable only by her solitude and secrecy. Implying as he does that this identity is linked as well to her femininity, Markham helps to introduce an important thematic of Brontë's novel: the tendentious relationship between privacy, personhood, and gender.

As the narrative unfolds, Brontë's readers gradually learn that the name of the woman in question is Helen Huntingdon, and that she is living with her young son as the tenant of Wildfell Hall under the assumed name of Mrs. Graham in order to prevent the husband she has left from finding them. Neither of these proper names, however, appears very often in the course of Markham's narrative, even after he has come to know the woman as Mrs. Graham or, more surprisingly, later in the narrative as Helen Huntingdon, her real name. Instead, he repeatedly resorts to labeling her with a series of epithets, referring to her variously as the "fair antagonist," the "fair tormentor," the "fair artist," the "fair hermit," or, more rarely, the "young mother." Markham's labels function in Brontë's narrative in several critical ways, not least of which is to emphasize the difficulty of knowing so reserved a person as Helen Huntingdon seems to him to be.

Yet if Helen's preservation of her privacy initially hinders Markham from feeling comfortable that he knows her, her reclusiveness does not completely account for his apparent unwillingness to directly name her in his narrative. His frequent use of "fair" to modify his epithets, for example, reveals the extent to which her womanhood contributes to and complicates his perception of the barriers to knowing her. Moreover, his efforts to identify Helen either according to one of the roles she plays (e.g., artist and mother) or in terms of how others see her (e.g., as antagonist, hermit, or recluse) imply that he is unable or unwilling to think of her as an autonomous individual with an existence independent of these roles.

Markham's narrative is just one of several ways in which *The Tenant of Wildfell Hall,* published in June 1848, calls attention to the problematic relationship between private and public dimensions of identity. His attention to Helen Huntingdon's solitude, silence, and secrecy—those hallmark thematic interests of Brontë's writing—becomes over the course of his narrative an obsession that leads him to trespass the boundaries of private life that she continually seeks to establish and defend. Yet the interest of Brontë's novel revolves as much around Markham's perceptions of Helen Huntingdon as around her self-perceptions and, as importantly, the extent to which this sense of self is influenced by those around her. Indeed, just as the title of Brontë's first novel, *Agnes Grey,* underscored the eponymous heroine's defiant declaration of individuality in the face of social conditions that thwarted her autonomy, so too does the title of her second novel suggest a continuing interest in the nature of subjectivity, self-conception, and the representation of self to others— issues in this instance made more complex by the narrative's simultaneous study of anonymity.

The Tenant of Wildfell Hall attends in more subtle and sophisticated ways than *Agnes Grey* to the process by which the heroine strives to establish and maintain an identity that is inconsistent with the expectations of those who surround her. In her second novel, Brontë works also with the idea that a woman can unwittingly compromise her attempt to establish autonomy by absorbing and accommodating the identity that others believe her to have. Brontë's focus on the dynamics of this process assumes an understanding of identity akin to that recently advanced by philosophers, such as Rom Harre, who propose that selfhood is fundamentally *intersubjective*—that is, that one's sense of self is informed by and in some sense a product of the concept of person invoked either directly or implicitly in interactions with others.[2] Harre distinguishes between "the concept of a person, the publicly recognized human individual who is the focus of the overt practices of social life" and "the sense that a person has of his own being" (1987, 110). The vexed relationship between these two reciprocally related dimensions of identity is the focal point of *The Tenant of Wildfell Hall,* the thematic bridge between Markham's narrative about Helen Huntingdon and the portion of Helen's self-narrative that Markham's letters enclose.

Brontë's narrative technique has been the locus of much critical controversy surrounding the novel. Yet read as a strategy with which to convey the intersubjective nature of self, the enclosed narratives of *The Tenant of Wildfell Hall* help stylistically to reinforce the novel's underlying assumptions about the relationship between psychological and social dimensions of identity.[3] Using the more traditional method of first-person narration throughout *Agnes Grey* enabled Brontë to foreground many of the issues that contributed to Agnes's problematic understanding of her self and equally vexed representation of her self to others. Brontë's narrative strategies in *The Tenant of Wildfell Hall* are considerably more complex. While readers are eventually granted indirect access to Helen's voice through the device of her diary, this diary is incomplete. The portions that are revealed are enclosed within and hence framed by Markham's own narrative. The diary functions as a private form of writing associated in the novel with the female protagonist, whereas the male protagonist, Markham, is associated with letter writing, a less private form of communication, as well as with the editorial control of Helen's diary.

Helen's diary thus enables Brontë to center the narrative on a woman who either cannot, because of her social situation, or will not, because of her psychological state, speak for herself. In this sense, *The Tenant of Wildfell Hall* continues a major interest in the idea of voice pursued by Brontë in her poetry and in *Agnes Grey,* and allows her to address the question of how women come to identify themselves through their writing when other dimensions of their experience deprive them of speech. In turn, Markham's account of meeting Helen and eventually being granted access to her diary is further framed within the novel by being transformed from "a certain faded old journal" (*TWH,* 34) and recast as a series of letters that Markham writes some years later to a friend under the guise of entertaining him with "an old-world story," one that he promises will be "a tale of many chapters" (*TWH,* 34).

Indeed, the letter with which Markham opens his account reveals an anxiety over the form his narrative will take: he first tells his correspondent he will "give him a sketch," but then corrects himself by writing "no, not a sketch,—a full and faithful account" (*TWH,* 34). Brontë's representation of Markham's anxiety over the generic status of his narrative—it is at once a sketch, a tale, a story, and an account—enables her to prepare her readers for the multiplicity of forms that will make up the narrative that follows. The narrative incorporates extracts from letters, diaries, and journals, and subsumes them within the novel.[4] The hybrid nature of the novel's textual identity in turn has a correlate in the heroine's personal identity, for Brontë's readers must construct their understanding of Helen Huntingdon from a variety of sources.

Narrative and Identity in *The Tenant of Wildfell Hall*

Not surprisingly, Brontë's narrative technique has attracted the puzzled attention of readers for years. Misunderstandings of her narrative strategies have led critics to describe *The Tenant of Wildfell Hall,* reductively, as a cautionary and didactic tale, a social problem novel, or an epistolary novel. Structural similarities between Emily Brontë's *Wuthering Heights* and *The Tenant of Wildfell Hall* have also led critics to argue, again reductively, that Brontë's novel was conceived as a rewriting of or an "antidote" to her sister's novel, published just one year before.[5]

George Moore was among the first of many to disparage the structure of the novel as an artistic failure on Brontë's part.[6] In his 1924 collection *Conversations in Ebury Street,* Moore claimed that "almost any man of letters would have laid his hand upon her arm and said: You must not let your heroine give her diary to the young farmer, saying 'Here is my story; go home and read it.' Your heroine must tell the young farmer her story, and an entrancing scene you will make of the telling" (254). Despite his patronizing tone, Moore's comments underscore an important issue within Brontë's novel—the function of "telling," of revelation and confession, within narratives of and about self.

Brontë's "Preface to the Second Edition" of *The Tenant of Wildfell Hall* reinforces the centrality of this thematic, emphasizing as it does the author's function as a confessor of social truths. In the preface, Brontë claims that her artistic goal was not to entertain her reader but rather "to tell the truth, for truth always conveys its own moral to those who are able to receive it" (*TWH,* 29). She goes on in the preface to say that she "would rather whisper a few wholesome truths therein than much soft nonsense" (*TWH,* 29), and to proclaim that:

> Such humble talents as God has given me I will endeavour to put to their greatest use; if I am able to amuse I will try to benefit too; and when I feel it my duty to speak an unpalatable truth, with the help of God, I *will* speak it, though it be to the prejudice of my name and to the detriment of my reader's immediate pleasure as well as my own. (*TWH,* 30)

Brontë's reference to her authorial duty to "tell," "whisper," and "speak" the truth emphasizes her function as a communicator and directs her reader's attention to the mechanisms of communication. The maneuver in turn suggests that Brontë's narrative strategies in the novel and particularly her decision to limit her heroine's opportunities to tell her story directly were deliberate efforts to represent the barriers to Helen Huntingdon's self-authorizing strategies—to her ability to construct and control her public identity.

Reading *The Tenant of Wildfell Hall* as a study in self-understanding and self-representation allows one to locate the faulty assumptions underlying George Moore's criticism of the novel.[7] In essence, Moore attributes the artistic faults of Brontë's novel to its misconceived preference for the written word over the spoken word. Since his remarks, many of Brontë's readers have sought to explain, if not to justify, her decision to confine her heroine's voice to the pages of a diary. To some readers, for example, her narrative method suggests that she desired to reinforce structurally an important theme of her work, the theme of addressing the myriad social conditions with the potential to mute woman's voice.[8] As Elizabeth Langland has summarized, "The woman's story must, it seems, be subsumed within the man's account, which is prior and originary" (1992, 111). This interpretation would suggest that by intentionally limiting her reader's access to Helen's feelings, Brontë represented and implicitly critiqued the domestic ideology that consigned women to the private sphere and hence to private forms of writing. While compelling, such an interpretation does not adequately account for the sophistication of Brontë's thinking, particularly when it came to issues of identity and self-representation and their relationship to narrative technique. In this light, Moore's comments are especially ironic, for he failed to recognize the frequency with which Brontë focused the attention of her novel on the act of "telling" as well as on its opposites—reticence, reserve, and concealment.

A decision on Brontë's part to have her fictional heroine directly and willingly narrate her story would have been incongruent with the novel's overarching emphasis on the complexities of all narrative acts and the problematic relationship between narrative, privacy, and identity. Probably no single act recurs more frequently in *The Tenant of Wildfell Hall* than that whereby one character commands another to "tell"—to account for an action or to reveal a secret. Indeed, Markham's first letter to Jack Halford opens with a reference to Halford's own narrated account of "remarkable occurences" and his correlary request for "a return of confidence" on Markham's part (*TWH,* 33). Markham goes on to attribute his initial refusal to the fact that he was not in "a story-telling humour" at the time and hence of declining under the pretense of "having nothing to tell" (*TWH,* 33). He apparently changes his mind because a subsequent "stiffness and reserve" on Halford's part have made him uncomfortable.

Far from being a simple device to begin the story, Markham's opening letter indirectly announces many of the issues that concern Brontë throughout the novel. It betrays, for example, Markham's remarkable confidence that he can penetrate another's identity and be certain in his knowledge. He chastises Halford for his ostensible overreaction as follows: "Are you not ashamed, old boy—at your age, and when we have known each other so intimately and so long, and when I have already given you so many proofs of frankness and confidence, and never resented your comparative closeness and taciturnity?" (*TWH,* 33). Claiming that he proceeds on a desire to "atone" for having offended his friend, Markham responds to Halford's request for a "return of confidence" by announcing that he will tell him "an old-world story" (*TWH,* 34). Yet readers soon discover that this story will be devoted primarily to his relationship with Helen Huntingdon and to the life Helen led before they met; moreover, it will culminate with his inclusion of parts of Helen's own private diary—which he unabashedly admits he had once promised her he would keep to himself. Opening her novel with Markham's letter, and thereby encouraging readers to question the reliability of his narrative, Brontë immediately makes the relationship between privacy and narration, which will be a central theme in the story that follows, problematic.

The command to tell a story, which opens Markham's letter, recurs throughout *The Tenant of Wildfell Hall,* creating in the process a novelistic meta-commentary on the function of narrative. Soon after Markham takes his reader, Halford, back to the story's beginning in 1827, he recounts an afternoon in which he returned home from his work as a "gentleman farmer" and was greeted with his mother's command to "shut the door . . . come to the fire . . . and tell [her] what [he had] been about all day" (*TWH,* 36). Markham soon discovers that his mother's request was little more than a ploy to elicit the same request from him, and that she really wants to tell her son about her visit to the home of the mysterious new neighbor. As the novel proceeds, Markham becomes more and more adept at manipulating the feelings of his mother and his sister by either tantalizing them with bits of information about "Mrs. Graham" or, more often, adamantly refusing to respond to their prompts. In these situations, Brontë reveals the ways in which stories are deployed not simply as idle gossip but as speech acts of a sort, as gestures intended to manipulate a response from another. Readers of the novel are already privy to the information that Markham has about Mrs. Graham, and hence his telling the information to his family does not further Brontë's plot, but rather helps to represent the dynamics of his interaction with his family. By having Markham convey or choose not to convey what he knows to his family, Brontë creates a situation in which narrative becomes a kind of property to be exploited at the expense of others.

Just as Markham revels in his ability to thwart the expectations of his family by withholding stories of Mrs. Graham from them, so too does he attempt to dominate her through the control of narrative. Initially he tries to establish a rapport with her by sharing information about how the neighborhood has been gossiping about her. Yet when he can no longer feel confident in their rapport, he attempts to discipline her by refusing to communicate. The first half of the novel culminates with a confrontation between the two in which she upbraids him for his willingness to believe the worst of her and for his inability to tell her on what information his feelings were based. Here again Brontë uses the situation to underscore the role of narrative in a play of power between two people. Helen says, "'Tell me . . . on what grounds you believe these things against me'" (*TWH,* 143), but Markham responds only with indirection, asking her a question about her relationship with Frederick Lawrence (her brother, but a man Markham mistakenly believes to be

her lover). Once his mistake becomes clear to Helen, she chastizes
Markham by saying, "'You should have told me all—no matter *how* bitterly—It would have been better than this silence" (*TWH*, 145). The
episode ends with Helen's transferral of her diary to Markham; significantly, she does so initially without speaking and then changes her mind,
to say only: "'Bring it back when you have read it; and don't breathe a
word of what it tells you to any living being—I trust to your honour'"
(*TWH*, 146). Although Markham initially is true to her request, he later,
of course, copies much of what he discovers in his letters to Halford.

Brontë's emphasis on the role that narrative plays in personal relationships is not just central to Markham's opening account but surfaces
in several ways within the portion of the novel devoted to Helen's diary
as well, thus providing another bridge between the two parts of *The
Tenant of Wildfell Hall*. In one sense, Helen defines her diary as a text
which is without the power to narrate, to "tell" or reveal a story. Early in
her relationship with Arthur Huntingdon, she writes:

> This paper will serve instead of a confidential friend into whose ear I
> might pour forth the overflowings of my heart. It will not sympathize
> with my distresses, but then it will not laugh at them, and, if I keep it
> close, it cannot tell again; so it is, perhaps, the best friend I could have for
> the purpose. (*TWH*, 169–70)

Brontë here reveals both the extent to which Helen embraces privacy
well before she becomes the tenant of Wildfell Hall and the extent to
which preservation of her privacy is a matter of survival. Her comment
implies that she is driven to write out of loneliness and insecurity as well.
Like Agnes Grey and many of the personae of Brontë's poetry, Helen
Huntingdon preserves her solitude as a defense mechanism, in this case
as a shield against the scorn with which she imagines others would react
to her emotional distress. Although her assumption that the diary "cannot tell again" proves false by the end of the novel, she indicates
nonetheless that this for her is its chief merit.

Helen's desire to keep her feelings to herself becomes increasingly
exacerbated as her relationship with Arthur Huntingdon develops.
Significantly, one of Huntingdon's first efforts to communicate with
Helen takes the form of a command to speak (*TWH*, 163). Later in her
diary she recounts in detail an episode in which he intrudes upon her
"favourite resort, the library" (*TWH*, 183), where she has gone to take
"refuge" from his harrassing behavior. Over the course of the encounter

in the library he commands her three times to tell him what is wrong, first by dictating that she "must and shall tell [him]" and subsequently by promising that if she will tell him he will "have something to say" in response (*TWH*, 183). When his coaxing her to admit to her love for him meets only with silence on her part, he threatens her by saying "If you deny it, I won't tell you my secret" (*TWH*, 184). Although the scene ends with her indirect admission of both jealousy and love, she never explicitly "tells" Huntingdon what he wants to hear, insisting instead that he already knows what he wants her to say. Their verbal struggle enables Brontë to stress the ways in which Helen's embrasure of privacy and silence frustrates Huntingdon. On another level, though, it illustrates the ways that narrative—specifically, the command to tell—can be deployed to manipulate the feelings of another and, ultimately, to engender further narrative.

Brontë's emphasis on these dimensions of narrative surface in Helen's diary in other ways as well. Once married and coping with a dissolute husband, Helen writes of her failed attempts to convince him not to degrade himself by drinking too much. After he returns exhausted from an extended visit to London, she asks him "'What *have* you been doing all this time?'" and he responds with "'You'd better not ask'" (*TWH*, 268). She retorts "'And you had better not tell—but you cannot deny that you have degraded yourself miserably'" (*TWH*, 268). Helen's response is significant because it seeks to exact from him a confession while it simultaneously insists that the confession be unspoken.

As the diary progresses, however, Brontë reveals Helen's increasing sense of discomfort with her own invocations to silence as well as with the silence of those around her. For example, when Huntingdon's friend Hargrave attempts to extract from his wife Millicent an explanation of her crying, she responds with "I'll tell you some other time . . . when we are alone" (*TWH*, 289). Unable to wait, he lashes out, "Tell me now!" and Helen—not Millicent—intercedes by crying out "*I'll* tell you, Mr Hattersley. . . . She was crying from pure shame and humiliation for you" (*TWH*, 290). In these and other episodes in the novel Brontë emphasizes the ways in which one's sense of privacy affects a willingness to respond to another's demand for verbal interchange. In the second instance, Helen's own private humiliation proves key to her adopting a new public persona—one decidedly more confident and commanding than she had previously seemed.

Brontë's novel attends in other ways as well to the relationship between her heroine's inner or private self and her command of narrative. As in *Agnes Grey,* Brontë calls attention to her heroine's interiority through the repetition of rhetoric highlighting Helen's thought processes.[9] The first portion of Helen's diary included in Markham's narrative illustrates Brontë's technique well. In the opening paragraph Helen writes of how well drawing suits her mood because she can think at the same time; she notes the "train of other wonderments" that course through her mind; and she speculates on what her aunt would tell her "if she knew what [she] was thinking about" (*TWH,* 148). Charting her subsequent involvement with Arthur Huntingdon, the diary reveals Helen's increasing reliance on what she calls "a secret something—an inward instinct" (*TWH,* 168). Later she writes of the "bitterness [she] felt within" that makes her feel "internally wretched" (*TWH,* 180). Brontë avoided simplistically representing Helen's interiority as a source of solace; instead, she used references to Helen's mind and thought processes as a way to explore the complex nature of subjectivity. When Helen first begins to doubt the solidity of her marriage, for example, she writes, "But I rebuke the inward questioner, and repel the obtrusive thoughts that crowd upon me" (*TWH,* 221), an admission that enables Brontë to illustrate the way that Helen consciously deceives herself and thereby limits her ability to take control of her life. As N. M. Jacobs has written, "Helen experiences her own mind as a structure within which her thoughts and feelings are confined, just as her narrative of secret misery is confined within Gilbert's less painful one in the structure of the novel" (1986, 210).

Self-deception is only one of many dimensions of subjectivity that *The Tenant of Wildfell Hall* depicts in its study of dilemmas of identity. Helen's account of her married life proceeds from this point to describe a range of situations in which she assumes a kind of power generated by her ability to reveal or withhold information. For example, at one point she chooses not to tell Lord Lowborough of his wife Annabella's infidelity, and later she decides to confirm his suspicions. Brontë stresses through these episodes the extent to which Helen controls her life through a series of events in which she decides either to conceal or to disclose information. Ironically, the ways in which she successfully exerts control through command of information complicate the story of her marriage, which emphasizes instead her lack of power.

With *The Tenant of Wildfell Hall,* then, Brontë produces a meta-commentary on the nature of narrative itself; narrative functions both as a topic and as a technique, and in both functions it proves instrumental to the construction of selfhood. Just as, in Helen's diary, the multiplicity of commands to tell make the nature and function of narrative itself a subject of interest, so too in Gilbert Markham's letters about Helen do readers find a range of references to telling, confession, and disclosure. Once Markham has finished copying out portions of Helen's diary for his correspondent, Halford, he returns to his own account of the evolution of his relationship with her. In this concluding portion of the novel Brontë again addresses the ways in which narrative—specifically the command or desire to narrate—helps to mark the dynamics of control undergirding interpersonal relationships. Once Helen's diary has succeeded in disclosing to Markham the truth of her identity, he assumes the very kind of control that she, in her life as Helen Huntingdon, had had: his access to her secret life provides him with information that he chooses initially to conceal and eventually to reveal. Similarly, he attempts to control her public identity by defending her from the gossip of others.

Although in the concluding portions of the novel Markham gains a limited amount of control through his access to and command of information about Helen's real identity, he is not free at the novel's end from the anxieties that characterized his earlier attempts to know her. Instead, Brontë shows the ways in which his understanding of her continues to be incomplete. In this sense as well, the two components of the novel—Markham's account of his relationship with Helen and her diary recounting her marriage—are linked, because both reveal the ways in which Helen both wittingly and unintentionally thwarts the efforts of others to know her.

Silence as Strategy in *The Tenant of Wildfell Hall*

In her depiction of male characters struggling to feel confident that they have access to Helen's inner feelings, Anne Brontë returns to the familiar thematic territory of secrecy, silence, and solitude. By invoking a variety of devices to create an interplay between the novel's emphasis on the narrative act and the central character's propensity to isolate herself and to be secretive and silent, she adds considerable complexity to issues of self-understanding and self-representation.

Throughout *The Tenant of Wildfell Hall,* Brontë represents the struggles of various characters to know Helen as emanating out of exasperation with her silent and secretive personality. The novel presents a complex dynamic: on the one hand, it emphasizes the narrative act through repetitious commands to tell and confess; on the other hand, the interest of its central character is generated by her quiet and often silent demeanor.

Indeed, Helen's first act of identifying herself to her inquisitive neighbors in Linden-Car is to refuse Markham's mother's offer to share household advice and recipes by proclaiming that she lived "in such a plain,
quiet way, that she was sure she should never make use of them" (*TWH,*
39). Soon after this, she responds to a question from Markham's brother
regarding the remoteness of her home by again identifying herself as
fundamentally quiet: "I am not sure the loneliness of the place was not
one of its chief recommendations—I take no pleasure in watching people pass the windows; and I like to be quiet" (*TWH,* 82).

No one is more perplexed by Helen's demeanor than Markham himself; even before he has met her, he is bothered by what he believes her
silence to represent. Recounting for Halford an episode in which Helen
discovers him to be watching her in church, Markham writes:

> Just then, she happened to raise her eyes, and they met mine; I did not
> choose to withdraw my gaze, and she turned again to her book, but with
> a momentary, indefinable expression of quiet scorn, that was inexpress-
> ibly provoking to me. (*TWH,* 41)

Throughout Markham's narrative, Brontë stresses the degree to which
he equates Helen's quiet with scorn, in essence interpreting her silence as
a personal affront. At one point Markham notes her "look of quiet, grave
surprise," and suggests that it "had the effect of a rebuke, whether
intended for such or not" (*TWH,* 94). In repeatedly emphasizing the
extent to which Helen's silence disturbs Markham, Brontë critiques the
Victorian domestic ideology that attempted to naturalize the association
of women with private life. Indeed, in both portions of *The Tenant of
Wildfell Hall,* Brontë illustrates the extent to which Helen's privacy
serves as a source of anxiety for the men in her life. Significantly, the only
person who encourages Helen's silence on any subject is her aunt, who
counsels her early on to be cautious about revealing her feelings.

Just as Markham's struggles with Helen's silence become a pervasive
topic of his narrative, so too do the same issues permeate Helen's
account of her relationship with her husband, again suggesting thematic
connections between the two components of the novel. Helen's account
of her courtship by Arthur Huntingdon and her life while married to
him is marked throughout by vacillation between quiet and disquiet.
Quiet is used either to distinguish Helen from Arthur or to characterize
her life without him: Whereas Helen is most satisfied when off on a
"quiet ramble" by herself in the countryside (*TWH,* 187), Huntingdon

tires of the "quiet life he leads" with her (*TWH*, 221). In a revealing moment, Huntingdon suggests that he prefers her to have a quiet demeanor, suiting her subordinate position as a woman: "'I must have some good, quiet soul that will let me just do what I like and go where I like, keep at home or stay away, without a word of reproach or complaint,'" he tells Helen (*TWH*, 234). Even after Helen returns to attend Arthur on his deathbed, his agitation seems to her something of a moral failing: To her brother she complains, "if [Arthur] would only be quiet and sincere, and content to let things remain as they are, but the more he tries to conciliate me the more I shrink from him and from the future" (*TWH*, 438).

Just as Brontë uses Huntingdon's disquiet to figure his moral ineptitude and ultimate incompatibility with Helen, so too does she represent Helen's own propensity for quiet as a source of agitation for him. Explaining to herself the way one plays into the other, Helen writes in her diary:

> I used to fly into passions or melt into tears at first, but seeing that his delight increased in proportion to my anger and agitation, I have since endeavoured to suppress my feelings and receive his revelations in the silence of calm contempt; but still, he reads the inward struggle in my face, and misconstrues my bitterness of soul for his unworthiness into the pangs of wounded jealousy. (*TWH*, 221)

The passage illustrates the multiple ways in which Brontë uses Helen's silence. Silence serves as a defense mechanism for Helen, as it does for Agnes Grey. For Helen, silence is a suppression of voice that she consciously invokes in emotional retaliation against her husband, yet it also marks what she calls "inward struggle," a phrase that suggests an uncomfortable repression of feelings. In either case, it is noteworthy that, as Markham does in the novel's frame portions, Arthur Huntingdon misreads Helen, this time interpreting her silence in the way most favorable to him.

Brontë uses Helen's silence in other ways as well. Throughout the portion of the novel devoted to Helen's relationship with her husband, Brontë emphasizes the connections between her heroine's penchant for a relatively reclusive life and her spiritual needs. Revealing to her diary how little satisfied are these needs, Helen at one point writes, "I have never, for a single hour since I married him, known what it is to realize that sweet idea, 'In quietness and confidence shall be your rest'" (*TWH*,

281–82), an allusion to a passage from the Book of Isaiah. While generations of readers of *The Tenant of Wildfell Hall* have found Markham an inadequate partner for Helen Huntingdon, Brontë suggests in the novel's conclusion that it is Markham's ability to appreciate the intensity of his wife's need for quiet seclusion that makes him capable of providing her with happiness. Markham's last gesture in the concluding portion of the novel is to anticipate his friend's leaving the "noisy, toiling, striving city" to join him and his family in the country for "a season of invigorating relaxation and social retirement"(*TWH*, 490). Indeed, in choosing the almost oxymoronic expression of "social retirement" as the phrase to describe the life Helen Huntingdon eventually leads with Markham, Brontë suggests that the second marriage has facilitated a balance between her heroine's public and private selves.

Although Brontë clearly distinguishes between Huntingdon and Markham, she uses the motif of Helen's quietness to stress disturbing similarities between the two. Both men equate penetrating Helen's mind with conquest. Brontë uses Helen's artwork to stress this connection, with the paintings themselves serving as visible manifestations of Helen's otherwise private thoughts. Just as Huntingdon taunted Helen into revealing her affection for him, so too does he on several occasions exploit her artwork as a revelation of her feelings and desires, insisting on looking at her work despite her pleas that he not do so. Later, in an effort to prevent her from leaving him, he takes her paintings from her.

Markham as well is attracted to Helen's artwork primarily as a medium through which to have access to otherwise private feelings. When first taken to her studio, he remarks "I see your heart is in your work, Mrs. Graham" (*TWH*, 68), and shortly after he elicits from her the information that she is concealing her true identity. On another occasion, Markham admits to himself that he felt "drawn by an irresistible attraction to that distant point where the fair artist sat and plied her solitary task" (*TWH*, 87). Despite her obvious discomfort, he insists on looking over her shoulder and watching as she works.

Artwork is only one of several devices that Brontë uses to represent the ways that Helen alternately presents her self to others and conceals it from others.[10] Her diary serves a similar function: as the "silent paper" to which Helen confesses her need for consolation (*TWH*, 256), it provokes in both Huntingdon and Markham an intense desire to invade her privacy. Both men equate their efforts to "read" Helen—whether via her written word, her artwork, or her facial expressions—with an emotional conquest. Helen's attempt to leave Huntingdon initially fails when he discovers her intentions in her diary, takes her papers from her, and destroys the accumulated artwork that she had intended to sell as a means to independence. Markham's relationship with Helen is characterized by similar, if less dramatic, efforts to encroach on her privacy. For both men, the artwork and the diary come to be valued after other attempts to comprehend Helen fail. For example, in an early encounter with her, Markham thinks he can read her thoughts; he comments, "I thought my hour of victory was come" (*TWH,* 110), only to subsequently realize that he can recognize but not understand the "inward conflict" he observes in her facial expression. Although Helen eventually gives her diary to Markham, it is hardly a willing gesture. Rather, it is a gesture marked by utter exasperation and made out of her conviction that nothing else will clear her reputation with him.[11] Significantly, Markham refers to her diary as his "prize" (*TWH,* 147), another sign on Brontë's part that access to Helen's interiority is treated as a conquest.

In a variety of ways, then, Helen's artwork and her diary are treated as personal, private property that becomes public property. For both Huntingdon and Markham, they represent concrete, tangible manifestions of Helen's interior feelings—of the side of her self that otherwise seems difficult or impossible to own. Brontë's use of Helen's artwork and her diary contribute to the theme of property and ownership running throughout the novel, most obviously through the story of Helen's lack of rights to her property.[12] The novel in fact begins with Markham pondering his father's directive to "transmit the paternal acres" to his children *(TWH,* 35*),* a passage that effectively encourages readers to consider the patriarchal ideology of ownership and inheritance framing the story that follows. Markham's thoughts occur to him as he identifies himself as his father's son, both "gentleman farmer[s]" *(TWH,* 35*).*

While Helen's story, enclosed within Markham's account, similarly underscores the extent to which she is defined by gender and class, it ultimately illustrates for Brontë how these mutually constitutive ideologies deprive Helen of an autonomous identity. Written well before the passage of the Matrimonial Causes Bill in 1857 and the Married Women's Property Acts later in the century, Brontë's novel calls attention to what Mary Poovey has described as "the paradoxical fact that in Britain, when a woman became what she was destined to be (a wife), she became 'nonexistent' in the eyes of the law" (1988, 52).[13] Brontë focuses especially on the ways in which marriage usurps Helen's rights to her "property," including her son, and in doing so forces her to cultivate other ways of establishing her independence.

One way that Helen maintains and exercises her personal rights is through her usage of what might be thought of as spiritual discourse.[14] Although throughout the narrative of her marriage to Arthur Huntingdon, Helen must rely on her husband for much of her security, she also sustains an identity independent of him by turning to her religious heritage. Her expression of her spirituality becomes Brontë's primary means of representing Helen's voice—the thematic alternative to her silence. In some respects, her narrative, although limited to the private form of her diary, charts the development of her public voice by recounting episodes in which she speaks out to and against others in an effort to define her self. Not surprisingly, this voice becomes increasingly strong as her need to find release from marital problems, and what she calls her "inward struggle" (*TWH*, 221), escalates. Brontë shows the ways in which Helen defines herself through a religious language and how she uses that language—her religious voice—to empower herself.[15]

Domestic Ideology, Self-Representation, and the Language of Salvation

From the very beginning of her relationship with Arthur Huntingdon, Helen desires to play the role of ministering angel. Before her marriage she tells her aunt, "If I hate the sins I love the sinner, and would do much for his salvation," promising that she will "save" Arthur from the spiritual ruin her aunt predicts for him (*TWH*, 166). Once married, she attempts to secure her husband's salvation by educating him, finding numerous occasions to remind him of his moral failings, and warning him of the implications for his ultimate redemption.

Her efforts as spiritual educator of her husband soon prove problematic. When her husband declares that he finds her "too religious," saying that "a woman's religion ought not to lessen her devotion to her earthly lord" (*TWH*, 217), Helen responds with a statement of spiritual equality that amounts to a declaration of independence:

> I will give my whole heart and soul to my Maker if I can . . . and not one atom more of it to you than He allows. What are *you*, sir, that you should set yourself up as a god, and presume to dispute possession of my heart with Him to whom I owe all I have and all I am. (*TWH*, 217)

This encounter sets the stage for subsequent battles over "ownership" of Helen's heart, which figures—as it does in Brontë's poetry—as a private

barometer of her emotional states. When Arthur challenges her by saying, "I know the heart within you," Helen responds by writing in her
diary "I was determined to show him that my heart was not his slave"
(*TWH*, 223). Here, as in other episodes in the novel, Brontë uses a
rhetoric of mastery and possession and their alternative, slavery, to
underscore the degree to which Helen's religiosity—particularly her
belief in duty to God first—allow her to articulate the individuality that
her marriage deprives her of.

Brontë does not oversimplify her treatment of the process by which
Helen learns to articulate her autonomy through religious language,
however. Instead, by linking Helen's spirituality with her ambiguous
authority as moral educator, Brontë analyzes the spiritual equality
granted to women through an evangelical understanding of their relationship to God. For Brontë, as for many Victorian thinkers, belief in a
personal relationship with and apprehension of God was the basis of
faith.[16] Yet, if religious rhetoric provides Helen with a means to identify
her independence from Arthur, it also provides her with a means to justify her dependency in the first place. As one critic has written, "Helen
is prepared to enter with zeal into her role as the good angel, the
woman specializing in goodness. It is her hubris, her special arrogance,
to suppose that she can be good enough for two, reform the rake, and
save the sinner's soul."[17] Although Arthur, through his frequent use of
such appellations as "angel monitress," "sweet enthusiast," "patron
saint," and "household deity" clearly enables Helen to act as his savior,
she accommodates the role, constructing herself, as Rom Harre would
argue, according to the concept of personhood invoked by those around
her.

Helen initially identifies herself as an instrument of God working to
reform her husband and secure his salvation. At one point in her marriage, for example, she writes of her disappointment that he stays so long
away from home as follows:

> And I had all along been looking forward to this season with the fond,
> delusive hope that we should enjoy it so sweetly together; and that, with
> God's help and my exertions, it would be the means of elevating his
> mind, and refining his taste to a due appreciation of the salutary and pure
> delights of nature, and peace, and holy love. (*TWH*, 236)

Through this rhetoric Brontë not only suggests the weaknesses of
Helen's assumptions regarding her marital role but also challenges the

domestic ideology that encouraged women to construct themselves as ethereal agents of morality and virtue.[18] In essence, Helen's religiosity and her understanding of her wifely duties rely on very similar vocabulary. Throughout the course of her narrative, Helen deplores her failure to "elevate and purify" her husband (*TWH*, 253) and her "fruitless efforts at conversion" (*TWH*, 271). In the end, her rebellion depends upon a rejection of these interrelated roles.

Brontë suggests that Helen's turning point comes when she disassociates her role from that of God, writing, "God might awaken that heart supine and stupified with self-indulgence, and remove the film of sensual darkness from his eyes, but I could not" (*TWH*, 271). Soon after she more directly rejects the domestic ideology that encouraged her to see herself as a savior in the first place, writing, "I am no angel and my corruption rises against it" (*TWH*, 279). Brontë stresses the degree to which Helen changes in Arthur's deathbed scene. When he pleads with her to act as his mediator and save him from hell, Helen responds by writing to her brother: "he clings to me with unrelenting pertinacity—with a kind of childish desperation, as if *I* could save him from the fate he dreads (*TWH*, 450). Helen later tells Arthur that "No man can deliver his brother, nor make agreement unto God for him," and instructs him instead to "let *Him* plead for you" (*TWH*, 451). Through her use of italic Brontë underscores the significance of Helen's disavowal of a redemptive role. Although at her husband's deathbed Helen agonizes about her inability to help him, she does not capitulate to his desperate request that she save him from hell; she tells him, up until his last moment, that he must pray for himself. Her disavowal of a redemptive role thus dovetails with Brontë's evangelical understanding that "the onus of interpreting God's Word . . . rests firmly upon the individual" and that "no human mediator is admitted to distance the relation between God and man" (Jay 1979, 51).

The deathbed scene near the conclusion of *The Tenant of Wildfell Hall* and the discussions between Helen and Arthur that lead up to it serve several additional purposes. They represent Brontë's attempt to incorporate in her work her belief in the doctrine of universal salvation, which she came to embrace after years of troubling consideration.[19] Believing that "no one could be predestined to eternal punishment" led Brontë to "the further idea that no punishment could be eternal" (Chitham 1979, 21). Perhaps the best articulation of this belief is to be found in the letter she wrote to the Reverend David Thom. Explaining that she had "cherished" the doctrine of universal salvation from childhood, Brontë wrote:

> We see how liable men are to yield to the temptation of the passing hour; how little the dread of future punishment—and still less the promise of future reward—can avail to make them forbear and wait; and if so many thousands rush into destruction with (as they suppose—the prospect of Eternal Death before their eyes—what might not the consequence be, if that prospect were changed for one of a limited season of punishment, far distant and unseen, however protracted and terrible it might be?[20]

After Arthur dies, Helen consoles herself that "whatever purging fires the erring spirit may be doomed to pass—whatever fate awaits it, still, it is not lost, and God, who hateth nothing that He hath made, *will* bless it in the end!" (*TWH*, 452).

Brontë also used this deathbed scene to grapple with a thorny problem of domestic ideology and the implications of that ideology for the development of selfhood. Brontë recognized the ways in which an "angel in the house" ideology, which seemed to empower women with moral responsibility, also proved debilitating.[21] She further attacked the ideology through her representation of Helen's developing assertiveness, an assertiveness that reaches its climax when she locks her husband out of their bedroom, thereby "shatter[ing] the Victorian icon of the submissive wife" (Margaret Smith 1993, xvi). In its devastating critique of the ideology of true womanhood and of the corollary notion that the home represented a safe haven and the natural place of the angelic middle-class woman, *The Tenant of Wildfell Hall* was far more radical than many works of women's fiction that were written later in the 19th century and are now recognized as feminist—works that, as Elaine Showalter has argued, "merely transposed" domestic ideology into "an activist key" (1977, 84).

In her recognition of the ways religious language seemed to endorse this domestic ideology, Brontë participated in a well-established tradition of women preachers and writers. As Christine L. Krueger writes, "From the women preachers of the eighteenth century to the Victorian novelists who were their heirs, women's writings testify to their ability to recognize the ideological conflicts in scripture that were suppressed in the patriarchal feminine ideal, and to interpret scripture as offering divinely sanctioned challenges to masculine authority."[22] Thus, the moment when Helen Huntingdon literally becomes free of her husband is interwoven in *The Tenant of Wildfell Hall* with the moment when she finally divests herself of the missionary role endorsed by her society's domestic ideology.

If Brontë's novel had focused exclusively on Helen's account of her marriage, one could conclude that the narrative charts the protagonist's growth from a state of subjugation to a state of independence and that this evolution can be measured by attending closely to the ways in which her use of religious language reveals her rejection of domestic ideology. But Brontë developed the frame narrative—Markham's account—to complicate this reading in two critical ways. Like Huntingdon, Markham refers on several occasions to Helen's angelic status. For example, he thinks of her diary as "too sacred for any eyes but her own" (*TWH*, 401), and, when she proposes to him by offering to him a rose as "an emblem of [her] heart" (485), he responds, "My darling angel—my *own Helen*" (*TWH*, 486). Markham's response suggests in part that Brontë wanted her readers to attend to the pervasiveness of language that inscribes women with redemptive potential. It is significant that this is one of the rare moments when Markham refers to Helen by her first name. Yet he subverts the very autonomy that his gesture would seem to confer by appropriating the person behind that identity as his own.

Just as Markham's language at the conclusion of *The Tenant of Wildfell Hall* suggests Brontë's rejection of simplistic solutions to the problems raised in her narrative, so too does Helen's language prove problematic, once again illustrating her complicity in constructing the identity that seems in some ways to thwart her development. If Brontë uses the diary to represent for readers the dilemmas Helen faces as a married woman, Markham's framing account provides a glimpse of similar problems that Helen faces as a mother. By using this approach, Brontë suggests that Helen's role as mother provides her with analogous opportunities to see her self as a savior. Just after her son's birth she ponders her duty "to guide him along the perilous path of youth, and train him to be God's servant while on earth, a blessed and honoured saint in heaven" (*TWH*, 252). Her decision to leave her husband in the first place is prompted by a fear that he will exert too much of an influence on her son. Speculating on this possibility, she writes "what *will* Arthur be, with all his natural sweetness of disposition, if I do not save him from that world and those companions" (*TWH*, 377). Even after she has managed to liberate her son from the influence of his father, she feels the need to shield him from worldly temptations. Explaining to Markham's mother the way she has educated her son to hate liquor, she says "I hope to save him from one degrading vice at least. I wish I could render the incentives to every other equally innoxious in his case" (*TWH,* 54).[23]

With this episode Brontë invites readers to consider several implications of Helen's role as moral educator. A reader whose position is akin to that of Helen's neighbors—that is, who does not yet know her story or her true identity—is likely to interpret her behavior as that of an overly zealous, extremely protective mother. A reader who reconsidered the episode after reading Helen's diary would be more likely to understand both Helen's reaction and Brontë's novelistic strategies. In a narrative that attends so frequently to Helen's solitude and silence, it is noteworthy that her first exchange with neighbors is characterized by the strength of her voice and the confidence of her self-assertion.[24] Brontë develops Helen's mode of self-presentation to mark her as distinctively different from the kind of fictional heroine who must camouflage her feminism. In her encounter with the Markhams, Helen vigorously defends herself as a mother and, in the process, asks them to consider the consequences of their views on education, views that she believes unjustly and dangerously distinguish between appropriate treatment of boys and girls. She says:

> You would have us encourage our sons to prove all things by their own experience, while our daughters must not even profit by the experience of others. Now *I* would have both so to benefit by the experience of others, and the precepts of a higher authority, that they should know beforehand to refuse the evil and choose the good, and require no experimental proofs to teach them the evil of transgression. I would not send a poor girl into the world unarmed against her foes, and ignorant of the snares that beset her path; nor would I watch and guard her, till, deprived of self-respect and self-reliance, she lost the power, or the will, to watch and guard herself. (*TWH,* 57)

Helen's speech, reminiscent of the "sermons" that Agnes Grey delivered to her readers near the end of her narrative, becomes one of several means that Brontë uses in *The Tenant of Wildfell Hall* to criticize her society's gendered standards of behavior.[25] In this case, she offers a feminist vision of education based on equality and on the assumption that women must learn to be independent.

Brontë's understanding of this equality was based, as Elizabeth Langland has written, on "an Enlightenment feminism," which "stressed woman's possession of a soul capable of redemption" (1989, 138).

Although Helen initially directs her remarks to Markham's mother, she turns at a critical point in the episode to Markham himself, implying that it is he who most needs to hear what she says. In doing so she distinguishes herself from the other women in the group who, in Markham's opinion, would have been far more likely to appease him. This distinction helps Brontë to advance her critique of domestic ideology. N. M. Jacobs wrote of the Markhams in this episode, "Their attitudes, which seem harmless traditionalism, are shown in Helen's diary to be essentially identical with those that produce the domestic hell at the center of the novel" (1986, 210). Thus, the episode accomplishes more than simply evidencing Helen's inability to fully relinquish her role as savior. It simultaneously illustrates the ways that her behavior as a mother is perceived by others and allows Helen the opportunity to interpret that behavior differently and, in doing so, to define her self accordingly. Brontë suggests in the process that Helen's identity is ultimately constituted by both her self and those around her.

Helen's gesture also enables Brontë to end the novel's opening chapter with an emphasis on communication and to associate communicative issues with the thematic of personal and social identity. Playing the fop, Markham tries to put an end to what he calls "her incomprehensible discourse" by saying "'Well! you ladies must always have the last word, I suppose,'" to which Helen replies "'You may have as many words as you please,—only I can't stay to hear them'" (*TWH*, 58). Markham responds, "'No; that is the way: you hear just as much of an argument as you please; and the rest may be spoken to the wind'" (*TWH*, 58). Through this encounter Brontë asks her readers to attend closely to the ways that language hinders or obstructs rather than facilitates self-knowledge and knowledge of others. Although the narrative that follows will bring revelation into the foreground through its commands to tell, speak, and confess, Brontë implies that refusals to listen are just as much a part of the story that follows.

The emphasis on speaking and hearing that distinguishes this opening episode resonates throughout the novel in its textual equivalent— writing and reading. In this way *The Tenant of Wildfell Hall* pursues in a variety of ways the interconnections between personal and textual identity. The two are linked most obviously through the character of Markham, who finally comes to believe he knows Helen Huntingdon from reading portions of her diary and letters to her brother. Halford, the recipient of Markham's letters, must interpret for himself the meaning of what he is presented with—Markham's notes, portions of Helen's diary, and portions of her letters to her brother—all of which make up what Markham significantly amends to call "not a sketch" but "a full and faithful account" of his relationship with Helen (*TWH*, 34). Structured as it is, Brontë's novel cannot be read linearly, for the potential meanings of its frame portions can be appreciated only after readers have, with Markham, been granted access to Helen's diary—to her own mode of representation.

The combination of the novel's narrative complexities with the circular mode of reading that is demanded by its narrative technique enables Brontë to suggest that textual identity, like personal identity, is multilayered, dialogically complex, and ultimately subject to appropriation and distortion. In this sense her achievement with *The Tenant of Wildfell Hall* goes far beyond the creation of "psychologically convincing" characters that critics have recognized her for.[26] Brontë's decision to continue publishing her work under the pseudonym Acton Bell and her statement in the "Preface to the Second Edition" of *The Tenant of Wildfell Hall* that "I would have it to be distinctly understood that Acton Bell is neither Currer nor Ellis Bell" (*TWH*, 31) represent attempts to preserve her own authorial identity from appropriation and distortion.[27] By writing in the preface that she "wished to tell the truth, for truth always conveys its own moral to those who are able to receive it" (*TWH*, 29), Brontë implied that her novel reflected her own spiritual calling and that it would exact from its readers the same kinds of interpretive demands that faced its characters.

Chapter Six

"A Close and Resolute Dissembler": Self-Representation and Anne Brontë's Artistry

In its treatment of the complex relationship between textual and personal identity, *The Tenant of Wildfell Hall* must be considered Brontë's most innovative treatment of the dynamics of self-development. Yet this achievement might not have been possible for Brontë had she not worked with the thematics of self-development in so many ways throughout her life. It is worthwhile reminding ourselves in conclusion of the import of the question Brontë posed to herself on the flyleaf of her Bible: "What, Where, and how shall I be when I have got through?"[1] The question, here addressed only to herself, echoes that which Brontë so often posed at the end of the diary papers written to be read by her sister Emily Brontë—questions such as "what changes shall we have seen and known; and shall we be much changed ourselves?" (*BLFC,* II, 53). These questions are also, of course, akin to those that Brontë had her poetic and fictional characters ask of themselves, as when Agnes Grey writes:

> Who can tell what this one month may bring forth? I have lived nearly three-and-twenty years, and I have suffered much, and tasted little pleasure yet: is it likely my life all through will be so clouded? Is it not possible that God may hear my prayers, disperse these gloomy shadows, and grant me some beams of heaven's sunshine yet! Will He entirely deny to me those blessings which are so freely given to others, who neither ask them nor acknowledge them when received? May I not still hope and trust? (*AG,* 137).

Agnes's speculations reveal the interplay between Brontë's fiction and her autobiographical writing, which also questions how much she should hope for change. Yet the similarities also suggest something of the depths of Brontë's ontological concerns with the nature of selfhood and with her own self-development.

Given Brontë's anxiety about how she would develop over time, it is ironic to consider the enormous changes that can be registered in her professional reputation in the nearly 150 years since she lived. Just how far critics have come in their estimation of her might best be measured by briefly reconsidering the impact of the famous indictment of Brontë, attributed in most critical and biographical accounts to Branwell Brontë, who was said to have once described his youngest sister as "Nothing, absolutely nothing—next to an idiot."[2] In actuality, the statement came not from Branwell himself, but from a fictional counterpart to him created by Charlotte Brontë in a youthful story titled "My Angria and the Angrians," written in October 1834. In it she creates a narrator named Lord Charles Wellesley and a figure named Patrick Benjamen Wiggins, a caricature of her brother Branwell. After responding to a question about his family posed by Wellesley, Wiggins is asked about his sisters, and the following conversation ensues:

> "What are your sisters' names?"
> "Charlotte Wiggins, Jane Wiggins, and Anne Wiggins."
> "Are they as queer as you?"
> "Oh, they are miserable silly creatures not worth talking about. Charlotte's eighteen years old, a broad, dumpy thing, Jane is sixteen, lean and scant, with a face about the size of a penny, and Anne is nothing, absolutely nothing."
> "What! Is she an idiot?"
> "Next door to it."[3]

Charlotte Brontë may presumably have intended in "My Angria and the Angrians" to portray her "real" brother's true sentiments. Yet, it is worth emphasizing that a statement about Anne Brontë that has been reproduced in numerous critical commentaries emanates from a hybrid source, at once fictional and biographical. The "source" of the comment was not Branwell Brontë directly but a caricature of him—the fictional character Patrick Wiggins. Perhaps more important, the subject of his comment was not Anne Brontë but "Anne Wiggins," another fictional caricature. The author of the piece was Charlotte Brontë, but she, too, distanced herself by speaking through the fictional narrator Lord Charles Wellesley, who engages Benjamin Wiggins in conversation about his sisters and their identities.

The comment, embedded as it is in Brontë lore and revealing multiple layers of narrative distance, functions as a paradigmatic example of the challenges that Anne Brontë faced in her effort to distinguish herself from her family and that her readers face in their efforts to interpret her writing. As this paradigm so readily reveals, interpretation of Brontë's writing involves first and foremost extricating her from the web of her family even while appreciating the extent to which she was situated in and contributed to the interplay of fictional and factual identities so central to all of their writing.

Even this interpretive task is further complicated by Brontë's own interest in disguise, an interest evident in all her writing. In her juvenilia, Brontë wrote poems "authored" by a variety of fictional creations, among them "Olivia Vernon," a "thinly veiled disguise" for Brontë herself (Chitham 1991, 86). In her last work, *The Tenant of Wildfell Hall,* Anne Brontë continued her exploration of the function of disguise through Helen Huntingdon, who for a significant portion of the narrative is disguised as the widow Mrs. Graham. Brontë's thinking about the role of disguise becomes particularly apparent in a crucial episode near the end of *Agnes Grey,* when Agnes pauses to explain herself to readers whom she imagines to be "well-nigh disgusted" with her disclosure of emotional weaknesses (*AG,* 121). Noting that they have been allowed to witness personal crises that she hid even from her family, Agnes writes, "I never disclosed it then, and would not have done so had my own sister or my mother been with me in the house. I was a close and resolute dissembler—in this one case at least" (*AG,* 121). Agnes's confession, couched as it is in the rhetoric of disclosure and self-control, illustrates Brontë's assumptions about the complexity of self-understanding and self-representation, as well as her approach to the writing process itself. The passage suggests that by having access to Agnes's private feelings readers are granted a more authentic view of her than that available to those with whom she is presumably most intimate. Yet by having Agnes then characterize herself as a "close and resolute dissembler," Brontë immediately undercuts the very trust between character and reader that the passage would seem to invoke and solidify. Agnes's maneuver enables Brontë to bring into the foreground the related roles that disguise, dissimulation, and secrecy play in any act of self-representation.

Such a gesture might initially seem to be incongruent with the pursuit of truth that Brontë claimed—at least in the "Preface to the Second Edition of *The Tenant of Wildfell Hall*"—was at the heart of her artistry. Nonetheless, her belief in the necessity of being truthful stemmed not from a desire for her work to achieve mimetic accuracy; rather, she endorsed a vision of truthfulness that encompassed a range of attitudes and behaviors—among them sincerity, candor, faithfulness, trustworthiness, and moral purity. In the "Preface"—Brontë's only public declaration of artistic purpose—she both committed herself to the evocation of "truth" and simultaneously put the burden of discovery and interpretation on her readers. She wrote:

> My object in writing the following pages was not simply to amuse the Reader, neither was it to gratify my own taste, nor yet to ingratiate myself with the Press and the Public: I wished to tell the truth, for truth always conveys its own moral to those who are able to receive it. But as the priceless treasure too frequently hides at the bottom of a well, it needs some courage to dive for it, especially as he that does so will be likely to incur more scorn and obloquy for the mud and water into which he has ventured to plunge, than thanks for the jewel he procures. (*TWH, 29*)

The key word in this passage might very well be "able," for Brontë points in particular to a select group of readers who share the capacity to apprehend the truth, and she implies that their ability entails having the courage to submit to public censure and abuse. Moreover, Brontë uses the preface to distance herself from the public world of "Press" and "Reader" and implies for herself a subordinate authorial position. Rather than representing her authorial role as that of crafter of truths, she suggests that she serves primarily as a liaison between the public world for which she writes and the private world of which she writes.

The authorial position Brontë constructs for herself is curiously deprived of agency. Instead, agency is reserved for a select group of readers, those ostensibly willing and able to confront the myriad challenges to moral learning that her subject matter poses. Brontë's interpretive paradigm implies, just as does Agnes Grey's confession of duplicity, that narratives of and about self are necessarily obscure: they inevitably implicate both those who project themselves on paper and those who in turn seek to comprehend the written self. They are narratives wrought with the "mud and water" that makes the readerly process of discovery as important as the final product heralded by the press.

Just as Brontë here clearly asks us to admire—and hence to *be*—readers willing to embark on an interpretive struggle for the truth, so too does she populate her work with characters engaged in acts of self-representation and corollary quests for truth. As chapter 3 of this book has suggested, "Self-Communion" (57)—perhaps Brontë's best-known poem—epitomizes the process of such an endeavor. The poetic persona of "Self-Communion" struggles to understand and "to see" her self despite the "mist," "smoke," and "clouds" that in the opening of the poem obscure her vision. Although she initially lacks the confidence to proceed (e.g., she writes of her life, "I cannot see how fast it goes" [l.26]), she comes to rely on an "inward spirit" (l.27) that leads her through the process of self-discovery to an acknowledgment of a synthetic unity of selfhood—the multiple selves implied by the title "Self-Communion." Brontë's persona reacts throughout the poem to a barrage of self-imposed prompts to investigate her past experiences, prompts to which she variously responds, "I see, far back, a helpless child" (l.43); "I see one kneeling on the sod" (l. 93); and "I see that time, and toil, and truth / An inward hardness can impart,—" (ll. 139–40). The poem constructs the identity that is at its center around this introspective *process* of self-investigation, rather than solely around its insights, its outcome. The poem concludes with the speaker's acknowledgment that the process of self-discovery has been arduous but necessary:

> O I have striven both hard and long
> But many are my foes and strong,
> My gains are light—my progress slow;
> For hard's the way I have to go,
> And my worst enemies, I know
> Are those within my breast. (ll. 297–302)

With its emphasis on unraveling what the speaker refers to as her "inner life" (l. 100), as well as with its use of multiple voices, all of which are understood to be dimensions of the single person addressing her readers, "Self-Communion" exemplifies Brontë's exploration of the nature of subjectivity, an investigation made more complex by her willingness to confront the idea that just as individuals disguise themselves from others, so too may they deceive themselves in their struggle toward self-knowledge.

Brontë's concern with the complex nature of subjectivity and with strategies of self-representation permeates all her writing—her juvenilia, her diary extracts and letters, the marginal and flyleaf notes made in her Bible, her poetry, and, finally, the fiction with which she ended her career. Whatever she grappled with—the nature of secrecy, silence, and solitude; the possibilities of autonomy and the problematics of anonymity; the interplay between public and private identities; the relationship of privacy to personhood; or the perplexities of human behavior and development—her writing underscores her awareness that individuals continually and sometimes inexplicably re-create themselves as they interact with others.

Brontë's earliest readers failed to recognize the sophistication of her innovative treatment of self-understanding and self-representation. Ironically, however, they were captivated by issues of identity. The identities of the Bell authors, the perplexing interplay of the fictional and the factual in their work, and the related issue of Brontë's position within her family commanded the attention of her first critics.[4] The literary critics who first encountered her novels were concerned primarily with distinguishing among the works of Currer, Ellis, and Acton Bell. Many critics concluded that the works emanated from a single author. In an unsigned notice that appeared in the *Spectator*, discussing the joint edition of *Wuthering Heights and Agnes Grey*, a reviewer wrote, "We know not whether the names of Ellis and Acton Bell, which appear on the title pages of this publication, have any connexion with Currer Bell, the editor of *Jane Eyre*; but the works have some affinity" (Allott 1974, 218). Similarly, an unsigned notice in the *New Monthly Magazine* began:

> Ellis Bell and Acton Bell appear in the light of two names borrowed to represent two totally different styles of composition and two utterly opposed modes of treatment of the novel, rather than to indicate two real personages. They are names coupled together as mysteriously in the literary, as the sons of Leda are in the asterial world; and there is something at least gained by being mysterious at starting. (Allott 1974, 229)

Even critics who acknowledged that the novels were written by different authors were fixated on establishing their similarities. For example, in a representative (unsigned) notice in the *Examiner*, one reviewer wrote:

> The authors of *Jane Eyre, Wuthering Heights, Agnes Grey,* and *The Tenant of Wildfell Hall* are evidently children of the same family. They derive their scenes from the same country; their associations are alike; their heroines are for the most part alike, three being thrown upon their own talents for self-support, and two of them being all-enduring governesses; and their heroes also resemble éach other, in aspect, and temper, almost in habits. We have, once or twice entertained a suspicion that all the books that we have enumerated might have issued from the same source; sent forth at different seasons, in different states of mind or humour, or at different periods or elevations of the intellect,—*Jane Eyre* having been achieved at

the culminating point. At all events, the writers are of the same stock, have undoubted marks of family resemblance. (Allott 1974, 254)

Although Anne Brontë's use of the pseudonym Acton Bell may have encouraged many of her readers to devote their attention to the identity of the author, she was evidently uncomfortable with the assumptions behind so many of the reviews. As previously noted, she wrote in her "Preface to the Second Edition of *The Tenant of Wildfell Hall*" that she "would have it to be distinctly understood that Acton Bell is neither Currer nor Ellis Bell" and that "it [could not] greatly signify . . . whether the name be real or fictitious" (*TWH,* 31). Brontë was undoubtedly reacting in part to American publications of works of the Brontë family that had incorrectly identified her as "Acton Bell, Author of 'Wuthering Heights'" (Allott 1974, 29). Her subsequent comments in the "Preface" may have further obscured the rationale for her use of a pseudonym, for she argued that all books, including her own, should be written for both men and women and hence that critics should not concern themselves with the sex of the author.

Brontë's comments in the "Preface" have led contemporary critics to assume that her choice of "Acton Bell" stemmed primarily from this concern with gender, authorship, and the reader. Yet, given her enduring interest in dilemmas of identity, it is imperative to point out the additional interpretive interest of her pseudonym. By using as the last name of her pseudonym the same name that her sisters were using, and indeed by submitting work for joint publication, she invited consideration of her work as part of a family parcel. The names Currer, Ellis, and Acton of course preserved the initials of Charlotte, Emily, and Anne, and all were names unrelated to the Brontë family and unidentifiable by gender. Brontë scholars will never know with any assurance exactly how the Brontë sisters deliberated on their pseudonyms. What remains clear, and what is ultimately most important to Anne Brontë scholarship, is that her pseudonym is, like her work, hybrid, simultaneously containing fictional and autobiographical components.

Brontë's plea to be distinguished from her sisters is ironic in one respect, because when her first critics did turn their attention from the issue of authorship to the substance and techniques of her work, they almost uniformly found it to be lacking. *Agnes Grey* was described pejoratively as "a simple tale," and *The Tenant of Wildfell Hall* was widely condemned for its ostensibly disreputable subject matter.[5] In a representative commentary, one reviewer for the *Spectator* wrote:

The Tenant of Wildfell Hall, like its predecessor, suggests the idea of considerable abilities ill applied. There is power, effect, and even nature, though of an extreme kind, in its pages; but there seems in the writer a morbid love for the coarse, not to say the brutal; so that his level subjects are not very attractive, and the more forcible are displeasing or repulsive, from their gross, physical, or profligate substratum. (Allott 1974, 250)

From the beginning, then, Brontë seems to have faced a double bind. When her works were interpreted in conjunction with those of her sisters, her achievements were devalued; yet when critics focused on her works alone, she was condemned.

There are, of course, many reasons why Brontë is now being increasingly recognized for her artistic achievement, but foremost among them is the sophistication of her study of self-understanding and self-representation. In a variety of ways, Brontë's work assumes an understanding of the intersubjective nature of identity very much like that promoted by scholars in such fields as the philosophy of mind and social psychology. While these fields treat the concept of the self as a historical and cultural construction, they also define the self both as an ever-changing product of interpersonal relationships and, simultaneously, as a "knowledge structure" that enables individuals to understand their experiences and to endow them with a synthetic unity.[6] The approach to self fostered by philosophers of mind and social psychologists illuminates Brontë's perceptive appreciation of the psychological and social dimensions of the writing process, as well as the innovative treatment of the dynamics of self-understanding and self-representation in her writing. These factors make her work more interesting to literary critics today than ever before.

Influenced by developments in a number of fields, literary critics have also challenged the notion of an essential, unified identity that once was believed to be central to authorship as well as to characterization. Instead, many critics today focus on the multidimensional and inevitably constructed qualities of selfhood. This focus provides for a Bakhtinian approach to meaning that emphasizes the heterogeneity of social voices, of the multiple "selves" fashioned and invoked by individuals. In turn, the advent of a variety of poststructuralist theories has made it fashionable to dismiss the notion of an organic, unified self entirely and to adopt in its place the less essentialist concept of subject positions. These trends, which in some measure account for recent redirections in Victorian studies, feminist criticism, and autobiographical theory, help us to appreciate the complexity of Brontë's treatment of self and identity as well as her emphasis on the dynamics of private and public life.[7]

That the contemporary literary critical community, emphasizing as it does the complex nature of subjectivity, would find Brontë's writing hospitable may initially seem unlikely, for her work has for many years been considered to be relatively transparent and therefore resistant to a variety of interpretations. To be fair, there is much about Brontë's writing that is decidedly traditional: her novels draw in many ways on a realist tradition typical of Victorian fiction, and her creation of characters engaged in self-reflection and struggling to achieve autonomy relies on a belief in the existence of self that initially seems at odds with some recent critical theory. Indeed, it is partly because Brontë's belief in the concept of selfhood is so evident in her work that much of her writing has been reductively treated as autobiography.

The interest of Brontë's work clearly extends well beyond its conformity to middle-class Victorian traditions. Distinguishing in a variety of ways between an individual's mind and his or her behavior, Brontë's work reveals her appreciation for the sociocultural dimensions of human psychology. Moreover, her writing suggests a perceptive understanding that selfhood adapts to and can be changed by experiences. The self that Brontë's writing constructs is hence something that an individual can become conscious of as heterogeneous and fragmentary even while he or she believes it to constitute and unify being.

One of Brontë's earliest readers—the reviewer for *The Spectator*—called attention to the "substratum" of her work to identify the point from which all that was "displeasing" in her writing originated. Yet it might be this very "substratum" that now, nearly 150 years later, accounts for renewed interest in her writing. The very fact that Brontë's work is multilayered—that it has recognizable substratums, underlayers of meaning that affect the surface of the text—allows for greater interpretive inquiry into her artistry. The multidimensional nature of Brontë's works emerged from her perception of human identity as equally multifaceted. Just as Brontë's use of the pseudonym "Acton Bell" suggests the complexity of her professional identity, so too does her self-described status as a "silent invalid stranger" remind us of the complexity of her personal identity. Her two selves—the personal and the professional—were of course related; they were projected, like the prisoners of her poetry and her alienated and exiled fictional heroines, from the perspective that her sister Charlotte Brontë once described as "a secret Sinai."

Notes and References

Chapter One

1. Emily Brontë's comment about her sister Anne is made in a diary paper dated 30 July 1841. It is printed in *The Brontës: Their Lives, Friendships, and Correspondence*, eds. T. J. Wise and J. A. Symington (Oxford: The Shakespeare Head Press, 1932; reprint, 4 vols. in 2, Philadelphia: Porcupine Press, 1980): vol. I, 238. All references are to these volumes; hereafter cited in text as *BLFC* with volume and page number.

2. Charlotte Brontë, "Biographical Notice of Ellis and Acton Bell," 19 September 1850, preface to the 1850 edition of *Wuthering Heights and Agnes Grey*. This phrase is taken from a passage excerpted in Edward Chitham's "Introduction" to *The Poems of Anne Brontë: A New Text and Commentary* (Totowa, N.J.: Rowman and Littlefield, 1979), 22.

3. The comment was indirectly attributed to Branwell Brontë by Charlotte Brontë in one of the stories written in her youth, "My Angria and the Angrians." It is reprinted in Winifred Gerin's *Branwell Brontë* (London: Thomas Nelson and Sons, Ltd., 1961), 7; hereafter cited in text. A detailed discussion of this comment is included in chapter 6 of this book.

4. The phrase "axiology of the self" comes from Regina Gagnier's *Subjectivities: A History of Self Representation in Britain, 1832–1920* (New York: Oxford University Press, 1991), 3; hereafter cited in text. She describes it as "the systems of values, expectations, and constraints that come into play when one represents oneself to others in the concrete circumstances of daily life" (3).

5. Lines 1–2 of "The Bluebell," which appears as poem 10 in Edward Chitham's *The Poems of Anne Brontë: A New Text and Commentary* (Totowa, N.J., Rowman and Littlefield, 1979), 73. All references to Brontë's poetry are from this edition and hereafter will be cited parenthetically in the text by poem number and line numbers.

6. Anne Brontë, *The Tenant of Wildfell Hall* (1848; reprint, Harmondsworth, England: Penguin, 1979), 314; hereafter cited in text as *TWH*.

7. For a good discussion of this issue, see Edward E. Sampson's *Social Worlds, Personal Lives: An Introduction to Social Psychology* (New York: Harcourt Brace Jovanovich, 1991), 218–20; hereafter cited in text.

8. Brontë refers in her preface to this slightly reworded accusation. The original accusation appeared in *The Spectator* on 8 July 1848 and now appears in *The Brontës: The Critical Heritage*, ed. Miriam Allott (London: Routledge & Kegan Paul, 1974), 250; hereafter cited in text.

9. Edward Chitham, *A Life of Anne Brontë* (Cambridge, Mass.: Basil Blackwell, 1991), 6; hereafter cited in text.

10. As P. J. M. Scott writes in *Anne Brontë: A New Critical Assessment,* "Anne was the pretty one; she was personable and appealing as Charlotte, all self-consciously, was not"(Totowa, N.J.: Barnes and Noble, 1983), 22; hereafter cited in text. Similarly, N. M. Jacobs dismisses the prevailing idea of a sisterly continuum—"Emily the wild pagan, Anne the mild Christian, with Charlotte somewhere in between"—only to propose an alternative basis of comparison based on a portrait of the sisters done by Branwell: this painting, which represents "Emily and Anne close together on the left and Charlotte keeping company with the ghost of Branwell's face on the right," is, according to Jacobs, "a true one." ("Gender and Layered Narrative in *Wuthering Heights* and *The Tenant of Wildfell Hall," Journal of Narrative Technique* 16 [Fall 1986], 204; hereafter cited in text.

11. Helena Michie, *Sororophobia: Differences among Women in Literature and Culture* (New York: Oxford University Press, 1992), 56; hereafter cited in text.

12. Typifying this tendency is Anne Smith, who writes, in her introduction to a recent edition of *Agnes Grey,* "This is not to claim that *Agnes Grey* [and] *The Tenant of Wildfell Hall* are better novels than *Jane Eyre, Villette,* or *Wuthering Heights,* though a case could certainly be made for their superiority to *The Professor* and *Shirley." (Agnes Grey* [1847; reprint, London: J. M. Dent & Sons, 1985], xv). All references to *Agnes Grey* are from this edition and are hereafter cited in text as *AG.*

13. Angela Leighton, *Victorian Women Poets: Writing Against the Heart* (Charlottesville: University Press of Virginia, 1992), 4–5; hereafter cited in text. Leighton goes on to argue that biography should be used not as a context for understanding writing but rather "side by side with it, in a suggestively interacting tension, rather than a determining sequence" (5).

14. The term "life writing" is explained in and used throughout Marlene Kadar's essay "Coming to Terms: Life Writing" in *Essays on Life Writing: From Genre to Critical Practice,* ed. Marlene Kadar (Toronto: University of Toronto Press, 1992); hereafter cited in text. Discussing the ways in which life writing can be considered a "critical practice" as opposed to a genre, Kadar explains, "It is best viewed as a continuum that spreads unevenly and in combined forms from the so-called least fictive narration to the most fictive" (10). Another contributor to Kadar's volume, Christl Verduyn, argues that life writing "enables its practioners to move beyond genre boundaries and disciplines, particularly with regard to narrative unity, 'objective' thinking, and authority," ("Between the Lines: Marian Engel's *Cahiers* and Notebooks," in Kadar, 1992, 29).

15. Winifred Gerin exemplifies this tendency, conflating as she does in the following passage the fictional character of Helen Huntingdon with Anne Brontë and the fictional character of Arthur Huntingdon with Branwell Brontë. Discussing Helen's sense of relief at her husband's death after years of dissolution, Gerin writes, "Helen Huntingdon, having watched her husband's terrible

end, proclaims the faith which it was Anne's only comfort to hold respecting Branwell" ("Introduction" to *The Tenant of Wildfell Hall* [1848; reprint, Harmondsworth, England: Penguin, 1979], 17; hereafter cited in text). Similarly, Herbert Rosengarten in his "Introduction" to a recent edition of *The Tenant of Wildfell Hall* confidently acknowledges Branwell's influence: "Branwell's counterpart in the book is Lord Lowborough, a man whose better self is almost destroyed by drink and by his wife's treachery" ("Introduction" to *The Tenant of Wildfell Hall* [1848; reprint, Oxford: Clarendon Press, 1992], xiv; hereafter cited in text).

   16.   Anne Brontë's critics have relied heavily as well on biographical information about shifting family loyalties, finding in her poetry and fiction "evidence" of changing relationships between Anne and her sisters and locating in *The Tenant of Wildfell Hall* evidence of her supreme frustration with the artistic failings of her sister Emily in *Wuthering Heights.*

   17.   Charlotte Brontë, "Biographical Notice of Ellis and Acton Bell," reprinted in Emily Brontë's *Wuthering Heights,* eds. Hilda Marsden and Ian Jack (London: Clarendon, 1976), appendix I; hereafter cited in text.

   18.   Elizabeth Langland summarizes the scholarly consensus in *Anne Brontë: The Other One:* "It is generally agreed that, however solicitous Charlotte may have been of Anne's health, she was often deprecatory of her talents. And it was Charlotte who early set the tone for evaluating Anne. While we should not underestimate the service Charlotte performed in galvanising her two younger sisters into print, we should note that once they were in print Charlotte seemed incapable of appreciating Anne's unique gifts as poet and novelist" (London: Macmillan, 1989), 1; hereafter cited in text.

   19.   Richard D. Altick, *Victorian People and Ideas* (New York: Norton, 1973), 190–202.

   20.   Sidonie Smith, *A Poetics of Women's Autobiography: Marginality and the Fictions of Self-Representation* (Bloomington: Indiana University Press, 1987), 5; hereafter cited in text. Smith offers an outline of a poetics of women's autobiography that encompasses psychoanalytic and historical approaches, addressing both the psychodynamics of an author's (or a fictional character's) emotional life and the social and cultural conditions that delimit the author's (or the character's) understanding of narrative and identity in the first place. See especially the chapter "Woman's Story and the Engendering of Self-Representation," where Smith identifies the phenomena that mark women's autobiographical texts. For another good discussion of issues related to women and self-representation, see Leigh Gilmore, *Autobiographics: A Feminist Theory of Women's Self-Representation* (Ithaca, N.Y.: Cornell University Press, 1994). According to Gilmore, there are not so much autobiographies as autobiographics—"those elements that instead mark a location in a text where self-invention, self-discovery, and self-representation emerge" (42).

   21.   Mary Jean Corbett has argued, in *Representing Femininity: Middle-Class Subjectivity in Victorian and Edwardian Women's Autobiographies,* that

"Concepts of the self and the forms that self-representations take are historically and culturally variable. . . . It is through cultural and historical analysis that
we can begin to understand not only the constitution of autobiographical subjects, but also the specific uses of autobiography for writers and readers and the
particular forms that subjectivities take" (New York: Oxford University Press,
1992), 4; hereafter cited in text.

22.   The phrase "exalted mission as mother" is from Margaret Homans's
*Bearing the Word: Language and Female Experience in Nineteenth-Century Women's
Writing* (Chicago: University of Chicago Press, 1986); hereafter cited in text. As
Homans writes, "Encomiums about woman's exalted mission as mother, which
we would today recognize as characteristically Victorian, indeed do not begin
appearing until the 1830s and 1840s, apparently in response to the perception
of women's growing independence from the home" (153).

23.   For an excellent study of the relationship between such media and
the development of the novel, see Nancy Armstrong's *Desire and Domestic
Fiction: A Political History of the Novel* (New York: Oxford University Press,
1987) hereafter cited in text.

24.   "Separate spheres" has come to denote the gendered bifurcation of
activity and behavior that many middle-class Victorians seemed to endorse, one
that defined women as naturally belonging to and existing within the confines
of the private household and home, and that correlatively associated men with
the public, cultured domain of the workplace. According to the ideology of separate spheres, women inhabited a distinct world of their own, one that revolved
around their nurturing role within the nuclear family. The idea of separate
spheres emanated out of cultural understanding of woman's psychological identity but extended beyond the psychological to advocate a corollary social behavior, one premised on the ideals of piety, purity, and submissiveness.

25.   The alternatives here are those delineated by Linda K. Kerber in
"Separate Spheres, Female Worlds, Woman's Place: The Rhetoric of Women's
History," *The Journal of American History,* 75 (June 1988), 17; hereafter cited in
text.

26.   One way to appreciate the historical complexity of the notion is to
acknowledge that the process by which the ideas we associate with "separate
spheres" came into focus took place concurrently—and not uncoincidentally—
with other important manifestations of cultural change. Many historians associate the period of the 1830s and 1840s primarily with widespread
industrialization and its attendant class conflicts, arguing that during this period the middle class became firmly entrenched in British society. Others stress
the ways in which Britain's imperial attitudes and actions were shaped just
before midcentury. The ideologies of class, race, and nation on which these
moments in British history depended were in a variety of ways inseparable from
the gender ideologies underwriting the notion of separate spheres. Indeed, so
deeply were notions of gender, class, race, and nation interwoven in Victorian
culture that they are often thought to be mutually constitutive.

27. In doing so she turns her heroine's diary into what Susan Lanser in her work on feminist narratology has called a "public 'display text,'" one that effectively collapses the public and private binary but exposes the emotional costs entailed in the process. See "Toward a Feminist Narratology," *Style* 20, 3 (Fall 1986), 351; hereafter cited in text.

28. In constructing a way of reading that can account for both perspectives, Lanser argues in her work on feminist narratology that works of literature should be studied "in relation to a referential context that is simultaneously linguistic, literary, historical, biographical, social, and political" (Lanser 1986, 345).

29. Joan Wallach Scott, "Women's History and the Rewriting of History," in *The Impact of Feminist Research in the Academy,* ed. Christie Farnham (Bloomington, Ind.: Indiana University Press, 1987), 44; hereafter cited in text.

Chapter Two

1. Branwell Brontë died in September 1848; Emily Brontë died in December of that year; and Anne Brontë died just five months later, in May 1849.

2. Charlotte Brontë, "Introduction" to "Selections from Poems by Acton Bell," first published in the 1850 edition of *Wuthering Heights and Agnes Grey* (London: Smith, Elder); hereafter cited in text as C. Brontë 1850. Reprinted in *Complete Poems of Anne Brontë,* ed. Clement Shorter (London: Hodder and Stoughton, 1920), v; hereafter cited in text.

3. The phrase "suffer and be still" was coined by Mrs. Sarah Stickney Ellis, who wrote in *The Daughters of England* (London: Fisher, Son, & Co., 1845) that a woman's "highest duty is so often to suffer and be still." Her phrase was used as the title of Martha Vicinus's important collection of essays, *Suffer and Be Still: Women in the Victorian Age* (Bloomington, Ind.: Indiana University Press, 1972).

4. Winifred Gerin, *Anne Brontë,* 1st ed. (London: Thomas Nelson and Sons, Ltd., 1959), 9; hereafter cited in text.

5. Juliet Gardiner, *The Brontës at Haworth: The World Within* (New York: Clarkson Potter, 1992), 30; hereafter cited in text.

6. Elizabeth Gaskell, *The Life of Charlotte Brontë* (1857; reprint, Harmondsworth, England: Penguin, 1985), 87; hereafter cited in text.

7. This is the school that Charlotte Brontë made infamous as Lowood in *Jane Eyre.* Maria Brontë died on 6 May 1825, and Elizabeth Brontë died on 15 June 1825. Both had returned home from school in ill health.

8. Biographers of Anne Brontë must rely heavily on information provided by Charlotte Brontë, and must assume that the relationship of the sisters was so close that all would have been aware of and involved in each other's activities. Juliet Gardiner reprints Charlotte's reworking of her mother's portrait and recounts that from rereading her mother's letters, Charlotte discovered "a mind of a truly fine, pure and elevated order'" (Gardiner 1992, 31). The descriptive phrase "independent-minded" comes from Gerin (1959, 5).

9. As Gerin has argued, "Religion was the mainspring of [Elizabeth Branwell's] life—though after much self torment it was not to be the religion of Anne Brontë" (1959, 39).

10. A photograph of the teapot and a transcription of its message appear in Gardiner (1992, 42).

11. A photograph of this sampler appears in Gerin (1959, 48). My transcription comes from a photograph of the sampler that is available at the Haworth Parsonage Library.

12. Although Fannie Elizabeth Ratchford is dismissive of Anne Brontë's contributions to the Gondal and Angrian chronicles, she provides the most complete available account of the evolution of the juvenilia in *The Brontës' Web of Childhood* (New York: Columbia University Press, 1941).

13. Ellen Nussey, "Reminiscences of Charlotte Brontë," *Scribner's Monthly,* II (May 1871). The comment refers to a time in 1833 when Nussey visited the Brontë family. Quoted in Chitham (1991, 34).

14. Chitham (1991) argues that while Emily and Anne Brontë worked together on the Gondal writing, Emily came gradually to dominate Anne, whose interest in the imaginary kingdom gradually diminished.

15. Gerin argues that "Unlike Charlotte's and Branwell's 'Angria'—the exotic empire into which the Great Glass Confederacy merged—the permanence of Gondal lay in the fact that it was *not* a world at several removes from reality but only a slightly blurred print of the landscape of home" (1959, 56).

16. For a more complete discussion of Anne Brontë's Gondal poetry, refer to chapter 3 of this book.

17. For more discussion, see Chitham (1991, 88–89). Chitham contends that "From December 1841 to mid-January 1842, we may see them as collaborating fully on systematizing Gondal, though the work was not finished by 1845, and was probably never finished" (89).

18. Quoted by Anne Smith in her "Introduction" to *Agnes Grey,* xviii. Smith goes on to make the good point that critical recognition of *Agnes Grey* suffered because it first appeared alongside the "more dramatic" *Wuthering Heights.*

19. Anne Brontë refers to herself as "a helpless child, / Feeble and full of causeless fears" in her 1847 poem "Self-Communion" (57, ll. 43–44). The many autobiographical elements of this poem make it an essential source of information for biographers.

20. For more discussion of Brontë's interest in music during her years as a governess, see Chitham (1991, 103 and 114).

21. Chitham writes, "Throughout the Brontës' childhood and beyond, they drew from copy-books, but they all enjoyed using live models too. . . . [A]ll the Brontës drew pictures of the animals and people around them" (1991, 36).

22. I refer specifically here to the untitled drawings designated A4.6 and A4.5 by the Brontë Society in its photographic file of Anne Brontë's drawings.

23.   For a discussion of possible interpretations of "Sunrise at Sea" and its relationship to Brontë's attitude toward William Weightman, see Chitham (1991, 64–66). For a discussion of possible interpretations of "What You Please," see Chitham (1991, 79).

24.   Reverend Patrick Brontë, "A Funeral Sermon for the late Reverend William Weightman, M.A." (Halifax: J. U. Walker, 1842). Reprinted in *Brontëana: The Reverend Patrick Brontë, A.B., His Collected Life and Works; and the Brontës of Ireland* (Bingley: T. Harrison & Sons, 1898), 256; hereafter cited in text.

25.   Chitham identifies seven "love" poems with a male subject who has "constant characteristics": numbers 9, 11, 12, 13, 20, 37, and 55. For a discussion of these poems, see Chitham (1979, 16).

26.   Anne Brontë, "Letter to the Reverend David Thom, D.D." 30 December 1848. Reprinted in appendix B of the second edition of Winifred Gerin's *Anne Brontë* (London: Allen Lane, 1976), 361. Brontë's letter was written shortly after the deaths of Branwell and Emily. Thom, a Liverpool minister, had read some of Brontë's poems and had responded favorably to her anti-Calvinist sentiments and her support of universal salvation.

27.   Because the papers were to be opened by Emily on her birthday, they are sometimes referred to as "birthday papers."

28.   Anne Brontë may well have picked up this phrase from Aunt Branwell. Winifred Gerin attributes such a phrase to Aunt Branwell in her biography of Branwell Brontë (1961, 45).

29.   Anne Brontë slightly misquotes Byron's Canto xv, stanza 99, of *Don Juan,* which reads: "How little do we know that which we are! / How less what we may be! The eternal surge / Of time and tide rolls on and bears afar / Our bubbles."

30.   Some Anne Brontë scholars believe that she originally intended *Agnes Grey* to be titled *Passages in the Life of an Individual.* Other scholars suggest that this title may refer to another work, or even to the beginnings of *The Tenant of Wildfell Hall.* Whatever the case, the title illustrates Brontë's interest in anonymity, a topic that permeates both of her published novels.

31.   The poetry seems likely to have been written by Anne Brontë. So faded now as to be nearly impossible to transcribe, it occurs just after a piece titled "An Elegy on the Death of Miss Warren, An amiable Young Lady, who died of a Consumption, in the Year 1771." In G. B. Wright's *Thoughts in Younger Life on Interesting Subjects* (London: J. Buckland, 1778), 49; hereafter cited in text.

32.   Above this entry is written "Begun about December 1841." On the end page of the Bible is the penciled date 30 April 1843. The Bible is an Authorized King James version (London: Longman, Hurst, Rees, Orne, and Browne, 1821). It is in the Brontë collection at the Pierpont Morgan Library in New York City (PML 17769).

33. The phrase "Create in me a clean heart" appears in Psalm 51: 10, and is one of the verses that Brontë made note of in the flyleaves to her Bible.

34. The extent of the relationship between Branwell Brontë and Mrs. Robinson, the way in which he was asked to leave Thorp Green, and the culpability of Mrs. Robinson in encouraging the relationship have been open to debate since Elizabeth Gaskell first tackled the problem in 1857 (Gaskell, 1985). The problem continues to plague Brontë scholars; see, for example, "Mildred Christian on the Lydia Robinson Affair," ed. Edward Chitham, in *Brontë Society Transactions,* 21 (1994), 71–77.

35. Kathryn Hughes, *The Victorian Governess* (London: Hambledon Press, 1993), xi; hereafter cited in text. Hughes argues that *Agnes Grey* reveals Brontë's "essentially conservative enquiry into the social and moral responsibilities of ladyhood" (6).

Chapter Three

1. For an excellent discussion of the way Victorian poets rebelled against inherited traditions, see Isobel Armstrong's *Victorian Poetry: Poetry, Poetics, and Politics* (New York: Routledge, 1993); hereafter cited in text.

2. Leighton (1992, 2). Leighton argues that "women's poetry of the nineteenth century, much more than the novel, was written and read as part of a self-consciously female tradition" (1).

3. See Germaine Greer's "Preface" to *Winged Words: Victorian Women's Poetry and Verse,* compiled by Catherine Reilly (London: Enitharmon Press, 1994), xv; hereafter cited in text.

4. For a full discussion of the rhetoric associated with Evangelicalism as well as with the literary usage of its doctrines, see Elisabeth Jay's *The Religion of the Heart: Anglican Evangelicalism and the Nineteenth-Century Novel* (Oxford: Clarendon Press, 1979); hereafter cited in text.

5. Elizabeth Langland summarizes this tradition well, writing in *Anne Brontë: The Other One,* "It has been common for critics to divide Anne Brontë's poetic output (a total of fifty-nine poems) into two groups: Gondal and non-Gondal. The former, a group of twenty-three poems, was produced almost entirely during periods of close intimacy with Emily. The latter, a group of over thirty poems, represents a spiritual and emotional autobiography that includes love poems, religious and didactic poems, hymns, and introspective and dialogue poems" (1989, 61).

6. Introducing this same passage in *The Poems of Anne Brontë,* Chitham writes,"Though *Agnes Grey* is a novel, not autobiography, the *attitudes* of the heroine (as opposed to the precise incidents related) appear to coincide in verifiable ways with those of the author" (1979, 28).

7. Originally untitled, this poem was given the title "Self-Congratulation" (9) for the 1846 publication of *Poems* by Currer, Ellis and Acton Bell. At the same time Brontë made several important revisions, among them

changing the opening mention of the anonymous "Maiden" to the more personal "Ellen." (See Chitham 1979, 71–73.)

8. Not all of Anne Brontë's poems are dated so precisely, so it is worthwhile paying attention to those that are. Her diary papers also reveal her interest in marking new beginnings in her development, as do the notes written on the fly-leaves of her Bible. For further discussion, see Chapter 2 of this book.

9. Chitham notes that "a much shorter hymn by Isaac Watts, beginning 'Eternal Power, whose high abode,' is in the same metre" (1979, 176).

10. Janis P. Stout, *Strategies of Reticence: Silence and Meaning in the Works of Jane Austen, Willa Cather, Katherine Anne Porter, and Joan Didion* (Charlottesville, Va.: The University Press of Virginia, 1990). Stout argues, "The woman writer may find another answer, however, to the multifarious problem of silencing by the male hegemony. That answer is to use silence, the very silence that has been imposed, as a tool to undermine the ascendancy that silenced her" (18).

11. Both Chitham and Langland have focused on the way the poem explores the predicament of separation from those one loves, a common theme for Brontë. Langland writes: "In these Gondal poems, Anne Brontë details a physical restraint that keeps suffering loved ones apart and that threatens to make the world a cold and loveless place" (1989, 65).

12. P. J. M. Scott argues of this portion of the poem that "By implication the proximity of a mate, 'one faithful dear companion,' would be compensation for its loss of liberty because one element in such fulfilments, not the whole" (1983, 64). I read the poem as on occasion moving between the dove and the speaker herself; the fifth stanza reveals the extent to which the speaker projects her own desires onto the dove.

13. Langland provides an exception to this rule of treating the poem as biographical evidence. She suggests a broader reading: "If these lines do refer to Weightman, then dead for several years, I would suggest that they express a more philosophical love—agape rather than eros—for an individual who had provided an image of Christian love, or caritas, in the world" (1989, 75).

14. Although Chitham argues that exact dating of this poem is impossible (1979, 179), Langland fruitfully compares "Home" (30) to "Lines Written at Thorp Green," which, as its title suggests, clearly was about longing for Haworth. For more discussion, see Langland (1989, 80–81).

15. Probably the single most frequently commented-upon poem of Brontë's, "Self-Communion" (57) has been heralded as her most deeply autobiographical work, one that invokes a "dialogue of Hope and Experience" to express "reconciliation of self to Life's disappointments" (P. J. M. Scott, 1983, 69).

16. According to many of her critics, Brontë is alluding here, as elsewhere in "Self-Communion," to changes in her relationship with Emily. What seems more important to emphasize is her acknowledgment in these portions of the poem of her own responsibility for adopting a new posture toward those outside her—a posture that she characterizes as only partially open.

17.   Line 328 of this stanza makes the second reference to "the narrow way" in "Self-Communion," the first being in line 98. Although untitled in its original form, Brontë's next poem (number 58), dated 24 April 1848, was named "The Narrow Way" by Charlotte Brontë for the 1850 edition. As Chitham notes, the phrase, popular for Christian hymns, had been used by Cowper in the Olney Hymn No. 52, and was a favorite image of Anne Brontë's, one that she "used in four of her other poems" (1979, 195).

18.   Isobel Armstrong argues that Victorian poetry evokes "two forms of utterance," one that represents unified selfhood and another that represents the "fracturing self awareness of the interrogating consciousness. . . . Victorian poetry does not swing between these two forms of utterance but dramatizes and objectifies their simultaneous existence" (1993, 12).

Chapter Four

1.   For an overview of how novelists worked with and transformed these reports, see "The Anathematized Race: The Governess and *Jane Eyre,*" in Mary Poovey's *Uneven Developments: The Ideological Work of Gender in Mid-Victorian England* (Chicago: University of Chicago Press, 1988), 126–163; hereafter cited in text.

2.   As Nancy Armstrong notes in *Desire and Domestic Fiction,* "It was by fulfilling the duties of the domestic woman for money that [the governess] blurred a distinction on which the very notion of gender appeared to depend" (1987, 79).

3.   I want to emphasize here that what I am labeling "psychological" would have been described in other terms in the period in which Anne Brontë wrote *Agnes Grey.* Anita Levy and Mary Poovey, among others, have attempted recently to explore the emergence of what Levy terms "proto-psychological writing" in 19th-century British history. Both critics associate this phenomenon—though in different ways—with developments in sociological writing and domestic fiction as well. See, for example, Anita Levy's "Ending Up at Home: Victorian Fictions of Family, Discipline, and Desire," a paper presented at the May 1994 conference of the Interdisciplinary Nineteenth-Century Studies organization.

4.   Elizabeth Langland's chapter on *Agnes Grey* stresses the novel's educational motivations, in its evocation of both Agnes's role as a teacher and Brontë's role as an author. For a good discussion of Brontë's treatment of the physical conditions of the governess, see chapter 4 of Langland (1989, 97–118).

5.   In "Toward a Feminist Narratology," Susan Lanser argues that women writers have created "semi-private" forms of narration as part of their effort to "redefine the simple distinction of public and private" (1986, 353).

6.   Quoted by Arnold Craig Bell in *The Novels of Anne Brontë: A Study and Reappraisal* (Braunton, Devon: Merlin Books, Ltd., 1992), 30; hereafter cited in text. Although many of Charlotte Brontë's statements about her sister

Anne's work are routinely dismissed as revealing little more than Charlotte's disregard for Anne's abilities, this particular comment, implying as it does Brontë's interest in psychology, seems to touch on a dimension of the novel that has received little critical attention.

7. Edward Chitham expresses a sensible approach to the relationship between Brontë's fiction and her own experiences in this regard. Looking primarily at Brontë's use of setting and at concrete features of Agnes's characterization, Chitham concludes, "It will not be legitimate to infer details of personalities, places and events in Anne's life from a reading of *Agnes Grey*. However, what does emerge, and has already been seen in the first pages, is a general consistency between the attitudes of Agnes and her creator" (1990, 8).

8. The connection between Agnes and her mother and their description of kindred willingness to approach their reduced conditions with enthusiasm are interesting in light of Anne Brontë's own connection to poverty via her mother. Maria Branwell Brontë wrote an essay titled "The Advantages of Poverty in Religious Concerns" that sought to disavow the association of poverty with moral evil and to advocate "the instruction and conversion of the poor" (27). Although this essay was never published in the Brontë's lifetime, it is printed in *BLFC*, I, 24–27.

9. Agnes's reference to New Zealand here may reflect Anne Brontë's family's affiliation with Mary Taylor, a schoolmate and friend of Charlotte's who traveled to New Zealand to find work. For more on this connection, as well as on the influence of Robert Southey's works on Brontë's use of New Zealand, see Jane Stafford's "Anne Brontë, *Agnes Grey* and New Zealand," *Brontë Society Transactions* 20, 2 (1990), 97–99.

10. For a thorough discussion of the ideological work performed by conduct and advice manuals in Victorian England, see Nancy Armstrong's *Desire and Domestic Fiction* (1987).

11. For an excellent overview of Victorian attitudes toward sexuality, see "Victorian Sexualities," a special issue of *Victorian Studies* edited by Andrew H. Miller. The quoted passages come from Miller's brief introduction to major aspects of the topic, entitled "Editor's Introduction," *Victorian Studies* 63, 3 (Spring 1993), 269–72.

12. The term "private speech" is drawn from literature on Bakhtin's Vygotskian psycholinguistics and has correlates in Bakhtin's theories of narrative and voice. For a good discussion that bridges Vygotskian psycholinguistics and literary theories, see James Wertsch's *Voices of the Mind* (Cambridge, Mass.: Harvard University Press, 1992).

13. Langland touches briefly on the same point in her study of Brontë, writing, "Through teaching, Agnes has plumbed her own strengths and honed her own understanding. . . . Agnes, as narrator, focuses on those episodes in which her education is being forwarded" (1989, 106).

14. P. J. M. Scott also writes, "The subject-matter and style of this book are of the first importance—in their very quietness" (1983, 43).

15.   Bell (1992, 30).

16.   For a discussion of autobiography, historical visibility, and feminism, see Mary Jean Corbett's introduction to *Representing Femininity* (1992, 3–16).

Chapter Five

1.   Linda Shires argues that Helen Huntingdon "is constructed by provincial neighbors as someone alien and threatening to cultural stability" and that their suspicions regarding her identity ultimately justify the rebelliousness that she comes to represent. See "Maenads, Mothers, and Feminized Males: Victorian Readings of the French Revolution," in *Rewriting the Victorians: Theory, History, and the Politics of Gender,* ed. Linda M. Shires (New York: Routledge, 1992), 160–162.

2.   Rom Harre, "Persons and Selves," in *Persons and Personality: A Contemporary Inquiry,* eds. Arthur Peacocke and Grant Gillett (New York: Basil Blackwell, 1987): 99–115; hereafter cited in text.

3.   Elizabeth Langland credits Brontë's "sophisticated technique of layered narratives" and sees it as "undergird[ing] the novel's preeminent theme." Her interpretations differ from mine in that she identifies this dominant theme broadly as Brontë's presentation of "'truth' or 'reality' as a complex interpretation, inevitably coloured by individual personalities" (1992, 118).

4.   For an excellent study of the novel's use of textual sources, see Jan B. Gordon's "Gossip, Diary, Letter, Text: Anne Brontë's Narrative *Tenant* and the Problematic of the Gothic Sequel," in *English Language History* 51 (Winter 1984), 719–45; hereafter cited in text.

5.   The term "antidote" is Robert Liddell's; from his study *Twin Spirits: The Novels of Emily and Anne Brontë* (London: Peter Owen, 1990), 10.

6.   George Moore, *Conversations in Ebury Street* (New York: Boni and Liveright, 1924); hereafter cited in text. For an overview of the critical reception of *The Tenant of Wildfell Hall* in Brontë's own time, see Margaret Smith's "Introduction" to the Oxford University Press edition of the novel (New York: Oxford University Press, 1993), ix-xiv; hereafter cited in text.

7.   Other critics also have found Moore's comments to be faulty. N. M. Jacobs notes that the displacement of narratives which troubled Moore and others "is exactly the point of the novel, which subjects its readers to a shouldering-aside of familiar notions and comfortable perceptions of the world. Both narrators, both narrations, and the jarring discrepancies of tone and perspective between them, are necessary to this purpose" ("Gender and Layered Narrative in *Wuthering Heights* and *The Tenant of Wildfell Hall,*" *Journal of Narrative Technique* 16 (Fall 1986), 208; hereafter cited in text.

8.   See Elizabeth Langland, "The Voicing of Feminine Desire in Anne Brontë's *The Tenant of Wildfell Hall,*" in *Gender and Discourse in Victorian Literature and Art,* eds. Antony H. Harrison and Beverly Taylor (De Kalb, Ill.: Northern Illinois University Press, 1992), 111–123; hereafter cited in text. As Langland

summarizes: "Within a traditional narrative analysis, then Brontë's *Tenant* may tell an untraditional tale of a fallen woman redeemed, but it tells it in . . . a way that reaffirms the patriarchal status quo of masculine priority and privilege, of women's subordination and dependency. The radical subject is defused by the form" (1992, 111). Langland goes on to offer a compelling analysis of what she calls "the transgressive nature of narrative exchange" (1982, 111).

9.   The novel's emphasis on Helen's interiority is another feature that has led critics to read the work autobiographically. For instance, Margaret Smith notes, "It was partly because Anne was outwardly still, but inwardly intense, that she was moved to express for a wider public what she could not say openly to her family" (1993, xi).

10.   See Sandra M. Gilbert and Susan Gubar, *The Madwoman in the Attic: The Woman Writer and the Nineteenth-Century Literary Imagination* (New Haven: Yale University Press, 1979); hereafter cited in text. Gilbert and Gubar argue that Helen serves as an example of the female artist who must "deny or conceal her own art, or at least deny the self-assertion implicit in her art" (81).

11.   Some critics have argued persuasively that Helen's decision to give her diary to Markham represents an important part of Brontë's feminist strategy. Jacobs, for instance, writes of this episode: "The effect on Gilbert of reading this document—of being admitted into the reality hidden within and behind the conventional consciousness in which he participates—is revolutionary, and absolutely instrumental to the partnership of equals their marriage will become" (1986, 211).

12.   Gordon discusses the ways in which history itself is treated as property through the motif of gossip in the novel (1984, 723). Gordon suggests as well that as a tenant, not an owner of property, Helen Huntingdon is immediately constituted within Markham's narrative as subversive (721).

13.   The Matrimonial Causes Act was designed to ease restrictions and simplify procedures for obtaining a divorce. As Poovey notes, it "was the first major piece of British legislation to focus attention on the anomalous position of married women under the law" (1988, 51).

14.   Many critics of *The Tenant of Wildfell Hall* have noted its attention to the legal status—or lack thereof—of married women like Helen Huntingdon and to the implications of their status as "nonpersons" for their relationships to their children. As Langland summarizes, "A full awareness of these inequities in British law informs Anne Brontë's novel *The Tenant of Wildfell Hall*, which also explodes the myth of domestic heaven and exposes the domestic hell, from which the protagonist ultimately flees into hiding" (1989, 24–25). The Married Women's Property Acts were passed in 1870 and in 1882, well after the publication of *The Tenant of Wildfell Hall*.

15.   For a fuller elaboration of this topic, see Maria Frawley, "The Female Saviour in *The Tenant of Wildfell Hall*," *Brontë Society Transactions* 20, 3 (1991), 133–143.

16. For a good discussion of evangelical doctrine in the 19th century, see Elisabeth Jay's *The Religion of The Heart* (1979).

17. Juliet McMaster, "'Imbecile Laughter' and 'Desperate Earnest' in *The Tenant of Wildfell Hall, Modern Language Quarterly* 43 (December 1982), 355; hereafter cited in text.

18. Langland notes that "the legion of female saviors in Victorian fiction testifies" to the novelist's desire to encode a woman's physical desires as spiritual reform (1992, 118).

19. As Jay points out, Brontë "had given earlier expression to her purgatorial theories in a poem entitled 'A Word to the Elect,' which as this title, and even more clearly its first title, 'A Word to the Calvinists', indicated was directed against those Evangelicals who wished to restrict heaven even further by their theories of predestination" (1979, 85). For an overview of Anne Brontë's religious beliefs, see Chitham (1979, 19–22).

20. Brontë's letter is reprinted in appendix B of the second edition of Winifred Gerin's *Anne Brontë* (London: Allen Lane, 1976), 361.

21. In *A Literature of Their Own: British Women Novelists from Brontë to Lessing* (Princeton, N.J.: Princeton University Press, 1977), Elaine Showalter notes, "This chivalrous vision of the sacred influence of women had been a central concept of the Victorian domestic ideal" (183–84); hereafter cited in text.

22. Christine L. Krueger, *The Reader's Repentance: Women Preachers, Women Writers, and Nineteenth Century Social Discourse* (Chicago: University of Chicago Press, 1992), 8.

23. In "The Villain of *Wildfell Hall:* Aspects and Prospects of Arthur Huntingdon," *The Modern Language Review* 88 (October 1993), 831–841, Marianne Thormahlen notes, "Helen's method of weaning her little boy off the varieties of alcohol his father had taught 'the little toper' to imbibe was one recommended by several writers on drunkenness in the 1820s and 1830s" (833). For more on the relationship of Brontë's novel to early 19th-century culture, see Thormahlen's essay.

24. Addressing this subject in *"The Tenant of Wildfell Hall:* Anne Brontë's *Jane Eyre"* and drawing on the work of Gilbert and Gubar (1979), Margaret Mary Berg argues that Helen's moments of self-assertion are paralleled in the novel by acts of concealment. *Victorian Newsletter,* no. 71 (Spring 1987), 10–15.

25. Juliet McMaster discusses Brontë's treatment of Regency morals in this light, focusing in particular on "Anne Brontë's vision of the disastrous divergence between the male and the female" in "her alignment of fun and laughter with the men, moral earnestness and tears with the women" (1982, 352).

26. Langland praises Brontë for "psychologically convincing" characterization (1989, 147). In the "Introduction" to *The Tenant of Wildfell Hall,* Margaret Smith notes the "psychological insight" Brontë brought to her creation of character (1993, xv).

27. As Gordon writes, "In this remarkable paragraph, Anne Brontë says, in effect, 'I am different from them, but you cannot know how because I am also different from my writing'" (1984, 736).

Chapter Six

1. Anne Brontë's Bible, Pierpont Morgan Library, New York, PML 17769.

2. For a full account of this incident, see Winifred Gerin's *Branwell Brontë* (1961).

3. Gerin (1961, 71).

4. Miriam Allott provides a good overview of the confusion regarding the authorship of the Brontë sisters' novels in her introduction to *The Brontës: The Critical Heritage* (Boston: Routledge & Kegan Paul, 1974), 28–35; hereafter cited in text.

5. See the January 1848 "Unsigned Notice" from the *New Monthly Magazine* and the 8 July 1848 "Unsigned Review," from the *Spectator,* respectively. Both are reprinted in Allott (1974, 229 and 249).

6. For a good overview of how social psychology views the self, see part 4 of Sampson's *Social Worlds, Personal Lives: An Introduction to Social Psychology,* 203–262. The idea of synthetic unity is explored fully in Harre's "Persons and Selves" (1987).

7. Individual chapters charting developments in the fields of Victorian studies and feminist criticism appear in *Redrawing the Boundaries: The Transformation of English and American Literary Studies,* eds. Stephen Greenblatt and Giles Gunn (New York: Modern Language Association, 1992).

Selected Bibliography

PRIMARY WORKS

Brontë, Anne. *Agnes Grey*. 1st ed., 3d of 3 vols. In Emily Brontë and Anne
Brontë. *Wuthering Heights and Agnes Grey*. London: T. C. Newby, 1847.
————. *The Poems of Anne Brontë: A New Text and Commentary*. Ed. Edward
Chitham. Totowa, N.J.: Rowman and Littlefield, 1979. An authoritative
edition of Brontë's poems that includes appropriate biographical informa-
tion as well as detailed analysis of Brontë's revisions.
————. *The Tenant of Wildfell Hall*. 1st ed., 3 vols. London: T. C. Newby,
1848.
Charlotte Brontë, Emily Brontë, and Anne Brontë, *Poems* by Currer, Ellis and
Acton Bell. London: Aylott and Jones, 1846.

LETTERS

T. J. Wise and J. A. Symington, eds. *The Brontës: Their Lives, Friendships and
Correspondence*, 4 vols. Oxford: The Shakespeare Head Press, 1932.
Reprint, Philadelphia: Porcupine Press, 1980.

SECONDARY WORKS

Allott, Miriam, Ed. *The Brontës: The Critical Heritage*. Boston: Routledge &
Kegan Paul, 1974. An essential reference source for early reviews of Anne
Brontë's works. Although it treats Anne Brontë as less gifted than her
sisters, Allott's introduction provides a valuable analysis of how reviewers
compared their novels.
Bell, Arnold Craig. *The Novels of Anne Brontë: A Study and Reappraisal*. Braunton,
Devon: Merlin Books, Ltd., 1992. Based largely on descriptions of
Brontë's plots, this study seeks to redress imbalances in the evaluation of
her works.
Berry, Elizabeth Hollis. *Anne Brontë's Radical Vision: Structures of Consciousness*.
No. 62, English Literature Studies Monograph Series. Victoria, B.C.:
University of Victoria, 1994. Berry examines image clusters, symbolism,
and thematic motifs in Brontë's poetry and fiction to reveal the spiritual
struggles of her characters. Berry suggests that Brontë's techniques reveal
her overarching concern with the repressive nature of her society's social
structures.
Chitham, Edward. *A Life of Anne Brontë*. Cambridge, Mass.: Basil Blackwell,
1991. A well-balanced biographical study of Brontë that attends careful-

ly to the problematic issue of using her works to deduce biographical information. This study has superseded Winifred Gerin's book as the standard biographical study of Brontë.

Gardiner, Juliet. *The Brontës at Haworth: The World Within*. New York: Clarkson Potter Publishers, 1992. A beautifully illustrated book that documents the history of the Brontë family and positions it in the family's Yorkshire environment. This book includes useful listings of Brontë family and friends as well as a section entitled "In the Footsteps of the Brontës" that describes local sites of importance to Brontë scholars.

Gerin, Winifred. *Anne Brontë*, 2d ed. London: Allen Lane, 1976. A pioneering study of Brontë, Gerin's biography includes invaluable descriptions of her formative years as well as the family and regional milieu that influenced her writing.

Gordon, Jan B. "Gossip, Diary, Letter, Text: Anne Brontë's Narrative *Tenant* and the Problematic of the Gothic Sequel," *English Language History* 51 (Winter 1984), 719–45. Even though she misspells Brontë's heroine's last name and tends to use jargon, Gordon provides an insightful analysis of Brontë's use of a range of forms, especially those associated with Gothic fiction, and links her narrative technique to a subversive feminist critique of history.

Jackson, Arlene M. "The Question of Credibility in Anne Brontë's *The Tenant of Wildfell Hall*." *English Studies* 63 (June 1982), 198–206. A study of the novel's narrative structure and dating that emphasizes the means Brontë uses to achieve psychological realism.

Jacobs, N. M. "Gender and Layered Narrative in *Wuthering Heights* and *The Tenant of Wildfell Hall*." *Journal of Narrative Technique* 16 (Fall 1986), 204–19. An extended analysis of the ways Anne Brontë's narrative structure enables her to depict oppositions between male and female versions of experience and to challenge the domestic ideology.

Jay, Elisabeth. *The Religion of the Heart: Anglican Evangelicalism and the Nineteenth-Century Novel*. Oxford: Clarendon Press, 1979. A major resource for understanding the importance of evangelical doctrine to Anne Brontë's works and culture. Jay includes much discussion of the Brontë family's writings.

Krueger, Christine L. *The Reader's Repentance: Women Preachers, Women Writers, and Nineteenth-Century Social Discourse*. Chicago: University of Chicago Press, 1992. Although she does not directly discuss Anne Brontë's writing, Krueger provides a good analysis of the relationship between evangelical doctrine and the emergence of women's issues in Victorian social discourse.

Langland, Elizabeth. *Anne Brontë: The Other One*. London: Macmillan, 1989. A useful and comprehensive analysis of Brontë's poetry and prose that emphasizes the ways in which a restrictive domestic ideology informs the feminist perspective of Brontë's work.

————. "The Voicing of Feminine Desire in Anne Brontë's *The Tenant of Wildfell Hall*." In *Gender and Discourse in Victorian Literature*. Eds. Antony H. Harrison and Beverly Taylor. De Kalb, Ill.: Northern Illinois University Press, 1992, 113–23. Invoking Roland Barthes's notion of narrative desire, Langland offers an alternative reading of *The Tenant of Wildfell Hall* that stresses the interactive relationship between narrative components of the novel, and emphasizes the "paradoxic voicing of feminine desire."

Liddell, Robert. *Twin Spirits: The Novels of Emily and Anne Brontë*. London: Peter Owen, 1990. An extended treatment of Anne Brontë's relationship with her sister Emily that pursues at length the idea that she sought in *The Tenant of Wildfell Hall* to rewrite *Wuthering Heights*.

McMaster, Juliet. "'Imbecile Laughter' and 'Desperate Earnest' in *The Tenant of Wildfell Hall*." *Modern Language Quarterly* 43 (December 1982), 352–68. A convincing analysis that reads Brontë's novel as a period commentary—a critique of the behavior and values associated with the reign of George IV.

Poole, Russell. "Cultural Reformation and Cultural Reproduction in Anne Brontë's *The Tenant of Wildfell Hall*." *Studies in English Literature* 33 (1993), 859–73. A study of the way that Brontë challenges patriarchal attitudes through her presentation of a theological debate. Poole argues that Brontë's theology is inextricably linked to her understanding of sexuality.

Rosengarten, Herbert. "Introduction" to Anne Brontë, *The Tenant of Wildfell Hall*. Ed. Herbert Rosengarten. Oxford: Clarendon Press, 1992, xi–xxxii. An excellent description and analysis of the textual history of Brontë's last novel.

Scott, P. J. M. *Anne Brontë: A New Critical Assessment*. Totowa, N. J.: Barnes and Noble, 1983. A comprehensive account of Brontë's interest in realism that includes a useful chapter on her letters and theology.

Sellars, Jane. "Art and the Artist as Heroine in the Novels of Charlotte, Emily and Anne Brontë." *Brontë Society Transactions* 20, 2 (1990), 57–76. Sellars provides an essential overview of the artistic output of the Brontë sisters, relating Anne Brontë's paintings both to episodes in her fiction and to traditions of 19th-century British painting.

Stafford, Jane. "Anne Brontë, *Agnes Grey* and New Zealand." *Brontë Society Transactions* 20, 2 (1990), 97–99. A brief discussion of the ways in which Brontë's association with Mary Taylor and her interpretation of Robert Southey combined to influence references to New Zealand in her first novel.

Index

The Author

Maria Frawley is an assistant professor of English at Elizabethtown College, Elizabethtown, Pennsylvania, where she teaches courses in Victorian literature, modern British literature, and women's literature. Her first book, *A Wider Range: Travel Writing by Women in Victorian England,* was published by Fairleigh Dickinson University Press in 1994. She is currently at work on studies of Emily Faithfull, editor of *Victoria Magazine,* and of the literature written by Victorian invalids about their experiences with illness. She lives in Lancaster, Pennsylvania, with her husband, son, and daughter.